Psychiatry

Psychiatry

FOURTH EDITION

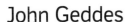

John Geddes
Professor of Epidemiological Psychiatry, University of Oxford

Jonathan Price
Clinical Tutor in Psychiatry, University of Oxford

Rebecca McKnight
Academic Clinical Fellow in Psychiatry, University of Oxford

with Michael Gelder and Richard Mayou

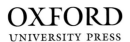

OXFORD
UNIVERSITY PRESS

OXFORD

UNIVERSITY PRESS

Great Clarendon Street, Oxford OX2 6DP

Oxford University Press is a department of the University of Oxford.
It furthers the University's objective of excellence in research, scholarship,
and education by publishing worldwide in

Oxford New York

Auckland Cape Town Dar es Salaam Hong Kong Karachi
Kuala Lumpur Madrid Melbourne Mexico City Nairobi
New Delhi Shanghai Taipei Toronto

With offices in

Argentina Austria Brazil Chile Czech Republic France Greece
Guatemala Hungary Italy Japan Poland Portugal Singapore
South Korea Switzerland Thailand Turkey Ukraine Vietnam

Oxford is a registered trade mark of Oxford University Press
in the UK and in certain other countries

Published in the United States
by Oxford University Press Inc., New York

© John Geddes, Jonathan Price, and Rebecca McKnight 2012

Third Edition 2005 © Michael Gelder, Richard Mayou, and John Geddes

Second Edition 1999

First Edition 1994

British Library Cataloguing in Publication Data

Data available

Library of Congress Cataloguing in Publication Data

Data available

Typeset by Techset Composition Ltd, Salisbury, UK
Printed and bound in China
on acid-free paper by
C & C Offset Printing Co. Ltd.

ISBN 978-0-19-923396-0

10 9 8 7 6 5 4 3 2 1

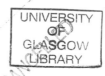

Preface

The fourth edition of *Psychiatry* has been thoroughly revised to reflect developments in the field, and case studies and 'science boxes' added to firmly pin theoretical study to clinical practice. However, we hope this new edition remains true to the principles and approach initiated by Professors Gelder, Mayou, and Gath.

With this edition we bid farewell to Professors Michael Gelder and Richard Mayou, who have now retired from the panel of authors. Michael and Richard began the successful series of *Psychiatry* textbooks almost 30 years ago, and their clinical expertise and wisdom, as well as their editorial skills, will be much missed.

John Geddes is delighted to welcome their replacements, Drs Jonathan Price and Rebecca McKnight, to the team. Jonathan has a particular interest in education and Rebecca brings the advantage of being at an earlier stage in her career. We believe that they have brought a welcome freshness and rigour to the writing of the book.

We are grateful to everyone who has helped us in the gestation of this book, from the identification and successful recruitment of the new blood all the way through to production and publication.

John Geddes, Jonathan Price, and Rebecca McKnight

Contents

PART SIX

Psychiatry and you 461

Introduction

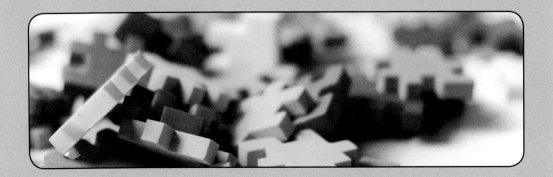

Introduction to psychiatry

Psychiatry is the branch of medicine that specializes in the treatment of those brain disorders which primarily cause disturbance of thought, behaviour, and emotion. These are often referred to as *mental*, or *psychiatric*, disorders. The boundary with the specialty of neurology, which also deals with disorders of the central nervous system, is therefore indistinct. Neurology mainly focuses on brain disease with clear physical pathology and/or obvious peripheral effects on, for example, motor function.

■ Mental disorders are complex but are yielding to scientific investigation

Mental disorders such as depressive disorder and psychoses have been recognized since antiquity. Modern epidemiological studies have demonstrated that they are both highly prevalent and widely distributed across all societies. Overall, mental disorders account for a very high proportion of the disability experienced by the human race (see Chapter 2). Unfortunately, in most societies mental disorders still do not receive the recognition or a level of health service commensurate with their public health importance. There are several reasons for this. Probably most importantly, the brain is a vastly complex organ and the neural systems underlying mental disorders remain poorly characterized. This inevitably means that our understanding of the pathophysiology is relatively poor compared with disorders such as diabetes or heart disease. The absence of a clear body of reliable scientific evidence means that competing unscientific views—and stigma—can flourish. Recently, however, our neurobiological techniques have improved in sophistication and sensitivity to the extent that mental disorders have become *tractable* problems. Phenomena such as mood symptoms, anxiety, and even psychosis seem to exist on a continuum in the population, and the absence of reliable neurobiological measures creates difficulties in determining where the thresholds lie in the gradual change from normality to illness. In clinical practice, the use of diagnostic criteria can increase the reliability of diagnoses and reduce the variations between clinicians. However, small changes in diagnostic criteria can have large effects on the resulting estimates of the prevalence of disorders. Unfortunately, the criteria themselves are based on very imperfect knowledge about the natural history or boundaries of the disorders.

■ Current treatments for mental disorders can be highly effective

This combination of limited understanding of pathophysiology, widespread prevalence, and efflorescence of competing unscientific or folk explanations (which a postmodern culture accords equal status) could lead to pessimism about the potential of psychiatry to help people suffering from the reality of mental disorders. It is remarkable, therefore, that such effective treatments *do* exist which, properly implemented, can produce worthwhile clinical benefits. We may not yet have arrived at the stage of rational therapies based on fundamental scientific understanding. Nonetheless, through a combination of speculative creativity and guided serendipity, coupled with rigorous evaluation in clinical trials, we have a range of valuable interventions. Moreover, although again not based on pathophysiological markers reflecting the underlying neurobiology, psychiatry has developed reliable diagnostic systems that create a common language to facilitate communication between clinicians and patients, clinicians and clinicians, and researchers.

There are compelling reasons for *all* doctors to have at least a basic awareness of mental disorders and their assessment and effective management. This text aims to provide that basic knowledge. We hope that students will be inspired to follow a career in psychiatry—which can be a rocky road, but one that amply repays the efforts expended by both satisfying intellectual curiosity and providing the unique reward of relieving the suffering of fellow humans.

The scale of the problem

One in four individuals suffer from a psychiatric disorder at some point in their life. In October 2009, the *British Medical Journal* estimated the 'economic, social and human cost of mental illness per year in the UK' as £100 billion ($1.6 billion). It is therefore clear that humans are highly vulnerable to mental health disorders, and that these impact significantly upon our society in many different ways.

Whilst most of medicine endeavours to fix physical aberrations, psychiatrists attempt to understand a patient within their context, and to alter their thoughts, behaviour, and neurobiology to help improve their quality of life. This is often a challenge, and one that is becoming more obvious as it becomes recognized that the prevalence of mental disorders worldwide is on the increase.

It is often difficult for the general public and clinicians outside psychiatry to think of mental health disorders as 'diseases' because it is harder to pinpoint a specific pathological cause for them. However, until recently most of medicine has been founded on this basis. For example, it was only in the late 1980s that *Helicobacter pylori* was linked to gastric/duodenal ulcers and gastric carcinoma. Still much of clinical medicine treats a patient's symptoms rather than objective abnormalities.

The World Health Organization (WHO) has given the following definition of mental health:

> *Mental health is defined as a state of well-being in which every individual realizes his or her own potential, can cope with the normal stresses of life, can*

work productively and fruitfully, and is able to make a contribution to her or his community.

This is a helpful definition, because it clearly defines a mental disorder as a condition that disrupts this state in any way, and sets clear goals of treatment for the clinician. It identifies the fact that a disruption of an individual's mental health impacts negatively not only upon their enjoyment and ability to cope with life, but also upon that of the wider community. The rest of this chapter will outline the prevalence of mental health disorders worldwide, the impact that these have on both individuals and society, and the public perception of psychiatry and the effect that this has on those with mental disorders.

■ Worldwide prevalence of mental disorders

Psychiatric disorders are amongst the most prevalent causes of ill health in humans. One in four adults will suffer from a diagnosable mental disorder at some time in their life, and one in five has one in any given year. This is true across the globe, in both economically developed and developing countries. Table 2.1 outlines the worldwide prevalence of the major psychiatric disorders, with some common physical disorders for comparison. Depression is one of the most prevalent diseases currently seen in humans, only superseded by conditions associated with poverty and poor access to healthcare (e.g. malnutrition, iron-deficiency anaemia, low vision). Approximately 6 per cent of the population have a severe, enduring psychiatric

Table 2.1 World prevalence of selected conditions (from WHO *The Global Burden of Disease: 2004 update* (2008))

Condition	World prevalence (millions)
Unipolar depressive disorders	151.2
Alcohol use disorders	125.0
Schizophrenia	26.3
Bipolar affective disorder	29.5
Alzheimer's and other dementias	24.2
HIV infection	31.4
Tuberculosis	13.9
Chronic obstructive pulmonary disease	63.6
Osteoarthritis	151.4
Symptomatic ischaemic heart disease	54.9
Diabetes mellitus	220.5

Table 2.2 Epidemiology of mental disorders in the USA in 2008 (from the US National Institute for Mental Health, www.nimh.nih.gov)

Condition	Prevalence (% population)	Median age of onset (years)
Anxiety disorders	18.1	21
All mood disorders	9.5	30
Unipolar depression	6.7	32
Post-traumatic stress disorder	3.5	23
Eating disorders	1–7 (females)	17
Bipolar disorder	2.6	25
Schizophrenia	1.1	20
Obsessive-compulsive disorder	1.0	19
ADHD	4.1	7
Autism	0.34	3
Alzheimer's disease	10% of over-65s	72

disorder which impacts upon their functioning in the long term. Schizophrenia, bipolar disorder, and unipolar depression make up the majority of these cases.

As an example of the relative prevalence of common mental health disorders seen in developed countries, Table 2.2 shows epidemiological data from the USA collected in 2008. Always remember that patients frequently fit the diagnostic criteria for more than one diagnosis—for example, social phobia and major depressive disorder—and that this is especially true for the mood, anxiety, and behavioural conditions. It is unclear at the moment whether the prevalence of many disorders is increasing, or if rising figures are merely a diagnostic artefact. Time will tell.

■ Global service provision for mental health disorders

As psychiatry is a medical specialty that affects such a large proportion of the population, it would seem logical for there to be health services at least equivalent to those for other medical conditions available. However, this is not the case. In 2008, the WHO published a report on the global provision of psychiatric services, concluding that those available currently are woefully inadequate. The following are key statistics from the report:

● Only 62.1 per cent of countries (including 68 per cent of the world population) have a specific mental health policy outlining provision of services.

- One-third of countries do not have a separate budget for mental healthcare.
- Thirty-one per cent of the world's population are not covered by a dedicated mental health law or legislation covering involuntary treatment and human rights.
- The mean number of psychiatric beds per 10 000 people worldwide is 1.69, compared with 8.9 for physical health conditions.
- There are just 1.2 psychiatrists per 100 000 population worldwide, of whom 90 per cent work in high-income countries.

Table 2.3 lists some drugs that are commonly used in psychiatry, and the percentage of countries with easy access to them. Most of the older typical antipsychotics are now widely available, but other 'basics' such as lithium and sodium valproate are still limited to two-thirds of the world. There are currently no data published for selective serotonin reuptake inhibitors (SSRIs) or atypical antipsychotics. Access to medications is a good marker for the level of development of health services. If a doctor does not have access to antidepressants, it is very unlikely that they will have other more complex treatments available, for example cognitive behavioural therapy.

In the UK, which has a National Health Service (NHS) funded from taxation, 13.8 per cent of the health budget is allotted to mental health services. This is the highest proportion in Europe, but still there is a distinct shortage of facilities, especially for psychological therapies and specialty services such as those for adolescents or eating disorders. There are 12.7 psychiatrists per 100 000 population, compared with 8.9 as a European average.

The impact of mental health disorders upon individuals and society

With so many people suffering from mental health disorders, it is unsurprising that these disorders have a major impact on society. Disability is defined as 'a loss of health', and is usually used to describe impairments in activities of daily living caused by physical or mental disorders. The disability-adjusted life year (DALY) is a measure of the overall burden of a disease, combining morbidity and mortality into one number. Table 2.4 shows the latest WHO data from the global burden of disease study, which has produced a list of the conditions giving rise to the greatest burden of disability worldwide. Depression is currently at number three, but is predicted to rise to first place by the 2012 edition of the report. Seven of the top 20 conditions are mental health disorders.

Whilst the majority of physical diseases tend to be more common in older people, psychiatric conditions predominantly affect the young and middle aged. Table 2.2 shows the median age of onset of various conditions in the USA; most are between 18 and 30 years. This means

Table 2.3 Availability of common psychiatric drugs worldwide (from *WHO Mental Health Atlas 2005, update* (2008))

Drug	Countries with availability (%)
Carbamazepine	91.4
Valproate	67.4
Amitriptyline	86.4
Diazepam	96.8
Haloperidol	91.8
Lithium	65.4
Levodopa	61.9
Chlorpromazine	91.4

Table 2.4 Disease and injury causes of disability in descending order by global prevalence: the 20 leading causes of disability worldwide (from WHO *The Global Burden of Disease: 2004 update* (2008))

1	Hearing loss
2	Refractive errors
3	**Depression**
4	Cataracts
5	Unintentional injuries
6	Osteoarthritis
7	**Alcohol dependence and problem use**
8	Infertility due to unsafe abortion and maternal sepsis
9	Macular degeneration
10	Chronic obstructive pulmonary disease
11	Ischaemic heart disease
12	**Bipolar disorder**
13	Asthma
14	**Schizophrenia**
15	Glaucoma
16	**Alzheimer's and other dementias**
17	**Panic disorder**
18	Cerebrovascular disease
19	Rheumatoid arthritis
20	**Drug dependence and problem use**

that mental health disorders tend to affect people when they are in the latter stages of education, starting a career and setting up home. In the UK, 44 per cent of claimants of incapacity benefit stated a mental health or behavioural disorder as the principle reason for their disability leading to an inability to work. The impact of psychiatric disorders on the economic success and social coherence of a country is therefore great.

Mortality associated with mental health disorders is very variable, depending upon the condition. The most important area is that of deliberate self-harm and completed suicide. Globally, it is estimated that 800 000 people complete suicide each year, 90 per cent of whom have a diagnosable mental health disorder. Two-thirds of those who commit suicide are aged between 15 and 44 years. Suicide is the leading cause of death in men aged 15–34 years in the UK, and for women it is the second most prevalent cause. Four times as many men die by suicide as women, although more women make attempts. Approximately 1 per cent of the population of economically more developed countries will die by completed suicide, a statistic usually unrecognized by most of the general public.

■ The public perception of mental health

It is an unfortunate truth that individuals with mental health disorders are subject to significant negative stigma within society. This also occurs in medicine. Those young doctors who express an interest in being psychiatrists are often deemed to be either mad themselves, or unable to get another specialty training post. The UK government has put some effort into identifying and tackling stigma surrounding mental health issues in recent years. In 2007,

it published a report entitled *Attitudes to Mental Illness*, based on the responses of 6000 randomly sampled adults to a short interview. Some of the more striking results included the following:

- Only 65 per cent of respondents thought that people with mental health problems should have the same right to a job as those without them.
- Six out of ten adults agreed with the statement 'one of the main causes of mental illness is a lack of self-discipline and will power'.
- Young people are the most prejudiced.
- Thirty-four per cent of respondents felt that 'all people with mental health problems are prone to violence'.
- Two-thirds of people said they were scared of those with psychiatric illnesses, and would not want to live next door to one of them.
- Eighty per cent of respondents underestimated the prevalence of mental health disorders in the UK by at least a factor of ten.

This survey is conducted every 2 years in Britain, and the results have been almost static over the last decade. Given that there is good evidence that some of the best outcomes for those with severe mental health problems come with the provision of appropriate housing, employment, and social support, this remains disappointing. One positive finding is that the majority of adults agree that community and outpatient-based interventions are preferable to prolonged hospitalizations. Education surrounding mental health is badly needed the world over, both to help the vast number of people with mental health disorders to cope with them more productively, and to allow the rest of society to include them in a cohesive manner.

 Further reading

Saraceno, B. (2009). *Oxford Textbook of Psychiatry*, 2nd edn. Ed. M. G. Gelder, J. J. Lopez-Ibor, N. C. Andreasen & J .R. Geddes, pp. 3–13. Oxford University Press, Oxford.

Waraich, P., Goldner, E. M., Somers, J. M. & Hsu, L. (2004). Prevalence and incidence studies of mood disorders: a systematic review of the literature. *Canadian Journal of Psychiatry* **49**: 124–38.

Henderson, C. & Thornicroft, G. (2009). Stigma and discrimination in mental illness: time to change. *Lancet* **373** (9679): 1928–30.

The World Health Organization website provides copious reading material on all aspects of mental health epidemiology, including a searchable database of psychiatric service provision for all countries.

www.who.int/topics/mental_health/en/
www.who.int/topics/global_burden_of_disease/en/

Mental disorder and you

■ Facts, beliefs, and prejudices

People's attitudes to mental disorder vary widely. Often this is because of the extent of their personal experience of mental illness. Some people have experienced a mental illness themselves, whilst others may well have experience of mental illness in a friend or relative. If you have been lucky enough to avoid these personal experiences, it is almost inevitable that you will be exposed to one or the other during your lifetime, and perhaps several times. Of course, because you are reading this book, it is likely that you are, or are intending to be, a healthcare professional. In whatever area of healthcare you work, you will encounter hundreds—if not thousands—of people with mental illness in your professional lifetime. The beliefs that you hold about mental illness and people with mental illness will influence how you respond to them. It is therefore important that you appraise your existing beliefs and, if necessary, consider changing some of them.

Appraising and altering our beliefs is difficult. We all tend to assume that what we believe—about ourselves, others, or the world around us—is true. However, only some of the beliefs that we hold are facts. Despite this, our beliefs tend to be 'static' and resistant to change, whether or not they are correct. One reason for this is the kind of biases that operate to maintain our system of beliefs. Cognitive therapists use a model which they call 'the prejudice model' to describe these biases. What they describe is that most evidence that conflicts with our core beliefs is either not noticed, or is altered in order to fit our core beliefs, whereas most evidence that fits with our core beliefs is noticed and used to bolster those beliefs. In this way, the beliefs that we hold tend to be relatively static through time.

Common prejudices

This section describes a short exercise for you to complete. There are three stages:

1 In Box 3.1, we list several common prejudices about mental illness. Rate each of these statements from 0 to 100 per cent, where the percentage is the extent to which you hold that belief. For example, if you believe that mental illness is indeed a sign of weakness in most cases, you might answer 80 per cent. It is important to be honest, rather than give what you believe to be the 'correct' answer.

2 Continue to read this chapter, where we challenge some of these prejudices, largely by comparing mental illness with physical illness. Think carefully about the comparisons and arguments that are offered, and how they fit with or contradict your own beliefs.

3 Re-rate the six statements in Box 3.1. Are there any differences from when you first rated them?

Mental illness is a sign of weakness

Is physical illness a sign of weakness? We do not commonly associate a fractured neck of the femur, a myocardial infarction, or diabetes mellitus with 'weakness', and yet people with mental illness may well be judged to be weak in some way. As you will see, the causes of mental illness are complex, involving physical, psychological, and social factors. In many cases, mental illness appears to have a strong genetic basis, and this is particularly likely in some illnesses, such as bipolar disorder. Furthermore, many people whose lives have demonstrated personal strength or extraordinary ability have also suffered from mental illness. These include Winston Churchill (who, besides his successes as a wartime politician, won the Nobel Prize for Literature), Florence Nightingale (pioneer of modern nursing), Vincent Van Gogh (artist), Isaac Newton (scientist), Linda Hamilton (actress), and JK Rowling (author). It is difficult, in these circumstances, to argue that mental illness is a sign of weakness. Indeed, one common mental illness—bipolar disorder—appears to be strongly represented among successful people, and it has been argued that mood disorder persists in populations because it may present a selective advantage in evolution.

Mental illness is something that affects other people

This is an important myth to dispel. Many of us are rather blasé about our health, both physical and mental. This may change when we receive an 'early warning' that something is wrong (such as high blood pressure or impaired glucose tolerance). Many of us have had short or mild periods of emotional distress, often in the context of personal difficulty such as the end of a relationship or the death of a close relative. Such an episode indicates that we are vulnerable. However, few of us, in those circumstances, seek help or advice, yet mental illness is often seen in healthcare professionals, including doctors and psychiatrists. Mood disorder, anxiety disorder, eating disorder, and alcohol and substance misuse are common. Unfortunately, healthcare professionals can be very slow in acknowledging that there is a problem and in obtaining effective assessment and care.

People with mental illness should just pull themselves together

If only this were possible. We know from personal experience that, when we have received some kind of setback, or when our energy or confidence are at a low ebb, achieving our goals is more difficult. By its nature, depression is associated with physical fatigue, mental fatigue, pervasive low mood, and negative biases about yourself, the world around you, and the future. Just imagine how difficult it must be to engage with treatment, and to continue with those aspects of life that are either essential or help to keep us going, during such an illness. The more depressed the person's mood, the more difficult it is for them to 'just pull themselves together', and the more dependent they are on others, including healthcare professionals, for support, tolerance, and the instillation of hope.

There are no effective treatments for people with mental illness

There is no doubt that mental illness can be difficult to treat and that, in some cases, the resulting distress and disability are chronic. However, this is a similar situation to the treatment and prognosis of physical disorders. Some physical illnesses, such as appendicitis, can be cured by a clear, discrete intervention. However, others,

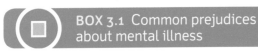

BOX 3.1 Common prejudices about mental illness

1 Mental illness is a sign of weakness

2 Mental illness is something that affects other people

3 People with mental illness should just pull themselves together

4 There are no effective treatments for people with mental illness

5 People with mental illness should be kept in hospital

6 People with mental illness are a risk to others

such as rheumatoid arthritis or multiple sclerosis, can often not be cured, and the focus of most physical interventions is on reducing disability rather than eliminating disease. Psychiatric treatments, such as selective serotonin reuptake inhibitors (SSRIs), have proven effectiveness for anxiety and depression, with a number needed to treat (NNT) of 5–8 versus placebo in panic disorder and 5 versus placebo for treatment response in moderately severe depression. Box 3.2 gives more details about NNTs.

People with mental illness should be kept in hospital

Perhaps it is helpful to ask, first, whether people with *physical* illness should be kept in hospital. Clearly, in some cases, they should. However, in most cases we will want to manage physical disorder in primary care, in outpatients, or through day care, with the patient spending most of their life at home. The treatment of mental illness is similar. Most psychiatric patients will at no time need to be admitted to hospital, and even those patients who need inpatient care will, for the vast majority of their lives, be managed as outpatients.

People with mental illness are a risk to others

The proportion of people with mental illness who present a risk to others is small. Even when a particular mental illness is associated with violence, the majority of people with that disorder are not violent. Indeed, people with mental illness are more likely to be the victims of violence than the perpetrators. The vast majority of people who are violent do not suffer from mental illness. Unfortunately, the public perception of this issue is maintained by some of the prejudices or cognitive biases that we mentioned earlier and, perhaps, by selective reporting in the media.

People with mental illness don't make good doctors

It is perfectly possible for people with diabetes, or hypertension, or asthma, to be good doctors, so why not people with anxiety disorder, or depressive disorder? Just as experience of physical illness may help to develop some important insights and skills, which can enhance good medical practice, so the experience of mental illness may help to develop individuals so that they can deliver particularly insightful and compassionate care. The General Medical Council accepts that doctors in training and qualified doctors may be or become ill, and offers guidance in *Good Medical Practice*.

■ Your mental health

It is quite possible that you have had a mental illness in the past, or that you are currently suffering from one. If so, you may well have sought help and advice from healthcare professionals. However, you may well have avoided seeking help. Perhaps you feared that your medical career would be in peril, that you couldn't be helped, that the problem was not very serious and you would be wasting someone's time, that you were too busy and could not afford the time, or that your fellow students, or others, might find out about your difficulties, and think badly of you. Whatever the reason or reasons, now is a good time to seek advice. Often, the experience of psychiatry as a trainee healthcare professional brings one's own emotions and emotional problems to the fore. Furthermore, you are early in your professional career, and seeking to understand and deal with your difficulties makes good sense at this stage. You will be able to learn the knowledge and skills to help to keep you well during the challenging early years of your career, and for the rest of your life. Finally, you may be able to consider important life and career decisions (such as location, choice of specialty, and choice of full- or part-time training) in the light of your greater understanding of your health.

Your first step should be to arrange to talk to your GP about your problems. This can be difficult, so it can be helpful to write down your concerns on paper, and take these with you. As you will see later in this textbook, our day-to-day concerns are maintained by avoidance—so facing up to your concerns is the first step towards managing

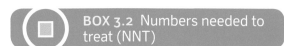

BOX 3.2 Numbers needed to treat (NNT)

The Number Needed to Treat is a potentially helpful way of presenting the comparative effectiveness of a treatment. It represents the number of patients who need to be treated with a treatment to achieve one additional good outcome. So, if we know, from randomized evidence, that a patient has a 60% chance of a bad outcome without the treatment, and that this decreases to 40% with the treatment, their Absolute Risk Reduction (ARR) is 20%, and we would need to treat 5 patients (100%/20%) to gain one whole additional good outcome. So, the NNT is 5.

If an NNT is quoted, it should relate to five specific pieces of context: (a) the patient group, (b) the experimental treatment, (c) the comparison treatment, (d) the time point at which the comparison is made, and (e) the outcome. So, for example, in a randomized controlled trial in adults with panic disorder (a), comparing individual CBT (b) with individual supportive therapy (c), at 8 weeks (d), the proportion of patients still with panic attacks (e) was 5/17 (29%) in the cognitive therapy group and 12/16 (75%) in the supportive group. The ARR is 46%, and so the NNT is 100%/46%, which is just over 2.

them effectively. Cognitive therapists know, through extensive experience with their patients (and themselves!), that fears about an event are often much greater than the reality of that event. By not avoiding, but rather by seeking help for your difficulties, you may well experience great relief that you have taken the first steps forward. So if you're concerned about your emotional health, don't delay—get in touch with your GP today.

Further reading

Moore, A. (2009). *What is an NNT?* Hayward Group Ltd. Available from www.medicine.ox.ac.uk/bandolier/pain-res/download/whatis/NNT.pdf.

Assessment

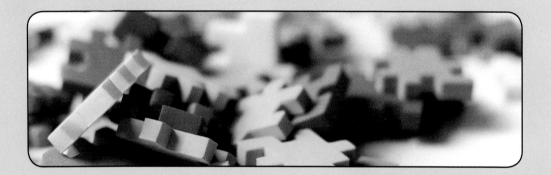

Setting up the assessment and taking a history

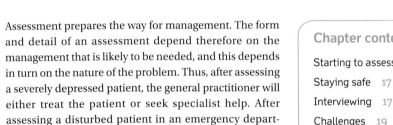

Assessment prepares the way for management. The form and detail of an assessment depend therefore on the management that is likely to be needed, and this depends in turn on the nature of the problem. Thus, after assessing a severely depressed patient, the general practitioner will either treat the patient or seek specialist help. After assessing a disturbed patient in an emergency department, the doctor's first action will be to calm the patient and ensure the safety of others. After assessing an elderly inpatient with severe memory loss, a physician will need to arrange appropriate aftercare. The length and focus of the assessment will differ in each case, although the basic structure will be the same.

Assessment begins as soon as the presenting problem is known—it does not wait until all the relevant data have been collected. From the start of the interview, the assessor begins to think what disorders could account for the presenting problem and what data will be required to decide. As the patient's personality and circumstances become known, further ideas will be generated about the plan of management that is most likely to succeed. Thus assessment is not a fixed procedure, carried out in the same way with every patient, but a dynamic process in which healthcare professionals make, test, and modify hypotheses as they gather information.

Although the details of the assessment vary in this way, the *general aims* are always the same. These are to:

- begin to form a therapeutic relationship with the patient;
- understand the problem, the symptoms, and their functional impact, from the patient's perspective, including their concerns;

- understand these issues from the perspective of the relatives/ other carers, if appropriate;
- compare the present condition of the patient with their former state, including any previous illnesses;
- enquire about current and past medication, and other treatments;
- learn about the patient's family and other circumstances, including sources of support.

Whenever possible, history from the patient is supplemented by history from another **informant** or **corroborant**. History taking is followed by an examination of the mental and physical state and, in some cases, by psychological or physical investigations. At this stage, the assessment may be complete or incomplete, depending on the complexity of the problem, the time available, and the information immediately accessible. The full assessment will inform the diagnosis and differential diagnosis (see Chapter 6), the aetiology of the disorder (see Chapter 7), the prognosis (see Chapter 8), the risks to the patient and others (see Chapter 9), and a plan of management (see chapters relating to specific disorders). When the assessment has been made, the results are discussed with the patient and often with a relative, and communicated to other relevant healthcare professionals (see Chapter 10).

The clinical skills required to elicit symptoms and signs and to make a diagnosis are similar to those used in other branches of medicine—careful **history taking**, systematic **clinical examination**, and sound **clinical reasoning**. The only substantial difference is that the clinical examination includes the mental as well as the physical state of the patient.

However, eliciting the signs and symptoms of mental disorder, and considering diagnoses, are only part of the assessment of patients. Interviewers should never lose sight of their patients as unique individuals. They need to understand how the disorder affects their patient's feelings about life, for example by making them feel hopeless, and how it affects their social roles, for example by affecting their caring for their small children. The more that interviewers gain insight into such personal experiences, the more they can help their patients. Because such understanding is equally important when caring for patients with physical illnesses, the experience gained during training in psychiatry is of value in every kind of clinical work. This understanding cannot be acquired solely from books—it is learned though listening to patients as they describe their lives. Some students are reluctant to do this, fearing that psychiatric patients may behave in odd, unpredictable, or alarming ways. In fact this is uncommon. Students should therefore take every opportunity to talk to patients—no textbook can replace this experience.

Indeed, students should also take every opportunity to talk to their friends and relatives about their emotional lives, and to consider their own emotional reactions and coping with adversity. This is because one of the most challenging tasks for any healthcare professional is deciding the boundary between 'normal' and 'abnormal'. To succeed in this task, it is vital to have an understanding of 'normal' emotional reactions to difficult circumstances, such as are usually found in the general population.

This Chapter and Chapters 5 to 10 are concerned primarily with the general assessment of adult patients. The assessment of children is described in Chapter 17, and of people with learning disability in Chapter 19. Assessment of suicide risk is described on p. 64, of alcohol problems on p. 387, and of sexual dysfunction on p. 410.

■ Starting to assess patients

Very early in your psychiatry attachment, you should feel confident enough to begin to interview patients, and to present your (initially very limited) findings in a structured and coherent way. Some of the language and the ideas will be new to you. You will not understand everything straight away, so don't be disgruntled. Most importantly, meet and talk to patients—like any medical specialty, psychiatry cannot be understood from a book or from lecture notes. Many of you will want to avoid seeing patients until you can do a 'good' assessment, but this is undoubtedly a mistake. We advise that you regard your initial meetings with psychiatric patients as being simply conversations with fellow human beings about their predicament—their experience of their illness, what led up to it, the impact that it has had on their life, and their experience of treatment, including admission. Subsequently, you should aim, with the help of this chapter, and Chapters 5 to 10, to be able to present a more comprehensive assessment summary.

We therefore suggest three stages when practising interviewing patients:

- First, meet several patients and become comfortable talking to them informally, enquiring about their life outside hospital, their life inside hospital, and their problems.

- Then, when you are comfortable talking to patients, steadily introduce more structure, and start to ask specific questions, until you are confident conducting a full psychiatric assessment.

- Finally, practise being flexible, so that you are equally confident conducting a very short screening assessment, a brief assessment, or a thorough assessment, depending on the circumstances.

■ Staying safe

Only a very small minority of patients with psychiatric illness are potentially dangerous, although this proportion depends on the setting (risk is greater in inpatients than outpatients) and subspecialty (greater in forensic psychiatry than old age psychiatry). Nevertheless, it is imperative that a brief risk assessment is done before seeing *any* patient, in *any* setting, no matter how busy you are. Only then will you get into the habit of thinking about, assessing, and managing the risk posed to you by patients and, of course, by their family and their acquaintances.

In some circumstances, it is obvious that risks need to be assessed and managed. For example:

- assessment of a disturbed patient, not known to health services, in an Accident and Emergency department;

- assessment of a man with a long history of violent offences who has presented to his GP surgery without an appointment as the surgery is closing for the evening and reception staff are leaving;

- assessment of a woman with schizophrenia, and a history of violence when unwell, who is thought to have relapsed, and needs to be seen at home;

- assessment late at night at her home of an elderly woman who is medically unwell, and who lives in an area where street robbery and assault are very frequent;

- assessment of a woman with severe abdominal pain, whose partner has a history of violence when stressed, at her home.

In many other cases, though, it is not clear that there are significant risks. If you do not prepare properly, you are at much greater risk if there is an incident. Simple risk management strategies should therefore be part of your daily routine, in whichever branch of medicine you practise. The simple approach outlined in Table 4.1 will ensure that you are considering the relevant issues.

■ Interviewing

Approach

The interview serves not only to collect information, but also to establish a therapeutic relationship. Thus the clinician's approach to the patient is important. This is described next, but it can only guide readers, who should take every opportunity to watch experienced interviewers at work and to practise under supervision. Psychiatric interviews are carried out in many different settings, including patients' homes, the wards of a general hospital, primary care clinics, and police station custody suites.

The advice that follows cannot be followed completely in every setting and situation, but it is nevertheless important to follow it whenever possible.

Starting the interview

It is important to work hard to form a successful working relationship with the patient. This will not always be possible, but if such a relationship is formed, the assessment will be easier and more will be revealed, such a relationship can be therapeutic in itself, and compliance (concordance) with treatment is enhanced. The approach below will help in this task.

The interview should be carried out in a place where it cannot be overheard and is, as far as possible, free from interruptions. If these requirements are difficult to meet, as in a medical ward, the interview should, if possible, be moved—for example to a side room. Patients should be seated comfortably, with the chairs arranged so that the interviewer sits at an angle to, and no higher than, the patient. Right-handed interviewers generally find it easier to attend to the patient while making notes if they seat the patient on their left.

Interviewers should welcome the patient, introduce themselves by name, and explain their role (e.g. medical student). They should greet anyone who is accompanying the patient, and explain how long they can expect to wait, and whether they too will be interviewed. It is usually better to see the patient on their own first, and to interview any accompanying person later. Exceptions are made if that person has to leave early, and when the patient is unable to give an account of the problems. Interviewers should explain briefly:

- how long the interview will last;

- in general terms, how it will proceed;

- the need to take notes;

- the confidentiality of these notes, but the need to share certain information with others directly involved in treatment.

Interviews are more likely to be effective if the interviewer:

- appears relaxed and unhurried, even when time is short;

- maintains appropriate eye contact and does not appear engrossed in the notes;

- is alert to non-verbal as well as to verbal cues of distress, and shows an understanding of the patient's feelings;

- attends to emotional problems and makes empathic responses to indications of distress, for example 'I'm sure that was very upsetting for you';

- intervenes appropriately when patients are over-talkative, or have departed from or avoided the subject;

- has a systematic but flexible plan.

Table 4.1 A plan to stay safe

Who?	Who is the patient?
	Ask someone who knows them, such as a member of nursing staff on the ward, and/or read medical notes/letters.
	Are they currently aggressive, irritable, or disinhibited? Do they have a history of harming others?
	Are they considered to be low risk to others?
Where?	Where will you interview?
	Which room? A room down a long corridor with no other offices nearby, or an interview room adjacent to the nursing station, with a viewing window so that other staff can observe proceedings while patient confidentiality is maintained?
	Where in the room? In a corner where your exit is obstructed by the patient, or adjacent to the door? Think about setting up the room to your requirements in advance, by moving furniture. If the patient sits in 'your' chair, politely ask them to move.
	With weapons or missiles? As part of your preparation of the room, consider removing objects that could be used as weapons, such as paperweights or letter-openers.
With whom?	With whom will you interview?
	You may be fine on your own.
	Alternatively, you may need to take another student, or a member of staff, so that if something does go wrong, one of you can go to fetch help.
With alarm?	Will you take an alarm?
	Many psychiatric wards now have 'pinpoint' alarm systems, where staff wear alarms on their belts, which can be activated when necessary and help other staff to locate (pinpoint) a staff member in trouble. An alarm is no use, however, if it is forgotten, it cannot be reached easily by the carrier, or the carrier does not know how to activate it.
	Some rooms, such as in Accident and Emergency departments, have alarm buttons fixed to walls. Again, this is of no use if staff members do not know where they are, or are not close enough to operate them.
	In the community, remember to carry a mobile phone, and consider carrying a personal attack alarm.
With knowledge?	Do other staff know where you are?
	This is particularly important in the community, where you should make sure that your team base knows (i) where you are going, (ii) who you are going to see, (iii) when you are due back, and (iv) how you are contactable (e.g. mobile phone number).
	On the ward, it can be as simple as saying to the patient's key worker that you will be interviewing patient X in room Y until time Z.
With insight?	Our communication, both verbal and non-verbal, within the assessment can 'wind up' or 'wind down' patients. Avoid actions that might provoke anger, such as approaching too close, prolonging eye contact, or avoiding eye contact altogether. Be aware of changes in the patient's emotional state and, in particular, their state of arousal.
	Finally, if in doubt, get out.

The interviewer *begins with a general question* to encourage the patient to express their problems in their own words: for example, 'tell me about your problem', 'tell me what you have noticed wrong', or 'tell me why you're here'. During the reply, interviewers should notice whether their patients are calm, or distressed despite their efforts to put them at ease. If the latter, interviewers should try to identify the nature of the difficulty and attempt to overcome it.

Continuing the interview

Having elicited the complaints, the next step is to enquire into them systematically. In doing this the interviewer should as far as possible *avoid closed and leading questions*. A closed question allows only a brief answer, usually 'yes' or 'no', whereas a leading question suggests the answer. 'Do you wake early?' is a closed leading question, but 'At what time do you wake?' is an open, non-leading question. If there is no alternative to a leading question, it should be followed by a request for an example. Thus, the only way to ask about an important symptom of schizophrenia is to use the leading closed question 'Have you ever felt that your actions were being controlled by another person?'. If the answer is yes, the interviewer should ask for one or more examples of the experience, and should conclude that the symptom is present only if the examples are convincing. Leading questions can be avoided by prompting the patient indirectly by:

- repeating what the patient has said, but in a questioning tone, for example: 'feeling low...?';
- restating the problem in other words, for example (after a patient has spoken of sadness): 'You say you have been feeling low';
- asking for clarification, for example: 'Could you say a little more about that?'

It is important to *establish when each symptom and problem began* as well as if and when it became worse or better. If a patient finds it difficult to remember these dates, it may be possible to relate the events to others that are more easily remembered, such as a birthday or a public holiday.

As the interview progresses, the interviewer has a number of tasks:

- **to help patients to talk freely** by interrupting only when necessary, by nodding, and by saying, for example, 'Go on', 'Tell me more about that', or 'Is there more to say?';
- **to keep patients to relevant topics** in part with non-verbal cues such as leaning forward or nodding to encourage the patient to continue with the topic;
- **to make systematic enquiries** but without asking so many questions that other—unanticipated—aspects of the problem are not volunteered;
- **to check their understanding** by summarizing key points back to the patient, and saying 'Is that right? Does that sum it up?';
- **to select questions according to the emerging possibilities** regarding diagnoses, causes, and plans of action. The choice of questions is modified progressively as additional information is gathered.

As explained above, *interviewing is an active and selective process, not the asking of the same set of questions for every patient*. The shorter the time available for the interview, the more important it is to proceed in this focused way. Occasionally, the patient is so disturbed that it is impossible to follow an orderly sequence of questioning. In such cases it is even more important to keep the diagnostic possibilities in mind so that the most relevant questions are selected and the most relevant observations carried out.

Ending the interview

Before ending the interview, the interviewer should summarize the main points and ask whether the patient has anything to add to the account that they have given. He should then explain what will happen next.

Taking notes

Whenever possible, notes should be taken during the interview because attempts to memorize the history and make notes later are time consuming and liable to error. Exceptions may, however, have to be made when patients are very restless or agitated. At the start of the interview, note taking should be deferred for a few minutes so that patients can feel that they have the undivided attention of the interviewer.

■ Challenges

Interviewing patients from another culture

If the patient and the interviewer do not speak a common language, it is obvious that an interpreter will be needed. However, language is not the only problem in such cases; cultural differences are also important, and interpreters may share the patient's language but not their culture. Issues such as the following may be understood best by talking with someone from the patient's cultural group.

- **Cultural beliefs** may explain why certain events are experienced as more stressful or shameful than they would be in the host culture.
- **Roles** within the family may differ from those in the host culture.
- **Distress may be shown in different symptoms.** In some cultures, distress is often expressed in physical rather than mental symptoms. Sadness may manifest as 'heartache', for example.
- **Distress may be shown in different behaviours.** In some cultures, unrestrained displays of emotion that would suggest illness in the host culture are socially acceptable ways of expressing distress.
- **Cultural beliefs** may include ideas that would suggest delusional thinking in the host culture, such as being under the influence of spells cast by neighbours.
- **Expectations about treatment** may be based on experiences of very different traditions of medical care.

Ideally, the interpreter should be a member of a health profession who knows both the language and the culture of the patient. This ideal arrangement is not easy to achieve and often the only available interpreter is a family member. Although a family member will know both the language and the culture, patients may not talk freely about personal matters through such a person, especially when their genders differ, or when there are problems within the family.

Patients who appear anxious or angry

The first step is to discover the reason for the anxiety or anger. The cause might be, for example, that the patient has come to the interview reluctantly, and at the insistence of another person (e.g. when there is an alcohol problem). Some patients are worried that their employers could learn about the interview. Once the problem is understood, appropriate reassurance usually reduces distress enough for the interview to proceed.

Patients who appear confused

Sometimes the patient's initial responses are muddled and confused. This problem can be caused by **anxiety**, **low intelligence**, or **cognitive impairment** (the latter due to delirium or dementia). If cognitive impairment seems possible, brief tests of concentration and memory should be carried out (see Chapter 5). If the results are abnormal, it is usually better to interview an informant before continuing with the patient.

■ Taking a history

Basic structure of the psychiatric history

As explained above, the amount of detail and the focus of the psychiatric history vary from case to case but the basic aims are the same—it is not necessary to learn a separate interview for each condition. These common aims are reflected in the basic structure of the interview shown in Table 4.2. When time is short, parts of the background history should be covered only in outline. It is important to be flexible and able to adopt any of the following three approaches: (i) to spend 2 minutes screening patients for mental disorder, (ii) to spend 5–10 minutes undertaking a shortened, focused history in an emergency, or (iii) to spend perhaps 30 minutes obtaining a full history. Note that the most important investigation in psychiatry is always obtaining a **corroborative history** from someone who knows the patient well.

Screening questions

In primary care and general hospital medicine, psychiatric disorder is common. When a patient complains of

Table 4.2 The elements of the psychiatric history

History of the presenting problems
Background history
Family history
Personal history
Social history
Past medical history
Past psychiatric history
Medicines
Personality
Corroborative history

symptoms of physical illness, for example, it is often appropriate to check for evidence of a psychiatric disorder, since this may be present as the cause or a consequence of the symptoms. For this purpose, a brief screening interview is required to detect any symptoms and problems that have not been complained of spontaneously. The following five domains are helpful:

- **General well-being:** fatigue, irritability, poor concentration, poor sleep, and a feeling of being under pressure/not coping.
- **Anxiety:** tension, sweating, palpitations, and repeated worrying thoughts. If replies are positive, go on to systematic questions about anxiety disorders.
- **Depression:** persistent low mood, low energy, loss of interest, loss of confidence, and hopelessness. If these questions are answered positively, go on to questions concerning depressive disorder, including suicidal ideas.
- **Memory:** difficulty in recalling recent events. If difficulties are reported or suspected, use simple tests of cognitive function (see Chapter 5).
- **Alcohol and illicit drugs:** the extent of use of alcohol and drugs is noted, and in appropriate cases the CAGE questions or the Alcohol Use Disorders Identification Test are used.

Shortened history taking in an emergency

When urgent action is required, the interview has to be *brief* (focused on the basic points set out above) and *effective* (leading to a provisional diagnosis and a plan of immediate action). The information needed includes, at the least, the following points:

- **the presenting problem** in terms of symptoms or behaviours, together with their onset, course, and present severity;
- **other relevant symptoms** with their onset, course, and severity, including an assessment of risks to self (e.g.

self-harm, suicide, neglect) and others (e.g. assault or homicide, childcare, driving, operating machinery);

- **stressful circumstances** around the time of onset and at the present time;
- **previous and current physical or mental disorders** and how the patient coped with them;
- **current medicines**
- **the use of alcohol and illicit drugs**
- **family and personal history**—covered with a few salient questions;
- **social circumstances** and the possibilities of support;
- **personality**—this is valuable, although it may be difficult to obtain this information in the circumstances of an emergency.

Throughout, the interviewer should think which questions need to be answered at the time and which can be deferred. If the patient has had previous treatment, efforts should be made to contact a professional who knows the patient. However short the time, the patient should feel that he has the interviewer's undivided attention and an opportunity to say everything that is important.

The full psychiatric history

The structure of the full psychiatric history is shown in Box 4.1. Readers may find it helpful to copy this page and refer to it when they interview their first patients. As explained already, the amount of detail required in a particular case varies with the diagnostic possibilities of the case and the time available. Experienced interviewers focus on the most relevant items, but students should practise the full history until they are confident in its use, before they learn the more selective approach. The following account explains some important points concerning the items in Box 4.1.

■ History of presenting problems

Patient's description of the presenting problems

The interviewer should allow patients adequate time to talk spontaneously before asking questions, otherwise

---

BOX 4.1 The psychiatric history

Name, age, and address of the patient; name of any informants, and their relationship to the patient.

History of presenting problems

- Patient's description of the presenting problems—nature, severity, onset, factors that are making the problem worse or better
- Other problems and symptoms
- Treatment received to date

Background history

Family history

- Parents: age (now or at death), occupation, personality, and relationship with the patient
- Similar information about siblings
- Social position; atmosphere of the home
- Mental disorder in other members of the family, abuse of alcohol/drugs, suicide

Personal history

- Mother's pregnancy and birth
- Early development, separation, childhood illnesses

- Educational history
- Occupational history
- Intimate relationships

Social history

- Living arrangements
- Financial problems
- Alcohol and illicit drug use
- Forensic history

Past medical history

Past psychiatric history

Medicines

Personality

Corroborative history

they may not reveal all their problems. For example, a patient who begins by describing depression may also have a marital problem that she is hesitant to reveal. If the interviewer asks further questions about depression as soon as this is mentioned, the marital problem may not be revealed. To avoid overlooking problems, when patients have finished speaking spontaneously the interviewer should summarize the problems that have been mentioned, and ask if there are any others. The interviewer's subsequent questions are designed to understand the following issues:

- **Nature** of the problem. For example, a patient who complains of worrying excessively could be describing anxiety, obsessional symptoms, or intrusive thoughts occurring in a depressive disorder.

- **Severity** of the problem, which will be related to (i) the amount of **distress** caused by the problem, and (ii) the amount of **functional impairment**/interference with day-to-day activities.

- **Onset**—how long ago it started, and whether this was spontaneous ('out of the blue') or related to stressful events.

- **Course** of the problem—whether it is static, worsening, improving, or fluctuating in severity, whether it has worsened gradually or in a stepwise fashion, and whether it is present continuously or intermittently.

- **Factors making the problem worse or better.** For example, low mood might be worse on work days, due to problems at work such as poor relationships with colleagues, and the presence of a supportive relationship at home. Alternatively, low mood might be better on work days, due to the structure and sense of purpose that work can bring, and the presence of a difficult marital relationship at home.

Other problems and symptoms

The interviewer should now enquire about the symptoms and problems that he judges relevant and that have not yet been volunteered by the patient. These further enquiries are guided by the interviewer's knowledge of the disorders in which the presenting symptoms and problems can occur (this information will be found in subsequent chapters). For example, if the presenting problem is poor sleep, the interviewer would ask about the symptoms of depressive and anxiety disorders, and about pain, all of which can cause insomnia. If the presenting problem is depression, a variety of physical, psychological, and social symptoms should be assessed (see Box 4.2).

The *date of onset* and *sequence* of the various symptoms should also be noted. For example, whether obses-

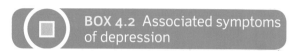

BOX 4.2 Associated symptoms of depression

Physical: low energy, poor (or increased) sleep, poor (or increased) appetite, loss (or gain) of weight, constipation, amenorrhoea

Psychological: diurnal mood variation, hopelessness, suicidal thoughts, helplessness, low self-esteem, reduced confidence, guilt, agitation, poor concentration

Social: social withdrawal, work absence, impaired work performance

sional symptoms began before or after depressive symptoms is relevant to diagnosis and treatment. The sequence of problems is similarly important, such as whether abuse of alcohol began before or after marital difficulties.

Treatment received to date

Finally, a note should be made of any *treatment already received*, its effectiveness or ineffectiveness, side effects, and adherence. For example, a patient may report that they took fluoxetine for low mood, for about 1 month, but this made them feel anxious and worsened their sleep, so they stopped taking it despite their GP advising them to continue, and that their GP also recommended that they read a named self-help book, but they have not yet obtained this.

Some specific symptoms

- **Pathological depression** is a pervasive lowering of mood accompanied by feelings of sadness and a loss of the ability to experience pleasure (**anhedonia**).

- **Pathological elation** is a pervasive elation of mood accompanied by excessive cheerfulness, which in extreme cases may be experienced as ecstasy.

- **Pathological anxiety** is a feeling of apprehension that is out of proportion to the actual situation. This is usually associated with autonomic changes, manifested by pale skin and increased sweating of the hands, feet, and axillae (see Chapter 24).

- **Depersonalization and derealization** are less easy to understand than anxiety and depression because they are less often experienced by healthy people. They are experienced occasionally by healthy people, sometimes when they are very tired. They occur as symptoms of many kinds of psychiatric disorder, especially anxiety disorders, depressive disorders, and schizophrenia, and occur also in temporal lobe epilepsy.

- **Depersonalization** is the experience of being unreal, detached, and unable to feel emotion. Paradoxically, this lack of emotional responsiveness can be extremely distressing. People who experience depersonalization often have difficulty in describing it and use similes such as 'it feels *as if* I were cut off by a wall of glass'. An 'as if' description of this kind must not be confused with a delusion (see p. 33), when the person lacks insight into their actual situation.

- **Derealization** is a similar experience, but occurs in relation to the environment rather than the self: for example, the feeling that other people seem 'as if made of cardboard' or that things no longer evoke any emotional response.

■ Background history

Family history

This part of the background history concerns the patient's father, mother, siblings, and other relatives. Enquiries about the patient's spouse or partner and children are made later. The family history is important for several reasons:

- Psychiatric disorder in other family members may point to *genetic causes*.
- Past events in the family, such as the divorce of parents, are the background to the patient's *psychological development*.
- Past events in the family may help to *explain the patient's concerns*. For example, the discovery that a brother died of a brain tumour may help to explain a patient's seemingly excessive concerns about headaches.
- Current events in the family may be *stressful*.
- A history of *completed suicide in a first-degree relative* increases the patient's risk of suicide.

A useful introduction to this part of the enquiry is: 'I would like to ask about the family into which you were born. Let us start with your father. Is he still alive?' If the father is alive, his age, state of health, and job are recorded. If the father has died, the cause of death, and his age and that of the patient at the time of the death should be determined. The father's personality and relationship with the patient can be elicited by asking 'What was your father like when you were a child?', 'What is he like now?', 'How did you get on when you were a child?',

and 'How do you get on now?' Similar enquiries are made about the mother, siblings, and other important figures in the patient's early life, such as a stepfather or a grandmother living with the patient.

The amount of detail required varies from case to case. It is unlikely to be profitable to spend time in detailed enquiries about the childhood of an elderly patient seeking help for poor memory, but it could be highly relevant to obtain this information about a young adult whose behaviour is unusual.

Personal history

The aims in taking the personal history are to describe and understand the following:

- the *life story*, including any influences that help to explain the patient's personality, concerns, and preferences. For example, sexual abuse in childhood may help to explain a woman's low self-esteem and sexual difficulties in adult life, and being the unwanted child of an unaffectionate mother may partly explain a man's fear of rejection;
- any *stressful circumstances*, including how the patient reacted to them.

The amount of detail required to achieve these aims varies from patient to patient.

Pregnancy and birth

The mother's health during pregnancy and the nature of the patient's delivery can be important in the context of learning disability. Information from the patient may be unreliable and should be checked whenever possible with the mother or with hospital records made at the time of the event. In most other cases, it is necessary to enquire only about any major problems.

Early development, separation, and childhood illnesses

The comments above about the relevance and reliability of information about pregnancy and delivery apply equally to developmental milestones, which are seldom important except when the patient is a child or an adult with learning disability. A note should be made of any *prolonged separation* from either parent for whatever reason. Since the effects of separation vary considerably, it is important to find out whether the patient was distressed at the time and for how long. If possible, this information should be checked with the parents. Serious and prolonged *childhood illnesses* may have affected the patient's emotional development. Diseases of the central nervous system in this period may be relevant to learning disability.

Educational history

The history of school and, if applicable, college and university education gives a general indication of intelligence and achievements, and contributes to an understanding of personality. As well as academic, artistic, and sporting achievement, enquiries are made about friendships, sociability, aggressive behaviour, bullying, leadership, and relationships with fellow students and with teachers.

Occupational history

The occupational history throws light on abilities and achievements, and on personality. Frequent changes of job, failure to gain promotion, or arguments with senior staff may reflect negative aspects of personality (although there are, of course, many other reasons for these events). Persistence with jobs or degrees that are poorly rewarded financially, and associated with frustrations and difficulties, may reflect more positive aspects of personality.

Intimate relationships

This part of the history includes the success and failure of intimate relationships, as well as sexual preferences and behaviour. Detailed enquiries are not needed in every case, but when they are relevant the interviewer should be able to make them sympathetically, objectively, and without embarrassment. Common-sense judgement and a knowledge of clinical syndromes will indicate how much to ask. If the patient is sexually active, questions about their attitude to pregnancy and contraception are relevant. Detailed questions about sexual preferences and behaviour may be relevant when one of the problems is a sexual one; in other cases it is usually enough to ask more generally whether there are any sexual problems. These are often relevant in patients with mental illness—for example, depression is associated with low sexual interest, and antidepressants can have sexual side effects, including delayed orgasm. Women should be asked about **menstrual problems** appropriate to their age, including psychological and other symptoms of the premenstrual syndrome and the menopause.

The interviewer should ask about long-term relationships, including marriage and other partnerships, including same-sex partnerships. Ask whether the partnership is happy, how long it has lasted, about the partner's work and personality, and about the sex, age, parentage, health, and development of any children. Similar enquiries are made about any previous partnership(s). If the partnership is unhappy, further questions should be asked about the nature and causes of this unhappiness, how the couple came together, and

any periods of separation or plans for future separation or divorce. These enquiries may also throw light on the patient's personality, which may be relevant to the management plan.

Social history

This section is important. Without the following topics being addressed, an overview of the patient's problems is not possible, and important aspects of the management plan will not be addressed.

- **Living arrangements.** Potentially relevant enquiries include the size and quality of the patient's home, whether it is owned or rented, who else lives with the patient, and how these people relate to one another, and to the patient.

- **Financial problems.** Does the patient have financial difficulties and, if so, what kind, and what steps are they taking to deal with them?

- **Alcohol and illicit drug use.** These are often associated with mental disorder, and a careful alcohol and drugs history should be taken in every case. A screening question will often suffice for illicit drug use.

- **Forensic history.** This concerns behaviour that breaks the law. Common sense should be used to judge its relevance, but it is important in all cases of alcohol or drug misuse. For example, a young man who binge drinks on Friday and Saturday nights may have convictions for assault and criminal damage while intoxicated with alcohol, and one or more convictions for drink driving, and yet be denying that he has an alcohol problem. If the patient has a criminal record, note the charges and the penalties, and find out whether other such acts have gone undetected.

Past medical history

Medical illnesses, past and current, should be asked about in every case. Medical problems are often a cause or a consequence of mental disorder. For example, in many cases, people with mental illness and physical illness receive poor-quality care for their physical illness, endocrine disorders such as hypothyroidism are associated with mental illness, and psychiatric medications such as antipsychotics have metabolic side effects.

Past psychiatric history

When there is a past psychiatric history, careful notes should be taken of the nature of the illness, the number and severity of episodes, any association with risks to self (e.g. self-harm) or to others, and success or otherwise of treatments, including inpatient admission.

Medicines

A careful medicine history should be recorded. Which medicines is the patient taking, at what dose, and at what frequency? Is the patient non-adherent and, if so, to what extent? Does the patient know why they are prescribed? Does the patient use tablets prescribed for someone else, such as using a relative's antidepressants as an occasional pick-me-up, or benzodiazepines to calm nerves? Does the patient buy other pills or remedies from the chemist, including herbal remedies such as St John's wort or valerian? St John's wort is a popular herbal remedy for depression, but it interacts with the metabolism of many medicines, including anti-AIDS drugs, the combined oral contraceptive, and immunosuppressants, and so potential risks include progression from HIV to AIDS, unwanted pregnancy, and organ rejection. A careful medicines history is essential.

Personality

Personality assessment is discussed more fully in Chapter 31, and only salient points will be mentioned here. Enquiries should begin by asking patients to describe their personality. Subsequent questions are concerned with education, work, social relationships, leisure activities, prevailing mood, character, attitudes and standards, and habits. Whenever possible, an informant should be interviewed since few people can give a wholly objective account of their own personality. Sometimes the interviewer's impressions of the patient formed during the interview are useful, but these impressions can be misleading, especially when the patient is very distressed or suffering from a psychiatric disorder. General practitioners are able to build up a picture of their patients' personalities over years of occasional medical contacts. This information is valuable and should be passed on if the patient is referred to a psychiatrist.

■ Corroborative history

What informants can contribute

In every case informants can provide useful information about the patient's personality. Their information is essential when the patient is unable or unwilling to

reveal important information, for example when the patient:

- is unaware of the nature and extent of his abnormality (e.g. a demented patient);
- knows the extent of the problem but is unwilling to reveal it (e.g. a patient with an alcohol problem);
- cannot say reliably when the disorder started.

The need for consent

With few exceptions, the patient's consent should be obtained before interviewing informants. The interviewer should explain that the interview is to obtain information that will help to decide how best to help the patient, and that information given to the interviewer by the patient will not be revealed to the informant unless the patient has agreed. The *exceptions to the need for consent* are when patients cannot provide an adequate history because they are: (i) confused, stuporose, extremely retarded, or mute; (ii) extremely agitated or violent; or (iii) depending on specific local mental health law, being assessed with a view to detention against their will. A further exception is usually made for children.

Arranging the interview

It is generally better to interview relatives or other informants after the interview with the patient. It is usually better to see them away from the patient so that they can speak freely: for example, a wife may be reluctant to talk in her husband's presence about his heavy drinking. The purpose of the interview should be explained because relatives sometimes expect that they are about to be blamed for the patient's problems, or asked to give help that they are not prepared to provide.

Confidentiality

Unless informants have agreed to disclosure, the interviewer should not tell the patient what they have said. This rule applies even when the relative has spoken of something that the interviewer needs to discuss with the patient, such as heavy drinking that has been denied. If the relative has refused permission for the information to be disclosed, the interviewer can only try to help the patient reveal the information himself. In view of this and because patients may ask to see their case notes, it is better to record the interview with the informant on a separate sheet. The law regarding access to notes is complex, and differs between countries, in some of which specific safeguards are in place to protect information given by relatives.

The informants' concerns

As well as asking for information about the patient, the interviewer should find out how the informants view the problem, how it affects them, and what help they are seeking.

Helping the informants

When the interview with informants reveals that they too have emotional problems, either as a result of the patient's illness or for other reasons, the interviewer should either offer help or assist them to obtain help from another professional.

 Further reading

Gelder, M., Harrison, P. & Cowen, P. (2006). *Shorter Oxford Textbook of Psychiatry*, 5th edn. Chapter 1, Symptoms and signs of psychiatric disorders, pp. 1–20. Chapter 3, Assessment, pp. 35–68. Oxford University Press, Oxford.

Conducting the assessment

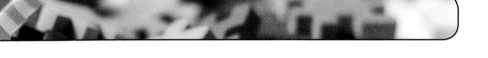

CHAPTER 5

■ Psychological ('mental state') examination

Terminology

In general hospital and community settings, the term '*physical* examination' is almost always applied to the procedures used by medical and other staff to examine the body, including the nervous system, of patients. In mental health settings, the terms '*psychological* examination' or '*mental* examination' might seem most appropriate for the procedures used to examine the mind. However, the lengthier term 'mental state examination' is usually used, often with initial capitals, for reasons of tradition. This term is often shortened to MSE.

You will find that effective communication of the results of the mental state examination requires familiarity with many new terms and with their precise meanings. It is important that you grapple with these issues early on in your training. Like specific diagnostic terms, the terms for specific abnormalities of mental state can become an effective shorthand, aiding communication between healthcare professionals.

Goals

The goal of the mental state examination is to elicit the patient's **current psychopathology**, that is their abnormal subjective experiences, and an objective view of their mental state, including abnormal behaviour. It therefore includes both **symptoms** (what *the patient reports* about **current** psychological symptoms, such as mood, thoughts, beliefs, abnormal perceptions, cognitive function, etc.) and **signs** (what *you observe* about the patient's behaviour during the interview).

Inevitably, the MSE (i.e. now) merges at the edges with history of the presenting problems (recently). Behavioural abnormalities that the patient reports as still present, but which cannot be observed at interview (e.g. disturbed sleep, overeating, cutting), are part of the history of the presenting illness. A symptom that has resolved, such as an abnormal belief held last week but not today, should usually form part of the history, but will not be reported in the MSE. In contrast, an abnormal belief held last week that is still held today will be reported in both history of the presenting problems and MSE.

How to conduct a mental state examination

The components of the mental state examination are listed in Box 5.1, and are explained further in this chapter. In taking the history, the interviewer will have learnt about the patient's symptoms up to the time of the consultation. Often the clinical features on the day of the examination are no different from those described in the recent past, in which case the mental state will overlap with the recent history.

Several aspects of the mental state examination do not require specific questions, and can be assessed by conversation with the patient and careful observation. These include appearance and behaviour, speech, the 'objective' assessment of mood, and the assessment of the 'form' and 'stream' of thoughts. however, other aspects do require specific questioning, including mood—subjective, thoughts—content, perceptions, cognition, and insight.

Mental state examination is a practical skill that can be learnt only by observing experienced interviewers and by practising alone and under supervision. This chapter can assist the reader with this training but cannot replace it. Do not be intimidated by the apparent complexity of the mental state examination. It is simply a structured conversation with a patient, with the aim of understanding their mental world in order to determine whether mental illness exists and, if it does, to characterize that illness. Students should learn how to conduct a *complete* mental state examination with every patient. With increasing experience, they will become able to focus on items judged from the history to be of particular relevance, so that their examination can focus on the necessary parts.

Form and content of psychiatric signs

Many psychiatric signs have two aspects: form and content. The distinction can be explained with three clinical examples. One patient may say that, when alone and out of hearing distance of other people, he hears voices telling him that he is changing sex. The *form* of his experience is an auditory hallucination (a sensory perception in the absence of an external stimulus, see p. 38), and the *content* is the idea that he is changing sex. Another patient may hear voices saying that he is about to be killed by persecutors. The form of this symptom is again an auditory hallucination, but the content is different. Finally, a third patient may experience repeated intrusive thoughts that he is changing sex but realize that these thoughts are untrue. The content of this symptom is the same as that of the first patient, but the form is different—it is an obsessional thought (see p. 36).

BOX 5.1 Mental state examination

Appearance and behaviour

- General appearance
- Facial expression
- Posture
- Movements
- Social behaviour

Speech

- Quantity
- Rate
- Spontaneity
- Volume

Mood

- Subjective
- Objective
  - Predominant mood
  - Constancy
  - Congruity

Thoughts

- Stream
- Form
- Content
  - Preoccupations
  - Morbid thoughts, including suicidality
  - Delusions and overvalued ideas
  - Obsessional symptoms

Perceptions

- Illusions
- Hallucinations
- Distortions

Cognition

- Orientation
- Attention and concentration
- Memory
- Language functioning
- Visuospatial functioning

Insight

In making a diagnosis, the form of the sign is important; delusions and obsessional features have a different diagnostic significance. In helping patients, the content is important as a guide to how they may respond (e.g. whether or not they might consider attacking a supposed persecutor) and in understanding their experience of the illness.

Difficulties in the mental state examination

Apart from the obvious problem of examining patients who speak little or no English—which requires the help of a skilled interpreter, preferably familiar with both cultures—difficulties can arise with patients who are unresponsive, overactive, or confused.

- **Unresponsive patients.** When patients are mute or stuporous (conscious but not speaking or responding in any other way) it is possible only to make observations of behaviour. Nevertheless, these observations can be informative. Since stuporous patients can sometimes become suddenly violent, it is prudent to be accompanied when examining such a patient.

  Before deciding that the patient is mute, it is important that the interviewer, (i) establishes that he is speaking a language that the patient understands, (ii) has allowed adequate time for reply (delay can be lengthy in severe depressive illness), (iii) has tried a variety of topics, and (iv) has found out whether the patient will communicate in writing.

  As well as making the observations of behaviour described above, the interviewer should note whether the patient's eyes are open or closed. If they are open, he should note whether they follow objects, move apparently without purpose, or are fixed. If the eyes are closed, the interviewer should note whether they are opened on request and, if not, whether attempts at opening them are resisted.

  Physical examination, including neurological assessment, is essential in all such cases, which should be seen, whenever possible, by a specialist who will look for certain additional, uncommon signs found in catatonic schizophrenia (e.g. waxy flexibility of muscles, negativism). In all such cases it is essential to interview an informant to discover the onset and course of the condition.

- **Overactive patients.** When the patient is overactive (e.g. because of mania) questions have to be limited to a few that seem particularly important, and conclusions have to be based mainly on observations of behaviour and on spontaneous utterances. Sometimes the overactivity has been made worse by attempts at physical restraint. A quiet, confident approach by the interviewer may calm the patient enough to allow adequate examination.

- **Confused patients.** When patients give the history in a muddled way, and especially when they appear perplexed or frightened, cognitive function should be tested early in the interview. If there is evidence of impairment, a corroborative history is essential. If consciousness is impaired, try to orientate the patient and reassure them, and then start the interview again in a simplified form.

■ Appearance and behaviour

Much can be learnt from general appearance, facial expression, posture, voluntary or involuntary movements, and social behaviour. Relevant features should be summarized in a few phrases that give a clear picture to someone who has not met the patient. For example, 'a tall, gaunt, stooping, and dishevelled man with a sad countenance, who looks much older than his 40 years, and who displays some parkinsonian features'.

General appearance includes physique, hair, make-up, and clothing. Manic patients may dress incongruously in brightly coloured or oddly assorted clothes. Signs of **self-neglect** include a dirty unkempt appearance and stained, crumpled clothing. Self-neglect suggests alcoholism, drug addiction, dementia, or schizophrenia. An appearance of **weight loss** is as important in psychiatry as it is in general medicine, suggesting **physical disorder** (e.g. cancer, hyperthyroidism), **psychological disorder** (e.g. anorexia nervosa, depressive disorder), or **social problems** such as financial difficulty or homelessness.

Facial expression. Mood states are accompanied by characteristic facial expressions and postures (Box 5.2). For example, turning down of the corners of the mouth and vertical furrows in the brow suggest **depression**; whereas horizontal furrows on the brow, wide palpebral fissures, and dilated pupils suggest **anxiety**. An unchanging 'wooden' expression may result from a **parkinsonian syndrome**, either primary or caused by antipsychotic drugs.

Posture may also give indications of prevailing mood. A depressed patient characteristically sits with shoulders hunched, and with the head and eyes 'downcast'. An anxious patient typically sits upright, with the head erect and the hands gripping the chair.

Movement. Manic patients are overactive, restless, and move rapidly from place to place and task to task. Depressed patients are inactive and move slowly. Rarely, a depressed patient becomes completely immobile and mute, a condition known as **stupor**. Anxious or agitated patients are restless, and sometimes tremulous. Any involuntary movements should be noted, including tics, choreiform movements, dystonia, or tardive dyskinesia.

BOX 5.2 Association between mood and appearance

- **Depression.** The corners of the mouth are turned down and the centre of the brow has vertical furrows. The head is inclined forward with the gaze directed downwards, and shoulders are bent. The patient's gestures are reduced.
- **Elation.** A lively, cheerful expression. Posture and expressive movements are normal.
- **Anxiety.** The brow is furrowed horizontally, the posture is tense, and the person is restless and sometimes tremulous. Often there are accompanying signs of autonomic overactivity, such as pale skin and increased sweating of the hands, feet, and axillae.
- **Anger.** The eyebrows are drawn down, with widening of the palpebral fissure, and a squaring of the corners of the mouth that may reveal the teeth. The shoulders are square and the body tense as if ready for action.

Social behaviour. Manic patients are disinhibited, and may break social conventions, for example by being unduly familiar. Some demented and some schizophrenic patients are disinhibited, while others are withdrawn and preoccupied. In describing these behaviours, a clear and accurate description of what is done or not done is more scientific than subjective terms such as 'disinhibited' or 'bizarre'.

Signs of impending violence include restlessness, sweating, clenched fists or pointed fingers, intrusion into the interviewer's 'personal space', and a raised voice.

Motor symptoms and signs such as mannerisms, sterotypies, and catatonic symptoms are briefly described in the chapter on schizophrenia (see p. 249) and more extensively in *The Shorter Oxford Textbook of Psychiatry*. Here we define three movement disorders:

- **Tics** are irregular repeated movements involving a group of muscles (e.g. a sideways movement of the head).
- **Choreiform movements** are brief involuntary movements that are coordinated but purposeless, such as grimacing or movements of the arms.
- **Dystonia** is a muscle spasm, which is often painful and may lead to contortions.

■ Speech

The physical characteristics of a patient's speech come under this heading; the 'form' and 'content' of the thoughts they express through the medium of speech are recorded later under 'Thoughts'. Here we describe changes to speech that are often seen in patients with depression or mania.

- **Quantity.** Depressed patients speak less than usual; manic patients speak more. Occasionally a patient does not speak at all (**mutism**).
- **Rate.** Depressed patients speak more slowly than usual. Manic patients speak faster. Copious rapid speech which is hard to interrupt is called **pressure of speech.**

- **Spontaneity.** Patients with depression or intoxicated patients may have a **long answer latency**; they are asked a question, but it can be many seconds, or longer, before an answer is forthcoming. Patients with mania will answer promptly, and often very quickly, if they are able to attend for long enough to the interview.
- **Volume.** Depressed patients may speak quietly; manic patients may often be heard far down the corridor.

Abnormalities of the **continuity** of speech, including any sudden interruptions, rapid shifts of topic, and lack of logical thread, should be recorded under 'Thoughts—form'.

■ Mood

Changes in mood are the most common symptoms of psychiatric disorder. They are the principal symptoms of depressive and anxiety disorders, but they may occur in every kind of psychiatric disorder, during physical illness, and in healthy people encountering stressful events. Terminology can be confusing. The term affect is used by some professionals instead of mood, and the term affective disorder is an alternative name for mood disorder. We recommend using the terms **mood** and **mood disorder**, as mood is a word which is in common use in the general population, and is therefore widely understood.

The patient's 'subjective' mood and the professional's 'objective' assessment of mood should be documented. Mismatch between the two can be useful in the assessment of diagnosis and risk.

Subjective mood

Ask the patient 'What is your mood just now?', or 'Can you tell me how you're feeling ... in your spirits?' or '... in yourself?'. Record the patient's responses without altering them, so record (for example) 'Great, never felt better', or 'OK, not too bad', or 'Awful, terrible, desperate'. Often, patients will need some encouragement to report their feelings, and you should be sensitive to this need.

Further questions can then be asked about the patient's recent mood, and about symptoms associated with particular mood states. These are aspects of history, and should be recorded there rather than within the MSE. However, it may help rapport within the interview to link questions about emotions here and now, within the interview, with questions about emotional experiences in recent days and weeks. If a **depressed** mood is reported, the associated symptoms may include a feeling of being ready to cry, lack of interest and enjoyment, and pessimistic thoughts, including thoughts of suicide. When **anxiety** is reported, associated symptoms include palpitations, dry mouth, tremor, sweating, and worrying thoughts. When **elevated mood** is reported, associated symptoms include excessive self-confidence, grandiose plans, and an inflated assessment of the person's own ability. These manic symptoms have, of course, to be elicited indirectly, for example by asking the patient about his plans and his assessment of his abilities.

Objective mood

The nature, constancy, and congruity of a patient's observed mood should be described:

1 **Nature of mood or moods.** What mood or moods appear to predominate within the interview? These might include *depression, elation, anger, anxiety, suspicion,* or *perplexity*. It is possible to record more than one; a patient might appear depressed and perplexed, for example. Of course, the patient may exhibit no particular emotions, and not appear, in particular, either depressed or elated. In this circumstance, many psychiatrists use the term '**euthymic**', but, as this term is unusual outside psychiatry, we prefer the term '**unremarkable mood**'. As described above, mood states are accompanied by characteristic facial expressions and postures, which can help to identify the mood of a patient who is denying emotion, for example denying that he is angry.

2 **Constancy of mood.** In healthy people, mood varies from day to day and hour to hour—it is normal for mood to fluctuate in reaction to internal circumstances (e.g. what the person is thinking about) and external circumstances (e.g. reminders of a failed relationship, or of recent exam success). However, this normal emotional reactivity is limited in extent and limited in time. This normal spectrum of change may be increased (**emotional lability),** such as in dementia, mania, or after a stroke, and, when it is extreme,

may be called **emotional incontinence.** Alternatively, it may be decreased (**reduced reactivity**, **blunting**, or **flattening**), such as in depression, when smiles or laughter do not follow a shift to a positive or amusing topic. **Irritability** is a term which spans two components of the objective assessment of mood—predominant moods (in irritability, this might include tension and anger) and variation in mood (in irritability, this would be labile, with anger triggered easily).

3 **Congruity of mood.** Normally, our *mood*, our *thoughts* and our *perceptions* are closely associated, and 'fit' together logically. For example, if we are watching news scenes from a natural disaster, we are *seeing* scenes of destruction and suffering, we are *thinking* about how difficult this must be for the people involved, and we are likely to be *feeling* subdued, contemplative, and maybe depressed. Equally, an elated person will be thinking happy thoughts and perceiving all the good, positive things in the world around them. In these cases, there is '**congruity of mood**', which is normal. Very occasionally, such as in schizophrenia, this linkage is lost, and there is '**incongruity of mood**', so that, for example, a person appears cheerful while describing sad events. This is different to the apparent cheerfulness that hides embarrassment (which is commonly experienced, and normal), and also different to the lack of outward show of emotion in people who feel it inwardly—a condition that occurs in some depressed patients.

■ Thoughts

Accessing thoughts

If we want to know what someone is thinking, we can work it out in several ways. The first and most obvious is to listen to what they are saying, either spontaneously or in response to our or someone else's questions. The next is to read what they are writing, whether that is on paper, on a computer, or in a text message. Finally, we can observe their appearance and behaviour, and use clues from that to guide our understanding of what might be in their mind (see Case Study 5.1).

Abnormalities of thought

Disorders of thinking can be of several kinds:

1 abnormality of the **stream** of thought (its amount and speed);

2 abnormality of the **form** of thought (the ways in which thoughts are linked together);

3 abnormality of the **content** of thought (preoccupations, morbid thoughts, delusions, overvalued ideas, obsessional and compulsive symptoms).

Case study 5.1 A patient's thoughts

John is a 21-year-old university physics student, who has been locking himself in his room, refusing to come out, except from time to time when he went around the house systematically switching off electrical items such as mobile phones, televisions, and computers. He refused to tell his housemates or his parents why he was doing this. His parents were called to his shared house by his housemates, and called his GP, Dr Jones, who has now attended for an assessment. On careful and supportive questioning by the GP, John explained his concern that he would be harmed by secret services from another country, which he would not name. He was wanted by them because of his new invention, which had arisen out of his final year project, and which would revolutionize warfare in the years to come. Switching off electrical devices was his way of preventing secret services locating him through electronic means. Dr Jones expressed some surprise that John's degree project had generated such an important finding, but John remained adamant that this was the case. Dr Jones asked if he might speak to John's research supervisor, to corroborate his account, and, after insisting on some safeguards, John reluctantly agreed.

Abnormalities of the stream of thought

In disorders of the stream of thought both the amount and the speed of thoughts are changed. There are three main abnormalities: **pressure**, **poverty** and **blocking** of thought.

1 **Pressure of thought.** Thoughts are unusually rapid, abundant, and varied. The disorder is characteristic of mania but also occurs in schizophrenia.

2 **Poverty of thought.** Thoughts are unusually slow, few, and unvaried. The disorder is characteristic of severe depressive disorder but also occurs in schizophrenia.

3 **Blocking of thought** refers to an experience in which the mind is suddenly empty of thoughts. The symptom of thought blocking should not be confused with the normal experiences of sudden distraction, the intrusion of a different line of thinking, or the experience of losing a particular word or train of thought while other thoughts continue. Thought blocking is the experience of an abrupt and complete emptying of the mind. It occurs especially in schizophrenic patients, who may interpret the experience in a delusional way (see below)—believing, for example, that their thoughts have been removed by another person (delusion of thought withdrawal).

Abnormalities of the form of thought

There are three main abnormalities of the ways in which thoughts are linked together: **flight of ideas, loosening of associations,** and **perseveration.**

1 **Flight of ideas.** In this abnormal state, characteristic of mania, thoughts and any accompanying spoken words move quickly from one topic to another, so that one train of thought is not completed before the next begins. Because topics change so rapidly, the links between one topic and the next may be difficult to follow. Nevertheless, recognizable and understandable links are present, though not always in the form of logical connections. Instead the link may be through: (i) **rhyme**, for example when an idea about chairs is followed by an idea about pears (rhyming links are sometimes called **clang associations**); (ii) **puns**, that is two words that have the same sound (e.g. male/ mail); and (iii) **distraction**, for example a new topic suggested by something in the interview room.

2 **Loosening of associations** is a lack of logical connection between a sequence of thoughts, not explicable by the links described under flight of ideas. This lack of logical association is sometimes called **knight's-move thinking** (referring to the sudden change of direction of the knight in chess). Usually the interviewer is alerted to the presence of loosening of associations because the patient's replies are hard to follow. This difficulty in understanding differs from that experienced when interviewing people who are very anxious or are of low intelligence. Anxious people become more coherent when put at ease, and people of low intelligence do so when questions are simplified. When there is loosening of associations, the links between ideas cannot be made more understandable in either of these ways. Instead, the interviewer has the experience that the more he tries to clarify the patient's thinking, the less he understands it. Loosening of associations occurs most often in schizophrenia. It is often difficult to distinguish loosening of associations from flight of ideas, and when this happens it is often helpful to tape-record a sample of speech and listen to it carefully.

3 **Perseveration** is the persistent and inappropriate repetition of the same sequence of thought, as shown in either speech or actions. It can be demonstrated by asking a series of simple questions; the patient repeats his answer to the first question as his response to all subsequent questions even though these require different answers. Perseveration

occurs most often in dementia, but may occur in other disorders.

Preoccupations

Preoccupations are thoughts that recur frequently but can be put out of mind by an effort of will. They are a part of normal experience—students, for example, who are concerned about an imminent exam are likely to be preoccupied with thoughts and concerns about their preparation, likely exam questions, and the consequences of a poor performance. They are clinically significant only if they contribute to distress or disability. They are commonly seen in psychiatric disorders, including (i) *depressive disorders*, where preoccupations about suicide should be explored carefully (see p. 65), (ii) *anxiety disorders*, where preoccupations may prolong the disorder (see p. 285), and (iii) *sexual disorders,* where preoccupations may influence behaviour (see p. 410). Some preoccupations are noticed during history taking; others may be revealed by asking 'What sort of things do you worry about?', or 'What sort of thoughts occupy your mind?'

Morbid thoughts

These are thoughts particularly associated with specific illnesses, through either their nature, for example *suicidality*, or their severity, for example *self-criticism*—it is normal, and can be helpful, to be self-critical, but in a depressive illness such self-criticism can be severe and pervasive, and help to maintain the disorder. Other morbid thoughts in depression include *hopelessness* (negativity about the future), *helplessness* (negativity about the prospects of being helped by healthcare professionals, medicines, or psychological treatment), *low self-esteem* (negativity about the self), and *guilt* (negativity about actions in the past, such as in relationships). The depressed patient is likely to consider their negative thoughts to be entirely reasonable, because they are interpreting evidence relating to themselves, the people around them, and the world around them, through 'grey-coloured spectacles', which emphasize the negative and minimize the positive. In contrast, the thoughts of a person with elated mood are distorted positively, through rose-coloured spectacles, which give them an overly positive view of themselves, the world, and the future.

Enquiring about **thoughts and plans of suicide** is an essential component of the MSE, and should always be asked about and recorded. Suicidal thoughts are a personal and sensitive matter, and it is important to practise asking about them in a supportive but rigorous way. Some interviewers are reluctant to ask about suicide, in case the questions should suggest the idea, but there is no evidence to support this. Approach the topic in stages:

1 Ask about feelings of depression, and then hopelessness ('Have you felt that you have lost hope for the future?'), before

2 Moving on to 'passive' suicidal ideas ('Have you thought life is not worth living?', 'Have you wished you might not wake up one morning?'), and finally

3 Asking about 'active' suicidal ideas ('Have you thought of taking steps to end your life?', 'Have you thought how you might do this?', 'What thoughts did you have?', and 'How close have you got to doing something about it?').

Delusions

A delusion is *a belief that is held firmly but on inadequate grounds, is not affected by rational argument or evidence to the contrary, and is not a conventional belief that the person might be expected to hold given his cultural background and level of education.* This rather lengthy definition is required to distinguish delusions, which are indicators of mental disorder, from other kinds of strongly held belief found among healthy people, such as religious or political views. A delusion is nearly always a false belief but not always so (see below). There are several problems surrounding the definition of delusions, and these are considered briefly in Box 5.3.

Conviction in the truth of a delusion does not necessarily influence all the person's feelings and actions, especially when the delusion has been present for a long time, as in chronic schizophrenia. For example, such a patient may have the delusion that he is a member of the Royal Family and yet live contentedly in a hostel for discharged psychiatric patients.

We distinguish between primary and secondary delusions. A **primary delusion** is one that *occurs suddenly without any other abnormal mental event leading to it.* For example, a patient may suddenly develop the unshakable conviction that he is changing sex, without ever having thought of this before and without any reason to do so at the time. Primary delusions are rare, and when they occur they strongly suggest schizophrenia. However, this is not very useful in practice because few patients can give a reliable account of how they first had a delusional idea. A **secondary delusion** *arises from some previous abnormal idea or experience*, which may be: (i) a *hallucination*, for example, a person hears a voice and believes he is being followed; (ii) a *mood*, for example, a person with deep depression feels worthless and believes that other people think the same about him; or (iii) *another delusion*. Secondary delusions occur in a variety of severe psychiatric disorders. When one

BOX 5.3 Some problems surrounding the definition of delusions

Delusions are arrived at through abnormal thought processes. This is the fundamental point that characterizes delusions but it cannot be observed directly. The various clauses in the definition of a delusion are intended to provide indirect criteria to establish the point, but there are some problems with each of them.

Delusions are held firmly despite evidence to the contrary. This is the key to the definition and it is often revealed through the person's words and actions. For example, a person with the delusion that persecutors are in the next room will not alter his belief when shown that the room is empty; instead, he may say that the persecutors left before he arrived. However, not all beliefs that are impervious to contrary evidence are delusions; some non-delusional beliefs are of this kind. For example, a convinced spiritualist hangs on to his belief in spiritualism when presented with contrary evidence that would convince a non-believer. These strongly held non-delusional beliefs are called **overvalued ideas**. When deluded patients recover, either with treatment or spontaneously, they pass through a stage of increasing doubt in the truth of their delusions. This stage of partial conviction in a belief that was previously a full delusion is called a **partial delusion**.

Delusions are false beliefs. Some definitions of delusion include this point. It is not included in our definition because very occasionally a delusional belief is either true from the onset, or subsequently becomes true. For example, a man may develop the delusional belief that his wife is unfaithful despite a complete lack of evidence of infidelity or of any other rational reason for holding the belief. The belief has been arrived at in an abnormal way and is delusional even if, unbeknown to him, his wife is unfaithful. The point is of mainly theoretical importance but it is sometimes brought up in discussions of delusion since it highlights the fact that the essential criterion for delusion is that it was arrived at in an abnormal way.

Delusions are usually odd and improbable beliefs. However, not all odd and improbable beliefs are delusional. Some people express seemingly improbable beliefs (e.g. that they are being poisoned by close relatives), which are subsequently proved to be true. Apparently odd beliefs should be investigated most carefully before they are accepted as delusional.

delusion gives rise to another in a sequence, the resulting network of interrelated ideas is known as a **delusional system,** in which many abnormal beliefs fit together into a coherent whole.

Other mental phenomena related to delusions

There are three mental phenomena that are closely related to delusions, but are not delusional in nature, despite their names incorporating the term 'delusional'. These are:

- **Delusional mood.** This is an inexplicable feeling of apprehension that is followed before long by a delusion that explains it. For example, a person is feeling inexplicably frightened, and then suddenly gains the belief that someone is following him with the intent to harm him.

- **Delusional perception.** This is the misinterpretation of the significance of something perceived normally. For example, a patient may suddenly be convinced that the particular arrangement of objects on his desk indicates that his life is threatened.

- **Delusional memory.** This is the retrospective delusional misinterpretation of memories of actual events. For example, the conviction that on a previous occasion when the patient felt ill his food had been poisoned by persecutors, though previously and at the time of the illness he did not believe this.

Shared delusions

Usually, other people recognize delusional beliefs as false and they argue with the deluded person in an attempt to correct them. Occasionally, a person who lives with or is otherwise in a close relationship with a deluded patient comes to share the delusional beliefs. This person is then said to have shared delusions or **folie à deux**. The affected person's conviction may be unshakable while they remain with the patient, but usually weakens quickly on separation.

Delusional themes

Delusions are usually grouped according to their main themes (Table 5.1). Since there is some correspondence between delusional theme and type of disorder, and since this is helpful in diagnosis, the main themes will be described briefly and will be related to the disorders in which they occur most often. The associations are described more fully in the chapters concerned with these disorders.

1 **Persecutory delusions** are often (but incorrectly) called **paranoid delusions**. Used strictly, 'paranoid' refers not only to persecutory but also to grandiose, jealous, amorous, and hypochondriacal delusions. However, this strict usage is seldom adopted. Persecutory delusions are

Table 5.1 Delusional themes

Persecutory (paranoid)
Reference
Grandiose and expansive
Guilt and worthlessness
Nihilistic
Hypochondriacal or dysmorphophobic
Jealousy
Sexual or amorous
Religious
Control
The possession of thoughts

ideas that people or organizations are trying to inflict harm on the patient, damage his reputation, or make him insane. It is important to remember that it is normal in some cultures to ascribe misfortunes to the malign activities of other people, for example through witchcraft. Such ideas are not delusions. Persecutory delusions are common in *schizophrenia*, and occur also in *organic states* and *severe depressive disorders*. When the delusions are part of a depressive disorder, the patient characteristically accepts that the supposed actions of his persecutors are justified by his own wickedness; in schizophrenia, however, he characteristically resents them.

2 **Delusions of reference** are concerned with the idea that objects, events, or the actions of other people have a special significance for the patient. For example, a remark heard on television is believed to be directed specifically to the patient, or a gesture by a stranger is believed to convey something about the patient. Delusions of this kind are associated with *schizophrenia*.

3 **Grandiose and expansive delusions** are beliefs of exaggerated self-importance. Patients may think themselves wealthy, endowed with unusual abilities, or in other ways special. Such ideas occur mainly in *mania* and sometimes in *schizophrenia*.

4 **Delusions of guilt and worthlessness** are beliefs that the person has done something shameful or sinful. Usually, the belief concerns an innocent error that caused no guilt at the time, for example a small error in an income tax return, which the patient now fears will be discovered and lead to prosecution. This kind of delusion occurs most often in *severe depressive disorders*.

5 **Nihilistic delusions** include beliefs that the patient's career is finished, that he is about to die or has no money, or that the world is doomed. Nihilistic delusions occur most often in *severe depressive disorders*.

6 **Hypochondriacal delusions** are false beliefs about the presence of disease. The patient believes, in the face of convincing medical evidence to the contrary, that he has a disease. Such delusions are more common among the elderly, reflecting the increasing concerns about ill health in later life. Related **dysmorphophobic delusions** are concerned with the appearance of parts of the body, for example the belief that the person's (normally shaped) nose is seriously misshapen. Patients with delusions about their appearance may seek the help of plastic surgeons. Hypochondriacal delusions occur in *depressive disorders* and *schizophrenia*.

7 **Delusions of jealousy** are more common among men. 'Morbid (pathological) jealousy' may lead to dangerously aggressive behaviour towards the person who is believed to be unfaithful.

8 **Sexual or amorous delusions** are more frequent among women. Usually, the woman believes that she is loved by a man who has never spoken to her and who is inaccessible—for example, an eminent public figure.

9 **Religious delusions** may be concerned with guilt (for example, divine punishment for minor sins) or with special powers. Before deciding that such beliefs are delusional, it is important to determine whether they are held by other members of the patient's religious or cultural group.

10 **Delusions of control** are beliefs that personal actions, impulses, or thoughts are controlled by an outside agency. This experience has to be distinguished from (i) voluntary obedience to commands given by hallucinatory voices, and (ii) culturally normal beliefs that human actions are under divine control. Delusions of control strongly suggest *schizophrenia*.

11 **Delusions concerning the possession of thoughts.** Healthy people have no doubt that their thoughts are their own and that other people can know them only if they are spoken aloud or revealed through actions. Delusions of thought possession are found most often in schizophrenia, and include:

(i) **delusion of thought insertion**—some of the person's thoughts have been implanted by an outside agency;

(ii) **delusion of thought withdrawal**—some of their thoughts have been taken away;

(iii) **delusion of thought broadcasting**—some of their thoughts are known to other people through telepathy, radio, or some other unusual way.

Asking about delusions

Often the first indication of the presence of delusions is during history taking, either from the patient or from an informant. When there is no such indication, judgement should be used about whether to enquire about delusions, because the questions may antagonize patients who have come for help for another problem. Questions should be asked whenever there is evidence of a *severe depressive disorder*, when *schizophrenia* enters the differential diagnosis, or in cases of doubt. It is often difficult to elicit delusions during mental state examination because the patient does not regard them as abnormal. A good way of starting the enquiry is to ask for an explanation of any unusual statements, unpleasant experiences, or unusual events that the patient has mentioned. For example, a patient may say that his headaches started when his neighbours caused him trouble; when asked why the neighbours should do this, he may say they are conspiring to harm him. Patients often hide delusions, and the interviewer needs to be alert to evasions, vague replies, or other hints that information is being withheld.

Having discovered an unusual belief, the interviewer has to decide three things:

1 **Is the belief true?** Some beliefs are clearly false; for example, that persecutors are damaging the patient's brain by beaming radiowaves on him. Other beliefs need to be checked—for example, that neighbours are collaborating in harassing the patient.

2 **How strongly are the beliefs held?** Considerable tact is required when finding out. The patient should feel that he is having a fair hearing, and that the interviewer's response is enquiring, rather than argumentative or dismissive. The interviewer should question the reasons for the beliefs gently but persistently.

3 **Are the beliefs culturally determined?** Are the beliefs accepted by others sharing the patient's cultural background or religious beliefs? In some cultures beliefs in evil forces or witchcraft are widespread. Doubt can usually be resolved by finding another person from the same religion or culture, and asking whether the patient's ideas are held by others from the same background.

Delusions of *thought broadcasting, thought insertion, thought withdrawal,* or *control* can usually be elicited only by asking direct questions. Since their presence strongly suggests schizophrenia, it is essential to check any positive answer by asking for examples. Appropriate questions include 'Do you ever think that other people can tell what you are thinking, even though you have not told them?', 'Do you ever think that thoughts have been put into your mind?', 'Why is that?', and 'How does that happen?'.

Overvalued ideas

An overvalued idea is an *isolated, preoccupying, and strongly held belief, that dominates a person's life and may affect his or her actions, but which (unlike a delusion) has been derived through normal mental processes*. For example, someone whose parents developed cancer within a short time of one another may be convinced that cancer is contagious, despite having been presented many times with evidence to the contrary. It is sometimes difficult to distinguish between overvalued ideas and delusions since the two may be equally strongly held, and the differentiation depends on a judgement of the way in which the idea developed. In practice, this difficulty seldom causes problems since diagnosis does not depend on a single symptom.

Obsessional and compulsive symptoms

Obsessions are *recurrent and persistent thoughts, impulses, or images, that enter the mind despite efforts to exclude them, that the person recognizes are senseless, and that the person recognizes as products of their own mind*. The obsessions usually concern matters that the person finds distressing or unpleasant, and often feels ashamed to tell others about. The person has no doubt that the intruding thoughts are their own, in contrast to a person with the delusion of thought insertion, who believes that the ideas have been implanted from outside. A sense of struggling to resist the intrusions is part of an obsessional symptom. Resistance distinguishes obsessions (in which it is present) from delusions (in which it is absent). However, when obsessions have been present for a long time, resistance may decrease so that this distinction becomes difficult to make. In practice, this decrease seldom leads to diagnostic problems because it takes place late in the course of the disorder, when the diagnosis has already been made.

Obsessional thoughts are repeated, intrusive words or phrases, which take many forms, including obscenities, blasphemies, and thoughts about distressing occurrences (e.g. that the patient's hands are contaminated with bacteria that will spread disease). There are several common themes (see Box 5.4). **Obsessional ruminations** are repeated sequences of such thoughts (e.g. about the ending of the world). **Obsessional doubts** are recurrent uncertainties about a previous action (e.g. whether or not the person has switched off an electrical appliance that could cause a fire). **Obsessional impulses** are urges to carry out actions that are usually aggressive, dangerous, or socially embarrassing (e.g. using a knife to stab someone, jumping in front of a moving train, or shouting obscenities in church). Whatever the urge, the person recognizes that it is irrational and does not wish to carry it out. This is an important point of distinction from delusions, which are regarded as rational by the patient and which may lead to action, such as aggression against a supposed persecutor. **Obsessional**

BOX 5.4 Themes of obsessional phenomena

Obsessional thoughts

- **Dirt and contamination**, for example the idea that the hands are contaminated with bacteria.

- **Aggressive actions**, for example the idea that the person may harm another person, or shout angry remarks.

- **Orderliness**, for example the idea that objects have to be arranged in a special way, or clothes put on in a particular order.

- **Disease**, for example the idea that the person may have cancer (some ideas of contamination refer to illness, e.g. ideas of contamination with harmful bacteria).

- **Sex**, usually thoughts or images of practices that the person finds disgusting.

- **Religion**, for example blasphemous thoughts, or doubts about the fundamentals of belief (e.g. 'Does God exist?') or about the adequacy of a religious practice such as confession.

Compulsions

- **Checking rituals**, which are often concerned with safety (e.g. checking repeatedly that a gas tap has been turned off).

- **Cleaning rituals**, such as repeated handwashing or domestic cleaning.

- **Counting rituals**, such as counting to a particular number or counting in threes.

- **Dressing rituals**, in which the clothes are always set out or put on in a particular way.

---

images are recurrent vivid mental pictures that are unexpected, unselected, usually unwelcome, and usually distressing (e.g. an image of oneself sick and dying in a hospital, or covered in human excrement from an overflowing sewer in the street, or standing mute and helpless while supposed to be giving an important talk to colleagues).

Obsessional symptoms are essential features of obsessive-compulsive disorder. They occur also in other psychiatric disorders, especially anxiety and depressive disorders. They should be distinguished from the following phenomena, which are not regarded by patients as unreasonable, and are not resisted:

- ordinary preoccupations of healthy people;
- intrusive concerns/preoccupations of anxious or depressed patients;
- recurring thoughts and images associated with sexual preference disorders/drug dependence;
- delusions.

Although compulsions are actions, not thoughts, it is appropriate to describe them here because most compulsions are associated with and motivated by obsessions. Compulsions are *recurrent and persistent stereotyped actions that the person feels compelled to carry out but resists, recognizes as senseless, and recognizes as a product of their own mind*. Compulsions are also known as **compulsive or obsessional rituals**. Sometimes the association between the action and the thought seems understandable, for example when

handwashing is associated with the idea that the hands are contaminated. In other cases there is no meaningful connection between the actions and the thoughts, for example when checking the position of objects is associated with aggressive ideas. Most compulsions are followed by an immediate lessening of the distress associated with the corresponding obsessional thoughts. However, the long-term consequence is that the thoughts persist for longer. Compulsions are sometimes accompanied by obsessional thoughts concerned with doubt that the compulsive behaviours have been executed correctly, and this can lead to further repetitions, which may last for hours.

Asking about obsessional phenomena

Ask 'Do any thoughts (images, impulses to act) keep coming repeatedly into your mind, even when you try hard to get rid of them?'. Patients who reply yes should be asked for examples. Patients are often ashamed of their obsessional thoughts (e.g. those with aggressive or sexual themes), so questioning needs to be sympathetic and patient. The interviewer should make certain that patients regard the thoughts as their own, rather than as being implanted from outside. Although not strictly disorders of thinking, compulsive rituals are driven by thoughts, and are therefore usually recorded with obsessional phenomena. The following questions are useful: 'Do you ever have to repeat actions over and over, which most people would do only once?' or 'Do you have to go on repeating the same action when you know this is unnecessary?'.

■ Perceptions

There are two important terms, perception and imagery, which need to be explained.

Perception is the process of becoming aware of what is presented to the body through the sense organs (the eyes, the ears, the nose, the tongue, the skin). You may, for example, go for a walk by a river, and *see* rowing boats, *hear* the chatter of the rowers, *smell* the fresh air, and *feel* the cool breeze on your face. These perceptions are experienced as real, and are real.

Imagery is an experience originating within the mind that usually lacks the sense of reality that is part of perception. After your walk, you may close your eyes and relive it in your *'mind's eye'* or imagination; it is *as if* you were walking, but the experience is clearly an internal one rather than being 'real'. Imagery differs from perception in that it can be initiated and terminated at will. Almost always, imagery is obliterated when something is perceived in the same modality. A few people experience **eidetic imagery**, which is imagery as vivid and detailed as perception.

Abnormalities of perception are of four kinds: (i) *changes in intensity*; (ii) *changes in quality*; (iii) *illusions*; and (iv) *hallucinations*. Each kind of abnormality will be described, but particular attention is paid to hallucinations, as they are of most significance in diagnosis. Sometimes, perception is *normal* in nature, but has a changed *meaning* for the person who experiences it. This phenomenon is called **delusional perception**. Despite this name it is not a disorder of perception; rather, it is a disorder of thinking and is described with other disorders of thinking.

Changes in the intensity of perception

In mania, perception seems more intense, and, for example, colours may be particularly bright and vivid, and the sound of a pin dropping can seem loud. In depressive disorder, perception may be less intense, with colours downgraded so that the world seems drab and grey.

Changes in the quality of perception

In some disorders, especially schizophrenia, perceptions may seem distorted or unpleasant; for example, food tastes unpleasant or flowers smell acrid.

Illusions

An illusion is a *misperception of a real external stimulus.* Illusions are likely if one or more of the following circumstances is present:

1 **sensory impairment**, such as at dawn or dusk, or if the person is visually or hearing impaired;

2 **inattention** on the sensory modality, such as when a person whose attention is focused on a book may mistakenly identify a sound as a voice;

3 **impaired consciousness**, such as delirium;

4 **emotional arousal**, usually fear.

Healthy people sometimes experience illusions, particularly when two or more of the above circumstances occur together. For example, a young person may be returning home late at night along an unlit rural road (visual impairment), on a windy night (hearing impairment), and become increasingly anxious about their personal safety (emotional arousal), such that they perceive a bush on the side of the road as a potentially threatening person.

Illusions may come to notice when the history is taken, or when the patient is being observed, for example in a medical ward. Visual illusions can be elicited with a question such as 'Have you seen anything unusual?' (or frightening, if the patient seems afraid). If the answer is yes, the interviewer should attempt to find out whether the experience is based on an actual visual stimulus (e.g. mistaking a shadow for a threatening person).

Hallucinations

A hallucination is a *perception experienced in the absence of an external stimulus to the corresponding sense organ*, for example, hearing a voice when no one is speaking within hearing distance, or seeing bright flashing lights when there is no light source. A hallucination has two qualities that distinguish it from imagery: (i) it is experienced as a true perception; and (ii) it seems to come from outside the head. Unless the experience has these two qualities it is not a hallucination. Experiences that possess one of these qualities, but not the other, are sometimes called **pseudohallucinations**.

Although hallucinations are generally regarded as the hallmark of mental disorder, healthy people experience them occasionally, especially when falling asleep (**hypnagogic hallucinations**) or when waking (**hypnopompic hallucinations**). These two kinds of hallucinations are brief and usually of a simple kind, such as a bell ringing or a name being called. Usually the person wakes suddenly and immediately recognizes the nature of the experience. These two kinds of hallucination do not point to mental disorder.

Modalities of hallucination

Auditory and visual hallucinations are the most frequent, but hallucinations can occur in all sensory modalities.

● **Auditory hallucinations** may be experienced as voices, noises, or music. Hallucinatory voices may seem to speak words, phrases, or sentences. Some address the patient as 'you' (**second-person hallucinations**). Others talk about the patient as 'he' or 'she' (**third-person hallucinations**), and these latter are characteristic of schizophrenia (see p. 248). Sometimes a voice seems to say what the patient is about to say and sometimes it seems to repeat what he has just been thinking (**thought echo**).

- **Visual hallucinations** may be simple, such as flashes of light, or complex, such as the figure of a man. Usually they are experienced as normal in size, but sometimes may seem unusually small or large. Visual hallucinations are associated particularly with organic mental disorders but can occur in other conditions.

- **Hallucinations of smell and taste** are uncommon. The taste or smell may seem to be recognizable, but more often it is unlike any smell or flavour that has been experienced before, and has an unpleasant quality.

- **Tactile hallucinations** are also uncommon. They may be experienced as superficial sensations of being touched, pricked, or strangled. Sometimes they may be experienced as sensations just below the skin, which may be attributed to insects or other small creatures burrowing through the tissues—in this way, a tactile hallucination may be associated with a delusional interpretation.

- **Hallucinations of deep sensation** are also uncommon. They may be experienced as feelings of the viscera being pulled or distended, or as sexual stimulation. Again, they may well be associated with delusional interpretation.

Diagnostic associations of hallucinations

Hallucinations occur in organic disorders, severe affective disorders and schizophrenia. Visual hallucinations occur particularly in organic psychiatric disorders, but also in severe mood disorders and schizophrenia. Although not specific to organic disorder, they should always prompt a thorough search for other symptoms of an organic disorder. Hallucinations of taste, smell, and deep sensation occur mainly in schizophrenia. Other associations between particular kinds of hallucination and individual disorders are described in the chapters on clinical syndromes.

Asking about hallucinations

Enquiries about hallucinations should be made tactfully, lest patients take offence. With experience, the interviewer will be able to judge when it is safe to omit these enquiries. If enquiry is indicated, questions can be introduced by saying 'When their nerves are upset, some people have unusual experiences'. Questions can then be asked about hearing voices or sounds when there is nobody within earshot, or about seeing unusual things. If patients say yes to either of these questions, they should

be asked whether the voice, sound, or vision appeared to be inside or outside the head. When the history makes it relevant, similar questions should be asked about other kinds of hallucinations. If the patient describes **auditory hallucinations**, further questions should be asked, to determine whether they are of a kind that is characteristic of schizophrenia (see p. 248). They should be asked whether they hear sounds or voices, if the latter, whether one voice or more, and whether the voices talk to them (second person) or to each other (third person). Hallucinations of voices discussing patients (**third-person hallucinations**) should be distinguished from the delusion that people at a distance are discussing them (**delusion of reference**). If the hallucinatory voices talk to the patient (**second-person hallucinations**), the interviewer should find out whether they give commands, and if so, what kind of commands, and whether the patient feels impelled to obey them. Such 'command hallucinations' can indicate a high risk of harm to self or others.

■ Cognition

Assessment of cognitive functioning can appear complex, as it seeks to assess several interrelated aspects of higher cortical functions. Nevertheless, it should be a standard part of the mental state examination, and it is relatively quick and easy to conduct screening tests. The usual domains which are assessed are *consciousness, orientation, attention and concentration, memory, language,* and *visuospatial functioning.*

Consciousness

Consciousness is awareness of self and the environment. Its level varies between the extremes of coma and alertness. Several terms are used for the intervening states of consciousness.

- **Clouding of consciousness** refers to a state of drowsiness with incomplete reaction to stimuli, impaired attention, concentration, and memory, and slow, muddled thinking.

- **Stupor** refers to a state in which the person is mute, immobile, and unresponsive, but appears conscious because the eyes are open and follow objects. Note that this is the use in psychiatry. In neurology the term is used when there is *some* impairment of consciousness.

- **Confusion** refers to muddled thinking. The resulting term, **confusional state,** can be qualified by the terms 'acute' or 'chronic', which are alternative terms for **delirium** and **dementia,** respectively.

Orientation

Orientation is assessed by asking about awareness of time, place, and person. **Disorientation** is an important symptom that indicates impairment of consciousness or impairment of new learning. Questions begin with the time, day, month, year, and season. In assessing responses to questions about time, the interviewer should remember that many people do not know the exact time of day (although they usually know it to the nearest hour) or the exact date (though they are usually accurate to a few days). Orientation in place is assessed by asking the name of the place in which the interview is being held. If the answer is inaccurate, further questions are asked about the kind of place (e.g. home, a hospital ward, or a home for the elderly), and the name of the town. Personal orientation is assessed by asking about other people present (e.g. relatives in the home, or the staff in a hospital ward). If patients give wrong answers, they should be asked about their own identity—their name, occupation, and role in life.

Attention and concentration

Attention is the ability to focus on the matter in hand, and **concentration** is the ability to sustain that focus. Attention and concentration can be impaired in many kinds of psychiatric disorder but especially in anxiety disorder, depressive disorder, mania, schizophrenia, and organic disorder. Detection of impaired attention or concentration does not help in diagnosis but is important in assessing the patient's disability; for example, poor concentration may prevent a person from working effectively in an office.

While taking the history, the interviewer should look out for evidence of impaired attention and concentration. In the mental state examination, specific tests are given. It is usual to begin with the '**serial 7s test**'. The patient is asked to subtract 7 from 100 and then to take 7 from the remainder repeatedly until it is less than 7. The interviewer assesses whether the patient can concentrate on this task. Of course, it is quite possible that poor performance could be due to poor arithmetic ability. If so, the patient should be asked to do a simpler subtraction, such as taking 3s from 30, or to avoid a mathematical task and say the months of the year in reverse order, or the simpler task of naming the days of the week in reverse order. Such tests of attention are given before tests of memory because poor attention can lead to poor performance on memory tasks, even when there is no memory deficit.

Memory

Memory problems may come to light during history taking. During the mental state examination, tests are given to assess **immediate, recent,** and **remote memory**. Note that, although this simple classification is useful in clinical practice, it does not correspond exactly with the types of memory identified through research. No 'memory test' is wholly satisfactory, and the results should be assessed cautiously and in relation to other information about the patient's ability to remember. If there is doubt, standardized psychological tests can be given by a clinical psychologist.

Assessment of immediate recall/working memory. This is assessed by asking patients to repeat sequences of digits immediately after they have been spoken slowly enough for them to register the digits (the '**digit span test**'). An easy sequence of three digits is given first to make sure that patients understand the task. Then a new sequence of four digits is presented. If patients can repeat four digits correctly, sequences of five, six, and seven are given. When patients reach a level at which they cannot repeat the digits, a different sequence of the same length is given to confirm the finding. Clearly it is important to use random series of digits, rather than (for example) telephone numbers. Healthy people of average intelligence can repeat seven digits correctly; five or less suggests impairment. Note that the test involves concentration and, therefore, cannot be used to assess memory when tests of concentration are abnormal.

This can also be assessed through a test of recall of a name and address. Say to the patient 'Please can you repeat back to me the following name and address ... (for example) John Peters, 22 Church Street, Oxford'. Common names and addresses likely to be familiar to a patient should be avoided. If the patient does not correctly repeat the name and address, the same name and address are repeated, and repeated, until the patient repeats all six elements of the name and address correctly. This is a test of immediate recall, and a requirement for several repetitions may indicate a deficit in attention and concentration, or in working memory.

Assessment of recent memory. This uses a continuation of the name and address test. When the patient has correctly registered the name and address, do *not* say to them 'Remember that name and address; I will ask you them later' – if you do this, the patient is likely to focus on that task, and performance on other tasks in the interim will be adversely affected. Other topics should then be discussed for 5 minutes, or other cognitive tests undertaken as distractors, and the patient is then asked to repeat the name and address that were given to them earlier. This task generates a score out of 6, of which 5 or 6 would be normal, 3 or 4 might indicate abnormality and would invite further testing, and 0, 1, or 2 would be abnormal. Responses should be recorded verbatim.

Recent memory can also be assessed by asking about news items from the last day or two, or about recent events in the patient's life that are known with certainty to the interviewer (do not ask the commonly used question about what the patient had for breakfast unless you know the answer). Questions about news items should be adapted to the patient's interests, and should have been widely reported in the media. Of course, if the patient has no interest in the news, or no access to newspapers or television, this is an inappropriate task.

Assessment of long-term memory. This can be assessed by asking the patient to recall personal events or well-known public events from some years before. Personal events could be the birth dates of the patient's children or grandchildren (provided these dates are known to the interviewer); public events could be political, sporting, or cultural.

Observations suggesting memory disorder. When a patient is in a general hospital, important information about memory is available from observations made by nurses or other staff. These observations include how rapidly patients learn the daily routine of the ward, and the names of staff and other patients, and whether they forget where they have put things, or cannot find their way about, although apparent deficits in visuospatial memory may indicate a disturbance in visuospatial functioning rather than memory *per se*. When the patient is at home, relatives may report comparable observations about the patient's ability to learn and remember.

Special tests of memory. Among elderly patients, questions about memory do not distinguish well between those who have cerebral pathology and those who do not. For cases of doubt there are standardized ratings of memory for recent personal events, past personal events, and general events, which allow a better assessment of severity. Standardized tests of learning and memory can also help in the diagnosis of organic mental disorder, and can be used for quantitative assessments of the progression of memory disorder. These tests are usually administered by a clinical psychologist. The Mini Mental State Examination (MMSE) is a useful screening test of cognitive functions.

Specific disorders of memory. Memory is affected in several kinds of psychiatric disorder, but is particularly suggestive of organic disorder. In *depressive disorder*, unhappy or guilt-laden memories are recalled more readily than other kinds of memory. In *organic disorder*, memory of remote events is impaired less than that of more recent memory. Total loss of memory, including memory for personal identity, occurs very rarely in organic conditions and strongly suggests psychogenic causes (see p. 310) or malingering (see p. 313). Some organic causes lead to an **amnesic syndrome,** in which short-term memory is severely impaired but longer-term memory is retained (see p. 327). Other abnormalities of memory include the following.

- **Anterograde amnesia.** This occurs after a period of unconsciousness. It is the impairment of memory for events between the ending of complete unconsciousness and the restoration of full consciousness.

- **Retrograde amnesia.** This is the loss of memory for events before the onset of unconsciousness. It occurs after head injury or electroconvulsive therapy (ECT), when patients will be unable to remember events such as waking and showering during the early morning before their treatment.

- *Jamais vu* is a failure to recognize events that have been encountered before, and ***déjà vu*** is the recognition of events as familiar when they have never been encountered before. Both abnormalities may occur in neurological disorders.

- **Confabulation** is the reporting as 'memories' of events that did not take place at the time in question. It occurs in some patients with severe disorders of recent memory (see amnesic syndrome, p. 327).

Language

Language functions can be tested in simple ways. These include the following.

- **Naming.** The patient is asked to name common objects, such as those in the interview room, e.g. pen, chair, window. It should be straightforward for a patient to name such objects, unless they have a severe deficit, but more obscure objects may pick up more subtle deficits—for example, rather than pointing to his shirt, the interviewer might point to his cuff, or cufflink.

- **Verbal instruction.** The patient is asked to carry out a command, which may have several components, such as 'Take this piece of paper, fold it, and place it on the table.'

- **Written instruction.** The interviewer writes a simple command on a piece of paper (e.g. 'Stand up'), shows it to the patient, and says 'Do what it says'.

- **Writing a sentence.** The interviewer hands the patient a pen and a piece of paper, and says 'Please write a sentence'.

Visuospatial functioning

This can be tested informally or formally. Informally, a patient's carers (whether relatives or healthcare staff such as nurses) can be asked to observe the patient's ability to find their way around, such as from their bed to the toilet and back again. More formally, a patient can be asked to:

- copy simple line figures, such as a star, a cube, and the front of a simple house, with windows and doors, as a simple test of visuospatial functioning;

- recall those simple line figures several minutes later, following distractor tasks (such as some of the language tasks described above), as a simple test of visuospatial memory;
- draw an old-fashioned clock face, with the time showing (for example) 'quarter to three'. This requires quite complex **visuospatial skills**, such as remembering that the '12' goes at the top of the clock, and spacing the numbers appropriately, and **executive functioning skills**, such as planning and sequencing the different actions—the circle must be drawn first, followed by the numbers, and then the hands. This is the 'clock drawing test', of which there are many variants and formal scoring schemes.

■ Insight

This is a term that is used more often in psychiatry than in other areas of medicine. It is akin to 'congruence', or *the extent to which the patient's view of their symptoms, illness, prognosis, and treatment is identical to that of their healthcare professional.* Assessment of insight is extremely important in determining a patient's likely cooperation with treatment. For example, a patient who believes that he is being persecuted and does not accept that his beliefs are a sign of illness is unlikely to accept treatment readily. Nonetheless he may be aware that he feels distressed and is sleeping badly, and may agree to accept help with these problems (which he ascribes to the persecution). Assessment of insight can therefore help in two ways. First, it suggests how far patients are likely to collaborate with treatment; the greater the degree of 'fit' between the patient's and professional's views, the better the prognosis is likely to be. Second, it provides information on where the patient's and professional's views differ, and where effort to change the patient's health and illness beliefs should be focused. Psychiatrists and other mental health professionals spend a high proportion of their face-to-face contact with patients working with them to change their attitudes to their symptoms, their illness, and their treatments.

At its briefest, insight can be described as 'good', 'moderate', or 'poor'. However, it is more helpful clinically to provide a short description of the areas in which the patient and professional hold similar views, and those in which they differ. These might include, for example:

1 **awareness of oneself as presenting phenomena that other people consider abnormal** (e.g. being unusually active and elated);
2 **recognition that these phenomena are abnormal** (versus, for example, being a desirable mental state, of which other people are jealous);

3 **acceptance that these abnormal phenomena are caused by mental illness** (versus, for example, being excited about and energized by a new project or idea, or having a physical illness);
4 **awareness that treatment is required** (versus treatment being unnecessary and undesirable);
5 **acceptance of the professional's specific treatment recommendations** (e.g. admission to hospital and sedative medication).

■ Physical examination

The extent of the physical examination is decided by considering diagnostic possibilities in the individual case. When there is doubt, a systematic physical examination should be performed, and should include a careful examination of the endocrine and nervous systems. In selected cases this examination should also include assessment of language, constructional apraxias, and agnosias. The methods of examination are described in textbooks of neurology, and are learnt during neurology training. Readers who have not had this training are advised to refer to *The Shorter Oxford Textbook of Psychiatry*, to consult a textbook of neurology, and to obtain supervised practice of the relevant clinical skills.

■ Investigations

Investigations are chosen according to the clinical features and the diagnostic possibilities. There is no single set of routine investigations appropriate for every patient.

A corroborative history

In psychiatry, the most important investigation is a corroborative history. If a corroborative history is not obtained, there must be a strong basis for this omission. Often, a corroborative history will give vital additional information or correct errors in the patient's account.

Physical investigations

Often, a focused physical history and examination are all that are needed to exclude the possibility of physical illness. However, sometimes physical investigations are appropriate. These are helpfully divided into near-patient tests which can be obtained quickly if the patient is cooperative (e.g. dipstick urinalysis for infection, dipstick urinalysis for illicit drugs, fingertip blood oxygen, weight and height) and non-near-patient tests (e.g. lab blood tests, imaging). Relevant physical investigations are discussed in subsequent chapters.

Psychological investigations

- **Questionnaires and rating scales.** These are used in certain cases to either (i) characterize the extent or nature of specific problems, e.g. the MMSE in the assessment of cognitive functioning, or (ii) follow the progress of a disorder, such as to monitor response to treatment, e.g. the Beck Depression Inventory in the assessment of depressive symptoms.

- **Neuropsychological tests.** A wide variety of structured, sophisticated tests are available for assessing specific aspects of cognitive function, such as frontal or parietal cortical functioning. These are usually conducted by clinical psychologists with specific training in this area. Although brain imaging methods are generally more useful in diagnosis, neuropsychological tests may be used to follow the progress of the disorder.

- **Tests of intelligence.** In most cases it is not necessary to have a precise assessment of intelligence. If a patient seems to be of low intelligence, or if his psychological symptoms could be a reaction to work beyond his intellectual capacity, intelligence tests can be helpful. In child psychiatry, tests of intelligence are often supplemented by tests of *reading ability*.

 ## Further reading

Gelder, M., Harrison, P. & Cowen P. (2006). *The Shorter Oxford Textbook of Psychiatry*, 5th edn. Chapter 1, Symptoms and signs of psychiatric disorders, pp. 1–20. Chapter 3, Assessment, pp. 35–68. Oxford University Press, Oxford.

Thinking about diagnosis

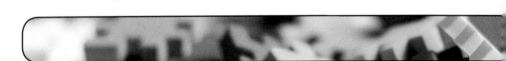

■ Why we diagnose

Rationale for diagnosis

Diagnosis performs a useful function because it allows us to classify patients into groups. This enables us to:

- **study** diagnostic groups, so that we can learn more about aetiology, prognosis, risks, and treatment through research;

- **communicate** briefly but effectively with other health-care professionals about a specific patient—rather than having to list the specific features in every case, we have a convenient shorthand;

- **predict** the likely aetiology, prognosis, risks, and effective treatments in a specific patient, based on evidence from other people with that diagnosis.

Objections to diagnosis

The process of diagnosis in mental health is not universally accepted as being appropriate. This stems from concerns that diagnosis:

- labels people with mental illness with names that may be unhelpful and stigmatizing, such as 'personality disorder' or 'schizophrenia';

- excessively simplifies the details of a particular person's predicament, so that the person's uniqueness is not acknowledged;

- relies upon an understanding of illness (existing classification systems) that does not reflect real illness categories, and therefore has low validity;
- relies upon the interpretation of the individual clinician, and therefore has low reliability—clinicians presented with the same information (the same patient) may draw different diagnostic conclusions.

We would argue that the rationale for diagnosis is strong, that no realistic alternative exists, and that the advantages of this approach far outweigh the disadvantages. When diagnostic assessment is conducted thoroughly and appropriately, it focuses very much on the *detail* of the patient's psychological, physical, and social situation, and emphasizes the *particular* aspects of an individual's case. It is therefore crucial that, when you are presenting a case, you stress those points, so that your case description is rich and individual, rather than being bland and general. The former reflects a real, unique person; the latter reflects a textbook description.

■ How to diagnose

Addressing complexity

In psychiatry, diagnosis is rarely just one simple term describing the patient's medical situation. As we have seen so far while considering assessment, there is usually more than one issue, and sometimes many, whether within the biological, psychological, or social domains. This complexity needs to be reflected in the shorthand of diagnosis. One way in which psychiatric diagnosis achieves this in an ordered way is by adopting a **multiaxial classification**, in which several axes reflect different aspects of the patient's situation. These axes may include:

- **main psychiatric diagnoses**—usually one or more mental illnesses;
- **other psychiatric diagnoses**—and, in particular, the presence of lifelong diagnoses such as *personality disorder* or *learning disability*, which may modify the presentation and prognosis of other psychiatric diagnoses;
- **physical disorder(s)**—especially those that are relevant to the presentation or prognosis of psychiatric diagnoses, such as cerebrovascular disease or endocrine disorder;
- **social problem(s)**—such as debt, unemployment, poor housing, social isolation, or abusive relationship(s);
- **extent of functional impairment**—the impact of the above psychological, physical, and social problems on day-to-day functioning and responsibilities, whether at home or at work/school/college, and whether to the self or to others, such as children. This may be formalized in a rating scale such as the Global Assessment of Functioning, which is a scale from 0 to 100, with written descriptions for each tenth. Whilst this approach is helpful in research, in clinical practice it is more common to describe functional impairment as nil, minimal, mild, moderate, or severe.

Diagnostic criteria

Typically, the diagnostic criteria for a particular disorder include five elements:

- **the main features**—those that define the core nature of the disorder and that are often required for the diagnosis to be made;
- **associated features**—those that are commonly seen in the disorder, but which may be absent, which are often shared with other disorders, and of which only a specific number or proportion may be required for diagnosis;
- **duration**—usually a minimum duration, but occasionally a maximum, or a minimum and a maximum;
- **severity**—often expressed as the extent of functional impairment; for a diagnosis to be made, it is usual for there to be functional impairment, although one important exception to this is when the patient has recovered from one or more episodes of illness, but they retain a diagnosis because of the increased risk of recurrence compared with the general population;
- **exclusions**—other diagnoses which might explain the presentation, and which need to be excluded in order for the diagnosis to be valid.

For example, in a depressive episode:

- main features include low mood, reduced enjoyment, and reduced energy;
- associated features are multiple, and include *physical* features such as poor appetite, weight loss, amenorrhea, and constipation, *psychological* features such as reduced concentration, guilt, low self-esteem, hopelessness, and suicidal thoughts, and *social* features, such as withdrawal from hobbies and interests, absence from work, and poor performance at work;
- the main features and associated features must last at least 2 weeks;
- there must be at least some functional impairment;
- several alternative causes of the depressive syndrome must be excluded, including harmful use of alcohol or other substances, physical disorder, prescribed medicines, and schizophrenia.

Variation in diagnostic criteria

There are two main classification systems used in psychiatry: the World Health Organization's International Classification of Diseases, version 10 (usually shortened to ICD-10) and the American Psychiatric Association's Diagnostic and Statistical Manual, version 4 (usually shortened to DSM-IV). Their descriptions of syndromes and associated diagnostic criteria are usually very similar. However, from time to time there is an important difference. These systems have been derived very carefully, through hard work by many mental healthcare professionals with extensive experience. When differences occur, they are often informative, as they may reflect core issues about diagnosis—areas where there are differences of opinion, where it has proved difficult to reliably categorize the complex natural phenomena that are mental illnesses.

The durational criterion of schizophrenia is one example. ICD-10 requires more than 1 month of the core symptoms before schizophrenia can be diagnosed, whereas DSM-IV requires 6 months of the core symptoms before the same diagnosis can be made. It is helpful to consider the impact that this change will make. In a large group of individuals with schizophrenia-like symptoms, ICD-10 schizophrenia will be more common, as it is diagnosed sooner. It will also be, on average, a better prognosis; the longer an illness continues, the more likely it is to continue, and so long duration is a predictor of poor prognosis. A rationale to diagnose early is to enable 'possible schizophrenia' to be identified early, and appropriate measures to be put in place to improve prognosis. On the other hand, a pressure to diagnose later is to avoid labelling patients with what is potentially a very stigmatizing illness, and to be more certain that the presenting illness is indeed 'schizophrenia' rather than something from which the patient will recover within weeks or months.

Lifetime diagnoses

Some patients retain a diagnosis even when they are symptom-free. For example, people who have had two or more discrete *depressive episodes* will retain the diagnosis of *depressive disorder* even when they are completely well. This is because the multiple depressive episodes bestow upon that person a lifetime risk of further depressive episodes that is significantly higher than if that person had not had those episodes. The multiple episodes therefore have prognostic significance. Making the diagnosis of depressive disorder, even in the absence of current symptoms, tells us as mental health professionals that we need to consider management approaches that will help to reduce the risk of recurrence.

How to make a diagnosis

When you first approach a patient, almost any diagnosis is possible. The aim of your assessment is to determine (i) your *preferred diagnosis*, (ii) other *differential diagnoses*, and (iii) *diagnoses which will not be considered further*. Within a minute or two, you may have been able to rule out several possibilities, and to start to focus your diagnostic radar. The aim is to systematically *rule out* some diagnoses, by which we mean that the chance of them being the 'real' diagnosis shifts progressively towards 0 per cent, although it is unlikely ever to reach 0 per cent. These diagnoses will not be considered further, unless there is a need for subsequent diagnostic review. Simultaneously, the aim is to *rule in* the preferred diagnosis, by which we mean that, by seeking specific, diagnostically relevant information, the chance of one diagnosis being the 'real' diagnosis shifts progressively towards 100 per cent, although it is unlikely ever to reach 100 per cent. Those diagnoses that are neither the preferred diagnosis nor excluded diagnoses form the small number of differential diagnoses. Typically, the differential diagnosis will include no more than two or three other mental illnesses. In addition, it is good practice to include the possibility of physical disorder, no matter how remote you consider this to be—this helps to keep the important possibility of physical disorder in mind.

Further reading

American Psychiatric Association (2000). *DSM-IV-TR: Diagnostic and Statistical Manual of Mental Disorders*, 4th edn, text revision. American Psychiatric Association, Washington, DC.

Kendler, K. & First, M. (2010). Alternative futures for the DSM revision process: iteration v. paradigm shift. *British Journal of Psychiatry* **197**: 263–265.

World Health Organization (1992). *The ICD-10 Classification of Mental and Behavioural Disorders: Clinical Descriptions and Diagnostic Guidelines*. WHO, Geneva.

Thinking about aetiology

Doctors need to be able to combine scientific knowledge with an empathic understanding of the patient to form a coherent account of their patients, their illnesses, and their predicaments. In this chapter, we will initially describe how this can be achieved in the assessment of the aetiology of a patient's disorder. We will then review ways of finding out the most up-to-date evidence for all kinds of clinical questions (but particularly methods of identifying the best treatments for specific clinical situations) by using the strategies of evidence-based medicine.

A knowledge of the causes of psychiatric disorders is important for two main reasons. First, in everyday clinical work it helps the doctor to evaluate possible causes of an individual patient's psychiatric disorder. Second, it adds to the general understanding of psychiatric disorders, which may contribute to advances in diagnosis, treatment, or prognosis. In this section we will only deal with the first of these—the *assessment of the causes of disorder* in the individual patient. The aetiology of specific disorders is considered when these conditions are reviewed in subsequent chapters.

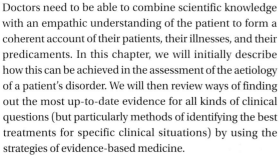

■ Aetiology and the individual patient

When assessing aetiology in a particular patient, we usually structure this by talking of **predisposing**, **precipitating**, and **perpetuating** (often called **maintaining**) factors. These terms are used most commonly in psychiatry and related disciplines, but the principles are applicable elsewhere.

Classification of causes

When there are multiple causes it is useful to group them into predisposing, precipitating, and perpetuating factors (see Figure 7.1 and Table 7.1).

Predisposing factors determine vulnerability to other causes that act close to the time of the illness. Many predisposing factors act early in life. Physical factors, for example, include genetic endowment, the environment *in utero*, and trauma at birth. Psychological and social factors in infancy and childhood are also relevant, such as bullying at school, abuse in its various forms, and family stability. Such factors lead to the development of a person's **constitution.**

Precipitating factors are events that occur shortly before the onset of a disorder and appear to have induced it. Again, these may be *physical*, *psychological*, or *social*. Physical precipitating causes include diseases such as hypothyroidism, myocardial infarction, breast cancer, or stroke, and the effects of drugs taken for treatment or used illegally. An example of a *psychological cause* is bereavement, while moving home is a *social cause*. Some causes may act in more than one way; for example, a head injury may induce a psychiatric disorder through physical changes in the brain and through psychological effects.

Perpetuating factors (often called maintaining factors) prolong a disorder after it has begun. Sometimes a feature of the disorder itself makes it self-perpetuating—for example, the thinking errors in anxiety disorders help to maintain them, as do the negative biases in thinking in depressive disorders. Social factors are also important (e.g. overprotective attitudes of relatives). Awareness of perpetuating factors is particularly important in planning treatment, because they may be modifiable even when little can be done about predisposing and precipitating factors.

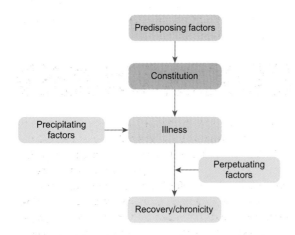

Fig. 7.1 Predisposing, precipitating, and perpetuating factors (see also Table 7.1).

Table 7.1 Predisposing, precipitating, and perpetuating factors in psychiatric disorder

Predisposing factors
Genetic endowment
Environment *in utero*
Trauma at birth
Psychosocial factors during childhood/adolescence
Precipitating factors
Physical diseases, medicines, use of illicit drugs, accidents
Psychological stressors
Social changes
Perpetuating factors
Intrinsic to the disorder, e.g. thinking errors
Poor compliance with treatment(s)
Use of alcohol and illicit drugs as self-medication
Avoidance of normal activities, at work and at home
Social isolation

An example from general medicine

In a 56-year-old man with poorly managed heart failure:

- predisposing factors include his male gender, his older age, and his obesity;
- precipitating factors include his recent myocardial infarction;
- perpetuating factors include his lack of adherence to cardiac medication due to associated side effects and lack of understanding of their role, the adverse impact of his breathlessness on his activity levels, and consequent further reductions in physical fitness and increase in weight.

Identified aetiological factors help to inform our view of prognosis and a management plan. In many cases, the perpetuating factors are particularly relevant, as their successful management enables a return to a higher level of functioning, and enables clinician and patient to address longer-term issues. In this cardiac case, prognosis is likely to be poor, with ongoing functional impairment and the likelihood of further cardiac events, unless the patient can be engaged to adhere to the treatment plan. Management might include an explanation of what heart failure is, and of the rationale for each cardiac medicine, an explanation of the role of exercise in training the heart and improving function, accompanied by rehabilitation with the aid of a physiotherapist or similar, and an appointment with a dietitian to help with healthy eating and define a plan for weight loss. In this way, specific management tasks are mapped on to specific aetiological factors.

An example from psychiatry

In assessing the causal significance of the events outlined in Case Study 7.1, the clinician can draw on his knowledge of scientific studies of depressive disorders, and on his understanding of human emotional reactions to life events. These enable the clinician to draw conclusions about likely *predisposing*, *precipitating*, and *perpetuating* factors.

Predisposing factors are those factors which increase an individual's risk above the population average. Genetic epidemiological studies have shown that a predisposition to depressive disorder is probably genetically transmitted (see p. 227). It is possible, therefore, that this patient inherited this kind of predisposition from his mother. Is the separation from his mother likely to have been significant? There have been several studies of the long-term effects of separating children from their parents, but they refer to people who were separated when younger than the patient was at separation. Nonetheless, extrapolation from this evidence and from human experience suggest that his mother's departure is likely to have been important.

Precipitating factors are those factors that appear to trigger the onset of illness in someone who may or may not have predisposing factors. In this case, it is understandable that a man should feel depressed when his wife leaves him, and this man is likely to be especially affected by this experience because the event recapitulates the similar distressing separation in his own childhood.

Perpetuating factors are those factors that keep an illness going, even in the absence of factors that might have precipitated it. In this case, empathy and common sense would suggest that the patient should have felt better when his wife came back, but he did not. This lack of improvement can be explained, however, by evidence that, once a depressive disorder starts, it is established through *physical* means (neurochemical changes are embedded, alcohol is used as self-medication, and helplessness means that compliance with medication is poor), *psychological* means (thinking is pervasively negative, with gloom and despondency affecting motivation and interest), and *social* means (reduced attendance at work, reduced hobbies and interests). Again, this can inform a simple management plan, in which the patient is informed about the nature of the illness and the role of persistence in its management, the depressant effect of alcohol, the antidepressant effect of medication, some simple cognitive techniques to make thinking more realistic, and staged return to work, hobbies, and interests.

This case study illustrates several important issues concerning aetiology in psychiatry:

- the interaction of different causes in a single case;
- the need to identify different causes through time—*predisposing*, *precipitating*, and *perpetuating*;
- the need to identify causes different in nature—*physical*, *psychological*, and *social*;
- the concept of stress and of psychological reactions to it;
- the roles of scientific evidence and of evaluation based on empathy and common sense;
- the link between an effective understanding of aetiology and an effective management plan.

Explanation and understanding

There are two ways of trying to make sense of the causes of a patient's problems. Both are useful, but it is important to distinguish between them.

- The first approach is quantitative and based on research findings. For example, a person's aggressive behaviour may be explained as the result of an injury to the frontal cortex sustained in a road accident. This statement draws on the results of scientific studies of the behaviour of patients with damage to various areas of the brain. It is conventional to refer to this kind of statement as **explaining** the behaviour.

 Case Study 7.1 Causes of psychiatric disorder

For 4 weeks a 38-year-old married man has become increasingly depressed. His symptoms started soon after his wife left him to live with another man. The following points in the history were potentially relevant to aetiology. The patient's mother had received psychiatric treatment on two past occasions, once for a severe depressive disorder and once for mania; on neither occasion was there any apparent environmental cause for the illness. When the patient was 14 years old, his mother went to live with another man, leaving the patient, his brother, and his sister with their father. For several years afterwards the patient felt rejected and unhappy but eventually settled down. He married and had two children, aged 13 and 10 at the time of his illness. Two weeks after leaving home, the patient's wife returned saying that she had made a mistake and really loved her husband. Despite her return the patient's symptoms persisted and worsened. He began to wake early, gave up his usual activities, and spoke at times of suicide.

- The second approach is qualitative and is based on an empathic understanding of human behaviour. We use this approach when we decide, for example, that a person was aggressive because his wife was insulted by a neighbour. The connection between these two events makes sense; it is convincing even though a quantitative study may not have shown a statistical association between aggression and this kind of insult. It is conventional to refer to this kind of statement as **understanding** the cause.

In every branch of medicine doctors need to explain and to understand their patients' problems. In psychiatry, understanding is often a particularly important part of the investigation of aetiology.

Remote causes, multiple effects, and multiple causes

In psychiatry, certain events in childhood are associated with psychiatric disorder in adult life; the causes are *remote* in time. For example, subjects who develop schizophrenia are more likely than controls to have been exposed to complications of pregnancy and labour. *One cause* can lead to *several effects*; for example, lack of parental affection in childhood has been reported to predispose to suicide, antisocial behaviour, and depressive disorder. Conversely, a *single effect* can have *several causes*, which act singly or in combination. For example, learning disability can be caused by any one of several distinct genetic abnormalities, whilst a depressive disorder can be caused by the combined effects of genetic factors and recent stressful events.

Models

In discussions of aetiology the word 'model' is often used to mean a way of ordering information. A model seeks to explain certain phenomena and to show the relationships between them. Several models are in use in psychiatric practice, and the following examples are not exhaustive.

- **The medical model** is an approach in which psychiatric disorders are investigated in ways that have proved useful in general medicine, such as by identifying regularly occurring patterns of symptoms (syndromes) and relating them to brain pathologies. This model has proved particularly useful in investigating organic psychiatric disorders, and in studying schizophrenia and mood disorders. It has proved less useful in the study of anxiety disorders and personality disorders, although rapid advances in functional neuroimaging may change this.

- **The behavioural model** is an approach in which psychiatric disorders are explained in terms of **adaptive** and **maladaptive** behaviours. For example, if a person is bullied at work by a particular individual, a strategy to discuss this with their manager, and to avoid that person when possible, might be considered *adaptive*, whereas taking time off work might be considered *maladaptive*. Equally, in a depressive illness, avoidance of the structure and enjoyment and sense of satisfaction that daily activities can bring is invariably maladaptive, unless those activities are placing unreasonable stress on the individual. By identifying adaptive and maladaptive behaviours, and by encouraging the adaptive and discouraging the maladaptive, progress can be made in treating psychiatric disorder and reducing the risk of relapse.

- **The cognitive model** is an approach in which psychiatric disorders are explained in terms of cognitive biases which influence our thoughts and beliefs. In depression, pervasive negative cognitive biases promote a negative, grey view of the person themself, including their illness, the people around them, and the world. In mania (elevated mood), pervasive positive biases lead to an inflated view of the person's abilities and their life's possibilities.

- **The biopsychosocial model** is an approach in which psychiatric disorders are explained by carefully integrating *physical* factors (such as those within the medical model), *psychological* factors (such as those within the behavioural and cognitive models), and *social* factors. It is helpful not only in psychiatry, but also in medicine in general, where physical factors derived from a medical model approach often dominate thinking about aetiology and treatment, but where significant improvements in functional outcome can be delivered by attending to psychological and social factors.

■ Methodological approaches

In this chapter, we will not provide an extensive review of the aetiology of psychiatric disorders; current knowledge about the causes of specific disorders is presented in the relevant chapters. Here, we provide a brief summary of the kinds of approach that have been, and are being, used to investigate the causes of psychiatric disorder. We suggest that the reader first reads the aetiology sections in the following chapters, using this section as a guide to allow them to keep up to date with advances in knowledge.

Epidemiology

Epidemiology is the study of the distribution of diseases in space and time within a population, and of the factors that influence this distribution. In psychiatry, epidemiology is used to provide information about prevalence (which is useful for planning services) and about causation.

BOX 7.1 Epidemiology: definitions

Case. A person in the population or study group identified as having the disorder. In psychiatry, the **case definition** is usually a set of agreed criteria or a cut-off point on a continuous scale.

Rate. The ratio of the number of cases to the number of people in a defined population.

Prevalence. The rate of all cases, new and old. Prevalence may be determined on a particular occasion (**point prevalence**) or over a period of time (e.g. 1-year prevalence).

Incidence. The rate of *new* cases. **Inception rates** represent the number of people who were healthy at the beginning of a defined period but became ill during it. **Lifetime expectation** represents the number of people who could be expected to develop a particular illness in the course of their whole life.

Information about the epidemiology of particular psychiatric disorders is given in other chapters in this book. Some important terms are defined in Box 7.1.

In psychiatry, the best method of *case definition* is usually by reference to the definitions in a standard system of classification, such as DSM-IV or ICD-10. The main types of study designs used in psychiatric epidemiology are shown in Box 7.2.

Genetics

Genetic studies in psychiatry are concerned with three issues: (i) the relative contributions of genetic and environmental factors to aetiology; (ii) the mode of inheritance of disorders that have a genetic basis; and (iii) biochemical mechanisms involved in hereditary disease. Three methods have been used to study these problems. **Epidemiological methods** of studying populations and families can evaluate the contribution of genetic factors to aetiology, and throw light on the mode of inheritance (e.g. whether dominant or recessive). The main study designs are shown in Box 7.3. **Cytogenetics** and **molecular genetics** provide information about chromosomal and genetic abnormalities and the mechanisms of inheritance (Box 7.4).

Biochemical studies

Biochemical studies in psychiatry are difficult to carry out for three main reasons.

● The living brain is inaccessible to direct study, post-mortem tissue is not often available (since most psychiatric disorders do not lead to death), and, even when it is, brain biochemistry may have been changed by old age or by the medical cause of death. To overcome this problem,

BOX 7.2 Study designs used in psychiatric epidemiology

Case–control study. This is an observational study comparing the frequency of an exposure in a group of persons with the disease of interest (**cases**) with a group of persons without the disease (**controls**). Case–control studies are commonly used to look for **risk factors** for psychiatric disorders. For example, a finding that a group of patients with schizophrenia had a higher rate of exposure to birth complications than a non-schizophrenic control group could be interpreted as meaning that birth complications predisposed to schizophrenia. Case–control studies are quick to do and relatively cheap, but are susceptible to biases.

Cohort study. This is an observational study in which a group of persons without the disorder is followed up to see which of them get the disorder. For example, a cohort of newly delivered babies could be followed through childhood and adolescence to see which of them developed schizophrenia—and if any birth characteristics are associated with a higher risk for the disorder. Cohort studies are potentially less susceptible to bias, but take a long time to do and are expensive.

Prevalence (or cross-sectional) study. This is an observational study in which the presence or absence of a disorder and any other variable of interest is measured in a defined population. For example, a sample of homeless people could be surveyed to estimate the prevalence of schizophrenia.

Ecological studies. These studies examine the rates of disorder in the population and relate them to other factors in the environment. For example, in the UK, it was observed that there was a reduction in the suicide rate following the change from coal gas to natural gas. This was interpreted as showing that reducing the availability of methods could prevent suicide, and has led to other initiatives in the UK, such as replacing bottles of paracetamol with blister packs.

BOX 7.3 Epidemiological study designs used in genetics

Family risk studies. The affected people (**probands**) are identified, rates of disorder are determined among various classes of relatives, and these rates are compared with those in the general population. From the observed prevalence, estimates are computed of the numbers of people likely to develop the condition subsequently. These corrected figures are called **expectancy rates** or **morbid risks**. Rates higher than those expected in the general population show that a familial cause is likely. Family studies can show whether a condition is familial, but they do not distinguish between the effects of inheritance and those of family environment.

Twin studies. Comparisons are made between concordance rates in uniovular (monozygotic, or MZ) twins and in binovular (dizygotic, or DZ) twins. If concordance is significantly greater among uniovular twins than among binovular twins, a significant genetic component is inferred. A more precise estimate of the contributions of heredity and environment can be made by comparing the rates of disorder among the rare cases of MZ twins reared apart with the rates among MZ twins reared together. If the rates are the same in those reared apart and those reared together, this indicates an important genetic component to aetiology.

Adoption studies. Children who, since early infancy, have been reared by unrelated adoptive parents are studied. Two comparisons can be made. The first is between adopted persons with a biological parent who had the disorder under investigation, and adopted persons with biological parents free from the disorder. A higher rate of the disorder among the former indicates a genetic cause. The second comparison is between the biological parents and the adoptive parents of adopted persons who have the disorder. A higher rate of the disorder among the biological parents indicates a genetic cause. Such studies can be affected by several biases; for example, adoptees may be assigned to adoptive parents on the basis of the socioeconomic status of the biological parents. In psychiatry, adoption studies have been applied to schizophrenia (see p. 254) and affective disorder (see p. 228), and the findings point to genetic causes in both conditions.

Mode of inheritance. This is assessed by using statistical methods to test the closeness of fit between the rates of disorder in various classes of relatives of the probands, and the rates predicted by various models of inheritance (e.g. dominant, recessive, sex-linked). When applied to psychiatric disorders, such studies have generally given equivocal results, suggesting that the mode of inheritance is not simple.

BOX 7.4 Study designs used in cellular and molecular genetics

Cytogenetic studies. These aim to identify abnormalities in the structure or number of chromosomes. **Karyotyping** is a commonly used technique in which chromosomal spreads are examined with a microscope. Cytogenetic abnormalities have been identified as causes of learning disabilities (e.g. Down's syndrome, in which there is a trisomy of chromosome 21). Chromosomal abnormalities have not been identified as a primary cause of functional psychiatric disorders although, occasionally, such abnormalities may give indirect clues to the aetiology of some disorders. For example, subjects with velocardiofacial syndrome (associated with a deletion on chromosome 22) have a high incidence of bipolar affective disorder.

Linkage studies. These studies seek to identify the chromosomal region likely to be carrying the genes responsible for a disorder in a family or group of families. Linkage studies have been successful in identifying the genes causing Huntington's disease and familial Alzheimer's syndrome. Their role is limited in disorders that are not due to single major genes, such as most psychiatric disorders. There are also problems in using linkage studies in psychiatric disorders due to uncertain phenotypes and statistical complexities. To date, no confirmed linkage has been found between a common psychiatric disorder and a single, specific chromosomal region.

Association studies. These are case–control studies (see Box 7.2) in which the frequency of a genetic variant (or polymorphism/ allelic variant) in a group of subjects with a disorder is compared with the frequency of the variant in a group of subjects without the disorder. The *advantages* of association studies compared with linkage studies are that they are easier to perform in complex disorders, they do not need familial samples, and they make fewer statistical assumptions. The *disadvantages* are that they require a **candidate gene** (a genetic marker that is close to or part of a gene that is suspected of being involved in the disorder) and that they are susceptible to **confounding** (a situation where an observed association with a gene or other cause is simply due to other differences between the cases and controls). So far, although encouraging, association studies have not produced unequivocal results in psychiatric disorders.

Table 7.2 Brain-imaging techniques

Structural imaging techniques	
Computed tomography (CT)	X-rays taken of the brain from many different angles are combined to produce a series of images or 'slices' through the brain. CT has demonstrated lateral ventricular enlargement in schizophrenia
Magnetic resonance imaging (MRI)	Non-ionizing radio waves are directed at the brain in the presence of a strong magnetic field. Asymmetrical nuclei align and resonate, producing signals which are converted into an image by a computer. MRI has demonstrated more subtle brain abnormalities in schizophrenia
Functional imaging techniques	
Positron emission tomography (PET)	Radiolabelled short-living isotopes (produced in a cyclotron) are injected and emit radiation, which is detected by a scanner and converted to an image by a computer. PET is used to measure regional cerebral blood flow and ligand binding
Single photon emission tomography (SPET)	This is simpler than PET and does not require a cyclotron. Photons emitted by injected radiochemicals are detected by a rotating gamma camera. SPET is used to measure regional cerebral blood flow and ligand binding
Functional magnetic resonance imaging (fMRI)	This is based on the sensitivity of MRI to magnetic effects caused by variations in the oxygenation of haemoglobin, which is induced by local changes in blood flow during task activation. Because it does not involve radiation, fMRI may be used repeatedly in the same subject
Magnetoencephalography (MEG)	This is based on the measurement of intensity, location, and change through time of the very weak magnetic fields generated by the brain's neural activity. The great advantage of MEG is its very high temporal resolution, milliseconds or faster, which allows it to track brain activity in real time

indirect approaches have been made through more accessible sites. Their value has been limited because concentrations of substances in cerebrospinal fluid, blood, and urine (especially the latter two) have uncertain relationships to their concentrations in the brain.

- Animal studies are of limited use because there are no obvious parallels in animals to the mental disorders found in humans. Animal studies have, however, proved useful in the study of the actions of drugs on the brain.

- It is difficult to prove that any biochemical abnormalities detected are causal and not secondary to changes either in diet or in activity induced by the mental disorder, or to the effects of drugs used in treatment.

Despite these problems, biochemical studies of post-mortem brain tissue have been moderately informative in Alzheimer's disease, schizophrenia, and affective disorder. In Alzheimer's disease there is a widespread decline in transmitter function; however, this decline could be no more than a consequence of the loss of cells in this disorder. In schizophrenia, the density of dopamine receptors is increased in the caudate nucleus and nucleus accumbens, but this increase could be the result of treatment with antipsychotic drugs, which block dopamine receptors and so might lead to a compensatory increase in their density. In severe affective disorder, some studies have found reduced 5-HT (serotonin) function in

the brainstem, but these findings were based on patients who had died by suicide, and they could result from terminal anoxia or the drugs used for suicide.

More recently, brain-imaging methods (see Table 7.2) have been used to study biochemical function in living brain tissue, and progress is being made.

Pharmacology

If a drug alleviates a disorder, and if the mode of action of the drug is known, then it might be possible to infer the biochemical abnormality underlying the disorder. This line of argument must be pursued cautiously, however, since effective drugs do not always act directly on the biochemical abnormality underlying the disorder. For example, anticholinergic drugs are effective in Parkinson's disease, but the symptoms of this disorder are caused by a defect in dopaminergic transmission, not by an excess of cholinergic transmission.

Progress is being made, however, by using psychiatric medicines such as antidepressants to study changes in brain mechanisms such as emotional processing in healthy volunteers. This has shown that antidepressants alter the way in which emotional information from faces is processed, thereby altering the person's perception of their social world, and that these changes are present almost immediately after injecting the antidepressant.

This provides a putative mechanism for antidepressant action, and, importantly, links *physical* intervention with *psychological* and *social* processes. Notably, this research is using mixed methods—**pharmacological manipulation** is being used alongside **neuropsychological testing** and **functional neuroimaging**—and this is an important trend in modern aetiological research in psychiatry.

Endocrinology

In psychiatric patients, tests of endocrine function have been used to study the following:

- Tests have been used to determine how hormonal activity changes in psychiatric disorder. For example, it has been shown that cortisol production is increased in depressed patients.

- Changes in endocrine function have been used as indirect measures of other processes. This usage is possible because many endocrine functions are controlled through neurotransmitters that could be involved in causing psychiatric disorder. Thus, if an abnormality in endocrine function is due to the disordered function of a particular neurotransmitter in one brain system, it is possible that the same neurotransmitter could be functioning abnormally in another brain system, and that this second malfunctioning could be the cause of the psychiatric disorder. For example, endocrine abnormalities indicating reduced 5-HT function have been found in depressive disorder, and it has been proposed that more widespread reduction of 5-HT is a cause of this disorder.

Neuropathology

Post-mortem brain studies have been carried out for over a century, yielding useful information about dementias and other organic disorders, but until recently they have shown no consistent abnormalities in the functional psychoses. Modern quantitative methods have demonstrated abnormalities in the medial temporal lobes and other brain areas of patients with schizophrenia, and these abnormalities could be relevant to the aetiology of this disorder. Advances in brain-imaging techniques have provided a method of investigating the structure and function of the brain before death.

Electrophysiology

Electrophysiological recordings made with electrodes on the skull surface (as in electroencephalography) do not give precise information about the nature and site of abnormal brain activity, and have contributed little to the understanding of psychiatric disorders, except for those related to epilepsy. More progress has already been made with the contemporary technique of magnetoencephalography (MEG) scanning (see Table 7.2.)

Psychology

Psychology is the study of normal behaviour, and is therefore highly relevant to the study of abnormal behaviour in mental disorders. Psychological studies have contributed to the understanding of causes of anxiety disorders, and, in particular, to the factors that maintain the disorders once started. The most relevant psychological mechanisms concern conditioning, social learning, and cognitive processing. A summary of each is given here, and more extensive information is available in textbooks of psychology or behavioural science.

Classic conditioning. Learning through association explains, for example, the development of situational anxiety in phobic patients following an initial attack of anxiety in the situation.

Operant conditioning. The reinforcement of behaviour by its consequences explains, for example, the maintenance of disruptive behaviour in some patients by the extra attention that is provided by staff or relatives when this behaviour occurs.

Cognitive processes are concerned with aspects of the ways in which patients select, interpret, and act on the information from the sense organs and memory stores. Some disorders are maintained, in part, by the ways that patients think about the physical symptoms associated with emotional arousal. For example, patients with panic disorder think that palpitations are a precursor of a heart attack and so become more anxious. Knowledge of these psychological mechanisms led to the development of the cognitive behaviour therapies.

Coping mechanisms are ways in which people attempt to deal with stressors. The term is used in both a wide and narrow sense. The *wide sense* includes any way of responding to stressors, whether or not the response reduces the stress reaction. The *narrow sense* refers only to ways of responding that reduce the stress reaction. To avoid confusion it is useful to apply the term **maladaptive** to responses that fail to reduce the stress reaction, or do so but cause other problems (e.g. taking an excessive amount of alcohol). Coping mechanisms have two components: (i) internal processes (usually thoughts) and (ii) external processes (usually behaviours). For example, after bereavement, a person's coping mechanisms might include thinking about religious beliefs (internal, thought) and joining a social club to combat loneliness (external, behaviour). Another internal coping mechanism is to change the meaning attached to an event; for example, an imposed alteration of job may be regarded at first as a threat (engendering anxiety) but later as a challenging opportunity (engendering excitement). Examples of maladaptive coping mechanisms are avoiding the problem or consuming alcohol to relieve distress.

Ethology

Ethology, which is concerned with the observation and description of behaviour, has contributed usefully to research into behaviour disorders of children. The methods provide quantitative observations that allow comparisons of an individual's behaviour with that of other people, and with relevant behaviour in animals. Thus the effects of separating human infants and infant monkeys from their mothers have been shown to be similar in certain ways; for example, infants of both kinds are distressed and active at first, and then call less and adopt a hunched posture. Such parallels help to distinguish between innate and culturally determined aspects of behaviour.

Sociology

Clinical observations indicate that psychiatric disorder may be provoked or influenced by factors in the social environment. Sociology, the study of human society, is therefore a potentially valuable source of information about the causes of psychiatric disorder. The main sociological concepts that have been applied to psychiatric disorders are listed below.

Social role: the behaviour that develops as a result of other people's expectations of, or demands on, a person. Most individuals have more than one role, for example as worker, mother, wife, and so on.

Sick role: the behaviour expected and required of an ill person. It includes rights and responsibilities. **Rights** include an exemption from some responsibilities, such as working, and the right to expect help from others. **Responsibilities** include the wish to recover, and an obligation to seek and comply with treatment.

Illness behaviour: the behaviour of the person in the sick role. It includes seeking help, consulting doctors, taking medicines, and giving up responsibilities. A person may adopt the sick role and show illness behaviour without having any illness, or may show illness behaviour that is out of proportion to the degree of ill health.

Socioeconomic status: status within society, determined usually on the basis of job or income. There is an association between schizophrenia and low socioeconomic status, and a debate about the extent to which this is cause or effect or both.

Life event: a stressful aspect of living that may be associated with changes in health status. Life events have been shown to contribute to the onset and maintenance of schizophrenia, affective disorder, and some other psychiatric disorders.

Culture: the way of life shared by a group of human beings. A **subculture** is the way of life shared by a subgroup within a wider cultural group. Culture affects the ways people behave when ill (the sick role and illness behaviour mentioned above), as well as the routines and values of carers and families. The presentation and course of mental disorders may be influenced by cultural factors.

Social mobility: a change of role or status in a society. Schizophrenia may lead to downward social mobility (decline to a lower social class), while upward mobility (e.g. promotion, movement away from one's social roots) may be a stressful experience provoking an adjustment disorder.

Migration: movement between societies. Migration can be a stressful experience, and it has been suggested as a cause of mental disorder including psychosis, although again there are challenging epidemiological issues relating to cause and effect.

Social institution: an established social organization, such as the family, school, or hospital, and the established way in which it goes about its business. The roles taken by the mother and father, and in the relationships between the 'nuclear' family of parents and children, and the 'extended' family of grandparents, aunts, and uncles may differ between cultures. These family differences are important in understanding the impact of one member's illness on other family members.

Total institution: an institution in which the inhabitants spend all their time in one place and have little freedom to choose their way of life; long-stay psychiatric hospitals can be total institutions. If life in the institution is unduly ordered, repetitive, and restrictive, the people living there may lose initiative, withdraw into fantasy, or rebel. In this way, institutional living can add further handicaps ('institutionalization') to those of the mental disorder. The term derives from the seminal text by Erving Goffman entitled *Asylums: Essays on the Social Situation of Mental Patients and Other Inmates*.

■ Keeping up to date: evidence-based medicine

Although every effort is made to ensure that textbooks are accurate, comprehensive, and up to date, inevitably, as knowledge increases, they become out of date. For example, questions about treatment arise frequently in clinical practice. Although the doctor will have learned about treatments during his training, rapid advances will occur and so it is difficult to keep up to date. New drugs, other kinds of treatment, and other clinical procedures are being introduced all the time, and it can be difficult to find unbiased information about them.

The doctor needs a way of quickly accessing the best available information—and also needs to know how to

Table 7.3 Types of clinical question and best study design

Type of question	Form of the question	Best study design
Diagnosis	How likely is a patient who has a particular clinical feature to have a specific disorder?	A **cross-sectional study** of patients suspected of having the symptom, sign, or diagnostic test result for the disorder, comparing the proportion of patients who really have the disorder and who have a positive test with the proportion of patients who do not have the disorder and who have a positive test result
Treatment	Is the treatment of interest more effective in producing a desired outcome than an alternative treatment (including no treatment)?	A **randomized controlled trial** (RCT) in which the patients are randomly allocated to receive either the treatment of interest or the alternative
Prognosis	How likely is a specific outcome in this patient?	A study in which an **inception cohort** (patients at a common stage in the development of the illness, especially first onset) are followed up for an adequate length of time
Aetiology	What has caused the disorder?	A study that compares the frequency of an exposure in a group of persons with the disease of interest (**cases**) with a group of persons without the disease (**controls**)—this may be an RCT, a case–control study, or a cohort study (see Box 7.1)
Screening	Is tool A or tool B better able to screen for patients with disease X in population Y, e.g. is the Hospital Anxiety and Depression Scale or the Whooley Two Question Test better able to screen for patients with depression in general hospital wards?	A randomized controlled trial (RCT), or, better still, a **systematic review** of several RCTs

BOX 7.5 Sources of evidence

The **NHS Evidence** (www.library.nhs.uk/) and, in particular, **NHS Evidence—mental health** (www.library.nhs.uk/mentalhealth/) web resources include their own content, such as Annual Evidence Updates, and act as portals to many other sources of high-quality evidence, including several of those listed below.

NICE, the NHS National Institute for Health and Clinical Excellence (www.nice.org.uk or via the NHS Evidence portal), produces and publishes high-quality clinical evidence on the management of a wide variety of disorders, including mental disorders, which are the accepted standards of care in the UK and, in many cases, internationally. Guidance, both completed and in development, on mental disorders is available at http://guidance.nice.org.uk/Topic/MentalHealthBehavioural. The full guidelines and NICE guidelines are extensive and, for most purposes, the quick reference guides are adequate.

The Cochrane Library. This is published quarterly on CD and the Internet (www.thecochranelibrary.com or via the NHS Evidence portal) and contains, among other resources, the authoritative *Cochrane Database of Systematic Reviews (CDSR)*. This is a continually updated database of high-quality systematic reviews maintained by the Cochrane Collaboration. The reviews are published in a uniform format. The CDSR is probably the next place to start searching for evidence about treatment, after NICE.

PubMed (www.ncbi.nlm.nih.gov/pubmed/ or via the NHS Evidence portal). This is the online portal to MEDLINE, the computerized index of biomedical journals maintained by the National Library of Medicine in the USA. It contains about 45% of relevant articles and is best at covering articles published in English. PubMed has a number of search filters that allow rapid searching for the most relevant articles.

PsycINFO (http://psycnet.apa.org or via the NHS Evidence portal). An electronic database similar to MEDLINE, but maintained by the American Psychological Association and specifically covering psychology and psychiatry journals.

EMBASE (www.embase.com or via the NHS Evidence portal). A European equivalent of MEDLINE, strong in biomedicine, and good for searching for drug trials.

Evidence-based Mental Health (http://ebmh.bmj.com/). This journal publishes systematically selected abstracts of the best mental health evidence research as it is published.

combine it with his understanding of the patient and their preferences. In the past, the doctor had to rely on potentially out-of-date or biased sources of information such as textbooks, authoritative reviews, promotional materials, or, most commonly, the opinions of colleagues. Recently, a number of techniques derived from advances in clinical epidemiology and information science have been introduced. Collectively, these strategies are called **evidence-based medicine** (**EBM**), and they are helpful for answering frequently arising clinical questions and keeping up to date.

It is sometimes thought that there is little evidence on which to base treatment decisions in psychiatry, and that psychiatry is too complex to be susceptible to this approach. Both of these assumptions are wrong. In fact, there is a great deal of evidence available about screening, diagnosis, aetiology, prognosis, and treatment in psychiatry (see Table 7.3). The aim of EBM is to allow the doctor to access the best available evidence as quickly as possible and to integrate it with his clinical expertise to best help a particular patient. Details of some of the most useful sources of evidence are provided in Box 7.5.

As we hope we have illustrated in this chapter, clinical decisions need to be based on other factors as well as sound scientific evidence. These factors involve an understanding of the patient and their circumstances and preferences. They also include an awareness of the costs of new treatments. Limited resources mean that there is an increasing requirement for new treatments to be at least as effective as existing treatments, but also to confer some additional added value, such as fewer adverse effects or reduced costs.

 ## Further reading

Geddes, J. (2009). From science to practice. In *New Oxford Textbook of Psychiatry*, 2nd edn. Ed. Gelder, M., Andreasen, N., Lopez-Ibor, J, & Geddes, J., pp. 122–9. Oxford University Press, Oxford.

The *New Oxford Textbook of Psychiatry* also includes an extensive section (Section 2) on the scientific basis of psychiatric aetiology, divided up into 22 subsections, each of which is easily digestible for those interested in a particular topic.

Thinking about prognosis

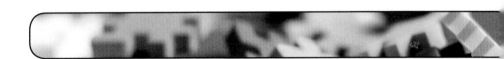

■ The role of prognostic assessment

The prognostic assessment aims to predict the future, using the evidence available. It results in an understanding of the following questions.

- **What outcomes are likely to happen?** These can be related to *the illness* (relapse and recurrence, for example—see below for definitions), to *treatments* (such as side effects or complications), to *risks* (to self or to others—see Chapter 9), or to *important social outcomes*, such as return to work, marital break-up, or permission to drive a motor vehicle.

- **How likely are they to happen, and when/over what time period?** An estimate of both **likelihood** and **time-line** is helpful. So, for example, in a patient with recurrent depressive episodes, who is now well, we may view that their lifetime risk of suicide is significantly higher than the population risk, that they are not currently at increased risk, and that suicide attempts are likely to occur in the context of depressive recurrence.

- **What can change the nature or likelihood of the outcomes?** For example, in the case above, we may view that the lifetime risk can be reduced by training the patient and family to spot the early warning signs of illness, by reducing daily consumption of alcohol, and by finding regular, stable employment.

The prognostic assessment is therefore closely linked to the assessment of diagnosis, of risks, of the patient's social situation, and of a suitable management plan. Indeed, the prognosis in a specific case helps to guide us in determining (i) whether any management is necessary, (ii) the nature and intensity of that management, and (iii) the health resources that it would be appropriate to use. It also helps to guide the patient to make decisions, based upon their own values and priorities. In an illness with minimal consequences that will be self-limiting, such as the common cold, the prognosis is good without medical management focused on the cause, and so symptomatic treatments are all that are required. In an illness with greater consequences, such as moderate depression, the illness is often not self-limiting, and there is evidence that medical treatments (whether physical or psychological) have an impact on prognosis.

■ Terminology

Specific terms are used by mental health professionals to describe the prognosis of psychiatric disorder. There is considerable debate about the precise definitions of these terms. For ordinary clinical practice, these issues are not relevant, but they need very careful thought and definition in clinical research. The following descriptions are intended to assist the reader in commenting on prognosis in specific cases, and in tackling the relevant literature, rather than to be an authoritative guide.

Response is some relief of symptoms and some improvement in functioning. The term 'response' implies that this improvement arises from treatment, usually because it is associated in time with that treatment. For example, 'Mr A appears to have responded to the introduction of an antidepressant', or 'I think that it is unlikely that she will respond to the antidepressant, due to her continued heavy drinking'.

Remission is a period of complete relief of symptoms and a return of full functioning, which may be brief. For example, 'Currently Mrs B appears to be in remission, with no depressive or anxiety symptoms, and is coping well at work'.

Recovery is a period of complete relief of symptoms and a return of full functioning, which is likely to be longer term. For example, 'Mr C appears to have recovered from his recent depressive episode, and has now been symptom free for 3 months'.

Relapse is the return of symptoms, satisfying the diagnostic criteria for the disorder, after a patient has either responded or remitted, but before recovery. For example, 'The patient was symptom free for 4 weeks, but in the last fortnight her mood has deteriorated significantly, and she is again unable to work', or 'There is a high probability of relapse, as Miss D has stopped taking her antidepressant, and her abusive partner has returned to her home after a period of time away'. In the mood disorders, relapse is usually conceived as being a return of the original mood episode, rather than the start of a new one.

Recurrence is the return of symptoms, satisfying the diagnostic criteria for the disorder, after the patient has recovered. The distinction from relapse is therefore temporal. In the mood disorders, recurrence is usually conceived as being a new mood episode. For example, 'Mrs E had been well for 1 year after her first depressive episode, but depressive symptoms have returned and she again meets criteria for a depressive episode', or 'Due to the high frequency of mood episodes in recent years, the likelihood of recurrence is high'.

Prognosis and treatment

Inevitably, consideration of the prognosis in a particular case is closely linked to consideration of treatment. In the last example above, the comment could have continued: 'Due to the high frequency of mood episodes in recent years, the likelihood of recurrence is high, but could be reduced significantly by improved compliance over a period of years with a mood stabilizer such as lithium carbonate'. This demonstrates the consideration of both static and dynamic factors. **Static factors** are those that cannot be changed—the recent high frequency of mood episodes, for example, or gender, or early onset. **Dynamic factors** are those that can be changed—compliance with medicines, for example, or reducing alcohol or substance use, or finding work.

There are two stages to thinking about prognosis and treatment. The first is to determine whether any treatment is necessary, by considering the prognosis without treatment. If this is good, then it may well be desirable to pursue a policy of 'active monitoring' (or 'watchful waiting'), watching for signs of deterioration, but without active treatment, therefore avoiding the side effects and risks associated with many treatments. If, on the other hand, the prognosis is moderate or poor, treatment should be considered. The second stage is to determine whether treatment will improve the prognosis and, by implication, which treatment will most improve the prognosis.

■ Communicating the prognosis

Communicating with health professionals

In day-to-day clinical practice, prognosis is usually mentioned only briefly, often by stating simply that the patient's prognosis is 'good', 'moderate', or 'poor'. This is unfortunate; high-quality clinical practice needs a rigorous approach to the assessment and communication of prognostic information, and we would urge you to practise a more comprehensive method. It is helpful to outline as many of the following as are appropriate in the time available:

- *overall*, whether the patient's prognosis is good, moderate, or poor;
- specifically *what* will be good or poor compared with their current situation, and *over what time period*;
- specific *risks*, if these have not been mentioned elsewhere;
- your *justification* of those views, citing evidence that is personalized to your particular patient, by combining evidence from the clinical assessment with evidence from textbooks or the scientific literature;
- *what can improve or worsen prognosis* (dynamic factors), e.g. starting a treatment, complying with a treatment, stopping drinking alcohol or using substances, finding or returning to work, being admitted to hospital, keeping a regular sleep–wake schedule, or engaging with the mental health team. Notably, these are all aspects that should be mentioned in your treatment plan, with which your prognostic assessment will therefore be closely linked.

Discussing the prognosis with patients

Before starting, ask the patient what they know about their prognosis—what might happen, how likely those things are to happen, and over what time period, and what they can do to improve their prognosis. From this, assess whether the patient understands the implications of their illness, and the impact that their own actions can have on their prognosis. Overall, form a view on whether the patient is *realistic* about their prognosis, *over-pessimistic*, or *over-optimistic*. Your approach will be different depending on your assessment of patient understanding. Your aim is for the patient to have a realistic understanding of their prognosis, and to understand how their own actions can improve their outcome.

Discussing prognosis can be difficult for patients and their relatives. Oncology and palliative care settings have set the pace in terms of considering the issues, and developing guidelines to assist clinicians in this area. Useful suggestions include the following.

- Arrange privacy and time.
- Develop rapport, and show empathy.
- Consider what the patient knows and doesn't know.
- Consider what the patient doesn't want to know.
- Take time, and avoid or explain jargon.
- Be realistic about uncertainty—your prognostic estimate is just that, and may well have wide 'confidence intervals'/significant uncertainty.
- Consider the family's/carer's needs, which may be distinct.
- Encourage questions and clarification.
- Consider the consistency of information from different mental health team/primary care team members.
- Record in the case notes what you have discussed.
- Write to other health professionals involved in the case, to let them know what you have said.

Risk assessment and management

Increased risk of harm to self and others occurs in several mental disorders, and the prediction and assessment of risk has become an important component of psychiatric practice.

Fatal self-harm—or suicide—is the most important risk to assess. At least a brief assessment of suicidal risk should be included in all psychiatric assessments. However, harm to others—both homicide and non-fatal harm—is increased in disorders such as schizophrenia, and a thorough assessment of the nature, severity, and likelihood of such risks will often form an important part of a psychiatric assessment. When assessing risk, it is useful to consider **static** and **dynamic** risk factors. Static risk factors cannot be changed, whereas dynamic risk factors change over time and include mental disorder.

Generally, the assessment of risk should include:

- the nature of the risk;
- the probability of the risk in the short and longer term;
- whether there are any factors that increase the risk;
- whether there are any factors that decrease the risk;
- whether there are any interventions that may reduce the risk.

A risk management plan will aim to:

- reduce the risk;
- review the risk.

Often, the most appropriate intervention to reduce risk will be to ensure that the patient is offered the most effective treatment for their specific condition. For example, a depressed person with suicidal ideation may be offered a low-toxicity antidepressant and regular follow-up. On the other hand, the management of a new mother with a postpartum psychotic depressive disorder who has thoughts of harming her new child may involve specific intervention to reduce the risk of harm to her baby as well as effective therapy for the depressive disorder.

■ Suicide

Many patients deliberately take drug overdoses or harm themselves in other ways. Some die (suicide); others survive (attempted suicide, parasuicide, or deliberate self-harm). The characteristics of those who kill themselves and those who harm themselves are rather different, although they overlap. The main clinical issues are the assessment of suicide risk and the management of deliberate self-harm.

Suicide accounts for about 1 per cent of deaths. It is rare among children and uncommon in adolescents. Rates increase with age and are higher in men than in women. There are two sets of interacting causes: social factors, especially social isolation, and medical factors, among which depressive disorder, alcoholism, and abnormal personality are particularly important.

The assessment of suicide risk depends on evaluating:

- the presence of suicidal ideas;
- the presence of psychiatric disorder;
- factors known to be associated with increased risk of suicide.

Referral to the specialist mental health services is usually appropriate when the suicidal intentions are strong, associated psychiatric illness is severe, and the person lacks social support. If the risk does not seem to require hospital admission, management depends on ensuring good support, telling the patient how to obtain help quickly if needed, and ensuring that all those who need to know are informed.

Deliberate self-harm is usually by drug overdose, but may be by self-injury, lacerations, and also more dangerous methods such as jumping from a height, shooting, or drowning.

Deliberate self-harm is commonest among younger people. **Predisposing factors** include childhood difficulties, adverse social circumstances, and poor health. **Precipitating factors** include stressful life events, such as quarrels with spouses or others in close relationships. Only a minority have psychiatric disorder. The motives are complex and often uncertain. Frequently there is no particular wish to die.

Up to a quarter of people who harm themselves do so again in the following year, and the risk of suicide during the year is about 1–2 per cent, a hundred times the risk in the general population.

Assessment must include:

- the risk of suicide;
- the risk of further deliberate self-harm;
- current medical and social problems.

Those with severe mental disorder may require admission, and others need continuing help from a mental health service or general practitioner. About a quarter require no special treatment.

■ Suicidal risk

Most completed suicides are planned and precautions against discovery are often taken. About one in six leaves a **suicide note**. Some notes are pleas for forgiveness. Other notes are accusing or vindictive, drawing attention to failings in relatives or friends. In most cases, some warning of intention is given to relatives or friends, or to doctors. There is a history of deliberate self-harm in between a third and a half of completed suicides.

An understanding of the epidemiology and causes of suicide is clinically useful for several reasons:

- as a basis for assessing suicidal risk;
- to help the relatives and others in the aftermath of suicide;
- as a guide to suicide prevention.

Epidemiology

In the UK, the suicide rate has decreased over recent years (Figure 9.1), and is about 10 per 100 000 per year in males and 3 per 100 000 in females (which is in the lower range of rates reported for developed countries). Suicide accounts for about 1 per cent of all deaths. However, official suicide statistics almost certainly underestimate the numbers of actual suicides because uncertain cases are not counted.

Suicide rates are highest in older people, in men, and those who are divorced or unmarried. In most countries, *drug overdoses* (especially analgesics and antidepressants) account for about two-thirds of suicides among women and about a third of those among men. The remaining deaths are by a variety of *physical means*, namely hanging, shooting, wounding, drowning, jumping from high places, and falling in front of moving vehicles or trains.

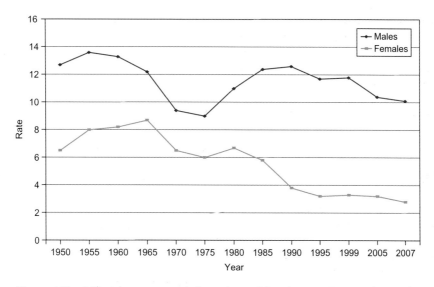

Fig. 9.1 UK suicide rates per 100 000 for males and females over the period 1950–2007. (Source: www.who.int/mental_health/media/unitkingd.pdf).

Causes of suicide

The large international, regional, and temporal variations in the prevalence of suicide reflect the importance of social causes. These causes interact with individual psychiatric and medical factors (see Box 9.1). Psychiatric disorder is an important cause of suicide; in contrast it is less important in deliberate self-harm (see Table 9.1).

 BOX 9.1 Causes of suicide

Social

- Old age
- Living alone
- Lack of family and other support
- Stressful events
- Publicity about suicides

Medical

- Depressive disorder
- Alcohol abuse
- Drug abuse
- Schizophrenia
- Personality disorder
- Chronic painful physical illness and epilepsy

Social causes

Social isolation. Compared with the general population, people who have died by suicide are more likely to have been divorced, unemployed, or be living alone. Social isolation is a common factor among these associations.

Stressful events. Suicide is often precipitated by stressful events, including bereavement and other losses.

Social factors influencing the method. Social factors also influence the means chosen for suicide. Thus a case that has attracted attention in a community or received wide publicity in newspapers or on television may be followed by others using the same method.

Psychiatric and medical causes

Many of the people who die from suicide have some form of *psychiatric disorder* at the time of death, most often a

Table 9.1 Comparison of those who die by suicide and those who harm themselves

	Suicide	Deliberate self-harm
Age	Older	Younger
Sex	More often male	More often female
Psychiatric disorder	Common, severe	Less common, less severe
Physical illness	Common	Uncommon
Planning	Careful	Impulsive
Method	Lethal	Less dangerous

depressive illness or alcohol dependence. Some have chronic, painful *physical illness.*

Depressive disorder. The rate of suicide is increased in patients with depressive disorder, with a lifetime risk of about 15 per cent in severe cases. Depressed patients who commit suicide differ from other depressed patients in being older, more often *single, separated, or widowed,* and having made more *previous suicide attempts.*

Alcohol abuse also carries a high risk of suicide. The risk is particularly great among (i) older men with a long history of drinking, a current depressive disorder, and previous deliberate self-harm, and (ii) people whose drinking has caused physical complications, marital problems, difficulties at work, or arrests for drunkenness offences.

Drug abuse also carries an increased risk of suicide.

Schizophrenia has a high risk of suicide, with a lifetime risk of about 10 per cent. The risk is particularly great in younger patients who have retained insight into the serious effect which the illness is likely to have on their lives.

Personality disorder is detected in a third to a half of people who die by suicide. Personality disorder is often associated with other factors that increase the risk of suicide, namely abuse of alcohol or drugs and social isolation.

Chronic physical illness is associated with suicide, especially among the elderly.

Causes among special groups

Rational suicide. Suicide is sometimes the rational act of a mentally healthy person. However, even if the decision appears to have been reached rationally, given more time and more information the person may change his intentions. For example, a person with cancer may change a decision to take his life when he learns that there is treatment to relieve pain. Doctors should try to bring about this change of mind, but some rational suicides will take place despite the best treatment.

Physician-assisted suicide has been an increasingly prominent matter of public and medical concern. It raises several important ethical and legal issues:

- a conflict between the duty to help the patient and the duty not to harm;
- competence of the patient to decide;
- differences between actively promoting death, withholding treatment which might prolong life, and the use of medication which as a side effect may shorten life.

Box 9.2 lists some of the clinical issues that may need to be considered and may need to be discussed with the patient and family.

Children and young adolescents. As noted above, suicide is rare among children, and uncommon in adolescents,

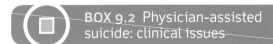

BOX 9.2 Physician-assisted suicide: clinical issues

- Need to discuss medical and other opportunities to minimize pain and suffering
- Importance of understanding the patient's and family's views on death
- Importance of treating depression as a cause of the wish to die
- Need to assess the patient's competence and/or review any advance directive
- Need to provide high-quality care and support to patient and family
- Awareness of pressure on patient from others, for instance those who may benefit financially

although rates in older adolescents have increased recently. In adolescence, suicide is associated with broken homes, social isolation, and depression, and also with impetuous behaviour and violence.

Doctors. The suicide rate among doctors is greater than that in the general population. The reason is uncertain although several factors have been suggested, such as the ready availability of drugs, increased rates of addiction to alcohol and drugs, the extra stresses of work, reluctance to seek treatment for depressive disorders, and the selection into the medical profession of predisposed personalities.

Suicide pacts. In a suicide pact, two people, usually in a close relationship in which one is dominant and the other is passive, agree that at the same time each will die by suicide. They are uncommon, and must be distinguished from murder followed by suicide (occurring sometimes when the murderer has a severe depressive disorder). When one person survives, a suicide pact has to be distinguished from the aiding of suicide by a person who did not intend to die, and also from an attempt to disguise murder.

The assessment of suicide risk

Every doctor will encounter, at some time, patients who express suicidal intentions, and must be able to assess the risk of suicide (see Box 9.3). This assessment requires:

- evaluation of suicidal intentions;
- assessment of any previous act of deliberate self-harm (see p. 71);
- detection of psychiatric disorder;
- assessment of other factors associated with increased risk of suicide;
- assessment of factors associated with a reduced risk;
- in some cases, assessment of associated homicidal ideas.

BOX 9.3 Risk factors for suicide

Intention

- Evidence of intent to die

Psychiatric factors

- Depression
- Schizophrenia
- Personality disorder
- Alcohol and drug dependence

Social and demographic factors

- Older age
- Severe social and interpersonal stressors
- Isolation

Medical factors

- Chronic, painful illness and epilepsy

Evaluation of intentions. Some people fear that asking about *suicidal intentions* will make suicide more likely. It does not, provided that the enquiries are made sympathetically. Indeed, a person who has thought of suicide will feel better understood when the interviewer raises the issue, and this feeling may reduce the risk. The interviewer can begin by asking whether the patient has thought that life is not worth living. This question can lead to more direct ones about thoughts of suicide, specific plans, and preparatory acts such as saving tablets. Box 9.4 shows a useful standard instrument—the Beck Suicide Intent Scale—which combines these and other informative questions.

When suicidal intentions are revealed they should be taken seriously. *There is no truth in the idea that people who talk of suicide do not enact it*; on the contrary, two-thirds of people who die by suicide have told someone of their intentions. A few people speak repeatedly of suicide so that they are no longer taken seriously, but many of these people eventually kill themselves. Therefore their intentions should be evaluated carefully on every occasion.

Previous deliberate self-harm of any kind is an indicator of substantially increased risk of suicide. Certain features of previous self-harm are particularly important predictors of suicide; these are summarized on p. 72 and in Box 9.8 below.

Detection of psychiatric disorder is an important part of the assessment of suicide risk. If possible an informant should be interviewed. *Depressive disorder* is highly important, especially when there is severe mood change with hopelessness, insomnia, anorexia, weight loss, or delusions.

BOX 9.4 Beck Suicide Intent Scale

(Reprinted with permission from Beck, A.T. *et al.* (1974). *The Prediction of Suicide*. Charles Press, Maryland.)

Circumstances related to suicidal attempt

1. Isolation
   - 0 Somebody present
   - 1 Somebody nearby or in contact (as by phone)
   - 2 No one nearby or in contact

2. Timing
   - 0 Timed so that intervention is probable
   - 1 Timed so that intervention is not likely
   - 2 Timed so that intervention is highly unlikely

3. Precautions against discovery and/or intervention
   - 0 No precautions
   - 1 Passive precautions such as avoiding others but doing nothing to prevent their intervention (alone in a room with unlocked door)
   - 2 Active precaution such as locked door

4. Acting to gain help during/after attempt
   - 0 Notified potential helper regarding the attempt
   - 1 Contacted but did not specifically notify potential helper regarding the attempt
   - 2 Did not contact or notify potential helper

5. Final acts in anticipation of death
   - 0 None
   - 1 Partial preparation or ideation
   - 2 Definite plans made (changes in will, giving of gifts, taking out insurance)

BOX 9.4 Beck Suicide Intent Scale (*continued*)

6. Degree of planning for suicide attempt	0 No preparation
	1 Minimal preparation
	2 Extensive preparation
7. Suicide note	0 Absence of note
	1 Note written but torn up
	2 Presence of note
8. Overt communication of intent before act	0 None
	1 Equivocal communication
	2 Unequivocal communication
9. Purpose of attempt	0 Mainly to change environment
	1 Components of '0' and '2'
	2 Mainly to remove self from environment

Self-report

10. Expectations regarding fatality of act	0 Patient thought that death was unlikely
	1 Patient thought that death was possible but not probable
	2 Patient thought that death was probable or certain
11. Conception of method's lethality	0 Patient did less to himself than he thought would be lethal
	1 Patient wasn't sure, or did what he thought might be lethal
	2 Act equalled or exceeded patient's concept of its medical lethality
12. 'Seriousness' of attempt	0 Patient did not consider act to be a serious attempt to end his life
	1 Patient was uncertain whether act was a serious attempt to end his life
	2 Patient considered act to be a serious attempt to end his life
13. Ambivalence towards living	0 Patient did not want to die
	1 Patient did not care whether he lived or died
	2 Patient wanted to die
14. Conception of reversibility	0 Patient thought that death would be unlikely if he received medical attention
	1 Patient was uncertain whether death could be averted by medical attention
	2 Patient was certain of death even if he received medical attention
15. Degree of premeditation	0 None; impulsive
	1 Suicide contemplated for 3 hours or less prior to attempt
	2 Suicide contemplated for more than 3 hours prior to attempt

It is important to remember that suicide may occur during recovery from a depressive disorder in patients who, when more severely depressed, had thought of the act but lacked initiative to carry it out. *Schizophrenia*, *personality disorder*, and *alcohol and drug dependence* also carry an increased risk of suicide.

Assessment of social and medical general factors associated with increased risk of suicide. These factors have been described above and summarized in Box 9.3, and include old age, loneliness, severe and intractable current life problems, and chronic painful illness or epilepsy.

Factors that may reduce risk. These include the availability of good support from the family and others to assist with social, practical, and emotional difficulties.

Homicidal ideas in suicidal patients. A few severely depressed suicidal patients have homicidal ideas; for example, the idea that it would be an act of mercy to kill the partner or a child, in order to spare that person intolerable suffering. If present, such ideas should be taken extremely seriously since they may be carried into practice. It is especially important to be aware of these dangers when assessing a mother of small children.

Management of a patient at risk of suicide

The risk of suicide should be considered in any patient who is depressed or whose behaviour or talk gives any suggestion of the possibility of self-harm. In hospital inpatient or emergency departments, evidence of suicidal intent should normally lead to obtaining advice from a specialist. However, other medical staff need to be aware of the general principles of assessment, especially with patients who are reluctant to stay and who are medically fit. Box 9.5 summarizes reasons for referral.

An exception to the general principle of admission when risk is judged to be high may be made when the patient lives with reliable relatives, who wish to care for the patient, understand their responsibilities, and are able to fulfil them. In these circumstances, a psychiatric opinion is very often useful. If hospital treatment is essential but the patient refuses it, compulsory admission will be necessary.

A number of patients remain at *long-term suicidal risk* despite specialist assessment that there are no indications that hospital treatment would be of benefit. An example would be a patient with longstanding problems who has had intensive psychiatric and social help without benefit, and for whom it is evident that further hospital admission would do nothing to help with the long-term problems in everyday life. Such a decision requires a particularly thorough knowledge of the patient and his problems, and should generally be made by a psychiatrist in conjunction with the general practitioner.

The main principles of treatment are as follows.

1 **Prevention of harm.** The obvious first requirement is to prevent the patient from self-harm by preventing access to methods of harm, and appropriately close observation. Most patients at serious suicidal risk require *admission to hospital*. The first requirement is the safety of the patient. To achieve this requires an adequate number of vigilant nursing staff, an agreed assessment of the level of risk, and good communication between staff. If the risk is very great, nursing may need to be continuous so that the patient is never alone. If *outpatient treatment* is chosen, the patient and relatives should be told how to obtain help quickly if the strength of suicidal ideas increases, for example an emergency telephone number. Frustrated attempts to find help can make suicide more likely.

2 **Treatment of any associated mental illness.** This should be initiated without delay.

3 **Reviving hope.** However determined the patient is to die, there is usually some remaining wish to live. These positive feelings can be encouraged and the patient helped towards a more positive view of the future. One way to begin this process is to show concern for the problems.

4 **Problem solving.** Initially overwhelming problems can usually be improved if they are dealt with one by one.

Help after a suicide

When a person has died by suicide, help is required by surviving relatives and friends who may need to deal with feelings of loss, guilt, or anger. They should have a full explanation of the nature and reasons for medical and other actions to assess the suicidal risk, to treat the causes, and prevent harm. They should also have an opportunity to discuss their own feelings, including guilt that if they had behaved differently the suicide could have been prevented. Those most directly involved in the previous care of the dead person should offer to meet the relatives as soon after the suicide as possible and to meet again at a later stage if the family and friends believe it would be helpful. The relatives' distress may be considerable and may be expressed indirectly in complaints about medical care. Some relatives suffer from longstanding or psychiatric or other problems which deserve treatment in their own right.

The doctor should also support other professional staff who had been closely involved with the patient. After suicide, the case should be reviewed carefully to determine whether useful lessons can be learnt about future clinical practice. This review should not be conducted as a search for a person at fault; some patients die by suicide however carefully the correct procedures have been followed.

BOX 9.5 Referral to a psychiatrist of patients at risk of suicide

In primary care, *referral* to a psychiatrist is usually appropriate when:

- suicidal intentions are clearly expressed;

- there is any change of presentation in a patient who has repeatedly self-harmed;
- associated psychiatric illness is severe;
- the person lacks social support.

Suicide prevention

There are two main approaches to prevention, namely *early recognition and help for those at risk,* and *modification of predisposing social factors.*

- **Identifying high-risk patients.** Many people who commit suicide have contacted their doctors shortly beforehand, and many of these have a psychiatric disorder, or alcohol dependence. Doctors can identify at least some of these patients as at high risk, and offer help.

- **Supporting those at risk.** This is mainly the responsibility of primary care and social agencies. Organizations such as the Samaritans give emergency 24-hour support to people who feel lonely and hopeless and express suicidal ideas, but it has not been shown convincingly that this support reduces suicide. In addition, it is possible that there are opportunities for modification of predisposing social factors.

- **Reducing the means** may help to reduce suicide (e.g. providing safety rails at high places, prescribing cautiously). However, people determined on suicide can find other means, such as overdoses of non-prescribed drugs.

- **Education** might be provided for teenagers about the dangers of drug overdosage and about ways of coping with emotional problems. However, there is little evidence that such education is effective.

- **Public health or social and economic policy.** Isolation and other social factors which increase the risk of suicide cannot be modified by the medical profession. They require public policy decisions.

■ Deliberate self-harm

Deliberate self-harm is not usually failed suicide. Only about a quarter of those who have deliberately harmed themselves say they wished to die; most say the act was impulsive rather than premeditated (see Figure 9.2). The rest find it difficult to explain the reasons or say that:

- they were *seeking unconsciousness* as a temporary escape or relief from their problems;

- they were trying to *influence another person* to change their behaviour (e.g. to make a partner feel guilty about threatening to end the relationship);

- they are *uncertain* whether or not they intended to die— they were 'leaving it to fate';

- they were *seeking help.*

Epidemiology

Deliberate self-harm is common and rates have risen progressively over the last 30 years. It now accounts for about 10 per cent of *acute medical admissions* in the UK. A further smaller number are seen by general practitioners but not sent to hospital because the medical risks are low, or attend emergency departments but are not admitted.

Epidemiological studies have shown the kind of people who are more likely to harm themselves and the methods that are common. Deliberate self-harm is more common among:

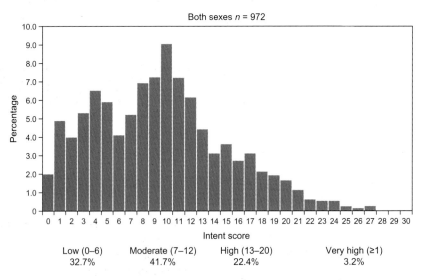

Fig. 9.2 Beck scores in deliberate self-harm attenders in 2001. (Reproduced with permission of Professor K. E. Hawton, Oxford University.)

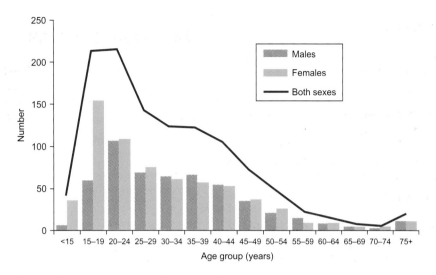

Fig. 9.3 The age groups of deliberate self-harm patients by sex in 2001. (Reproduced with permission of Professor K. E. Hawton, Oxford University.)

- **younger adults** (see Figure 9.3): the rates decline sharply during adult life (they are also very low in children under the age of 12 years);
- **young women**, particularly those aged 15–20 years;
- **people of low socioeconomic status**;
- **divorced individuals, teenage wives, and younger single adults**.

Methods of deliberate self-harm

Drug overdosage. In the UK, about 90 per cent of the cases of deliberate self-harm treated by general hospitals involve drug overdose. The drugs taken most commonly in overdose are **anxiolytics, non-opiate analgesics**, such as salicylates and paracetamol, and **antidepressants**. Paracetamol is particularly dangerous because it damages the liver and may lead to delayed death, sometimes in patients who had not taken the drugs with the intention of dying.

Antidepressants are taken in about a fifth of cases. Of these drugs, tricyclics are particularly hazardous in overdosage since they may cause cardiac arrhythmias or convulsions. Despite these and other dangers, most deliberate drug overdoses do not present a serious threat to life.

The use of alcohol. About half of the men and a quarter of the women who harm themselves have taken alcohol within 6 hours before the act. This often precipitates the act by reducing self-restraint. Its effects interact with those of the drugs.

Self-injury. In the UK, between 5 and 15 per cent of all cases of deliberate self-harm treated in general hospitals are self-inflicted injuries. Most of these injuries are lacerations, usually of the forearm or wrist. Most patients who cut themselves are young, have low self-esteem, impulsive or aggres-

sive behaviour, unstable moods, difficulty in interpersonal relationships, and often problems of alcohol or drug abuse. Usually, the self-laceration follows a period of increasing tension and irritability which is relieved by the self-injury. The cuts are usually multiple and superficial, often made with a razor blade or a piece of glass.

Less frequent and medically more serious forms of self-injury include deeper lacerations, jumping from heights or in front of a moving train or motor vehicle, shooting, or drowning. These highly dangerous acts occur mainly among people who intended to die but have survived.

Causes

Deliberate self-harm is usually the result of multiple social and personal factors (see Box 9.6), including

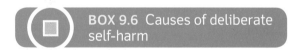

BOX 9.6 Causes of deliberate self-harm

Psychiatric disorder
Personality disorder
Alcohol dependence
Predisposing social factors
Early parental loss
Parental neglect or abuse
Long-term social problems: family, employment, financial
Poor physical health
Precipitating social factors
Stressful life problems

BOX 9.7 Factors that predict the repetition of deliberate self-harm

Previous deliberate self-harm before the current episode	History of violence
Previous psychiatric treatment	Low social class
Alcohol or drug abuse	Unemployment
Personality disorder	Age 25–54 years
Criminal record	Single, divorced, or separated

national and local attitudes. Overall, rates appear to be affected by awareness of the occurrence and methods of self-harm in a population (for example, television and press reports and local knowledge of suicide and attempted suicide in the neighbourhood). Psychiatric disorder is less important than in suicide.

Social and family factors

Predisposing factors. Evidence of childhood emotional deprivation is common. Many patients who harm themselves have long-term marital problems, extramarital relationships, or other relationship problems, and may have financial and other social difficulties. Rates of unemployment are greater than in the general population.

Precipitating factors. Stressful life events are frequent before the act of self-harm, especially quarrels with or threats of rejection by spouses or sexual partners.

Association with psychiatric disorder

Although many patients who harm themselves are anxious or depressed, relatively few have a psychiatric disorder other than an acute stress reaction, adjustment disorder, or personality disorder. The latter is found in about a third to a half of self-harm patients, and dependence on alcohol is also frequent. (In contrast, psychiatric disorder is common among patients who die by suicide; see p. 64.)

The differences between factors associated with suicide and deliberate self-harm are summarized in Table 9.1.

Outcome

Since deliberate self-harm results from long-term adverse social factors and is associated with personality disorder, it is not surprising that a significant proportion of subjects have a poor overall outcome in terms of personal and social adjustment. More specifically, outcome is assessed in terms of repetition of self-harm and of suicide. Between 15 and 25 per cent of people who harm themselves do so again in the following year and 1–2 per cent commit suicide. Of those who harm themselves again:

- some repeat the act only once;
- some repeat it several times within a period in which there are continuing severe stressful events;

- a few repeat it many times over a long period as a habitual response to minor stressors.

The factors associated with repetition of deliberate self-harm are shown in Box 9.7.

People who have deliberately harmed themselves have a much increased risk of later suicide (Figure 9.4). In the year after the self-harm, the risk of suicide is about 1–2 per cent, that is, about 100 times the risk in the general population. The risk factors for suicide after deliberate self-harm are shown in Box 9.8.

It is important to note that a *non-dangerous method of self-harm does not necessarily indicate a low risk of subsequent suicide* (although the risk is higher when a violent or dangerous method has been used).

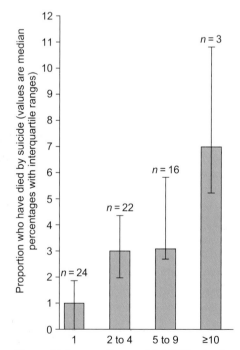

Fig. 9.4 Suicide after non-fatal deliberate self-harm (DSM) according to duration of follow-up. *n* refers to the number of published studies in each group. (Reproduced with permission from (1998) Deliberate self-harm. Effective Health Care 4(6).)

BOX 9.8 Factors predicting suicide after deliberate self-harm

Evidence of intent

- Evidence of serious intent (see Box 9.5)
- Continuing wish to die
- Previous acts of deliberate self-harm

Psychiatric disorder

- Depressive disorder

- Alcoholism or drug abuse
- Antisocial personality disorder

Social and demographic

- Social isolation
- Unemployment
- Older age group
- Male sex

Assessment

Every act of deliberate self-harm should be assessed thoroughly. For many patients seen in primary care, the physical consequences of the act and concern about the risk of repetition will lead to hospital referral. In other cases, referral may not be necessary, for instance, when the act was not reported until some time later, when the results are clearly not medical serious, where suicidal intent was low, and where the patient and family are known to the doctor.

All deliberate self-harm patients seen in hospital emergency departments should have a psychiatric and social assessment (Figure 9.5). This assessment can be carried out by a psychiatrist, by general medical staff, or by psychiatric nurses or social workers with appropriate special training, or by a psychiatrist. All patients found on this assessment to be suffering from psychiatric disorder or with a high risk of further self-harm should be seen by a psychiatrist. Since many patients who are medically fit do not wish to stay for specialist assessment, it is essential

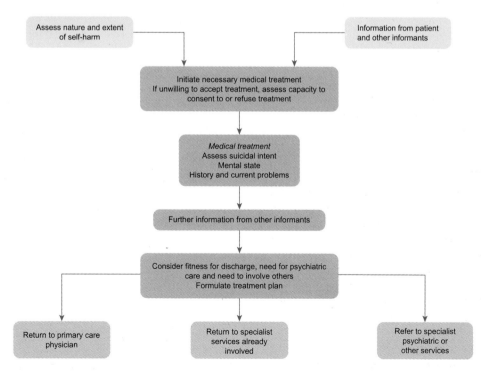

Fig. 9.5 Action that should be taken in the emergency department for deliberate self-harmers.

that all emergency department medical staff are competent to assess risk.

Steps in assessment

The assessment should be carried out in a way that encourages patients to undertake a constructive review of their problems and of the ways they can deal with them. If patients can then resolve their problems in this way, they may be able to do so again in the future instead of resorting to self-harm again.

When to assess. When patients have recovered sufficiently from the physical effects of the self-harm they should be interviewed, if possible, where the discussion will not be overheard or interrupted. After a drug overdose, the first step is to determine whether consciousness is impaired. If so, the interview should be delayed until the patient has recovered further and can concentrate on the questions.

Sources of information. Information should be obtained also from relatives or friends, the general practitioner, and any other person (such as a social worker) already involved in the patient's care. Such information frequently adds significantly to the account given by the patient. The following issues should be considered.

Information required

1 **What were the patient's intentions before and at the time of the attempt?** Patients whose behaviour suggests that they intended to die as a result of the act of self-harm are at greater risk of a subsequent fatal act of self-harm. Intent is assessed by considering the following.

- Was the act *planned* or carried out on impulse?
- Were *precautions* taken against being found?
- Did the patient seek *help after the act*?
- *Was the method dangerous*? Not only should the objective risk be assessed, but also the risk anticipated by the patient, which may be different (e.g. if he believed that he had taken a lethal dose of a drug even though he had not).
- *Was there a 'final act'* such as writing a suicide note or making a will?

2 **Does the patient now wish to die?** The interviewer should ask directly whether the patient is relieved to have recovered or wishes to die. If the act suggested serious suicidal intent, but the patient denies such intent, the interviewer should try to find out by tactful but thorough questioning whether there has been a genuine change of resolve.

3 **What are the current problems?** Many patients will have experienced a mounting series of difficulties in the weeks or months leading up to the act of self-harm. Some of these difficulties may have been resolved by the time the patient is interviewed, but if serious problems remain, the risk of a fatal repetition is greater. This risk is particularly great if the problems are of loneliness or ill health. Possible problems should be reviewed systematically, covering *intimate relationships* with the spouse or another person, *relations with children and other relatives, employment, finance,* and *housing, legal problems, social isolation, bereavement,* and *other losses.*

4 **Is there psychiatric disorder?** This question is answered with information obtained from the history, from a brief but systematic examination of the mental state, and also from other informants and from medical notes.

5 **What are the patient's resources?** These include the capacity to solve problems, material resources, and the help that others may provide. The best guide to future ability to solve problems is the past record of dealing with difficulties such as the loss of a job, or a broken relationship. The availability of help should be assessed by asking about the patient's friends and relatives, and about support available from medical services, social workers, or voluntary agencies.

6 **Is treatment required and will the patient agree to it?** Management aims to:

- treat any psychiatric disorder;
- manage high suicide risk;
- enable the patient to *resolve difficulties* that led to the act of self-harm;
- *deal with future crises* without resorting to self-harm.

Of the patients referred to hospital for treatment of deliberate self-harm:

1 About 1 in 10 need immediate inpatient psychiatric treatment, usually for a depressive disorder or alcohol dependency, or for a period of respite from overwhelming stressors.

2 About two-thirds need care from a psychiatric outpatient team or from the primary practitioner (but many do not accept this help).

3 About a quarter require no special treatment because their self-harm was a response to temporary difficulties and carried little risk of repetition.

Management

The mainstay of treatment is **problem solving** (see p. 134) based on the list of problems compiled during the assessment. The patient is encouraged to consider what steps he could take to resolve each of these problems, and to formulate a practical plan for tackling one at a time. Throughout this discussion, the therapist helps the patient to do as much as possible to help himself. When there are interpersonal problems, it is often helpful to have a joint or family discussion.

The results of treatment

Successful treatment of a depressive or other psychiatric disorder reduces the risk of subsequent self-harm. There is less strong evidence that problem solving and other psychological methods reduce repetition, although they do reduce personal and social problems. This lack of strong evidence may be due, in part, to the methodological difficulties of randomized trials in this heterogeneous population. Particular types of psychological or social problem have been shown to benefit from specific treatments, such as couple therapy for problems between couples, problem solving for practical and everyday difficulties, and cognitive behaviour treatment for longstanding personal difficulties.

Management of special groups

Certain subgroups of patients pose special management problems. In most cases, specialist advice should be obtained.

Mothers of young children. Because there is an association between deliberate self-harm and child abuse, it is important to ask any mother with young children about her feelings towards the children, and to enquire from other informants, as well as the patient, about their welfare. If there is a possibility of child abuse or neglect, appropriate assessment action should be carried out (see p. 166). There is also an association between depression and infanticide.

Children and adolescents. Deliberate self-harm is uncommon among young children, but becomes increasingly frequent after the age of 12, especially among girls. The most common method is drug overdosage; in only a few cases is there a threat to life. Self-injury also occurs, more often among boys than girls.

The motivation for self-harm in young children is difficult to determine, but it is more often to communicate distress or escape from stress than to die. Deliberate self-harm in children and adolescents is associated with broken homes, family psychiatric disorder, and child abuse. It is often precipitated by difficulties with parents, boyfriends or girlfriends, or schoolwork.

Most children and adolescents do not repeat an act of deliberate self-harm, but an important minority do so, usually in association with severe psychosocial problems. These repeated acts of deliberate self-harm carry a significant risk of suicide. Children or adolescents who harm themselves should be assessed by a child psychiatrist. Treatment is not only of the young person but also of the family.

Patients who refuse assessment and treatment. Some patients try to leave hospital before emergency gastric lavage and other treatment. Others seek to do so before psychological assessment can be completed.

In most countries, there is a legal power to detain those who require potentially life-saving treatment and whose competence or capacity to take an informed decision about discharge is likely to be impaired by their mental state. The doctor should obtain as much information about mental state and suicidal risk as time allows. The patient should only be allowed to leave hospital when serious suicidal risk has been excluded (Box 9.9).

In taking decisions about emergency treatment, the doctor is likely to be helped by relatives, inpatient medical notes, and by telephoning the primary care doctor and any other doctor, social worker, or person who has

BOX 9.9 Patients who harm themselves and refuse treatment

- There are wide differences in national procedures, practice, and legislation.

- The patient who has harmed himself and is alert and conscious should be presumed to be competent to refuse medical advice and treatment unless there is evidence to the contrary.

- The most senior experienced doctor available should be prepared to discuss the need for treatment, the alternatives, and the patient's anxieties. It is often appropriate to involve relatives. Calm, sympathetic discussion is often effective in enabling the patient to decide to consent to treatment.

- Capacity should be assessed (see p. 102), preferably by a psychiatrist.

- If the patient is competent and continues to refuse consent, the consequences should be clearly outlined to the patient and the discussion fully recorded. The patient should be allowed to go, but encouraged to return. Where possible, an alternative plan should be agreed with the patient and, if possible, relatives or friends. If the patient is assessed as being incompetent, then the reasons should be recorded fully. Emergency treatment should proceed and a compulsory order under mental health legislation should be sought.

been involved with the patient in the past. It is essential to write detailed notes and to be aware of the legal requirements about both emergency treatment and confidentiality.

Frequent repeaters. Some people take overdoses repeatedly, often at times of stress in circumstances that suggest that the behaviour is to reduce tension or gain attention. These people usually have a personality disorder and many insoluble social problems. Although sometimes directed towards gaining attention, repeated self-harm may cause relatives to become unsympathetic or hostile, and these feelings may be shared by professional staff as their repeated efforts at help are seen to fail. Usually, little can be done to change the pattern of behaviour. Neither counselling nor intensive psychotherapy is effective, and management is limited to providing support. Sometimes a change in life circumstances is followed by improvement, but unless this happens the risk of death by suicide is high.

Deliberate self-laceration. It is difficult to help people who lacerate themselves repeatedly. They often have low self-esteem and experience extreme tension. They also often have difficulty in recognizing feelings and expressing themselves in words. Efforts should be made to increase self-esteem and to find an alternative, simple way of relieving tension, for example, by taking exercise. Anxiolytic drugs are seldom helpful and may produce disinhibition. If drug treatment is needed to reduce tension, a phenothiazine is more likely to be effective.

■ Risk to others

The assessment of risk to others is an important part of clinical practice. It is, however, important to get the magnitude of the risk to others into perspective. Although several mental disorders are associated with increased risk of violence to others, the vast majority of violent crime is committed by people who are not mentally unwell. Furthermore, people with mental disorders are much more likely to be victims of crime than perpetrators.

Assessment of risk to others

Several psychiatric disorders are known to be associated with an increased risk of violence to others:

- substance abuse: relative risk (RR) compared with general population 8
- schizophrenia: RR approximately 5
- bipolar disorder: RR approximately 5.

The risks associated with these disorders interact— thus the RR of schizophrenia with substance abuse comorbidity is around 22.

Violence may result directly from the psychopathology of the disorder itself. For example, hallucinatory voices may command the patient to act in a specific way—which may be aggressive or homicidal. It may also arise from the combination of frustrations, difficulties, and disabilities that result from chronic mental disorder. Furthermore, there are a number of specific clinical situations which are known to be high risk in psychiatry:

- morbid jealousy (see p. 261)
- misidentification syndromes
- depressive disorder with suicidal ideation in mothers of small children
- stalking.

The clinical prediction of risk to others has become a major focus of interest in recent years and extensive risk assessment tools have been developed. A commonly used example is the Psychopathy Checklist–Revised, which is used to measure psychopathic attributes and has reasonable predictive characteristics in some settings. The main difficulty with the general application of these tools to low-risk situations is that the performance remains limited and both the positive and negative predictive values of an assessment are low. This means that very few of those patients assessed as high risk will be violent, and most cases of violence will occur in those patients who are judged low risk. This is simply an epidemiological fact due to the limitations of the prediction and the low absolute risk of a violent event.

Nonetheless, there are two things always worth considering. First, it appears that *risk estimates are more accurate in the short term* and it is always worth considering the likelihood of immediate harm to others. Secondly, the *past is the best predictor of the future* and so patients with a past history of violence to others should be considered at relatively high risk of reoffending.

All assessments should be clearly recorded in the clinical notes.

Management of risk to others

The goal of managing risk to others is to do all that can be reasonably done to reduce the risk of harm. Psychiatric disorder should be diagnosed and treated, if necessary in hospital using compulsory detention. If there is clear evidence of harm to a particular person, consider warning them—this may mean compromising confidentiality.

Further reading

Mullen, P. E. & Ogloff, J. R. P. (2009). Assessing and managing the risks of violence towards others. In *New Oxford Textbook of Psychiatry*, 2nd edn. Ed. Gelder, M. G., Andreasen, N. C., Lopez-Ibor, J. J. & Geddes, J. R., pp. 1991–2002. Oxford University Press, Oxford.

Communicating your findings

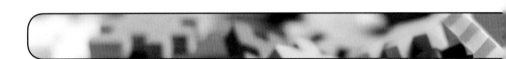

In recent years, there has been increased emphasis on improving communication between healthcare professionals and their patients, and rightly so. This chapter will offer some guidance on how to explain to patients and their carers the results of your assessment. However, during the same period there has been little change to training in communication between healthcare professionals. In our view, this represents a missed opportunity. Communication between healthcare professionals is a vital part of modern healthcare. No longer can one nurse or one doctor, working in geographical and professional isolation, seek to deliver effective health interventions to a population. Instead, healthcare is delivered in complex systems, incorporating primary, secondary and tertiary care, different disciplines, such as doctors, nurses, psychologists, and occupational and physiotherapists, and different specialties. It is vital that every healthcare practitioner is able to *transmit* and *record* information about patients in a way that is understandable by others, and is equally able to *receive* information from others about shared patients. We would urge all who are interested in the management of mental disorder to focus considerable effort on developing their skills to communicate with their colleagues about patients with mental disorder.

■ Communicating with the patient and their relatives

Confidentiality

Interviewers should be aware of the ethical and legal principles that govern the giving of information to people other than the patient. These principles are summarized in Box 10.1. Sometimes, a relative or another person telephones the interviewer to ask for information about the patient. As a general rule, no information should be given over the telephone. Instead the patient should be told of the request. If he agrees that the information should be given to the enquirer, an interview should be arranged with that person. The clinician should never allow a conspiratorial atmosphere to develop in which he conceals from the patient conversations with family, friends, or others.

Explaining the diagnosis and management plan

Patients and relatives need to know more than the diagnosis and the basic facts about treatment. It is useful to begin by finding out what they know already, and what help they are expecting. This information makes it easier to meet their requirements, help with their concerns, and explain the treatment plan. It is useful to keep in mind the list of frequently asked questions shown in Box 10.2. The plan should be explained in an unhurried way, avoiding jargon, checking from time to time that the patient (or relative) has understood, and seeking questions. If, after a full discussion, the patient does not accept some part of the plan, or the relatives do not accept the role proposed for them, a compromise should be negotiated. It is now usual to copy the assessment letter to the patient, so that they have a written record of what has been decided, and so that they can be more aware of their care and more active in it.

■ Communicating verbally with healthcare professionals

Structure and content of the case presentation

Psychiatry is a medical specialty, and the presentation of the psychiatric assessment is structured in a similar way to that in medicine and surgery, with a brief **introduction** to set the context, followed by a description of the **history**, the **examination**, and any **investigations** carried out to date (Table 10.1). However, there are two important ways in which the presentation of the psychiatric assessment will differ from that seen elsewhere. First, the physical examination is supplemented by the mental examination or, as it is usually called, the **mental state examination** (MSE).

 BOX 10.1 Ethical issues of confidentiality

General rule. Confidentiality is vital in psychiatry because patients often reveal highly personal information, and they need to know that it will be held and used in confidence, for their benefit. Doctors have a general duty to maintain confidentiality unless the patient gives informed consent to disclosure. In the UK, the General Medical Council gives useful guidance on this matter at www.gmc-uk.org/guid-ance/ethical_guidance.asp.

Exceptions to the rule. This general duty is overridden in two circumstances: (i) in response to a court order; or (ii) when disclosure may assist the prevention, detection, or prosecution of a major crime such as a serious assault or the abuse of children. In both circumstances every effort should be made to obtain the patient's informed consent to disclosure. If, despite this, consent is withheld, the case should be discussed with an experienced colleague and the need for medicolegal advice should be considered.

Confidentiality and the treatment team. Psychiatric treatment often involves not only the interviewer but also other members of a treatment team. To do their job effectively, these members need at least a part of the information given by the patient to the interviewer. Interviewers should explain the need to share information and seek the patient's agreement to this way of working. The other members of the team must, of course, respect the confidence of the information. The sharing of information with other members of the team for the purpose of providing best treatment is not generally viewed by the law as a breach of confidence. Problems may arise when the treatment plan involves other professions whose members may have slightly different practices about confidentiality. If these problems seem possible, they should be discussed with the patient and appropriate consent should be sought.

Consent to obtaining further information. Generally, patients' consent should be obtained before eliciting information from other people. The exception to this rule is when patients who are unable to give an account of themselves are unable to give consent to seeking information from others, and the information is needed to assist them. The same considerations apply when information is given to relatives or others concerning a patient who is unable to give consent. In such cases, where the patient lacks capacity, the professional must always be guided by the best interests of the patient, and must think carefully about what those are.

BOX 10.2 Communicating with patients and relatives

When giving information to patients and their relatives, it is useful to keep in mind relevant questions from the following list.

The diagnosis

- What is the diagnosis? If it is uncertain, what are the possibilities?
- Is further information or special investigation required?
- What may have caused the condition?
- What are the implications of the diagnosis for this patient's life?

The care plan

- What is the plan, and how far is it likely to help the patient and the family?
- What can the patient do to help him- or herself?
- What can the family do to help the patient?
- If medication is included:
  - What is its name, and why has it been chosen?
  - What is the dosage schedule?
  - What are the benefits, and when might they be seen?
  - What are the side effects, and will they settle down with time?

- Are there any possible toxic effects, and what should be done if they are noted?
- Has the patient any concerns (e.g. that antidepressants are addictive)?
- How long is the planned course of treatment?
- If psychological treatment is included:
  - What is involved, and who is involved?
  - How often will it take place and how long will it last?
  - When should improvement be expected?

Who does what?

- Will the general practitioner carry out the treatment alone, or will another person be involved (e.g. practice nurse, consultant psychiatrist, member of community mental health team)?
- If others are involved, what is their role?

Emergencies

- Are they likely, how can they be avoided, and if one occurs what should be done?
- Are there possible warning signs of a crisis?
- Who should be approached in an emergency, and how can they be found urgently?

Second, the most important investigation is to obtain a **corroborative history**, to corroborate the patient's report.

Additionally, some psychiatrists will present the background history *before* the history of the presenting complaints, which is the opposite of usual practice in medicine and surgery. This different approach may help the listener to understand the temporal relationship of events, as a more narrative approach is possible. The assessment needs to obtain both a *longitudinal* (the past) and *cross-sectional* (the present) view of the patient's problems. Think of the assessment as moving from the distant past (background history), to recent past (history of presenting problems), to the present (mental and physical examination). As you describe relevant features from your assessment, make sure that you mention them at the appropriate stage. For example, 'The patient suffered from a depressive episode about 10 years ago ...' (*background history*: past psychiatric history), 'has suffered the onset of low mood and other depressive symptoms including hopelessness in recent weeks ...' (*history of presenting problems*), and 'appeared depressed today,

and reported feeling hopeless with some thoughts of ending his life' (*mental state examination*: appearance and behaviour, mood, and thought content).

Diagnosis is considered next, with the evidence for and against each possible diagnosis being assessed. First, the **preferred diagnosis** is presented, together with evidence for it and against it; clearly the former will outweigh the latter. Then **alternative diagnoses** are presented, again alongside evidence for and against each. To obtain a full, biopsychosocial picture of the patient's clinical condition, several other aspects also need to be detailed. These include the presence, nature, and extent of any *physical disorder(s)*, and the presence, nature, and extent of any *social problem(s)*. Finally, the extent of *functional impairment* arising from physical, psychological, and social problems should be assessed, either using a formal scale such as the Global Assessment of Functioning, or by simply recording 'mild', 'moderate', or 'severe' functional impairment.

The order of the following elements of the assessment varies, depending on local traditions and preferences.

Table 10.1 The presentation of the psychiatric assessment

Introduction

History

  Background

  Of presenting problems

Examination

  Mental state

  Physical

Investigations

  Corroborative history

  Near-patient tests

  Other investigations

Diagnosis

  Preferred psychiatric diagnosis

  Differential psychiatric diagnosis

  Relevant physical diagnoses

  Social problems

  Extent of functional impairment

Aetiology

  Predisposing factors

  Precipitating factors

  Perpetuating factors

Prognosis

Risks

  To self

  To others

Management

  Short-term and long-term

  General, physical, psychological, and social aspects

There is no 'correct' order, but it is helpful to individual practitioners if they practise delivering summaries in a consistent way, and it is helpful for all members of the same mental health team to share the same approach.

Aetiology is described next, after diagnosis. Its division into predisposing, precipitating, and perpetuating factors has been addressed in Chapter 7. In order for the case presentation to be coherent, it is important that key conclusions about aetiology and, especially, about perpetuating factors map on to and are echoed in the management plan.

Prognosis is described next, and has been discussed in Chapter 8. General comments should be included on prognosis in the short term (recovery from this episode) and longer term (risk of further episodes), alongside comments on what will impact on prognosis, for better (e.g. adherence

to medication, support from family members) or worse (e.g. further marital infidelity).

Risks are described next, and have been considered in Chapter 9. It is important to consider the full range of risks, including risks to self and others, and those risks that are very often relevant but are usually neglected, such as the risk of driving.

Management is described finally. The management of particular disorders is described in subsequent chapters on clinical syndromes. The management plan should address the required:

- **general** aspects of treatment, such as inpatient or outpatient care, support from family, or support from specific professionals;

- **physical** aspects of treatment, such as abstinence from alcohol and illicit drugs, medicines such as antidepressants, exercise, and specific treatments such as electroconvulsive therapy;

- **psychological** aspects of treatment, such as educating the patient and their relative(s) about their illness and how to manage it, formal psychological treatments such as cognitive behaviour therapy, and how such treatments might be delivered, for example individual or group;

- **social** aspects of treatment, such as a phased return to work, involvement in voluntary activities that can help to restore a sense of worth and purpose, or day hospital attendance that can help to bring structure to the patient's day.

The management plan should also consider *short-term* aspects of treatment, which are usually those focused on achieving remission and subsequently recovery from the current episode, and *longer-term* aspects of treatment, which are focused on maintaining recovery and reducing the likelihood of recurrence.

Flexibility in your case presentation

Psychiatric assessment can involve the collection and integration of a great deal of information. It is not usually appropriate to present all of this information. We would urge readers to be able to deliver several different levels of case presentation, depending on the circumstances, as follows.

Long case presentation. Occasionally, it is helpful to present the bulk of the information that is known about a particular patient. However, this is a lengthy process, taking perhaps 15 minutes. There must therefore be a clear rationale for it, such as when a patient has not responded to treatment after some time, and the case is being thoroughly reviewed to determine whether an important factor has been missed.

Short case presentation. This is the usual way in which a case will be presented. The results of the assessment are summarized, in a standardized way, so that they can be presented in less than 5 minutes. An example is shown in Box 10.3. This approach is often called 'formulation', but we are not keen on this term, because it is not in common use outside mental health settings, and may therefore mystify observers of psychiatric practice in a way that is unnecessary and unhelpful.

Brief summary. This is a very brief summary of a case, presenting only the most salient features. This is commonly used when introducing a patient on a ward round, for example, so that those in attendance are aware of the context, are orientated to the case, and can contribute appropriately.

In our experience, students are often very good at collecting large quantities of information and presenting it in an organized and coherent way. However, they are often not very good at cutting down that information

such that it is usable in ordinary clinical practice. It is vital to practise prioritizing the information that you have, making decisions about what is 'essential' to understanding a case, what is 'important' to understanding a case, and what is 'interesting' but probably not important. This is the same type of process as reducing a very large number of diagnostic possibilities to only three or four—at each stage, there are advantages (increasing focus) and disadvantages (possibility of eliminating the 'real' diagnosis) associated with reducing the size of the list. It is only through practice that you will be able to do this.

Helping the listener to hear what you're saying

It is easy to think that presenting is the hard part, and that listening is easy. However, effective listening is easy only

---

 BOX 10.3 Example of a short case presentation

Mrs AB is a 30-year-old married woman who has been feeling increasingly depressed for 6 weeks and is now unable to cope adequately with the care of her children.

Regarding **diagnosis**, my *preferred diagnosis* is of a depressive episode, of moderate severity. Mrs AB has several typical symptoms of a depressive episode: she wakes unusually early, feels worse in the morning than in the evening, and has lost appetite and libido. She blames herself unreasonably, feels guilty, and does not think that she can recover, though she has no ideas of suicide or of harming the children. Her functioning is impaired to a moderate degree. None of the findings is incompatible with this diagnosis.

There are three *other diagnoses* that I have considered but excluded at this stage.

The first is adjustment disorder. Although Mrs AB has experienced several stressful events, including her husband's recent infidelity, the presence of clear symptoms of a depressive disorder and their duration overrule the diagnosis of adjustment disorder.

The second is personality disorder. There is no evidence for personality disorder. Mrs AB is normally a resilient, caring, and sociable person who is a good mother.

The third is physical disorder. Mrs AB has no significant past medical history, and there are no new physical symptoms on systematic enquiry.

Regarding **aetiology**, although she has not been depressed before, both her mother and sister have had depressive disorders, so it is possible that she is

predisposed to develop a depressive disorder. The symptoms were *precipitated* by her husband's infidelity. The disorder may be *maintained* by continuing quarrels with her husband, concerns about her mother's health, and active negative cognitive biases.

Regarding **risk**, suicide risk and risk of harm to the children are currently both low, but need monitoring.

Regarding **prognosis**, provided that the marital problems and her mother's health improve, Mrs AB should recover. The possible predisposing factors indicate that she may develop further depressive disorder.

Regarding **management**, Mrs AB does not currently need inpatient care, but her mental state will need monitoring by the primary care team, especially with a view to risk of suicide. Her sister has offered to provide short-term help with the care of the children, and Mrs AB is normally a good mother and should be able to take full care of her children when her condition improves. An SSRI antidepressant is appropriate. SSRIs occasionally cause increased agitation during the first few days of treatment, and Mrs AB will need to be warned of this, and of other common side effects. To prevent relapse, medication should be continued for about 6 months and, again, it is important that Mrs AB is aware of this. Her husband regrets his infidelity and is now supportive. If problems continue in their relationship, marital counselling through Relate or a similar organization will be appropriate. This management plan should be reviewed in 1 week, and regularly thereafter.

if the presenter helps. The following techniques can be employed by the presenter:

- **Pace yourself.** When anxious, or when there is a lot to present, most presenters will speed up, so that they become more difficult to hear, more difficult to follow, and more difficult to understand. Quicker isn't necessarily better. A more measured, considered pace allows the listener to keep up, and to weigh the information presented himself.

- **Use pauses as punctuation.** In written communication, we use commas, full stops, and paragraph breaks to indicate the beginning and end of clauses and sentences, and to provide emphasis. In verbal communication, these cues are absent and, instead, verbal and non-verbal cues must be deployed. A powerful cue is the pause. It alerts the listener to a change, and arouses their interest. A pause can be particularly powerful when used just before a signpost.

- **Signpost.** This is exactly what it says on the tin—a verbal signpost to what is coming next. So, for example, the presenter finishes talking about the findings on examination, pauses for a second or two to alert the listener, and says 'on investigation', to orientate them to what is about to be said.

- **Summarize.** It's easy to get bogged down in a wealth of detail. Summarize whenever possible—the listener can always ask for more detail or for clarification. So, for example, rather than reading a long list of individual biological symptoms of depression, simply state that the patient reported several biological symptoms.

- **Think rather than read.** Case presentations generally make sense when we are forced to think about what we are saying, rather than reading what we are saying. In other words, don't focus on the patient's case notes or your presentation notes. Instead, think about the key messages that you are attempting to put across, and refer to the notes for clarification only if needed.

- **Attend to your listeners.** Look up rather than down, and look at them in turn. If you are presenting in front of the patient, be sure to attend to the patient as well, especially when relating particularly sensitive or emotional aspects of their case. Show that you are on their side, and that you understand their predicament.

- **Have an obvious ending.** It can be unclear when someone has finished talking. Avoid this uncertainty by making it clear, with non-verbal and verbal cues.

■ Communicating in writing with healthcare professionals

Communication is either **verbal** (such as on ward rounds, or on the telephone) or **written** (such as referral letters, assessment letters, psychiatric notes, or general hospital notes). In each of these situations, a problem list can be helpful for prioritizing care and facilitating communication.

Problem lists

A problem list is a useful way of summarizing any case other than the very simplest. It is particularly useful in cases with both medical and psychiatric aspects, and is therefore suitable for use in primary care and in general hospital medical practice. The problem list makes the active problems and components of management clear to anyone who sees the patient when their usual healthcare professional is not available.

A summary of a case is shown in Case study 10.1, together with its associated problem list. Importantly, the problem list also incorporates a list of what will be done, and by whom, and when the status of that problem will be reviewed.

Letters of referral to psychiatrists

A referral letter should make it clear to the recipient why the patient is being referred, and how the referrer would like to be helped by this referral. For example, 'the patient's depressive illness has not responded to citalopram 20 mg, rising to 40 mg daily, despite good compliance during a period of 6 weeks, and I would welcome your advice on further pharmacological management'. The letter should be concise, but should also include as a minimum:

- the *course and development* of the disorder, with the dates on which problems began or changed;

- the *mental state* at the time of writing;

- any *abnormal behaviour that may be concealed or denied* by the patient when interviewed by the psychiatrist (e.g. excessive use of alcohol) or not recognized by the patient (e.g. lapses of memory);

- relevant points in the *medical history*, and current *medications;*

- details of any *treatment*, together with a note of the therapeutic response and side effects;

- *family relationships*, including marital problems and difficulties between parents and children;

- *personality* as known to the referring doctor from previous contacts with the patient.

Assessment letters from psychiatrists

It is important that assessment letters from mental health professionals to non-specialists:

- are brief;

- focus on the issues that triggered the referral or presentation;

Case study 10.1 Making a problem list

Case study

A 54-year-old woman consulted her general practitioner because of mixed anxiety and depressive symptoms. The diagnosis was depressive disorder, and the immediate cause appeared to be the stress of caring for an elderly debilitated mother (also the general practitioner's patient), whose condition had worsened in the last 2 months. Important contributory factors were menorrhagia and chronic agoraphobia, which prevented the patient from visiting friends and relatives. The immediate plan was to treat the patient's depressive disorder with an SSRI, and to obtain respite care for her mother. In the longer term, the agoraphobia would be treated with behaviour therapy, and a gynaecological opinion would be obtained about the menorrhagia.

Problem list

Problem	Action	Agent	Review
Anxiety and depression	Citalopram 20 mg (an SSRI) in the morning	GP	Check response weekly for 3 weeks, then review
Caring for elderly mother	Obtain respite care for mother	Geriatrician/elderly care social worker	3 weeks
Chronic agoraphobia	Behaviour therapy	Clinical psychologist	3 months
Menorrhagia	Gynaecological opinion	GP	1 month

- avoid psychiatric jargon, unless it is explained;
- make it clear what treatment is proposed, and who will be responsible for delivering that treatment;
- make it clear if and when the patient will be seen again by psychiatric services, and for what purpose.

Unfortunately, assessment letters are often used not only to *communicate* with the referrer, but also to *record* the much more extensive information that forms the background history, history of presenting complaint, and examination. While this may assist the person who has conducted the assessment, it is rarely helpful either to the referrer or to the patient. The more copious the information included, the more likely is the 'action list' for the referring doctor and the patient to be lost or ignored.

Recording in psychiatric case notes

Good case notes are important in psychiatry, as in other branches of medicine, for both clinical and medicolegal reasons. Case notes are not only an aide-memoire for the writer but are also an essential source of information for any other person called to help the patient in an emergency. The results of the assessment and the progress

Table 10.2 Example of a life chart

Year	Age (years)	Events	Physical illness	Psychiatric illness
1967	Born			
1968	1			
1969	2			
1970	3			
1971	4			
1972	5	Started school	Bed-wetting	
1973	6			
1974	7			
1975	8			
1976	9			
1977	10	Grandmother died		School refusal

Table 10.2 Example of a life chart (*Continued*)

Year	Age (years)	Events	Physical illness	Psychiatric illness
1978	11			
1979	12			
1980	13	Father's illness	Unexplained abdominal pain	
1981	14			
1982	15			
1983	16			
1984	17			
1985	18	Started at university		Adjustment disorder
1986	19			
1987	20			
1988	21			
1989	22	Married		
1990	23			
1991	24	First child born		
1992	25			
1993	26	Second child born (Caesarean section)		
1994	27			
1995	28			
1996	29		Cone biopsy	
1997	30			
1998	31			
1999	32			
2000	33			
2001	34	Mother died		Depressive episode
2002	35			
2003	36		Intestinal obstruction	
2004	37			
2005	38			
2006	39	Husband's illness		Depressive episode
2007	40			
2008	41	Son started university		Depressive episode
2009	42			
2010	43	Husband died		Adjustment disorder
2011	44			Depressive episode

notes should be recorded with this purpose in mind. Since patients may ask to read their notes, any information that informants have refused to make available to the patient should be recorded distinctly and separately.

A **life chart** can be a useful way of summarizing information in the case notes, which are often unwieldy in patients with long histories of mental disorder. A life chart summarizes life events, both 'good' and 'bad', alongside the occurrence of episodes of medical and psychiatric illness. The chart has five columns: the year, patient's age, life events, physical illness, and psychiatric disorder. The example in Table 10.2 is of a woman with a depressive disorder. She has had two episodes of emotional disorder in childhood (bed-wetting and school refusal), a third at the age of 18 (adjustment disorder), and a depressive disorder at age 34. The chart shows that the episodes of emotional disturbance were related in time to separations (starting school and going to university) and loss (the deaths of her grandmother and mother). The present illness is related in time to the death of her husband. None of the episodes were related to physical illness or childbirth.

Recording in general hospital case notes

When patients on general hospital wards are seen by mental health professionals, it is important that written communication in the notes has the same characteristics as assessment letters to non-specialists (see above), and in addition is:

- whenever possible, supplemented by a conversation with the person who made the referral to psychiatric services;

- 'topped' by a clear heading indicating that this is a summary of a mental health assessment;

- 'tailed' by a clear record of the name, status, and contact details of the person who has conducted the assessment, so that the general hospital team can make contact again should the need arise.

Management

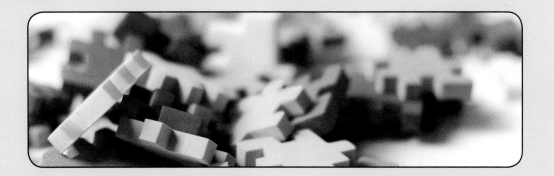

PART THREE

General aspects of care: settings of care

Current mental healthcare services in most of the developed world are unrecognizable compared with those of the mid-twentieth century. There has been a major shift from long-term institutional to community care. This chapter describes current approaches to providing mental health services, particularly for people between the ages of 18 and 65 (services for children are discussed in Chapter 17, and services for the elderly in Chapter 18). It is important for all medical students and doctors to have a basic understanding of the structure of services for three main reasons.

1 It will help you to get the most out of clinical rotations in psychiatry, either at undergraduate or postgraduate level.

2 All clinicians need to know when and how to refer their patient to appropriate services.

3 As 25 per cent of the population have mental health problems at some point, patients seen in all medical specialties may be being treated within psychiatric services. To liaise appropriately and manage a patient in their context, all those involved must understand what types of treatment they are receiving.

Mental health services are organized in different ways from country to country. This chapter describes mainly the provision of services in the UK, but the principles apply generally.

■ Epidemiology: the need for mental healthcare services

To understand the range of psychiatric services that are required for a specific community it is necessary to know:

1 the frequency of mental disorders in the population;

2 the severity of these conditions and the impact they have upon a person's ability to function;

3 how patients with these disorders come into contact with the health services;

4 what type of services people engage with and find effective.

The local prevalence of mental disorders will vary, but approximate estimates can be obtained from national surveys (Table 11.1). Approximately 20 to 25 per cent of the population experience a mental health problem in any given year. In the UK, estimates of psychiatric bed requirement are 50–150 per 250 000 people of working age. A more detailed discussion of the epidemiology of mental health as a whole can be found in Chapter 2, pp. 6–7, and for specific disorders in their individual chapters.

■ The principles of providing mental healthcare

The basic principles of the provision of mental health services are the same as for any other health service. Services should be accessible, comprehensive, appropriate to the needs of the community, offering up-to-date treatments, and effective and economical. Patients should be offered a choice in the treatment they receive, although the caveat to this is when an individual is being treated under the Mental Health Act.

What makes mentally ill people seek help?

Not everyone with a psychiatric disorder seeks medical advice. Some people with minor emotional reactions to stress obtain help from their family and friends, religious groups or non-medical counselling or support agencies. Internet websites, message boards, and chat sites have become a huge source of support for many people with mental illness. The majority of people with problems of substance abuse do not seek help of any kind. Nevertheless, in Britain, about 9 in 10 people with mental disorder attend a general practitioner, although many do not complain directly of psychological symptoms. Whether a person with *clinically significant psychiatric disorder* consults a general practitioner depends on several factors (Table 11.2). Mental disorders are stigmatized and there is much misunderstanding about them among the general population.

It is commonly believed that people with mental health problems are more likely to make use of, and to benefit from, services that take fully into account the views of those who use them. For this reason, patients are encouraged to be involved in all stages of service development.

Table 11.1 Epidemiology of mental disorders in the USA (2008); from the US National Institute for Mental Health, www.nimh.nih.org

Condition	Prevalence (% population)
Anxiety disorders	18.1
All mood disorders	9.5
Unipolar depression	6.7
Post-traumatic stress disorder	3.5
Eating disorders	1–7 females, 0.1 males
Bipolar disorder	2.6
Schizophrenia	1.1
Obsessive-compulsive disorder	1.0
ADHD	4.1
Autism	0.34
Alzheimer's disease	10% of over-65s

Table 11.2 Factors influencing a person's decision to seek medical advice

- Severity and duration of the disorder
- The person's attitude to psychiatric disorder; some people feel ashamed of the disorder and embarrassed to ask for help
- Attitudes and knowledge of family and friends—if these people are unsympathetic the affected person may be less likely to admit the problem or seek help for it
- The person's knowledge about possible help; if he does not know that help can be provided or if he has false expectations about the likely treatment he may not seek help
- The person's perception of the doctor's attitude to psychiatric disorder—if the doctor is viewed as unsympathetic, the person is less likely to ask for help
- The person's previous experiences of mental healthcare services
- Financial issues (this is more or less relevant, depending on the type of healthcare system in a particular country)

■ The structure of mental healthcare services

A very simplified diagram of the structure of services is shown in Figure 11.1. The first point to consider is how patients actually come to the attention of psychiatric services. The prevalence of mental health problems in primary care is approximately 200 per 1000 patients of working age, although only about half of these will require any intervention for their symptoms. The majority of patients seen in secondary care psychiatric services are referred from primary care, although a few may be seen as emergencies or referrals from other specialties.

The role of primary care

Although in the UK primary care is very separate from secondary services, it is an essential part of psychiatric service provision for three main reasons.

1 Primary care is where most mental illness is first detected.
2 The majority of people who suffer from a mental health problem can be successfully treated by their general practitioner (GP), and do not need specialist input.
3 The GP can be invaluable in coordinating care between different agencies and specialties.

The majority of patients presenting to primary care with psychological or somatic manifestations of mental disorder are suffering from anxiety and/or depression.

General practitioners vary in their ability to detect these undeclared psychiatric disorders. Two factors will help:

1 always considering the *possibility of mental disorder* in consultations;
2 having good *interviewing skills*. The key skills are the ability to gain the patient's confidence (and so enable them to disclose any psychiatric symptoms) and the ability to identify any psychological factors that are contributing to physical symptoms.

GPs can improve their ability to detect common psychiatric disorders, such as depression, by using screening questions or questionnaires, for example the two-question screening for depression, or the SCOFF questions for eating disorders.

Once a psychiatric disorder has been identified in primary care, it is usually treated by GPs themselves. They deal with nearly all adjustment disorders, the majority of the anxiety and depressive disorders, and many problems of alcohol abuse. The treatment of these conditions is discussed in the individual chapter for each disorder. GPs refer to psychiatrists about 5–10 per cent of the patients identified as having psychiatric disorders, selecting particularly those with severe mood disorders, psychosis, eating disorders, and other disorders when severe and persistent.

In the UK, almost all GP surgeries now have access to counsellors and/or clinical psychologists. This has allowed basic psychological therapies (e.g. CBT for depression or OCD, counselling for bereavement) to be

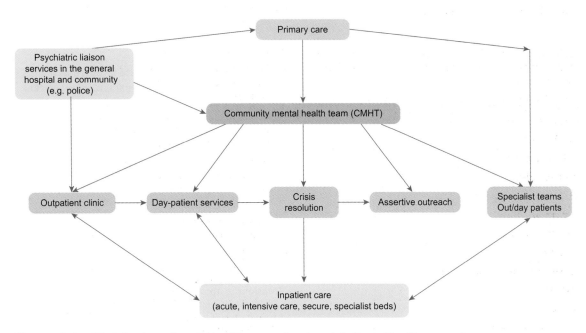

Fig. 11.1 A simplified structure of mental healthcare services in a state-funded health care system.

Table 11.3 Factors influencing a general practitioner's decision to refer to the specialist psychiatric services

- Uncertainty about diagnosis
- Failure to respond to treatment in primary care
- Severity of the condition; need for hospital admission
- Safety of the patient, family, and community
- Need for treatment that is unavailable in primary care
- Willingness of the patient to see a psychiatrist
- Accessibility of psychiatric services, how far the patient has to travel, and how promptly patients are seen by the psychiatrist
- Local guidelines regarding referrals

delivered in primary care. Polyclinics or **community mental health clinics**, which are centres in which several GP surgeries pool their mental health resources, are becoming an increasing source of treatment in the community.

Patients who do not respond to treatment, have severe illnesses, or need treatments not available in primary care need to be referred to the specialist psychiatric services. The decision to refer to a psychiatrist is determined by several factors (Table 11.3). In the UK, the common point of referral for the majority of psychiatric diagnoses is the **community mental health team (CMHT)**.

Specialist mental healthcare services

All psychiatric services must provide for patients with serious psychiatric disorders, some of whom may be suicidal or dangerous to others because of their illness. Managing the whole spectrum of severity of mental illness has led to the development of a tiered service, with a common entry for assessment, followed by providing treatment at the least intensity appropriate for the patient.

The main components of the adult psychiatric services include (Figure 11.1):

- CMHTs—assessment of new patients, decisions regarding appropriate care, and coordination of services;
- outpatient clinics;
- day services;
- crisis resolution teams;
- inpatient facilities;
- assertive outreach teams;
- specialist teams (e.g. complex needs, eating disorders);
- rehabilitation resources;
- liaison with general hospitals, the voluntary and the private sectors.

Community mental health teams (CMHTs)

The CMHT model was developed with the following aims:

1 to provide a single point of referral for primary care or refer from hospital specialties;

2 to avoid unnecessary admission to hospital by providing intensive treatments in the community;

3 to include a multidisciplinary team, providing a coordinated care package for each patient;

4 to provide services as close as possible to the patient's home;

5 to provide continuity of care for patients with chronic psychiatric disorders.

In the UK, a CMHT usually covers a geographical area including 20 000–50 000 people, of whom 200–250 will be on the caseload at any given time. The multidisciplinary team (MDT) typically consists of 12–20 people, including psychiatrists, clinical psychologists, social workers, mental health nurses, and occupational therapists. Their various roles are described in Table 11.4. In a well-functioning CMHT, the members work flexibly as well as performing tasks specific to their profession. The team will meet one or two times per week to:

- allocate new referrals for assessment;
- discuss patients assessed since the last meeting;
- discuss patients on the existing caseload;
- manage the waiting list.

It is usual for a routine referral to be assessed within 4 weeks, an urgent referral within 1 week, and an emergency to be seen the same day.

The model of community care favoured in the UK is **case management**. For every patient, a **key worker** is identified, who may be any member of the MDT but is most frequently a community psychiatric nurse. It is their responsibility to make sure that the patient's needs are met and clinical status is regularly assessed. When a patient is initially referred to the service, a psychiatrist will assess them. They will make a diagnosis, discuss the case with the whole team, and together make a plan as to the best form of management. A formal **care plan** is then drawn up, in which members of the team are assigned specific tasks to carry out. An example of a care plan is shown in Box 11.1. The team meet regularly and review the care plan. This way of working is known as the **Care Programme Approach (CPA)**. Every 5–6 weeks there is a larger formal CPA review, after which a copy of the care plan is distributed to all concerned parties, including the patient and their GP.

Table 11.4 Mental health professionals in a community mental health team (CMHT)

Profession	Role
Psychiatrist	The clinical leader of the team and responsible for psychiatric assessments. Initiates and supervises drug treatments and provides brief psychological interventions. Supervises outpatients, inpatients, and day patients
Community psychiatric nurse (CPN)	The core members of the team who usually work exclusively in the CMHT. Act as key workers for patients with chronic mental disorders, monitor medication and side effects, and provide some psychological treatments
Clinical psychologist	Performs psychological assessments and provides a full range of psychological treatments
Occupational therapist	Performs functional assessments, provides social skills training, some psychological treatments, and assists the patient in finding employment
Social worker	Performs social and Mental Health Act assessments and assists the patient in meeting accommodation and financial needs. May also provide some psychological treatments

BOX 11.1 An example Care Programme Approach Review

Name of patient: John Smith

Address: 42 West Street

CMHT: North East City

Diagnoses: 1. Bipolar disorder I

                2. ....

GP: Dr Robinson

Mobile number: 0000000000

Key worker: Jane (social worker)

Team members present at meeting: Dr Brown, Sarah, Katie, Jane, Martin and 2 medical students.

Problem	Intervention	Team member allocation
1 Mania	Take regular medications (olanzapine and lithium)	Dr Brown (psychiatrist)
	Attend outpatient appointments	
	Be at home when team members visit	
2 Too much spare time	Activity planning	Sarah (CPN)
	Attend day centre	
	When stable, look for a part-time course in photography	Katie (occupational therapist)
3 Fighting with family	Attend early-intervention training course with parents	Dr Brown to organize Sarah (CPN)
	Phone daughter's mother weekly	
4 Money	Complete and send off social benefit forms	Jane (social worker)
	Complete free school meals form for daughter	
5 Avoiding relapse	Medication adherence	Martin (psychologist)
	Attend CBT for bipolar disorder	
	When stable, attend local support group	
	Phone Jane when feeling unwell	

Risks considered? Yes—self-neglect

Date of next review: 01/06/2010 at 4pm

Signature of care coordinator: ....

Signature of patient: ....

The key to the CMHT approach is *effective collaboration between all those involved in care.* Team members should meet regularly and between meetings should communicate effectively with each other and with the patients, relatives, or carers and any others involved in the patient's care, such as social services and the general practitioner. One major advantage of this approach is that as a patient moves between care settings (e.g. outpatient clinic to inpatient), the MDT remains the same.

Outpatient clinics

Psychiatric outpatient clinics function in exactly the same way as those in other medical specialties, and are an efficient way of providing psychiatric assessment and treatment. They provide the majority of specialist mental healthcare services; most patients do not need more intensive treatment. They are suitable for stable patients, or those whose mental illness is not severe enough to put themselves or others in danger. Patients are typically seen by a psychiatrist, but may also have appointments with their community mental health nurse or psychologist. The frequency of appointments is variable; CBT is usually delivered weekly by clinical psychologists, but a psychiatrist reviewing a stable patient may only see them every 3 months or so.

Day hospitals

Day hospitals—called **partial hospitalization** in some countries—provide a step between the outpatient clinic and hospitalization. They usually run for 4 or 5 days a week, from 8 am–4 pm (or equivalent), but there has been a move to provide evening sessions (6–10 pm) to cater for those in education or employment. Day hospitals are usually based in a psychiatric hospital, and provide assessment and treatment for patients who need intensive treatment but can sleep safely at home or in a hostel. An example might be of a patient whose depression has not responded to an antidepressant and outpatient CBT, and whilst it is preventing them from working, they are not suicidal. Day hospitals provide supervised drug treatment, a range of psychological treatments (in group and individual formats), occupational therapy, art/music therapy, and support from peers. They can also act as a form of rehabilitation. An example of a daily timetable is shown in Table 11.5. Day treatment is suitable for patients with moderately severe mood disorders, chronic schizophrenia, severe and chronic neuroses, and any other patient who would be deemed to benefit from it. Eating disorders lend themselves particularly well to day hospitals, but this is usually delivered in a specialist unit. Day hospitals can shorten the length of inpatient stay and avoid admission altogether for some patients.

Table 11.5 An example of a mood disorders day hospital timetable

Time	Activity
8.45–9.30	Arrival and morning review group *(Group discussion of how their evening/weekend went)*
9.30–10.30	Therapy group *(e.g. CBT for mood disorders, art therapy, creative writing)*
10.30–11.00	Coffee break and free time
11.00–12.00	Individual therapy
12.00–13.00	Lunch and free time
13.00–14.00	Community group *(Discussion of issues pertaining to life in the group)*
14.00–15.00 *Tues–Fri*	Therapy group
15.00–16.00	Evening planning and home
14.00–17.00 *Mondays only*	Ward round, CPA reviews *20–30 minute slots per patient*

Crisis resolution

The crisis resolution (or **home treatment**) teams aim to provide a rapid response and accessibility to intensive psychiatric services. Their aim is to keep patients who would otherwise be admitted to hospital in the community. The team usually consists of specially trained community psychiatric nurses, social workers, and, occasionally, psychiatrists. The team receive referrals from primary care, CMHTs and other specialist teams and see all the referrals within 24 hours. They have a small number of patients at a time, visiting each at least once per day, and providing 24-hour phone support for the patient and their family. The crisis team is particularly useful for patients with severe mood depression, anxiety disorders, or schizophrenia. An adolescent version focusing on managing eating disorders in the community has been very successful.

Assertive outreach

Assertive outreach (AO) (called **assertive community treatment** in the USA) is another method of reducing hospitalization, but has been designed especially for patients with chronic psychoses. It focuses on those patients who are difficult to engage, non-compliant with medications, and have frequent relapses. The service works on a proactive basis—they do not wait for patients, to attend appointments and make decisions for themselves but visit them at home regularly, trying to enhance motivation and compliance with treatment. Community psychiatric nurses and social workers take the main role, not only doing home visits but also taking patients out shopping, to the cinema, to job interviews, or to GP appointments. This can be provided over the longer term (months to years), and there is good evidence that it reduces the risk of relapse considerably.

Inpatient facilities

Although every effort has been made to treat as many patients in the community as possible, there are situations where hospitalization is the safest option. All specialist psychiatric services require an inpatient unit, capable of treating patients with severe mental disorders (voluntarily or involuntarily), and able to admit patients promptly in an emergency. Admission to hospital is needed when:

- patients need a level of assessment that cannot be provided elsewhere;
- patients need a treatment that cannot be provided in any other setting;
- patients have insufficient social support;
- patients might put themselves or other people at risk;
- arrangements for care outside hospital break down and a comprehensive care plan needs to be put in place.

Psychiatric inpatient units serving a large area used to be grouped together in a single psychiatric hospital; now they are often smaller, dispersed, and accommodated in general hospitals serving smaller areas. Units in specialist hospitals have the advantage that a wider range of treatments can be made available (e.g. specialized occupational and rehabilitation facilities). Units in a general hospital have the advantages of reduced stigma, early liaison with other specialties, and, usually, closeness to the patient's home. There are four main types of adult inpatient wards in most countries:

Acute psychiatric wards. These are the mainstay of inpatient beds, and treat severe mental illness in the relatively short term, for example acute psychosis, mania, and severe depression with suicidal intent. They are provided relatively locally (e.g. a psychiatric hospital in a large town) and can include patients being treated under the Mental Health Act. They provide 24-hour nursing care and observation (Box 11.2), and typically run a therapeutic programme similar to that in day hospitals, but full-time. The average inpatient stay in the UK is 6 weeks.

Psychiatric intensive care units. These are low-security units, or locked sections of the general psychiatric hospital, usually only catering for a few patients at a time. They have 1:1 nursing and manage acutely disturbed patients who cannot be safely treated on an open ward.

Specialist inpatient units. These provide specialist care for particular conditions—the majority cater for alcohol/drug problems or eating disorders. The advantage of these wards is that they have a specialist team who intensely focus on the behavioural problems that the patients have, away from the challenging environment of the acute psychiatric ward. In set-up they are similar to acute wards, with 24-hour nursing care and highly structured timetables providing therapy and activities.

Medium- and high-secure units. These provide a secure environment for the treatment of patients with mental

---

 BOX 11.2 Levels of observation on a psychiatric ward

Observations refer to the level of monitoring that patients receive on a psychiatric ward, and are usually undertaken by nursing staff. They are designed to keep each patient safe, preventing primarily self-harm and suicide attempts, but also aggressive or disruptive behaviour. Observations can be individually tailored—for example, to help reduce behaviours such as vomiting after meals in bulimia nervosa or hand washing in OCD. A decision will be made during the admission assessment or interview as to which level to start at, and this will be regularly reviewed (often daily) by staff.

Level	Frequency of observation
1	Constant observation: within sight and constant close proximity to staff at all times
	'At arm's length'
2	Constant observation: within sight of staff at all times
3	Observations at defined time intervals
	Typically 15 minutes, but can be 5 10, or 30
4	Hourly observations

disorders who have committed crimes and/or are deemed to be a danger to the public. Patients are admitted from prisons, the courts, or less secure units. High-security hospitals usually treat patients indefinitely, but the medium-secure units aim to rehabilitate the patient to move back into the community in a number of years.

In the past, patients often remained in inpatient units long after the acute stage of illness had passed; when recovery was incomplete some patients remained for many years. Now patients with residual problems are usually discharged from hospital and are given continuing treatment. The advantage of remaining in hospital ('asylum') is easier provision of accommodation, treatment, rehabilitation, and protection; the disadvantage of a prolonged stay in hospital can be institutionalism that adds to the handicap produced by the disorder. If community care can meet patients' needs it is generally better than prolonged inpatient care, and is preferred by patients and their carers. However, when patients are discharged from hospital without adequate provision for their needs for accommodation and treatment, community care can be worse for the patient than long-term care in hospital. The **stepped model of care** is used to try and safeguard against this happening. For patients who have received intense treatments (i.e. inpatient or day-patient care), they are stepped down to the next level prior to discharge. Typically, a patient will be discharged from the ward, but attend the day hospital for some time. For patients being treated in units a long way from home, or who do not have access to a day hospital, periods of leave are granted whilst still an inpatient.

Early intervention

It is well recognized that early intervention and treatment of patients with psychosis improve outcome. One initiative that has been set up is the early intervention teams, who specialize in the early diagnosis and treatment of these patients. They have three main roles:

1 to identify and monitor high-risk patients;

2 to raise awareness of psychoses in the wider community;

3 ongoing patient care.

Frequently, early intervention and family education can avoid hospital admission and reduce the morbidity associated with psychosis.

■ Liaison with other medical services

Liaison psychiatry (or **consultation psychiatry**) is the specialty of treating mental health disorders in the general hospital population. This includes pre-existing psychiatric conditions and new diagnoses which may be related to physical health problems. The liaison service may be provided by the mental health trust, with psychiatrists based elsewhere going into the general hospital, or it may be a separate unit within the acute hospital trust itself. The role of the liaison service is to:

- assess patients with new psychiatric symptoms;
- manage pre-existing mental health problems;
- manage behavioural disturbance;
- provide advice on treatments, especially medications;
- assess and manage patients presenting with deliberate self-harm or parasuicide;
- assist with management of patients under the care of the mental health teams, but who need medical stabilization or treatment in the general hospital;
- provide a link between the acute hospital and the CMHT.

As well as the dedicated liaison service, there are other links to medical specialties which are essential to providing a comprehensive mental health service. A good example is the link between an eating disorders unit and the local gastroenterology/acute medical department. Many patients who need inpatient care will need admission for medical stabilization (e.g. for hypokalaemia or dehydration), and the occasional one will need nasogastric feeding. Having an organized set-up whereby patients in the general hospital receive regular reviews and visits from their specialist team is essential for a good outcome.

■ Culturally specific approaches to treatment

It is important to recognize that patients from varying cultural and religious groups have markedly different beliefs surrounding mental illness. In many cultures, mental illness is not recognized, and this can make cooperation with treatment (especially from the wider family and community) very challenging. Specialist help may be needed to overcome problems of denial, and a patient advocate or professional with knowledge of the relevant culture can be an invaluable member of the team. Many people of African origin rarely experience the typical psychological symptoms of depression or anxiety, instead presenting with somatic symptoms (e.g. pain). An open mind needs to be kept when assessing patients. In some areas with a high population of particular ethnic groups, support groups and treatment are available within that community.

There are situations where patients, especially women, may not be free to visit a doctor or attend appointments without their family (usually husband) present. This can make regular follow-up and patient confidentiality very difficult. It is usually necessary for these patients to be visited at home, with appropriately trained staff present.

Some treatments are more efficacious in particular ethnic groups, and psychiatrists should be aware of that. Large, randomized controlled trials of medications frequently include a subgroup analysis of efficacy in different ethnic groups; for example, it has been reported that antipsychotics for psychosis are more effective in black Africans than in Caucasian males. Psychological therapies are also more effective in some cultures, but this seems to have more to do with acceptance of mental illness than inherent physiological differences.

■ The role of the voluntary and private sectors

In most countries, there are voluntary organizations that provide a variety of services for those with mental health problems. Some UK examples include:

- Alcoholics Anonymous;
- Cruse (a charity providing bereavement counselling and services);
- Mind (a national mental health charity providing accommodation, employment, and advice);
- Relate (provides marriage guidance counselling).

Many referrals received by these organizations are from psychiatrists or other mental health professionals.

In a state-funded health service, there are always limitations on the care that can be provided. In the UK, there is a growing private sector providing specialist treatment for most psychiatric conditions. This includes office-based outpatient psychiatrists and psychologists, and day/inpatient units. There are specialist units for all major psychiatric illnesses, but especially for those areas which have been less provided for by national services, for example adolescent inpatient care, eating disorders, and alcohol and drug problems.

■ Accommodation and employment

The vast majority of those with a mental health disorder live with their families, in owned or rented accommodation, and can care for themselves. However, some others need more help, and can benefit from specialized accommodation. This is provided from a variety of sources,

including the voluntary sector, social services, health services, or private companies. There are four main types of assisted accommodation:

1 **Group homes.** Some relatively independent patients are able to live in group homes, which are houses in which four or five patients live together. These houses are often owned by a charitable organization. Patients perform all the essential tasks of running the house together, even though separately they could do only some of them.

2 **Day staffed hostels.** Patients with greater handicaps can live in hostels where members of staff are present throughout the day to provide support. These are usually not nursing staff, but trained individuals who help with activities of daily living and encourage medication compliance.

3 **Night staffed hostels.** These houses are staffed 24 hours a day, ensuring greater supervision and assistance.

4 **24-hour medically staffed homes.** This form of accommodation is usually in the private sector, and is for those patients with long-term, uncontrolled, severe mental illness. It includes those with severe and profound learning disabilities. There is specialist nursing care on hand, and they are run more in the style of a nursing home for older adults.

Provision of appropriate occupation

Some patients with chronic psychiatric disorder can undertake normal employment or, if beyond retirement age, can take part in the same activities as healthy people of similar age. Other patients require **sheltered work**, in which they can work productively, but more slowly than would be possible elsewhere. Patients who are too handicapped to undertake sheltered work need **occupational therapy** to avoid boredom, under-stimulation, and lack of social contacts.

Adequate support for carers

Family and friends are the main carers of most patients living outside hospital. It is their role to encourage suitable behaviours, provide psychological support, and encourage adherence with treatment. They have to tolerate unusual and challenging behaviour or social withdrawal. Prolonged involvement in care is stressful, and the impact of mental illness on both carers and the extended family should not be underestimated. The welfare of carers should be considered within a patient's care plan, and appropriate counselling or respite organized if necessary. Many inpatient and day-patient units run carers groups, in which families/carers can come together to discuss the challenges of living with someone with psychiatric problems.

■ Involvement of the patient in service provision

All patients who have the capacity to make decisions for themselves should be included in the decision-making processes surrounding their care. This includes agreeing to referrals, which professionals they see, and the type of treatments they receive. The situation for those being treated under the Mental Health Act is slightly different, but efforts should always be made to help the patient to agree to treatment. However, a busy complicated health service can be difficult for patients to negotiate (especially if acutely unwell), or they may have problems or complaints to make about the service. In the UK, the **Patient Advice and Liaison Service (PALS)** has been created to provide information to patients and deal with complaints. Most other countries have similar schemes, with privately run hospitals managing their own internal complaints. The aims of PALS are to:

- provide patients with information about the national health service (e.g. what mental health services are available in a given area);

- help resolve concerns and problems;
- provide information about making complaints;
- provide a link to agencies and supportive groups outside the health service;
- improve services by gathering suggestions and listening to patient experiences;
- give feedback to health trusts about the positive and negative aspects of the services they provide, from the patient's perspective.

All patients also have access to patient advocates, some of whom are linked to PALS, but mostly from charitable organizations, which provide an independent liaison between the patient and health services. These can be especially helpful when patients are being treated non-voluntarily.

Many hospital foundation trusts in the UK now run schemes by which any member of the public can become a member of the trust. The idea is that this group will represent all areas of society, and will provide a voice for patients within the structure of the trust. Members can share their experiences, sit on advisory panels, and even become non-executive members of the board of directors.

Further reading

Muijen, M. & McCulloch, A. (2009). Public policy and mental health. In *New Oxford Textbook of Psychiatry*, 2nd edn. Ed. M. G. Gelder, J. J. Lopez-Ibor, N. C. Andreasen & J. R. Geddes, pp. 1425–502. Oxford University Press, Oxford.

Patient Advice and Liaison Service (PALS) www.pals. nhs. uk/

Mind, The UK national charity for mental health. www. mind.org.uk/ This website has a lot of useful links to other voluntary organizations providing mental healthcare.

The World Health Organization website provides copious reading material on all aspects of mental health epidemiology, including a searchable database of psychiatric service provision for all countries. www.who.int/topics/mental_health/en/

CHAPTER 12

Psychiatry and the law

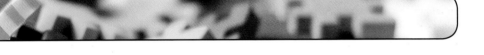

■ Psychiatry and civil law

The interface between psychiatry and the law

Psychiatry is closely connected with the law, and for most psychiatrists the legal aspects of their work represent a large part of their everyday practice. This is quite a different situation from most other medical specialties, which may only encounter legal issues when they surround complaints or difficult ethical challenges. There are three main areas of law which are relevant to psychiatry:

1 civil law relating to the involuntary admission and treatment of patients with mental disorders (in the UK, this is outlined in the **Mental Health Act 2007**);

2 civil law concerning issues of consent and capacity (the **Mental Capacity Act 2005**);

3 criminal law as it relates to individuals with mental disorders.

In most circumstances mental health legislation will only be relevant to those working within mental health services; however, the relationship of psychiatry and the law is of importance to all doctors for the following reasons.

● Laws, regulations, and official guidelines provide backing to some aspects of ethical decision making within medicine.

● The law regulates the circumstances under which treatment can be given without patients' consent, and the compulsory admission of patients with a mental disorder to hospital. Primary care and hospital doctors may encounter situations in which patients refuse essential treatment, and may have to decide whether to invoke powers of compulsory admission and/or best interest treatments.

- Doctors may be asked for reports used in legal decisions, such as the capacity to make a will or to care for property, and claims for compensation for injury. They may be asked for reports that set out the relationship between any psychiatric disorder and criminal behaviour.
- A minority of patients behave in ways that break the law. Doctors need to understand legal issues as part of their management of care.
- Victims of crime may suffer immediate and long-term psychological consequences.

This chapter will describe the main principles of mental health legislation with particular reference to UK law. While some of the detail discussed (e.g. particular definitions or legislative act numbers) may not be relevant to international readers, legal frameworks across the globe are broadly similar. The latter part of the chapter will provide an overview of the relationship between mental disorders and crime. For more detailed information, readers should use the references in the further reading section on p. 109.

The Mental Health Acts 1983 and 2007

In the UK, the key legislation covering involuntary admission and treatment of individuals with mental health problems is the Mental Health Act 1983 (MHA 1983), and its recent amendments in the Mental Health Act 2007 (MHA 2007). These laws have three purposes:

1 **to ensure essential treatment** is provided for patients with mental disorders who do not recognize that they are ill, and refuse treatment. Three criteria are used to decide whether treatment is essential: the safety of the patient, the safety of others, and the need to prevent deterioration in health that would lead to one of the former categories;

2 **to protect other people**—for example, from the violent impulses of a paranoid patient;

3 **to protect individuals from wrongful detention.**

Mental health laws tend to provide legislation covering all of the areas shown in Table 12.1. There will be differences between countries, but this is a reasonably comprehensive summary.

Definition of mental disorder

Under the MHA 2007, mental disorder is defined as *any disorder or disability of the mind*. The four categories of mental disorder described in the MHA 1983 are no longer included. The only exclusion criterion is that dependence on alcohol or drugs alone is not considered to be a

Table 12.1 What is included in mental health legislation?

- Definition of mental disorder
- Procedures for the assessment of patients with mental disorders who may need involuntary admission and treatment
- Urgent admission procedures for patient with mental disorders who are not in hospital
- Criteria for and procedures of providing involuntary treatment
- Emergency treatment by doctors (psychiatrists or generalists)
- Emergency procedures for compulsory detention of patients already in hospital (general or psychiatric)
- Police powers to detain for medical assessment
- Criminal or forensic detainment and treatment
- Safeguards: patient advocacy and mental health tribunals
- Discharge and follow-up community treatment
- Capacity and consent (*in the UK, covered by the Mental Capacity Act*)

mental disorder. Similarly, a person with a learning disability is not considered to be suffering from a mental disorder simply as a result of that disability unless it is *associated with abnormally aggressive or seriously irresponsible conduct.*

Professional roles within the MHA 2007

In order to understand the conditions by which the various parts of the MHA can be instigated, various pieces of terminology need to be explained. Many of them have been redefined between the MHA 1983 and MHA 2007 in order to allow a broader range of health professionals to carry out parts of the act.

- Approved Mental Health Professional (AMHP) is the term that has replaced Approved Social Worker (ASW). An AMHP may be any mental health professional (e.g. social worker, nurse, psychologist) who has undergone specific training in assessing and dealing with patients with mental disorder. They can apply for patients to be assessed or treated under sections of the MHA.
- The term Approved Clinician (AC) used to be confined to doctors, but has been widened to include other health professions with the relevant training.
- The term Responsible Clinician (RC) has replaced the Responsible Medical Officer (RMO). Any Approved Clinician can act as an RC. Each patient being treated under the MHA has an RC who is responsible for their overall care.
- A 'Section 12 Approved' doctor (usually a consultant psychiatrist or senior registrar) is a doctor with appropriate

training and approval to certify patients under the MHA. The requirement for at least two doctors, one Section 12 approved, to make recommendations for use of the MHA in patients under Section 2 and 3 (see below), has not changed.

- The nearest relative (NR) of a patient can now include any of the following (in order): spouse or civil partner, child, parent, sibling, grandparent, grandchild, uncle or aunt, nephew or niece. A patient is now allowed to apply to the courts for dismissal of their nearest relative if they feel they are not a suitable person for the job.

Commonly used sections of the MHA 2007

The most commonly used sections of the MHA in England and Wales are summarized in Table 12.2; abbreviations are as outlined in the section above. At any one time, approximately 10–15 per cent of psychiatric inpatients in the UK are admitted under the MHA; the majority of patients are therefore admitted voluntarily—this comes as a surprise to many people.

Section 2

When psychiatrists are asked to go out into the community to do an MHA assessment, it is usually with a view to admitting the patient under Section 2 of the MHA. This is an assessment order, allowing detention of the patient for up to 28 days for assessment of their mental disorder. At the end of this time, the section must either be converted to a treatment order (Section 3) or the patient discharged; it cannot be renewed. Application for a Section 2 is made by an AMHP, and two doctors (one of whom must be Section 12 approved) are needed to recommend use of the section. The criteria that the patient must fulfil to be held under a Section 2 are as follows:

- *The person must be suffering from a mental disorder of a nature or degree that warrants their detention in hospital for assessment* and

- *The person ought to be detained in the interests of their own health or safety or with a view to the protection of others.*

The word **nature** refers to the exact mental disorder from which the patient is suffering, and the **degree** refers to the current manifestation and severity of the disorder.

Section 3

Section 3 is a treatment order and is the section under which most detained inpatients are held. It lasts up to 6 months, after which it may be renewed for another 6 months, and then after that for a year at a time. If a patient is deemed well enough to no longer require involuntary treatment, the section may be lifted at any time. As with Section 2, an AMHP must make an application for use of the section, and two doctors (one Section 12 approved), who must have seen the patient within 24 hours, recommend its use for the patient. The criteria are as for Section 2, plus one additional criterion which is a new addition to the law from 2007. This is that there must be *appropriate medical treatment available* for the mental disorder from which the patient is suffering. This can include nursing, psychological interventions, provision of new skills, rehabilitation and care, as well as traditional medical treatments. When applying for the section, the RC must have a definite treatment and management plan for the patient.

Section 4

Section 4 allows the emergency admission of patients not already in hospital for whom waiting for the paperwork or personnel to complete Section 2 would cause a dangerous delay. An application from an NR or AMHP is made on recommendation from one doctor, who does not need to be Section 12 approved. It is usually converted to a Section 2 upon arriving at hospital. Section 4 can last up to 72 hours, and is non-renewable.

Table 12.2 Mental Health Act 2007 for England and Wales

Section number	Order	Duration (maximum)	Application	Authorization
2	Assessment order	28 days	AMHP	2 doctors (at least one Section 12 approved)
3	Treatment order	6 months	AMHP	2 doctors (at least one Section 12 approved)
4	Emergency order	72 hours	NR or AMHP	1 doctor
5(2)	Holding order for patient already in hospital	72 hours	Not needed	1 doctor or RC
5(4)	Holding order for an informal psychiatric inpatient	6 hours	Not needed	1 registered mental health nurse or AMHP
136	Police order to remove a person to a place of safety	72 hours	Not needed	Police officer

Section 5(2)

This section provides a means of detaining a patient who is already in hospital; this includes general and psychiatric hospitals, but not the emergency room. Any doctor can detain a patient for up to 72 hours, during which time they should liaise with a psychiatrist to plan for admission under Section 2.

Section 5(4)

Popularly known as the 'nurses' holding power', Section 5(4) allows a registered psychiatric nurse (and since the MHA 2007, any AMHP) to detain an informal patient for up to 6 hours. This is used when an informal patient is attempting to discharge against medical advice, and might cause serious harm to themself or others (e.g. commit suicide). During the 6 hours, the nurse should contact the members of staff needed to place a Section 2.

Section 136

This section allows police officers to remove a person believed to be suffering from a mental disorder from a public place and take them to a place of safety. This is usually the local psychiatric ward/hospital, a designated room in the police station, or an emergency room. Once there, a doctor and AMHP must assess the patient; 90 per cent are then detained under Section 2 or 3.

Other sections of the MHA 2007

Some less commonly used sections include:

- **Section 7 (guardianship):** This enables patients to receive community care which could not otherwise be provided without the use of another MHA section. The guardian—an AMHP—can require the patient to live in a particular place, attend specific treatment, and allow authorized persons to visit. Application is by an AMHP or NR and needs two medical recommendations.
- **Section 17:** This section permits patients being treated under Section 3 to go on leave from hospital whilst still under the section. It requires the RC and a doctor to agree and sign the section.
- **Section 17A-G (compulsory treatment order, CTO):** The CTO used to be called a 'supervised discharge' and was under Section 25, but has been incorporated into Section 17 by the MHA 2007. This requires a patient discharged from inpatient care to have to attend for/comply with treatment in the community (e.g. attend for depot antipsychotic doses or therapy). There is also a power to recall the patient to hospital if they do not comply with restrictions.
- **Section 117 (aftercare):** This is a legal requirement that all patients detained on longer-term sections (3, 37, 47, or 48) are provided with formal aftercare. All patients must have regular reviews of health and social needs, an agreed care plan, an allocated health worker, and regular progress reviews.

- **Sections 35 and 26 (criminal pre-trial orders):** These are allied to Sections 2 and 3, but are for individuals with a mental disorder that warrants treatment in hospital, but who are awaiting trial for a serious crime. The patient will then be held in a secure hospital rather than a prison.
- **Section 37 (criminal post-trial order):** This applies to patients who have a mental disorder that warrants treatment in hospital, but who have already been convicted of an offence punishable with imprisonment by the courts. There does not need to be a link between the offence and illness. The procedure is then as for Section 3.

Safeguarding patients

Individuals with mental health disorders are by definition a vulnerable group, and those who are acutely unwell are at high risk of exploitation by others. In order to ensure that patients are not wrongfully detained, or kept under a Mental Health Act section for longer than necessary, the law contains various safeguards.

Appeals against detention

An important safeguard against misuse of the power to detain is a system of independent review. In England and Wales, all patients detained under a Section 2, 3, or CTO must be referred to a **Mental Health Review Tribunal (MHRT)**, at the latest by 6 months from the date the initial application was made for use of the MHA, if the patient has not already applied themselves. A patient can also ask for a hearing at any time. In the USA, these proceedings are very similar, and are called 'commitment hearings'. The review panel consists of three people:

1 a legal member—chairs the panel, usually a lawyer with experience of mental health cases;
2 a doctor—typically an independent consultant psychiatrist, who must have examined the patient before the tribunal takes place;
3 a lay member—this is a member of the public who has volunteered to sit on these panels. The majority have practical experience of working in social or mental health.

The tribunal happens in a designated room within the hospital, and the patient, their NR, and members of the clinical treatment team all attend. The patient may have their own legal representative with them. The panel questions the patient about why they feel they do not need to be in hospital any longer and the team for evidence to the contrary. If the panel decides the criteria for discharge have been met, the section is lifted and the patient must be discharged. The reality is that the majority of decisions recommend that the patient needs further involuntary treatment.

Advocacy

Advocacy ensures patients do not face discrimination or unfairness due to their mental health problems. It provides the patient with a voice to express their views and defend their rights. An advocate is an independent person who represents the patient's wishes non-judgmentally, and without putting forward their own opinion. Whilst advocacy has been widely available throughout the UK for some years, the 2007 amendments to the MHA 1983 placed a duty on local authorities to provide an independent advocate for patients detained involuntarily. They typically help the patient understand the process of what is happening to them (e.g. explaining the law), help them to complete paperwork (e.g. preparing for a MHRT), and stand up for their rights (e.g. to have vegetarian food provided in hospital).

Other relevant parts of the MHA 2007

Consent to certain treatments

Generally, the legal authority to detain a patient carries with it the authority to give basic treatment even without the patient's consent (e.g. intramuscular sedation). Under a Section 3, medications can be given for up to 3 months of detention. After this time, either the patient has to consent or an independent doctor must provide a second opinion to confirm that the treatment is still in the patient's best interests. In some other countries, additional authority has to be obtained before any treatments may be given without consent.

Electroconvulsive therapy (ECT) has specific guidance relating to its usage. ECT may not be given to a refusing patient who has the capacity to refuse it, and may only be given to an incapacitated patient where it does not conflict with any advance directive, decision of their NR, or decision of the courts. The only exception to this is emergency (life-threatening) situations, in which the RC can authorize up to two ECT treatments for patients detained under Section 3.

Treating physical illness

The MHA 1983/2007 relates only to the treatment of mental disorders, not physical disorders. It does not permit the treatment of any physical co-morbidity that a detained psychiatric patient may have. There are only two exceptions to this rule:

- enforced refeeding of a severely emaciated patient suffering from anorexia nervosa. This is allowed because anorexia nervosa is a mental disorder, and refeeding constitutes a necessary first stage of its treatment sequelae;
- treatment of physical sequelae of an attempted suicide, which was direct result of an underlying mental disorder.

Patients with co-morbid physical conditions, who are deemed not to have capacity, may be treated under the Mental Capacity Act 2005 (see below).

Age-appropriate services

The law now requires that for patients aged under 18 who are admitted to hospital, an environment suitable to their needs is provided. In practical terms, this is supposed to prevent the treatment of adolescents on adult wards. It was previously the case that if a child aged 16 or 17 refused hospital admission, their parents could consent for them. Under the MHA 2007, this is no longer the case. In this situation, the MHA would need to be used as for an adult.

Laws concerning capacity and consent to treatment

Across medicine it is essential that a patient's consent is gained before a health practitioner treats them; without consent this treatment is an assault. Consent must be informed, given voluntarily without undue influence, and be given by the patient. It is good practice to document consent. There are a variety of different groups of people within society who may not be in a position to make decisions for themselves, and various other (often emergency) situations in which gaining consent can be problematic. Some of these are shown in Table 12.3.

The Mental Capacity Act 2005 (MCA 2005)

In the UK, the MCA 2005 provides the first definite legislation to protect vulnerable individuals who are deemed not to have capacity to make their own decisions. The act provides the means to assess whether or not an individual has capacity, and, if not, how those caring for them can make decisions in their best interests. It applies to people aged 16 or over, as those below the age of 16 can have consent given by their parents. The act is underpinned by five principles.

1 An adult is assumed to have capacity unless it is established that they lack capacity.

Table 12.3 Situations in which problems of consent to treatment are likely to arise

- Emergency life-threatening situations
- Increasing or severe cognitive impairment
- Mental disorder impairing ability to give informed consent to treatment of a physical disorder
- Unwilling or unable to give consent to treatment of major mental disorder
- Children
- People with learning disability

2 A person is not to be treated as unable to make a decision unless all practicable steps to help them to do so have been taken without success.

3 A person is not to be treated as unable to make a decision merely because they make an unwise decision.

4 Anything done for, or on behalf of, the person must be in their best interests.

5 Anything done for, or on behalf of, the person should be the least restrictive option with respect to their basic rights and freedoms.

Assessing capacity

The MCA 2005 sets out a clear test for assessing whether a person lacks capacity to make a particular decision at a particular time. The person must have been shown to have 'an impairment of the mind or brain, or a disturbance of mental function'. To have capacity to make a decision a person must:

- have a general understanding of the decision and why they need to make it;
- have a general understanding of the likely consequences of making, or not making, the decision;
- be able to understand, retain, use, and weigh up the information presented to them;
- be able to communicate their decision to others.

If it is decided that the person does not have capacity to make the particular decision, the rest of the act applies.

Best interests

Everything that is done for the patient who lacks capacity must be in their best interests. The act contains a checklist of factors which must be worked through to make a best interests decision. All patients have the right to make a written statement, which must be considered, as must the feelings of family and carers.

Acts in connection with care or treatment

The act offers statutory protection from prosecution where a person is performing an act in connection with care or treatment of someone who lacks capacity. For example, if a doctor was to decide that examining a patient was in their best interests, it would not be assault to do so. Individuals who neglect or ill treat a person who lacks capacity can be imprisoned for up to 5 years.

Advance decisions to refuse treatment

The act makes it possible to make an advance decision to refuse treatment should a person lack capacity in the future. Advance decisions can only be made by those aged 18 years or older, and only when the person is deemed to have capacity to make the decision. Any treatment may be refused, except for those needed to keep them comfortable (e.g. warmth, offering food and water by mouth).

Lasting Power of Attorney (LPA)

This allows a person to appoint an attorney to act on their behalf if they should lose capacity in the future. The LPA can then make financial, property, health, and welfare decisions for them. There is a formal legal protocol to register an attorney.

Safeguards

A number of safeguards have been put in place to ensure that individuals lacking capacity are treated in the rightful manner. These include a court of protection, a public guardian (who is responsible for creating all LPAs), and independent mental capacity advocates (IMCAs). The latter are individuals appointed to speak for a person who lacks capacity and has no one to speak for them.

Other aspects of civil law relevant to psychiatry

Making a will

Doctors are sometimes asked to advise whether a patient is capable of making a will—that is, whether he has 'testamentary capacity'. The requirements are that the person:

- understands what a will is;
- knows the nature and extent of his property (although not in detail);
- knows who his close relatives are and can assess their claims to his property;
- does not have any mental abnormality that might distort his judgement (e.g. delusions about the actions of his relatives).

Most patients with mental disorder are wholly capable of making a will.

Fitness to drive

Questions about fitness to drive arise quite often in relation to psychiatric disorder. Patients may drive recklessly if they are manic, depressed and suicidal, or aggressive, or if they abuse alcohol or drugs. Concentration on driving may be impaired in many kinds of psychiatric disorder, and also by the sedative side effects of drugs used in treatment. The issue should be considered in all cases in which a patient drives a motor vehicle. Advice to stop driving should be given if necessary and the patient reminded of his duty to report illnesses to the licensing authority. In the UK, the DVLA publishes a guide for clinicians as to which conditions should be reported, and with which the patient's license is invalid. Examples include mania, acute psychosis, and severe depression with suicidal ideation. Particular caution is required for patients who drive public service vehicles or goods vehicles.

Compensation for personal injury

Doctors are often asked to write medical reports about disability following accidents or other trauma and in relation to claims of medical negligence. Such reports are concerned mainly with the nature and outlook of physical disability, but they should include any psychiatric consequences directly attributable to the trauma or induced by the physical disability. The conclusions should summarize the psychological and social consequences of the trauma and the extent to which they appear to be attributable to it.

In many cases there is evidence that there were psychological problems or social difficulties before the event, and it is important to decide how far the psychological and social changes found after the trauma represent a continuation of these previous difficulties rather than new developments. Evidence from a close relative or other informant, interviewed separately, should be obtained whenever possible.

■ Psychiatry and criminal law

Originally, the term 'forensic psychiatry' referred to the interaction between psychiatry and the law. However, as the first half of this chapter explained, psychiatry is intricately connected with the law. Forensic psychiatry now mostly deals with two types of patient:

1 individuals with mental disorders who have broken the law, i.e. **mentally disordered offenders**;

2 individuals with mental disorders who are, or may be, violent.

In most developed countries, forensic psychiatry is a distinct subspecialty of psychiatry, but in some other countries all psychiatrists may be involved in the management of mentally disordered offenders.

There are two UK legal concepts relevant to mentally disordered offenders—the defence of 'insanity' and that of 'diminished responsibility'.

- **The defence of insanity** can be used as a defence against any crime of which the defendant is charged. In order to 'qualify' for insanity, the defence must prove not only that the defendant had a disease of the mind at the time of the offence, but also that this led to a defect of reason. This

leads to the supposition that the defendant did not know that what he was doing was wrong at the time. The defendant is then acquitted on grounds of insanity.

- **Diminished responsibility** is a defence that can only be used for a charge of homicide. If the defence convince the jury that due to their underlying mental illness they were not fully to blame for their crime, the charge may be reduced to manslaughter.

This section provides a brief overview of the links between mental disorders and crime, and the structure of forensic psychiatry. For more detailed information, see the further reading section on p. 109.

Current patterns of crime

The prevalence and pattern of criminal offending change over time in most countries. Figures for the prevalence of crime must be viewed cautiously as they depend on reporting and upon definitions of crime. Typically, the public perception of the quantity and type of crimes is markedly different from official statistics (Figure 12.1). The public tend to overestimate both the number of and severity of crimes committed in their neighbourhood. Much criminal behaviour goes unreported; this is especially true of domestic violence.

In the UK, crime has been steadily reducing for the past two decades. The latest British Crime Survey figures show an overall decline of 5 per cent for the period 2008–2009 compared with the previous year. The risk of being a

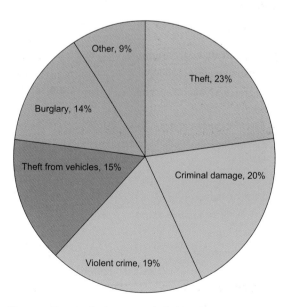

Fig. 12.1 Types of crime as recorded by the British Crime Survey 2008–2009. Numbers are the proportion as a percentage of total crime recorded. (Reproduced by permission of the Home Office.)

victim of crime in any given year is currently 26 per cent, down from 40 per cent in the mid 1980s.

Risk factors for criminal offending

Although this chapter is mainly concerned with the links between mental disorders and crime, it is worth considering the general risk factors for criminal offending. This is because most of them are the same for offenders with and without a mental health problem. They are best considered within the biopsychosocial model (Table 12.4); from the table, it is clear that family and social factors are by far the most important risk factors.

Mental disorders and crime

Contrary to public perception, few psychiatric patients break the law, and when they do, it is usually in minor ways. Although serious violent offences by psychiatric patients receive much publicity, they are infrequent and committed by an extremely small minority of patients. It is, however, important that doctors are aware of the risk of criminal behaviour amongst those who are mentally ill. Threats of violence to self or to others should be taken seriously, as should the possibility of unintended harm resulting from disinhibited, reckless, or ill-considered behaviour.

As mentioned above, the risk factors for someone with a mental disorder committing a crime are primarily those in Table 12.4, but there is a particular concern about violent behaviour. There is a small but significant association between mental disorder and violence; 5 per cent of violent crimes in the UK are committed by an individual with a severe psychiatric illness. The prevalence of violent behaviour in those with mental disorders compared with the general population is as follows:

- The prevalence of violent behaviour in the general population (without mental disorder) is 2 per cent.
- The prevalence in those with a *major* mental illness is 7 per cent.
- The prevalence in individuals with a substance abuse disorder is 20 per cent.

There are a few specific risk factors associated with violent behaviour (these are further described for individual diagnoses below); these are shown in Table 12.5. Remember that no matter what the underlying diagnosis is, a past history of violent behaviour is the greatest predictor

Table 12.4 Risk factors for criminal offending

Biological

- Male gender
- Low IQ
- Age (peak 10–25 years)
- Genetics: in monozygotic twins concordance for committing crime is 80%
- Ethnicity (Afro-Caribbeans > Caucasians > Asians)
- Hyperactivity and impulsivity
- Teenage mother

Psychological

- Personality traits: lack of empathy
- Poor parental supervision and poor attachment
- Harsh discipline in childhood
- Aggression, violence, or criminal activity within the family
- Parental conflict and/or 'broken homes'
- Separation from biological parents before 10 years of age

Social

- Larger family size
- Lower socioeconomic status
- Poor housing
- Unemployment
- Peer influences: school, neighbourhood (especially gang culture)
- Spouse or partner is an offender
- Inner-city living
- Alcohol and substance abuse

Table 12.5 Risk factors for violent behaviour in patients with mental disorders

Major psychoses (especially if associated with the following):

- Paranoia (with increased perception of threat to self)
- Command hallucinations
- Passivity phenomena

Puerperal psychosis—increased risk to the child

Delusional disorders (especially delusional jealousy towards a partner)

Severe depression (increased risk of infanticide and arson, but not most other crimes)

Antisocial, impulsive, or narcissistic personality traits (increases risk by 16-fold)

Poor impulse control

Co-morbid use of alcohol or substances

Prior history of conduct disorder

Poor insight into illness or behaviour

of future behaviour, and that all the general risk factors in Table 12.4 are relevant. It is worth noting that whilst manic patients are at high risk of disinhibited behaviour, reckless spending/driving and agitation, violence towards others or property is rare.

It is widely appreciated that mental disorders are massively over-represented amongst the prison population of most countries, and several large meta-analyses have been undertaken which confirm this (see Table 12.6.). The prevalence of psychosis and major depression appears to be at least twice as high as in the general population, and the prevalence of personality disorders about 10 times as high.

The UK Ministry for Justice publishes yearly figures of the number of mentally disordered offenders detained in specialist secure psychiatric hospitals. At the time of writing, the latest figures (2008) were that 3970 mentally disordered offenders were detained. This represents 5 per cent of the total population in prison. Although the prison population has been steadily growing in recent decades, the number of mentally disordered offenders detained has been almost static.

Associations between specific psychiatric disorders and types of offence

It is difficult to directly link specific psychiatric diagnoses with particular offences. Mental disorders are not like many medical conditions (e.g. appendicitis) in that they rarely have a typical presentation. There is great clinical heterogeneity and this is represented in the variety of offences that may be committed. The following provides a brief overview of some associations between crime and particular disorders.

Schizophrenia

Overall, crime is uncommon and usually minor. However, threats of violence should be taken seriously. Compared with the general population, there is a two- to fourfold increase in risk of violence in men with schizophrenia, and a six- to eightfold increase in women. The individuals who are violent are often suffering from persecutory delusions, command hallucinations, or passivity phenomenon—typically the patient perceives others to be a threat to their safety. Violence is almost always towards family members; stranger attacks are uncommon. Whilst these positive symptoms are risk factors, they are outweighed by the increased risks associated with using alcohol and drugs.

Delusional disorders

Individuals with delusional disorders are significantly over-represented in secure psychiatric hospitals, but uncommonly commit serious crime. The particular conditions that are involved are delusional jealousy, delusions of love, querulous delusions, and misidentification delusions. Sixty per cent of those with delusional jealousy are violent towards their partners. Stalking is a particularly interesting condition, which may be associated with a delusional disorder. There is an increased risk of homicide (both in the stalker and their victim) associated with stalking.

Mood disorders

There is a low risk of offending in mood disorders. An association between shoplifting and depression was suggested but systematic review has not confirmed this. Very rarely, patients with severe depression may become violent. Approximately 5 per cent of UK homicides are followed by suicide of the perpetrator; in this situation depression is a common finding, although nihilistic delusions as a possible trigger are extremely rare. More often, marital breakdown and other socioeconomic problems are evident.

Manic patients occasionally commit petty crime due to their exuberant, unpredictable behaviour. Charges such as indecent exposure, disrupting the peace, and minor theft are not uncommon. Violent or serious crimes are rare.

Personality disorders

The association between personality disorders and all types of crime is much stronger than for mental disorders. Antisocial, paranoid, and borderline traits are particularly likely to lead to crime. As previously mentioned, up to two-thirds of prison inmates have a personality disorder, most frequently antisocial personality disorder. The combination of a personality disorder and alcohol/drug misuse increases the risk of offending by 16 times. Official figures from Sweden reported 50 per cent of individuals convicted of homicide in 2005 had a diagnosis of a personality disorder. As well as violence, there is also an increased risk of sexual offences.

Table 12.6 Prevalence of mental disorders amongst prison inmates

Diagnosis	Males (%)	Females (%)
Psychosis	3.7	4
Major depression	10	12
Personality disorder	65	42
Antisocial personality disorder	47	21

Reproduced with permission from Fazel, S. & Danesh, J. (2002). Serious mental disorders in 23 000 prisoners: a systematic review of 62 surveys. *Lancet* **359**: 545–550.

Alcohol and drug abuse

Both of these addictions are commonly associated with offending of all types. There is an added risk of driving under the influence, with alcohol playing a role in about 20% of traffic-related deaths. Alcohol is also identified as a factor in over half of interpersonal assaults in England and Wales. In the USA, 40 per cent of homicides are related to drugs or alcohol, and 17 per cent are committed by someone who has a mental disorder and is under the influence of substances. Much petty theft, fraud, and other minor crimes are committed to fund drug habits.

Learning disability and autistic spectrum disorders

These are rarely associated with offending, and when they are it is usually a minor crime by an individual lacking understanding of the legal implications of their actions.

Crimes of violence

Homicide

The rate of homicide varies enormously between countries, but it is clear that only a minority are committed by mentally disordered people. In the UK, there are 500–600 homicides each year, in 80 per cent of which the victim is known to the perpetrator. In the USA, the majority are by shooting. Approximately 10 per cent of homicides are committed by a person in touch with mental health services, only half of whom have a 'severe' mental illness. Of these, one-third have had admissions under the Mental Health Act. Five to ten per cent of homicide convictions are reduced to manslaughter due to a plea of diminished responsibility, or acquitted on grounds of insanity.

Infanticide

Infanticide is the killing of a child below the age of 12 months by the mother. When the killing is within 24 hours of birth, the baby is usually unwanted, and the mother is often young, distressed, and ill equipped to cope with the child, but not usually suffering from psychiatric disorder. When the killing is more than 24 hours after the birth, the mother usually has a mental disorder, most commonly untreated puerperal psychosis or postnatal depression. About a third of mothers in this second group try to kill themselves after killing the child.

Family violence

Violence within the home is common but often undetected. It may affect children, the partner, or an elderly relative living in the house. Violence is strongly associated with excessive consumption of alcohol. A quarter of women experience domestic violence, which leads to serious injuries (e.g. broken bones) in 10 per cent of cases. Wife battering is associated with aggressive personality, alcohol abuse, and sexual jealousy. Marital therapy may be attempted to reduce factors provoking the violence, but often alternative safe accommodation has to be found for the woman and any children.

Sexual offences (Box 12.1)

A sex offender is *an individual whose sexual behaviour contravenes the law*. The most frequent offences are indecent exposure, rape, and unlawful intercourse. Most sexual offences are committed by men; the common sexual offence among women is prostitution. Severe mental disorders are rare amongst sex offenders, but personality disorders are over-represented.

BOX 12.1 Sexual offences

Indecent exposure. Indecent exposure of the genitalia is mainly an offence of men between 25 and 35 years of age. The offence is usually a result of the psychiatric disorder known as exhibitionism, although in a minority exposure is a prelude to a sexual assault or disinhibition caused by alcohol or drug intoxification.

Voyeurism. This is the sexual interest of watching people engaged in intimate activities (e.g. undressing, having sex). The perpetrators are commonly known as 'peeping Toms'.

Rape. Rape is forceful sexual intercourse with an unwilling partner. The degree of force varies: in some cases force is threatened either verbally or with a weapon; in others there is extreme brutality. Few rapists have a psychiatric disorder.

Unlawful intercourse. This is sexual intercourse with a child under the age at which legal consent can be given. The sexual acts vary from minor indecency to seriously aggressive penetrative intercourse, but most do not involve violence. The offence is common. An adult who repeatedly commits sexual offences against children is known as a paedophile. Most are male. Some are timid and sexually inexperienced, some learning disordered, and some have difficulty in finding a sexual partner of their own age. Others prefer intercourse with children to that with adults. Although most offences do not involve major assault and most convicted offenders do not reoffend, an important minority persist in their behaviour, and a few progress to more serious and damaging forms of sexual behaviour with children.

Incest. Incest is sexual activity between members of the same family, most often between father and daughter, or between siblings. When incest has been discovered the family needs much specialist support to deal with guilt and recriminations.

Other offences

Shoplifting. Most shoplifters act for gain but a minority do so when mentally disordered. Patients with alcoholism, drug dependence, and chronic schizophrenia may shoplift because they lack money, and patients with dementia may forget to pay. Among middle-aged female shoplifters it is common to find family and social difficulties and depression.

Arson is setting fire to property, an act that may also endanger life. Most arsonists are male. Usually, there is no obvious motive for the act and many arsonists are referred for a medical opinion. However, few have a psychiatric disorder.

Repeated gambling (pathological gambling). This term is used to describe a condition in which a person has an intense urge to gamble and a preoccupation with thoughts about gambling. Gambling is not, in itself, an offence but large debts can accumulate and may result in stealing or fraud. Some psychiatrists regard this condition as a disorder akin to addiction to alcohol, and offer treatment similar to that used for substance abuse.

The role of doctors

There are a variety of legal issues on which doctors may be asked to advise the police, most commonly by providing a factual medical report. This is usually the remit of specialist forensic psychiatrists, but other psychiatrists, and occasionally general practitioners may be asked for their input. Box 12.2 provides an overview of the role of doctors in relation to crime. It is an important ethical principle that both doctors and those they are assessing are clear that *acting for a third party*, such as a court, involves different obligations and responsibilities to usual clinical practice, where the relationship is between the doctor and patient. Box 12.3 provides some guidance on the writing of a medical report for the courts.

Treatment of mentally disordered offenders

The fundamental aspect of treating mentally disordered offenders is that the principles of treatment are the same as for any other patient. However, it may need to be undertaken in a more secure environment. Forensic psychiatrists tend to treat these patients, be they in prison, a secure psychiatric hospital, or in the community.

The prison psychiatrist

As already outlined earlier in this chapter, a vast proportion of individuals within prisons have psychiatric disorders. The majority of forensic psychiatrists work in 'normal' prisons, and only a few in secure psychiatric hospitals. There are four main situations in which a psychiatrist may be asked to see a prisoner:

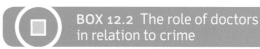

BOX 12.2 The role of doctors in relation to crime

- Assessment of offenders who may have a mental disorder.
- Advice to the police when they are deciding whether to proceed with charges against mentally disordered offenders.
- Fitness to plead. To be fit to plead, a person must be able to understand the nature of the charge and the difference between a plea of guilty and a plea of not guilty, instruct lawyers and challenge jurors, and follow evidence presented in court. A person can suffer from severe mental disorder and still be fit to plead. A person judged unfit to plead is not tried but detained in a hospital until fit to plead, at which time (if it comes) the case is tried.
- Assessment of responsibility; providing evidence and/or an opinion as to whether the defence of insanity or diminished responsibility is appropriate.
- Giving evidence in court, or writing a formal report for the criminal court.
- Treatment of offenders whilst in custody or prison, in hospital, or in the community.
- Providing risk assessments of offenders anywhere within the criminal legal system.

1 to provide a court report before a trial;

2 to assess a patient in prison;

3 to provide treatment for prisoners;

4 to provide a report for the parole board.

Prisoners should be assessed as for any other patient, and offered the same range of treatments as would be available in the community.

Secure psychiatric hospitals

Patients may be admitted to secure psychiatric hospitals from the courts, prisons, or less secure hospitals. The majority of mentally disordered offenders are sentenced to undertake a prison sentence in the mainstream system or compulsory treatment in the community. However, when there is a continuing risk to other people of aggression, arson, or sexual offences, treatment is arranged in a unit providing greater security to ensure the protection of society.

There are several parts of the MHA 1983/2007 which provide specific legislation for mentally disordered offenders.

- Sections 35 and 36 are equivalent to Sections 2 and 3 in civil law, and are used for patients awaiting trial for a

BOX 12.3 Preparing a medical report for criminal proceedings

When a doctor is asked for a written medical report on a person it is sensible to (as far as possible) avoid technical language, explain any technical terms that are essential, and not use jargon. The report should be concise, have a clear structure, and be limited to matters relevant to the reason for the report. The following headings are recommended:

1 The doctor's particulars: full name, qualifications, and present appointment.

2 When the interview was conducted and whether any third person was present.

3 Sources of information, including any documents that have been examined.

4 Relevant points from the family and personal history of the defendant.

5 The accused person's account of the events of the alleged offence, whether they admit to the offence or have another explanation of the events, and if they admit to it, their attitude and expressed degree of remorse.

6 Other relevant behaviour such as the abuse of alcohol or drugs, the quality of relationships with other people, general social competence, and personality traits or behaviour indicating ability to tolerate frustration.

7 Mental state at the time of the assessment, mentioning only positive findings or specifically relevant negative ones.

8 A decision as to whether or not the person has a mental disorder as defined by the Mental Health Act. A more specific diagnosis can be added (such as dementia or schizophrenia) but the court is unlikely to be helped by the finer nuances of diagnosis.

9 Mental state at the time of the alleged offence. As explained above, this question is highly important in law but difficult to answer on medical evidence. A judgement is made from the present mental state, diagnosis, the accused person's account, and accounts from any witnesses. If the person has a chronic mental illness (such as dementia) it is less difficult to infer his mental state at the time of the alleged offence than it is if he has a depressive disorder, which could have been more or less severe at the former time than it was at the assessment. To add to the difficulty, the court does not simply require a general statement about the mental state at the time, but a specific judgement about the accused person's intentions.

10 Fitness to plead is referred to when this is relevant.

11 Assessment of criminal responsibility. For most offences, a person is not regarded as culpable unless they were able to choose whether or not to perform the unlawful action, and unless they were able to control their behaviour at the time. Again a judgement has to be made on the available evidence, and may not be clear cut. This is especially important in cases where a defence of insanity or diminished responsibility is being made.

12 Advice on further treatment is likely to be particularly helpful to the court. It is not the doctor's role to advise the court about sentencing, although sometimes it is helpful to indicate the likely psychiatric consequences of different forms of sentence that might be considered by the court (e.g. custodial vs. non-custodial).

serious crime. They are an alternative to sending the patient to prison whilst awaiting trial.

- Section 37 is a treatment order (similar to Section 3) which can be used for mentally disordered offenders who have been convicted of a serious crime and sentenced to imprisonment. After 6 months, the patient may request an MHRT in the usual way, but if the patient is found to have recovered from the mental disorder they are transferred to prison rather than discharged home.

- Patients who pose an extremely high risk to others may have a Section 41 added to their Section 37. This imposes further restrictions, most importantly that only the Home Secretary can decide that the person can leave hospital.

- Section 47 allows for prisoners to be transferred from a prison to a psychiatric hospital for treatment.

In the UK, there are three tiers of secure psychiatric hospitals; high-, medium-, and low-security facilities. There are five high-security hospitals in the UK:

1 England: special hospitals at Broadmoor, Rampton, and Ashworth;

2 Scotland: the state hospital at Carstairs;

3 Northern Ireland: the central mental hospital at Dundrum.

These facilities take patients who pose *grave imminent danger to the public,* and are extremely secure. There are at least two high perimeter fences outside the hospital walls, and maximal security within. The ratio of staff to patients is very high. The average stay in Broadmoor is 8 years, and contrary to popular belief, most patients who receive treatment in a high-security facility are eventually rehabilitated sufficiently to move back into the community. In the UK, there are now also special high-secure units for patients with **dangerous severe personality disorders (DSPD)**, encompassing 300 beds. Two of these are located on the sites of high-security hospitals, and two at high-security prisons. A large part of the treatment in these units is targeted at rehabilitation, and helping the patient towards moving back into the community.

Medium-secure facilities fall somewhere between the 'escape-proof' secure facilities and locked wards. The majority of patients in these facilities move there due to behaviour that is unmanageable in lower-security environments. The length of stay is much shorter—2 years on average—and then most patients are well enough to return to a less restrictive environment. There are several facilities in the UK that take adolescents needing a medium level of security.

Low-security units are mainly based in large general psychiatric hospitals or on the same site as a medium-secure facility. They are essentially locked wards, with similar security to that which is provided in intensive care units for patients who have not offended. Most patients are admitted for a relatively short time, until their illness is under better control and they are able to return to a non-secure environment.

Community treatment

As in the rest of psychiatry, treating a mentally disordered offender has two parts: managing the acute psychiatric disturbance and then rehabilitating the patient to life in the community. Once a mentally disordered offender is deemed fit for discharge from hospital, and has completed their mandatory sentence, it is essential they receive appropriate community follow-up. This is provided in a similar way to that in the general services, with community psychiatric nurses, social workers, occupational therapists, and many other professionals providing input. For a patient to be successfully reintroduced into society and to reduce the chance of reoffending it must be clear that their mental state is appropriate, and that they have the skills required for community living. This includes help finding somewhere to live, employment, hobbies, financial assistance, and reintegration with family. The latter can be extremely difficult, and family therapy plays a vital role.

 Further reading

Fazel, S. & Grann, M. (2006). The population impact of severe mental illness on violent crime. *American Journal of Psychiatry* **163:** 1397–1403.

Stone, J. H., Roberts, M., O'Grady, J., Taylor, A. V., & O'Shea, K. (2000). *Faulk's Basic Forensic Psychiatry.* Blackwell, Oxford.

www.dh.gov.uk/en/Healthcare/Mentalhealth/DH_078743. UK Department of Health website; a useful summary of the changes in the Mental Health Act 2007 (accessed April 2011).

www.legislation.gov.uk/ukpga/2005/9/contents. UK Department of Health website page covering the Mental Capacity Act (accessed April 2011).

Drugs and other physical treatments

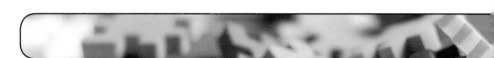

This chapter is about the use of drugs and electroconvulsive therapy. Psychological treatment is considered separately in Chapter 14. This is a convenient way of dividing the subject matter of a book, but in practice these *physical treatments are always combined with psychological treatment*, most often supportive or problem-solving counselling, but also one of the specific methods described in Chapter 14.

The account in this chapter is concerned with practical therapeutics rather than basic pharmacology, and it will be assumed that the reader has studied the pharmacology of the principal types of drug used in psychiatric disorders. (Readers who do not have this knowledge should consult a textbook—for example, *The Oxford Textbook of Clinical Pharmacology and Drug Therapy* by D. G. Grahame-Smith and J. K. Aronson.) Nevertheless, a few important points about the actions of psychotropic drugs will be considered, before describing the specific groups of drugs.

■ General considerations

Pharmacokinetics of psychotropic drugs

To be effective, psychotropic drugs must reach the brain in adequate amounts. How far they do this depends on their absorption, metabolism, excretion, and passage across the blood–brain barrier.

Absorption

Most psychotropic drugs are absorbed readily from the gut, but absorption can be reduced by intestinal hurry or a malabsorption syndrome.

Science box 13.1 Drug discovery in psychiatry

The first generation of effective drugs for mental disorders were, in the main, identified by acute clinical observation of the effects of drugs that were originally developed for different purposes. Thus, the monoamine oxidase inhibitors were originally investigated as antituberculosis agents, chlorpromazine began life as an antihistamine, and the effectiveness of lithium was discovered when it was used to increase the solubility of uric acid, which had been hypothesized to cause mania.

Second-generation drugs tended to be refined, more selective versions of first-generation drugs. So, for example, selective serotonin reuptake inhibitors (SSRIs) were developed to target the 5-hydroxytryptamine (5-HT) system and, by avoiding the broader effects of tricyclic drugs, caused less side effects and toxicity. Second-generation antipsychotics were designed to replicate the dopamine-blocking effects of first-generation antipsychotics without causing motor side effects.

By the early 2000s, a large number of 'me-too' compounds had been developed in the major areas of antidepressants and antipsychotics, but there were no major breakthroughs in treatment to lead to fundamental control of mental disorders. Rational development was inhibited by the slow pace of increasing knowledge on the basic mechanisms of the disorders.

At the time of writing, the difficulty of discovering new drugs has led to the withdrawal of several major drug manufacturers from active drug development in psychiatry. We hope (and predict), however, that this will act as a spur to the international academic community to take up the challenge to fill the black hole left by the withdrawal of industry. A key challenge will be the development of reliable experimental models of psychiatric disorders to allow the efficient development of promising agents. Perhaps the next step will be to aim to repeat the successes of the early pioneers by investigating existing agents for potential benefits.

Metabolism

Most psychotropic drugs are metabolized partially in the liver on their way from the gut via the portal system to the systemic circulation. The amount of this so-called **first-pass metabolism** differs from one person to another, and it is altered by certain drugs, taken at the same time, which induce liver enzymes (e.g. barbiturates) or inhibit them (e.g. monoamine oxidase inhibitors (MAOIs)). Although first-pass metabolism reduces the amount of the original drug reaching the brain, the metabolites of some drugs have their own therapeutic effects.

Because many psychotropic drugs have active metabolites, the *measurement of plasma concentrations of the parent drug is generally a poor guide to treatment*. Such measurement is *used routinely only with lithium carbonate*, which has no metabolites (see p. 123).

Distribution

In plasma, psychotropic drugs are bound largely to protein. Because they are lipophilic, they pass easily into the **brain**. For the same reason they enter into **fat stores** from which they are released slowly, often for many weeks after the patient has ceased to take the drug. They also pass into **breast milk**—an important point when a breast-feeding mother is treated.

Excretion

Psychotropic drugs and their metabolites are excreted through the kidneys, so smaller doses should be given when renal function is impaired. Lithium is unique among the psychotropic drugs in being filtered passively in the glomerulus and then partly reabsorbed in the tubules by the mechanism that absorbs sodium. The two ions compete for reabsorption so that when sodium levels fall, lithium absorption rises and lithium concentrations increase—potentially to a toxic level.

Drug interactions

When two drugs are given together, one may either interfere with the other, or enhance its therapeutic or unwanted effects. Interactions can take place during absorption, metabolism, or excretion, or at the cellular level. For psychotropic drugs, most pharmacokinetic interactions are at the stage of liver metabolism, the important exception being lithium, for which interference is at the stage of renal excretion. An important pharmacodynamic interaction is the antagonism between tricyclics and some antihypertensive drugs. When prescribing a psychotropic and another drug it is good practice to consult the *Summaries of Product Characteristics* (*SPC*, online at www.medicines.org.uk) or a work of reference such as the *British National Formulary* (*BNF*) to determine whether the drugs interact.

Drug withdrawal

When some drugs are given for a long period, the tissues adjust to their presence and when the drug is withdrawn there is a temporary disturbance of function until a new adjustment is reached. This disturbance appears clinically as a withdrawal syndrome. Among psychotropic drugs, anxiolytics and hypnotics are most likely to induce this effect (see p. 114).

General advice about prescribing psychotropic drugs

Use well-tried drugs. When there is a choice of equally effective drugs (as is often the case in psychiatry), it is generally good practice to use the drugs whose side effects and long-term effects are understood better. Also, well-tried drugs are generally less expensive than new ones. Clinicians should become familiar with a few drugs of each of the main types—antidepressants, antipsychotics, and so on. In this way they will become used to adjusting dosage and recognizing side effects.

Change drugs only for a good reason. If there is no therapeutic response to an established drug given in adequate dosage, it is unlikely that there will be a better response to another from the same therapeutic group. The main reason for changing medication is that side effects have prevented adequate dosage. It is then appropriate to change to a drug with a different pattern of side effects — for example, from an antidepressant with strong anticholinergic effects to another with weaker ones.

Combine drugs only for specific indications. Generally, drug combinations should be avoided (see drug interactions above). However, some drug combinations are of proven value for specific purposes, for example, lithium and antidepressant for drug-resistant depressive disorder (see p. 233), or lithium and valproate for preventing relapse in bipolar disorder. Usually, drug combinations are initiated by a specialist because the adverse effects of such combinations can be more hazardous than those of a single drug. However, general practitioners may be asked to continue prescribing.

Adjust dosage carefully. Dose ranges for some commonly used drugs are indicated later in this chapter; others will be found in the SPC or BNF. Within these ranges, the correct dose for an individual patient is decided from the severity of the symptoms, the patient's age and weight, and any factors that may affect drug metabolism or excretion.

Plan the interval between doses. Less frequent administration has the advantage that patients are more likely to be reliable in taking drugs. The duration of action of most psychotropic drugs is such that they can be taken once or twice a day while maintaining a therapeutic plasma concentration between doses.

Decide the duration of treatment. The duration depends on the risk of dependency and the nature of the disorder. In general, anxiolytic and hypnotic drugs should be given for a short time—a few days to 2 or 3 weeks—because of the risk of dependency. Antidepressants and antipsychotics are given for a long time—several months—because of the risk of relapse.

Advise patients. Before giving a first prescription for a drug, the doctor should explain several points:

1 the likely **initial effects** of the drug (e.g. drowsiness or dry mouth);

2 the **delay** before therapeutic effects appear (about 2 weeks with antidepressants);

3 the likely **first signs of improvement** (e.g. improved sleep after starting an antidepressant);

4 **common side effects** (e.g. fine tremor with lithium);

5 any **serious effects** that should be reported immediately by the patient (e.g. coarse tremor after taking lithium);

6 any **restrictions** while the drug is taken (e.g. not driving or operating machinery if the drugs reduce alertness);

7 **how long** the patient will need to take the drug: for anxiolytics, the patient is discouraged from taking them for too long; for antidepressants or antipsychotics, the patient is encouraged to continue taking the drug after symptoms have been controlled.

Adherence to treatment

Many patients do not take the drugs prescribed for them. Their unused drugs are a danger to children and a potential source of deliberate self-poisoning. Other patients take more than the prescribed dose, especially of hypnotic or anxiolytic drugs. It is important to check that repeat prescriptions are not being requested before the correct day. (Adherence to prescribed treatment was previously referred to as **compliance,** and the agreement between doctor and patient on a course of treatment is sometimes called **concordance**.)

To adhere to prescribed treatment, a patient must be:

1 **convinced of the need to take the drug.** Schizophrenic or seriously depressed patients may not be convinced that they are ill, or may not wish to recover. Deluded patients may distrust their doctors;

2 **free from fears or concerns about its dangers.** Some patients fear that antidepressant drugs will cause addiction; some fear unpleasant or dangerous side effects;

3 **able to remember to take it.** Patients with memory impairment may forget to take medication, or take the dose twice.

Time spent at the start of treatment in discussing reasons for drug treatment and the patient's concerns, and explaining the beneficial and likely adverse effects of the drugs, increases adherence. Adherence should be checked at subsequent visits and, if necessary, the discussion should be repeated and extended to include any fresh concerns of the patient.

What to do if there is no therapeutic response

The first step is to find out whether the patient has taken the drug in the correct dose. If not, the points described above under 'adherence' should be considered. If the prescribed dose has been taken, the diagnosis should be reviewed: if it is confirmed, an increase of dosage should be considered. Only when these steps have been gone through should the original drug be changed.

■ Review of drugs used in psychiatry

Psychotropic drugs are those which have effects mainly on mental symptoms. They are divided into six groups according to their principal actions. Several have secondary actions used for other purposes. For example, antidepressants are sometimes used to treat anxiety (Table 13.1).

1 **Anxiolytic drugs** reduce anxiety. Because they have a general calming effect, they are sometimes called **minor tranquillizers** (major tranquillizer is an alternative name for antipsychotic drugs; see below). In larger doses these drugs produce drowsiness and for this reason are sometimes called **sedatives**.

2 **Hypnotics** promote sleep; many hypnotics are of the same type as drugs used as anxiolytics.

3 **Antipsychotic drugs** control delusions, hallucinations, and psychomotor excitement in psychoses. Sometimes they are called **major tranquillizers** because of their calming effect, or **neuroleptics** because of their parkinsonian and other neurological side effects. (**Antiparkinsonian** agents are sometimes employed to control parkinsonian side effects.)

4 **Antidepressants** relieve the symptoms of depressive disorders but do not elevate the mood of healthy people. Antidepressant drugs are also used to treat chronic anxiety disorders, obsessive-compulsive disorder, and, occasionally, nocturnal enuresis.

5 **Mood-stabilizing drugs** are given to prevent recurrence of recurrent affective disorders.

Table 13.1 Psychotropic drugs

Type	Indications	Classes of drug
Anxiolytic	Acute anxiety	Benzodiazepines
		Zopiclone
Hypnotic	Insomnia	Benzodiazepines
		Cyclopyrrolones
		Zopiclone
Antipsychotic[a]	Delusion and hallucinations	Conventional: Phenothiazines
	Mania	Butyrophenones
	To prevent relapse in schizophrenia	Substituted benzamides
		Atypical
Antidepressant	Depressive disorders	Tricyclics
		MAOIs
	Chronic anxiety	SSRIs
	Obsessive-compulsive disorder	
	Nocturnal enuresis	SNRIs
Mood stabilizer	To prevent recurrent mood disorder	Lithium
		Carbamazepine
		Valproate
		Lamotrigine
Psychostimulant	Narcolepsy	Amphetamine
	Hyperkinetic disorder in children	
Cognitive enhancers	Dementia	Donepezil
		Rivastigmine
		Galantamine

[a] Antiparkinsonian drugs are used to control side effects of antipsychotics.
MAOIs, monoamine oxidase inhibitors; SSRIs, selective serotonin reuptake inhibitors.

6 **Psychostimulants** elevate mood but are not used for this purpose because they can cause dependence. Their principal use in psychiatry is in the treatment of hyperactivity syndromes, particularly in children (see p. 446).

The main groups of drugs will be reviewed in turn. For each group, an account will be given of important points concerning therapeutic effects, the compounds in most frequent use, side effects, toxic effects, and contraindications. General advice will also be given about the use of each group of drugs, but *specific applications to the treatment of individual disorders will be found in the chapters dealing with these conditions.* Drugs with a use limited to the treatment of a single disorder (e.g. disulfiram for alcohol problems) are discussed solely in the chapters dealing with the relevant clinical syndromes.

Anxiolytic drugs

Anxiolytic drugs reduce anxiety, and in larger doses produce drowsiness (they are **sedatives**) and sleep (they are also **hypnotics**). (Hypnotics are discussed on p. 115.) These drugs are prescribed widely, and sometimes unnecessarily for patients who would improve without them. Anxiolytics are used most appropriately to reduce severe anxiety. They should be prescribed for a short time, usually a few days, and seldom for more than 2–3 weeks. Longer courses of treatment may lead to tolerance and dependence.

Buspirone (see below) seems to be an exception to the general rule that anxiolytics produce dependency, but its anxiolytic effect develops more slowly and is less intense than that of the benzodiazepines. The drugs called anxiolytics are not the only ones that reduce anxiety. Antidepressant and antipsychotic drugs also have anxiolytic properties. Since they do not induce dependence, they are sometimes used to treat chronic anxiety. Beta-adrenergic agonists are used to control some of the somatic symptoms of anxiety (Table 13.2).

Benzodiazepines

These bind to the benzodiazepine-receptor site on GABA$_A$ (gamma-aminobutyric acid) receptors and thereby potentiate inhibitory transmission. As well as anxiolytic, sedative, and hypnotic effects, benzodiazepines have muscle relaxant and anticonvulsant properties. Benzodiazepines are rapidly absorbed and metabolized into a large number of compounds, many of which have their own therapeutic effects.

Compounds in frequent use. The many benzodiazepines are divided into short- and long-acting drugs (Table 13.3). Short-acting drugs are useful for their brief clinical effect, free from hangover. Their disadvantage is that they are more likely than long-acting drugs to cause dependence.

Table 13.2 Drugs used to treat anxiety

Primary anxiolytics
Benzodiazepines
Buspirone
Other drugs with anxiolytic properties
Some antidepressants
Phenothiazines
Beta-adrenergic antagonists

Table 13.3 Long- and short-acting benzodiazepines

Group	Approximate duration of action	Examples
Short-acting	<12 hours	Lorazepam
		Temazepam
		Oxazepam
		Triazolam
Long-acting	>24 hours	Diazepam
		Nitrazepam
		Flurazepam
		Chlordiazepoxide
		Clobazam
		Chlorazepate
		Alprazolam

Side effects are mainly *drowsiness*, with ataxia at larger doses (especially in the elderly). These effects, which may *impair driving skills* and the operation of machinery, are potentiated by alcohol. Patients should be warned about both these potential hazards. Like alcohol, benzodiazepines can *release aggression* by reducing inhibitions in people with a tendency to this kind of behaviour. This should be remembered, for example, when prescribing for women judged to be at risk of child abuse, or anyone with a history of impulsive aggressive behaviour.

Toxic effects are few, and most patients recover even from large overdoses which produce sedation and drowsiness. Benzodiazepine effects can be reversed with the benzodiazepine receptor antagonist flumazenil. There is no convincing evidence of teratogenic effects; nevertheless, these drugs should be avoided in the first trimester of pregnancy unless there is a strong indication for their use.

Withdrawal effects occur after benzodiazepines have been prescribed for more than a few weeks; they have been reported in up to half the patients taking the drugs for more than 6 months. The frequency depends on the dose and the type of drug. The withdrawal syndrome is shown in Table 13.4. Seizures occur infrequently after rapid withdrawal from large doses. The obvious similarity between benzodiazepine withdrawal symptoms and those of an anxiety disorder makes it difficult, in practice, to decide whether they arise from withdrawal of the drug or the continuous presence of the anxiety disorder for which treatment was initiated. A helpful point is that withdrawal symptoms generally begin 2–3 days after withdrawing a short-acting drug, or 7 days after stopping a long-acting one, and diminish again after 3–10 days. Anxiety symptoms often start sooner and persist for longer. Withdrawal symptoms are less likely if the drug is withdrawn gradually over several weeks. (For the treatment of benzodiazepine dependence, see p. 398.)

Table 13.4 Benzodiazepine withdrawal syndrome

- Apprehension and anxiety
- Insomnia
- Tremor
- Heightened sensitivity to stimuli
- Muscle twitching
- Seizures (rarely)

Buspirone

This anxiolytic, which is an azapirone, has no affinity for benzodiazepine receptors but stimulates 5-HT_{1A} receptors and reduces 5-HT transmission. It does not cause sedation but has side effects of headache, nervousness, and light-headedness. It does not appear to lead to tolerance and dependence. Its action is slower than that of benzodiazepines and less powerful. It cannot be used to treat benzodiazepine withdrawal.

Beta-adrenergic antagonists

These drugs do not have general anxiolytic effects but can relieve palpitation and tremor. They are used occasionally when these are the main symptoms of a chronic anxiety disorder. An appropriate drug is **propranolol** in a starting dose of 40 mg daily increased gradually to 40 mg three times a day. The several **contraindications** limit the use of these drugs. These are: *asthma* or a history of *bronchospasm*, or *obstructive airways disease*; incipient *cardiac failure* or *heart block*; *systolic blood pressure below 90 mmHg*; *a pulse rate less than 60 per minute*; metabolic acidosis, for example in *diabetes;* and after prolonged fasting, as in *anorexia nervosa*. Other contraindications and precautions are listed in the manufacturer's literature. There are **interactions** with some drugs that increase the adverse effects of beta-blockers. Before prescribing these drugs, it is important to find out what other drugs the patient is taking, and consult a work of reference about possible interactions.

General advice about use of anxiolytics

- **Use sparingly.** Usually, attention to life problems, an opportunity to talk about feelings, and reassurance are enough to reduce anxiety to tolerable levels.
- **Brief treatment.** Benzodiazepines should seldom be given for more than 3 weeks.
- **Withdraw drugs gradually** to reduce withdrawal effects. When the drug is stopped, patients should be warned that they may feel more tense for a few days.
- **Short- or long-acting drug.** If anxiety is intermittent, a short-acting compound is used; if anxiety lasts throughout the day a long-acting drug is appropriate.

- **Consider an alternative.** As explained in the section on anxiety disorders (p. 291), some antidepressant and antipsychotic drugs have secondary anxiolytic effects and are useful alternatives to benzodiazepines.

Hypnotic drugs

An ideal hypnotic would increase the length and quality of sleep without changing sleep structure, leave no residual effects on the next day, and cause no dependence and no withdrawal syndrome. No hypnotic drug meets these criteria, and most alter the structure of sleep: rapid eye movement sleep is suppressed while they are being taken and resumes once they have been stopped.

Benzodiazepines are the most frequently used hypnotic drugs. A short-acting drug such as temazepam is suitable for cases of initial insomnia and less likely to cause effects the next day than long-acting compounds such as nitrazepam. These hangover effects can be hazardous for people who drive motor vehicles or operate machines.

Non-benzodiazepine drugs acting on GABA receptors. These drugs include **zopiclone, zolpidem, and zaleplon,** which bind selectively to omega 1 benzodiazepine sites on GABA receptors but not to the omega 2 sites involved in cognitive functions, including memory. They are short-acting and have theoretical advantages over benzodiazepines, although these have not been clearly shown to be clinically significant in patients with insomnia.

Chloral hydrate is less commonly used than previously. It may also affect hepatic enzymes and should be avoided in people with severe renal, hepatic, or cardiac disease.

Patients should be warned that **alcohol** potentiates the effects of hypnotic drugs, sometimes causing dangerous respiratory depression. This effect is particularly likely to occur with chlormethiazole and barbiturates, which should not be prescribed to people taking excessive amounts of alcohol, except under careful supervision in the management of withdrawal (see p. 391).

Hypnotic drugs are prescribed too frequently and for too long. Some patients are started on long periods of dependency on hypnotics by the prescribing of night sedation in hospital. These drugs should be prescribed only when there is a real need, and should be stopped before the patient goes home. (The management of insomnia is discussed on p. 362.)

Prescribing for special groups

For *children* the prescription of hypnotics is not justified except occasionally for the treatment of night terrors or somnambulism. For *the elderly,* hypnotics should be prescribed with particular care since they may become confused and thereby risk injury.

Antipsychotic drugs

Antipsychotic drugs reduce psychomotor excitement, hallucinations, and delusions occurring in schizophrenia, mania, and organic psychoses. Antipsychotic drugs block dopamine D_2 receptors to varying degrees. The degree to which they do so may account for their therapeutic effects, and certainly explains the propensity of individual drugs to cause extrapyramidal side effects. Several drugs, particularly the newer 'atypical' antipsychotics, are also serotonin 2_A receptor antagonists and this may explain their different clinical effects. Antipsychotic drugs also block noradrenergic and cholinergic receptors to varying degrees, and these actions account for some of their many side effects.

Antipsychotic drugs are well absorbed and partly metabolized in the liver into numerous metabolites, some of which have antipsychotic properties of their own. Because of this metabolism to active compounds, measurements of plasma concentrations of the parent drug are not helpful for the clinician.

Types of antipsychotic drugs available

There are many antipsychotic drugs, with different chemical structures. The following grouping is clinically useful, although it should be recognized that the classification is not based on formal pharmacological class.

First-generation (also known as 'typical' or 'conventional') antipsychotic drugs (FGAs) bind strongly to postsynaptic dopamine D_2 receptors. This action seems to account for their therapeutic effect but also their propensity to cause movement disorders (see p. 116).

Second-generation (also known as 'atypical') antipsychotic drugs (SGAs) vary in the extent to which they bind to dopamine D_2/D_4, 5-HT_2, alpha$_1$-adrenergic, and muscarinic receptors. It is thought that the balance between the D_2 and 5-HT_2 antagonism may account for their therapeutic actions. SGAs are less likely to cause movement disorders than the typical antipsychotics and do not cause hyperprolactinaemia. SGAs include **clozapine, olanzapine, risperidone, quetiapine, sertindole, zotepine,** and **ziprasidone.**

Clozapine was the first SGA and it binds only weakly to D_2 receptors and has a higher affinity for D_4 receptors. It also binds to histamine H_1, 5-HT_2, alpha$_1$-adrenergic, and muscarinic receptors. At the time of writing, clozapine is the only antipsychotic which has been demonstrated to be effective in patients who are unresponsive to FGAs. Clozapine does not cause extrapyramidal side effects, but it causes neutropenia in 2–3 per cent of patients, which progresses to agranulocytosis in 0.3 per cent of patients. For this reason, it is used only when other drugs have failed, and then with regular blood tests, and an explanation of the risks and benefits.

Dopamine system stabilizers. One current target for new drug development is the production of molecules that 'stabilize' the dopaminergic system. These drugs are partial agonists and can increase dopamine transmission in D_2 receptors when it is low and lower it when high. Thus, it may be possible to achieve relief of psychotic symptoms without inducing parkinsonism. **Aripiprazole** is the prototype of this class of drugs, although older drugs such as sulpiride and amisulpiride may have some of the same characteristics.

Slow-release depot preparations are given by injection to patients who improve with drugs but cannot be relied on to take them regularly by mouth. These preparations are esters of the antipsychotic drug, usually in an oily medium. Examples include fluphenazine decanoate, flupenthixol decanoate, risperidone, and olanzapine. Their action is much longer than that of the parent drug, usually 2–4 weeks after a single intramuscular dose. Because their action is prolonged, a small test dose is given before the full dose is used.

Adverse effects

The numerous adverse effects of antipsychotic drugs are related mainly to the antidopaminergic, antiadrenergic, and anticholinergic effects of the drugs (Table 13.5). They are common even at therapeutic doses and so are described in some detail. When prescribing, the general account given here should be supplemented with that found in the SPC or BNF.

Antidopaminergic effects give rise to four kinds of **extrapyramidal** symptoms and signs (Table 13.6). These effects often appear at therapeutic doses and are most frequent with conventional antipsychotic drugs.

1 **Acute dystonia** occurs soon after the treatment begins. It is most frequent with butyrophenones and phenothiazines with a piperazine side chain. The clinical features are shown in Table 13.7. The term **oculogyric crisis** is sometimes used to denote the combination of ocular muscle spasm and opisthotonus. The clinical picture is dramatic and sometimes mistaken for histrionic behaviour. Acute dystonia can be controlled by an anticholinergic drug such as biperiden, given carefully by intramuscular injection following the manufacturer's advice about dosage.

2 **Akathisia** is an unpleasant feeling of physical restlessness and a need to move, leading to inability to keep still. It starts usually in the first 2 weeks of treatment but can be delayed for several months. The symptoms are not controlled reliably by antiparkinsonian drugs but generally disappear if the dose is reduced.

3 **Parkinsonian effects** are the most frequent of the extrapyramidal side effects. They are listed in Table 13.8. The syndrome often takes a few weeks to appear. Parkinsonism

Table 13.5 Unwanted effects of first-generation antipsychotic drugs

Effect	Comments
Antidopaminergic effects	
Acute dystonia	
Akathisia	See text
Parkinsonism	
Tardive dyskinesia	
Antiadrenergic effects	
Postural hypotension	Hypotension particularly likely after intramuscular injection and in the elderly
Nasal congestion	
Inhibition of ejaculation	
Anticholinergic effects	
Dry mouth	
Reduced sweating	
Urinary hesitancy and retention	Especially important in the elderly
Constipation	
Blurred vision	
Precipitation of glaucoma	
Other effects	
Cardiac arrhythmias	
Hypothermia	Especially important in the elderly
Weight gain	
Hyperprolactinaemia (leading to amenorrhoea and galactorrhoea)	Chlorpromazine and some other drugs
Hypothermia	
Worsening of epilepsy (some)	
Photosensitivity (some)	
Accumulation of pigment in skin, cornea, and lens (some)	
Neuroleptic malignant syndrome	See Table 13.9 and text

Table 13.6 Extrapyramidal effects of antipsychotic drugs

Effect	Usual interval from starting treatment
Acute dystonia	Days
Akathisia	Days to weeks
Parkinsonism	A few weeks
Tardive dyskinesia	Several years

Table 13.7 Clinical features of acute dystonia

- Torticollis
- Tongue protrusion
- Grimacing
- Spasm of ocular muscles
- Opisthotonus

Table 13.8 Clinical features of parkinsonism

- Akinesia
- Expressionless face
- Lack of associated movements when walking
- Stooped posture
- Rigidity of muscles
- Coarse tremor
- Festinant gait (in severe cases)

can sometimes be controlled by lowering the dose. If this cannot be done without losing the therapeutic effect, an antiparkinsonian drug can be prescribed. With continued treatment, parkinsonian effects may diminish even though the dose of the antipsychotic stays the same. It is appropriate to check at intervals that the antiparkinsonian drug is still required, since these compounds may increase the risk of tardive dyskinesia.

4 **Tardive dyskinesia** is so called because it is characteristically a late complication of antipsychotic treatment. The clinical features are shown in Table 13.9. The condition may be due to supersensitivity of dopamine receptors resulting from prolonged dopamine blockade. Tardive dyskinesia occurs in about five patients per 100 patients treated with FGAs per year—affecting about 15 per cent of patients on long-term treatment. Since it does not always recover when the antipsychotic drugs are stopped, and responds poorly to treatment, prevention is important. This is attempted by keeping the dose and duration of dosage of antipsychotic drugs to the effective minimum and by limiting the use of antiparkinsonian drugs (see above). Usually, the best treatment for tardive dyskinesia is to stop the antipsychotic drug when the state of the mental illness allows this. At first the dyskinesia may worsen, but often it improves after several drug-free months. If the condition does not improve, or if the antipsychotic drug cannot be stopped, an additional drug can be prescribed in an attempt to reduce the dyskinesia. No one drug is uniformly

Table 13.9 Clinical features of tardive dyskinesia

- Chewing and sucking movements
- Grimacing
- Choreoathetoid movements
- Akathisia

successful and specialist advice should be obtained. (The specialist may try a dopamine-receptor antagonist such as sulpiride or a dopamine-depleting agent such as tetrabenazine.)

Antipsychotic drugs may cause *depression,* but as this symptom is part of the clinical picture of chronic schizophrenia, it is not certain whether antipsychotic drugs have an independent effect.

The neuroleptic malignant syndrome (NMS) is a rare but extremely serious effect of neuroleptic treatment, especially with high-potency compounds. The cause of NMS is unknown. The symptoms, which begin suddenly, usually within the first 10 days of treatment, are summarized in Table 13.10. Treatment is symptomatic. The drug is stopped, the patient cooled, fluid balance maintained, and any infection is treated. There is no drug of proven effectiveness. NMS is a serious condition and about 20 per cent of patients die. If a patient has had NMS, specialist advice should be obtained before any further antipsychotic treatment is prescribed.

Weight gain. Both FGAs and SGAs, but particularly clozapine, olanzapine, and quetiapine, can cause substantial weight gain and this can limit their acceptability to patients. It is important to inform the patient about the possibility of weight gain and to monitor their weight while taking the drugs.

Hyperglycaemia. There is evidence that several of the atypical drugs, including olanzapine and risperidone, can induce hyperglycaemia and diabetes. They should therefore be used with caution in patients at risk of developing diabetes, and blood sugar should be routinely monitored in such patients. It should be noted that many patients with schizophrenia have risk factors for developing diabetes.

Specific adverse effects of clozapine. About 2–3 per cent of patients taking clozapine develop leucopenia, and this can progress to agranulocytosis. With regular monitoring leucopenia can be detected early and the drug stopped; usually the white cell count returns to normal. (Monitoring is usually weekly for 18 weeks and twice weekly thereafter.)

Clozapine may also cause excessive salivation, postural hypotension, weight gain, and hyperthermia, and, in high doses, seizures. Clozapine is sedating and respiratory

Table 13.10 Neuroleptic malignant syndrome

Principal features	
Fluctuating level of consciousness	
Hyperthermia	
Muscular rigidity	
Autonomic disturbance	
Associated symptoms	
Mental symptoms	Fluctuating consciousness
	Stupor
Motor symptoms	Increased muscle tone
	Dysphagia
	Dyspnoea
Autonomic symptoms	Hyperpyrexia
	Unstable blood pressure
	Tachycardia
	Excessive sweating
	Salivation
	Urinary incontinence
Laboratory findings	Raised white cell count
	Raised creatinine phosphokinase (CPK)
Consequent problems	Pneumonia
	Cardiovascular collapse
	Thromboembolism
	Renal failure

depression has been reported when it has been combined with benzodiazepines.

Teratogenesis. Although these drugs have not been shown to be teratogenic, they should be used with caution in early pregnancy.

Contraindications. There are several contraindications to the use of antipsychotic drugs. They include myasthenia gravis, Addison's disease, glaucoma, and past or present bone marrow depression. Caution is required when there is liver disease (chlorpromazine should be avoided), renal disease, cardiovascular disorder, parkinsonism, epilepsy, or serious infection. The manufacturer's literature should be consulted for further contraindications to the use of specific drugs.

Choice of drug

Of the many compounds available, the following are among the appropriate choices:

- a more sedating drug— olanzapine, chlorpromazine
- a less sedating drug—risperidone, trifluoperazine, or haloperidol

- a drug with fewer extrapyramidal side effects—sulpiride or risperidone

- an intramuscular preparation for rapid calming—chlorpromazine or haloperidol

- a depot preparation—fluphenazine decanoate or risperidone

- for patients resistant to other antipsychotics—clozapine (to be initiated by a specialist).

Antiparkinsonian drugs

Although these drugs have no direct therapeutic use in psychiatry, they are used to control the extrapyramidal side effects of antipsychotic drugs. For this purpose the anticholinergic compounds used most commonly are benzhexol, benztropine mesylate, procyclidine, and orphenadrine. An injectable preparation of biperiden is useful for the treatment of acute dystonia (see p. 116).

Although these drugs are used to reduce the side effects of antipsychotic drugs, they have side effects of their own. Their anticholinergic side effects can add to those of the antipsychotic drug to increase constipation, and precipitate glaucoma or retention of urine. Also, they may increase the likelihood of tardive dyskinesia (see p. 117). *Benzhexol and procyclidine have euphoriant effects, and are sometimes abused to obtain this action.*

Antidepressant drugs

Antidepressant drugs have therapeutic effects in depressive illness, but do not elevate mood in healthy people (contrast the effects of stimulants such as amphetamine). Drugs with antidepressant properties are divided conveniently into specific serotonin reuptake inhibitors (SSRIs), tricyclic antidepressants, modified tricyclic and related drugs, serotonin (5-HT) and noradrenaline reuptake inhibitors (SNRIs), specific noradrenaline uptake inhibitors (NARIs), and monoamine oxidase inhibitors (MAOIs). There are some differences in efficacy between the drugs which, although minor, may be clinically important, especially when considered alongside the more substantial differences in adverse effects.

Antidepressant drugs increase the monoamines 5-HT and/or noradrenaline (NA). The development of SSRIs suggested that the antidepressant effects result from increased 5-HT function. SNRIs such as reboxetine are also better than placebo although they seem to be less effective than SSRIs in indirect meta-analyses. Thus, both 5-HT and NA may be involved in the mechanism of action of conventional antidepressants although neither is necessary. The antidepressant efficacy of other drugs, such as SGAs and new antidepressants with different pharmacological actions (such as agomelatine, which acts as an agonist at melatonergic MT1 and MT2 receptors and an antagonist at 5-HT_{2C} receptors), demonstrates that innovative approaches to drug development may produce useful results.

Most antidepressants have a long half-life and so can be given once a day. Antidepressants should be withdrawn slowly, because sudden cessation may lead to restlessness, insomnia, anxiety, and nausea. Antidepressant action seems to commence very quickly, although it may be 10–14 days before it is easily detectable clinically.

Specific serotonin reuptake inhibitors (SSRIs)

These drugs selectively inhibit the reuptake of serotonin (5-HT) into presynaptic neurons. Examples are fluoxetine, fluvoxamine, paroxetine, and sertraline. Their antidepressant effect is comparable to that of the tricyclic antidepressant drugs, and because they lack anticholinergic side effects they are safer for patients with prostatism or glaucoma, and when taken in overdose (Table 13.11). They are not sedating. Their side effects are listed in Table 13.12. SSRIs may induce suicidal thoughts or behaviour in some patients, particularly younger people. SSRIs should be avoided in children and adolescents. It is important to monitor all patients who start antidepressant drugs of any kind for the emergence of suicidal thoughts.

Drug interactions. The combination of SSRIs with **MAOIs** should be avoided since the combination may produce a 5-HT toxicity syndrome with hyperpyrexia, rigidity, myoclonus, coma, and death. **Lithium** and **tryptophan** also increase 5-HT function when given with SSRIs—this combination can be useful clinically but needs to be closely monitored. Combinations of lithium and SSRIs are effective for depressive disorders resistant to other treatment. Other interactions are listed in the manufacturer's literature.

Toxic effects. Overdosage leads to vomiting, tremor, and irritability.

Serotonin and noradrenaline reuptake inhibitors (SNRIs)

Venlafaxine blocks 5-HT and noradrenaline reuptake but does not have the anticholinergic effects that characterize

Table 13.11 Indications for SSRI treatment for depressive disorder

Concomitant cardiac disease[a]
Intolerance to anticholinergic side effects
Significant risk of deliberate overdose
Excessive weight gain with previous tricyclic treatment
Sedation undesirable
Obsessive-compulsive disorder with depression

[a] SSRIs are safer than tricyclics but caution is required.

Table 13.12 Side effects of SSRIs

Gastrointestinal	Nausea
	Flatulence
	Diarrhoea
Central nervous system	Insomnia
	Restlessness
	Irritability
	Agitation
	Tremor
	Headache
	(Acute dystonia, rarely)
Sexual	Ejaculatory delay
	Anorgasmia

Table 13.13 Side effects of tricyclic antidepressants

Anticholinergic effects	Dry mouth
	Constipation
	Impaired visual accommodation
	Difficulty in micturition
	Worsening of glaucoma
	Confusion (especially in the elderly)
Alpha-adrenoceptor-blocking effects	Drowsiness
	Postural hypotension
	Sexual dysfunction
Cardiovascular effects	Tachycardia
	Hypotension
	Cardiac conduction deficits
	Cardiac arrhythmia
Other effects	Seizures
	Weight gain

tricyclic antidepressants and is not sedative. Side effects resemble those of SSRIs; in full doses it may cause hypotension. Venlafaxine appears to be slightly more effective than SSRIs in comparative trials but less well tolerated than drugs such as sertraline and citalopram.

Specific noradrenaline reuptake inhibitors

Several tricyclic antidepressants are relatively specific noradrenaline reuptake inhibitors (e.g. desipramine and lofepramine). Reboxetine is a specific noradrenaline reuptake inhibitor. Meta-analysis shows that it is less effective and less well tolerated than most other antidepressants.

Tricyclic antidepressants

These drugs are so named because their chemical structure has three benzene rings. They have many adverse effects (see below) and toxic effects on the cardiovascular system. Because of these effects, tricyclics are being replaced for most purposes by SSRIs. However, they are still important because they are of proven effectiveness in severely depressed patients.

Adverse effects. Tricyclic antidepressants have many side effects which can be divided into the groups shown in Table 13.13. Most of the effects are common and those that are infrequent are important, so the list should be known before prescribing. The following points should be noted.

- Difficulty in micturition may lead to retention of urine in patients with prostatic hypertrophy.
- Cardiac conduction deficits are more frequent in patients with pre-existing heart disease. If it is necessary to prescribe a tricyclic drug to such a patient, a cardiologist's opinion should be sought (it is often possible to choose a drug of another group without this side effect; see below).

- Seizures are infrequent but important. Antidepressant drugs should be avoided if possible in patients with epilepsy; if their use is essential, the dose of anticonvulsant should be adjusted—usually with the advice of the neurologist treating the case.
- Toxic effects: in overdosage, tricyclic antidepressants can produce serious effects requiring urgent medical treatment. These effects include: ventricular fibrillation, conduction disturbances, and low blood pressure; respiratory depression; agitation, twitching, and convulsions; hallucinations, delirium, and coma; retention of urine and pyrexia.
- Teratogenic effects have not been proved, but antidepressants should be used cautiously in the first trimester of pregnancy and the manufacturer's literature consulted.

Contraindications. These include *agranulocytosis*, severe *liver damage*, *glaucoma*, and *prostatic hypertrophy*. The drugs should be *used cautiously in epileptic patients* because they are epileptogenic, in the elderly because they cause hypotension, and after myocardial infarction because of their effects on the heart.

Modified tricyclics and related drugs

The chemical structure of the tricyclics has been modified in various ways to produce drugs with fewer side effects. Of the many drugs, two will be mentioned.

1 **Lofepramine** has less strong anticholinergic side effects than amitriptyline and is less sedating; however, it may

cause anxiety and insomnia. In overdose it is less cardio-toxic than conventional tricyclics.

2 **Trazodone** also has few anticholinergic effects, but has strong sedating properties.

Monoamine oxidase inhibitors

Monoamine oxidase inhibitors (MAOIs) are seldom used as first-line antidepressant treatment because of their side effects and hazardous interactions with other drugs and foodstuffs (described below). They are usually started by a specialist, but since general practitioners and hospital doctors may treat patients who are taking MAOIs, their hazardous interactions should be known.

Monoamine oxidase inhibitors inactivate enzymes that metabolize noradrenaline and 5-HT, and this action probably accounts for their therapeutic effects. They also interfere with the metabolism of tyramine, and certain other pressor amines taken medicinally. MAOIs also interfere with the metabolism in the liver of barbiturates, tricyclic antidepressants, phenytoin, and antiparkinsonian drugs. When the drug is stopped, these inhibitory effects on enzymes disappear slowly, usually over about 2 weeks, so that the potential for food and drug interactions outlasts the taking of the MAOI. MAOIs with more rapidly reversible actions have been produced. Reversible MAOIs are less likely to give rise to serious interactions with foodstuffs and drugs. The various MAOIs differ little in their therapeutic effects.

Commonly used drugs include phenelzine, isocarboxazid, and tranylcypromine. The latter has an amphetamine-like stimulating effect in addition to its property of inhibiting monoamine oxidase. This additional effect improves mood in the short term but can cause dependency. Moclobemide is a *reversible* MAOI.

Adverse effects. The common adverse effects of MAOIs are listed in Table 13.14.

Table 13.14 Side effects of MAOIs

Autonomic	Dry mouth
	Dizziness
	Constipation
	Difficulty in micturition
	Postural hypotension
Central nervous system	Headache
	Tremor
	Paraesthesia
Other	Ankle oedema
	Hepatotoxicity (hydrazines)

Interactions with tyramine in food and drinks. Some foods and drinks contain tyramine, a substance that is normally inactivated in the body by monoamine oxidases. When these enzymes are inhibited by MAOIs, tyramine is not broken down and exerts its effect of releasing noradrenaline, with a consequent pressor effect. (As noted above, with most MAOIs the inhibition lasts for about 2 weeks after the drug has been stopped. With the 'reversible' MAOI, moclobemide, inhibition lasts for a shorter time, usually about 24 hours.) If large amounts of tyramine are ingested, blood pressure rises substantially with a so-called **hypertensive crisis** and, occasionally, a cerebral haemorrhage. An important early symptom of such a crisis is a severe, usually throbbing, headache. The main tyramine-containing foods and drinks to be avoided are listed for reference in Table 13.15. About four-fifths of reported interactions between foodstuffs and MAOIs, and nearly all deaths, have followed the consumption of *cheese*. It is important to consult this list

Table 13.15 Interactions of MAOIs with drugs and food

Due to inactivation of monoamine oxidase
Foods and drinks with high tyramine content
Most cheeses
Extracts of meat and yeast
Smoked or pickled fish
Hung poultry or game
Some red wines
Drugs with pressor effects
Adrenaline, noradrenaline
Amphetamine, ephedrine
Fenfluramine
Phenylpropanolamine
L-Dopa, dopamine
Due to effects on other enzymes
Morphine, pethidine
Procaine, cocaine
Alcohol
Barbiturates
Insulin and oral hypoglycaemics
Drugs that promote brain 5-HT function
SSRIs
Clomipramine
Imipramine
Fenfluramine
L-Tryptophan
Buspirone

and the manufacturer's literature before prescribing MAOIs. Patients should be given a list of foodstuffs and other substances to be avoided (available usually from the manufacturer).

Drug interactions. Patients taking monoamine oxidase inhibitors should not be given drugs metabolized by enzymes inhibited by MAOIs or those that enhance 5-HT functions. The former fall into three groups:

1 **Drugs metabolized by amine oxidases and with pressor effects.** Of these, ephedrine is a constituent of some 'cold cures', and adrenaline is used with local anaesthetics.

2 **Drugs metabolized by other enzymes affected by MAOIs.** The most important of these drugs are listed for reference in Table 13.15. Sensitivity to oral antidiabetic drugs is increased, leading to the risk of hypoglycaemia.

3 **Drugs that potentiate brain 5-HT function** (see Table 13.15). Combinations of these drugs with MAOIs may produce a **5-HT syndrome** with:

   (i)   hyperpyrexia;

   (ii) restlessness, muscle twitching, and rigidity;

   (iii) convulsions and coma.

Combinations of MAOIs and tricyclics. In *specialist practice* combinations of MAOIs and tricyclic antidepressants are sometimes used for resistant depression. Other doctors are unlikely to start this treatment, but they may treat patients already taking the combination.

Treatment of hypertensive crises. Hypertensive crises are treated by parenteral administration of phentolamine or to block alpha-adrenoceptors, if this drug is not available, by intramuscular chlorpromazine. Blood pressure should be followed carefully.

Treatment of the 5-HT syndrome. All medication should be stopped and supportive measures given. Drugs with 5-HT antagonist properties may be tried but their benefits have not been proved: propranolol and cypropeptadine are possible choices.

Contraindications to MAOIs

These include liver disease, phaeochromocytoma, congestive cardiac failure, and conditions which require the patient to take any of the drugs that react with MAOIs.

Management

Because the drugs have so many interactions, MAOIs should not be prescribed as the first drug for the treatment of depressive disorders, and usually specialist advice should be obtained when they appear to be indicated.

Information for patients. The dangers of interactions with foods and other drugs should be explained carefully, and a warning card should be provided. Patients should be warned not to buy any proprietary drugs except from a qualified pharmacist, to whom the card should always be shown.

Choice of drug. Phenelzine is a suitable choice, starting with 15 mg twice daily and increasing cautiously to 15 mg four times a day. Tranylcypromine, which has amphetamine-like effects as well as MAOI properties, is often effective but as noted above some patients become dependent on its stimulant action.

Changing drugs. As noted above, if an MAOI is not effective, *at least 2 weeks* must pass between ceasing the MAOI and starting another kind of antidepressant. As MAOIs should be discontinued slowly, the time for changeover is even longer. These periods are shorter for the reversible MAOI, moclobemide (see above).

Choice of antidepressant

The clinician should become familiar with the use of a small number of drugs from each of the following three groups, in each of which a possible choice of drugs is shown:

1 two SSRIs which are both effective and reasonably well tolerated (we suggest sertraline and citalopram);

2 a drug of optimal efficacy—venlafaxine;

3 a sedating tricyclic—amitriptyline or trazodone;

4 a less sedating tricyclic—imipramine or lofepramine.

Although there are small but quantifiable differences between antidepressants in efficacy and speed of onset of action, the choice depends on an assessment for each patient of the likely importance of side effects, toxic effects, and interactions with other drugs. Of course, given a number of reasonable generic choices, cost should be taken into account.

Side effects. Sedating effects may useful when depression is accompanied by anxiety and insomnia, but may be troublesome for drivers of motor vehicles or other forms of transport, and for operators of machinery. Anticholinergic side effects need to be avoided for patients with prostatism or glaucoma.

Toxic effects. Cardiotoxic effects should be considered especially when there is an increased risk that the patient may take a deliberate overdose, or there is cardiac disease.

Epilepsy. All antidepressants have the potential to provoke seizures and so the dose of antiepileptic drugs may have to be increased in patients with epilepsy.

Interaction with other drugs used to treat medical disorders. Consult the BNF or SPC if the patient is taking or is likely to commence medication for another condition, and a choice should be made to prevent drug interactions.

Cost. It is appropriate to choose the least expensive drug within the group that is clinically appropriate.

Advice to patients

Before prescribing, the following points should be explained and discussed with the patient:

Delayed response. A noticeable therapeutic effect is likely to be delayed for up to 2 or 3 weeks, but side effects will appear sooner. The improvement in symptoms may not be linear over time and there may be temporary setbacks on the road to recovery.

Adverse effects. The common effects should be described, including drowsiness, and a warning given of the dangers of driving a motor vehicle or using machinery even when only slightly drowsy. Patients taking SSRIs may feel irritable or restless. With tricyclics, dry mouth and accommodation difficulties are common side effects.

Effects of alcohol. The effects of alcohol are increased when antidepressants are taken.

Older patients. Older patients should be warned about the effects of postural hypotension and told how to minimize these (e.g. by rising slowly from bed). Effects of tricyclics on bladder function should be explained. Reassurance can be given that most of these effects are likely to decrease with time.

Starting treatment

Drugs with sedative side effects can be given in a single dose at night, so that sedative effects help the patient to sleep and the peak of other side effects occurs during sleep. SSRIs and other drugs that cause insomnia should be given in the first half of the day, usually in a single dose.

Doses should be reduced for elderly patients, those with cardiac disease, or prostatism, or other conditions that may be exacerbated by the drugs, and those with disease of the liver or kidneys. If agitation, as a symptom of depressive disorder, is not controlled by a sedative antidepressant, a phenothiazine can be added.

Since patients feel the side effects of the drug before experiencing its benefits, they should be seen again after a week, or earlier if the disorder is severe. At this interview, the severity of depression is reassessed, side effects are discussed, and encouragement given to continue taking the medication until the therapeutic response occurs.

When tricyclics are prescribed, the starting dose should be moderate; for example, amitriptyline 50 mg per day increased gradually to 150 mg per day according to the urgency. The dose may be increased further if there is no response, after the extent of the side effects has been observed.

Non-response

The management of depressed patients who fail to respond to antidepressant medication is discussed on p. 235.

Mood-stabilizing drugs

Drugs that prevent recurrence of bipolar disorder are often called **mood stabilizers**. The term is simply descriptive and does not denote a pharmacological class. The main mood stabilizers are lithium and a number of antiepileptic drugs including sodium valproate, carbamazepine, and lamotrigine. Mood stabilizers may also be effective at treating acute mood episodes. For example, lithium and sodium valproate are used to treat acute mania, and lithium and lamotrigine are used in depressive disorders, especially those occurring in bipolar disorder.

Lithium

Pharmacology

It is not known which of lithium's many pharmacological actions explains its therapeutic effects, but its effect in increasing brain 5-HT function may be relevant. Lithium also acts on secondary messenger systems within neurons—in particular it inhibits inositol monophosphatase and glycogen synthase kinase 3 (GSK-3), and current research is investigating these actions as potential approaches to developing new versions of lithium.

Lithium is absorbed and excreted by the kidneys where, like sodium, it is filtered and partly reabsorbed. Lithium concentrations rise, sometimes to dangerous levels, in three circumstances:

1 **Dehydration.** When the proximal tubule absorbs more water, more lithium is reabsorbed.

2 **Sodium depletion.** Lithium is carried by the mechanism that carries sodium, and more lithium is transported when there is less sodium.

3 **Thiazide therapy.** Thiazide diuretics increase the excretion of sodium but not of lithium, and plasma lithium rises.

Dosage and plasma concentrations

General practitioners are often asked to supervise continuing treatment with lithium started by specialists, and hospital doctors treat these patients for other conditions. Because the therapeutic and toxic doses are close together, it is essential to measure plasma concentrations of lithium regularly during treatment. Measurement is made first after 4–7 days, then weekly for 3 weeks, and then, provided that a satisfactory steady state has been achieved, once every 12 weeks.

The *timing of the measurement* is important. After an oral dose, plasma lithium levels rise by a factor of two or three within about 4 hours and then fall to the steady-state level. Since the steady-state level is important in therapeutics, concentrations are normally measured *12 hours after the last dose*, usually just before the morning dose, which can be delayed if necessary for an hour or two. It is the steady-state level 12 hours after the last dose, not the 'peak', which is the level referred to when discussing the concentrations aimed at in treatment and prophylaxis. If an unexpectedly high concentration is found, the first step is to find out whether the patient has inadvertently taken the morning dose before the blood sample was taken.

The required plasma concentrations are:

- for prophylaxis: 0.5–1.0 mmol/litre, increased occasionally to a maximum of 1.2 mmol/litre;
- for treatment of acute mania: 0.8–1.5 mmol/litre.

Toxic effects begin to appear over 1.5 mmol/litre and may be serious over 2.0 mmol/litre. Although the therapeutic effect is related to the steady state concentration of lithium, any renal effects caused by the drug (see below) may relate to the peak concentrations. For this reason, the drug is often given twice a day. Delayed-release tablets have been introduced for the same reason, but the time-course of plasma levels resulting from these tablets is not substantially different from that of standard preparations.

Adverse effects. These effects are listed in Table 13.16.

Table 13.16 Side effects of lithium

1 Early effects
Polyuria
Tremor
Dry mouth
Metallic taste
Weakness and fatigue
2 Later effects
Fine tremor[a]
Polyuria and polydipsia
Hair loss
Thyroid enlargement
Hypothyroidism
Impaired concentration
Weight gain
Gastrointestinal distress
Sedation
Acne
Impaired memory (see text)
ECG changes[b]
3 Long-term effects on the kidney
See text

[a] Coarse tremor is a sign of toxicity.
[b] T wave flattening and QRS widening (reversible when drug is stopped).

The following points should be noted.

- **Polyuria** can lead to dehydration with the risk of lithium intoxication. Patients should be advised to drink enough water to compensate for the fluid loss.
- **Tremor.** Fine tremor occurs frequently. Most patients adapt to this; for those who do not, propranolol 10 mg three times daily often reduces the symptom. *Coarse tremor is a sign of toxicity.*
- **Enlargement of the thyroid** occurs in about 5 per cent of patients taking lithium. The thyroid shrinks again if thyroxine is given while lithium is continued, and it returns to normal a month or two after lithium has been stopped.
- **Hypothyroidism** occurs commonly (up to 20 per cent of women patients) with a compensatory rise in thyroid-stimulating hormone. Tests of thyroid function should be performed every 6 months, and a continuous watch kept for suggestive clinical signs, particularly lethargy and substantial weight gain. If hypothyroidism develops and lithium treatment is still necessary, thyroxine treatment should be added.
- **Impaired memory.** Usually this takes the form of everyday lapses such as forgetting well-known names. The cause is not known.
- **Long-term effects on the kidney.** A few patients develop a persistent impairment of concentrating ability. A few patients develop nephrogenic diabetes insipidus due to interference with the effect of antidiuretic hormone. This syndrome does not respond to antidiuretic treatments but usually recovers when the drug is stopped. Provided doses are kept below 1.2 mmol/litre, renal damage is rare in patients whose renal function is normal at the start. Nevertheless, it is usual to test renal function every 6 months.

Toxic effects

The toxic effects of lithium (Table 13.17) constitute a serious medical emergency, as they can progress

Table 13.17 Toxic effects of lithium

- Nausea, vomiting
- Diarrhoea
- Coarse tremor
- Ataxia, dysarthria
- Muscle twitching, hyper-reflexia
- Confusion, coma
- Convulsions
- Renal failure
- Cardiovascular collapse

through coma and fits to death. If these symptoms appear, lithium should be stopped at once and a high intake of fluid provided, with extra sodium chloride to stimulate an osmotic diuresis. Lithium is cleared rapidly if renal function is normal but in severe cases renal dialysis may be needed. Most patients recover completely, some die, and a few survive with permanent neurological damage.

Teratogenesis

Lithium crosses the placenta, and there are reports of increased rates of **fetal abnormalities,** most affecting the heart. Therefore, the drug should be avoided in the first trimester of pregnancy if possible. Lithium should be stopped a week before delivery or otherwise reduced by half and stopped during labour to be restarted afterwards. However, lithium is **secreted into breast milk** to the extent that plasma lithium concentrations of breast-fed infants can be half or more of that in the maternal blood. Therefore, bottle-feeding is usually advisable.

Drug interactions

There are several important interactions between lithium and other drugs. The manufacturer's literature or a book of reference should be consulted whenever lithium treatment is started and a second drug is prescribed for a patient taking lithium. The principal interactions are listed for reference in Box 13.1.

Contraindications

These are not absolute but include *end-stage renal failure* or *recent renal disease, cardiac failure* or *recent myocardial infarction*, and *chronic diarrhoea* sufficient to alter electrolytes. Lithium should not be prescribed if the patient is judged unlikely to observe the precautions required for its safe use.

Management of lithium treatment

Lithium is usually continued for at least 2 years, and often for much longer. In patients taking long-term therapy, the need for the drug should be reviewed every 5 years. Review should take into account any persistence of mild mood fluctuations which suggest the possibility of relapse if treatment is stopped. Continuing medication is more likely to be needed if the patient has previously had several episodes of mood disorder within a short time, or if previous episodes were so severe that even a small risk of recurrence should be avoided. There should be compelling reasons for continuing treatment for more than 5 years, although patients have taken lithium safely for much longer periods.

Lithium should be withdrawn gradually over a few weeks; sudden withdrawal may cause irritability, emotional lability, and, occasionally, relapse (more often into mania than depression).

The management of patients on lithium. Treatment with lithium is usually started by a specialist, but general practitioners are often involved in continued treatment. Careful management is essential because of the potential effects of therapeutic doses of lithium on the thyroid and, possibly, the kidneys, and the toxic effects of excessive dosage.

Before starting lithium, a note should be made of any other medication taken by the patient and a *physical examination* including weight and ECG should be done. Thyroid function tests, electrolytes and urea, blood creatinine levels (and creatinine clearance test if indicated), haemoglobin, ESR, and a full blood count are often done as well. If indicated, pregnancy tests should be done.

Advice to the patient. The doctor should explain:

1 the common side effects;

2 early toxic effects which would indicate an unduly high blood level of lithium;

 BOX 13.1 Principal interactions between lithium and other drugs

1 Lithium concentrations may be increased by several drugs, including:

- *haloperidol;*
- *thiazide diuretics* (potassium-sparing and loop diuretics seem less likely to increase lithium levels but should be used cautiously);
- *muscle relaxants*: when a patient on lithium is to have an operation the anaesthetist should be informed in advance because the effect of muscle relaxants may be potentiated; if possible, lithium should be stopped 48–72 hours before the operation;
- *non-steroidal anti-inflammatory drugs* (NSAIDs);

- *some antibiotics:* metronidazole and spectinomycin;
- *some antihypertensives:* angiotensin converting enzyme inhibitors and methyldopa.

2 Interaction with antipsychotics:

- potentiation of extrapyramidal symptoms;
- occasionally, confusion and delirium.

3 Interaction with specific serotonin reuptake inhibitors (SSRIs):

- 5-HT syndrome (see p. 122).

4 Later action with ECT may cause a reaction similar to a 5-HT syndrome.

3 the need to keep strictly to the dosage prescribed;

4 the arrangements for monitoring blood levels of lithium;

5 the circumstances in which unduly high levels are most likely to arise—low salt diet, unaccustomed severe exercise, gastroenteritis, renal infection, or dehydration secondary to fever;

6 the need to stop the drug and seek medical advice if these conditions arise.

If the patient consents, it is usually appropriate to include another member of the family in these discussions. An explanatory leaflet should be provided, repeating the same points for reference.

Starting lithium prophylaxis. Lithium carbonate is usually given in a single night-time dose. The commonest dose for adults is 800 mg per day, tapered as indicated. The dose is adjusted until a lithium level of 0.5–1.0 mmol/litre is achieved in a sample taken 12 hours after the last dose. The optimal level is usually the highest level within this range tolerated without significant adverse effects. Levels between 1.0 and 1.5 mmol/litre may be used in the treatment of acute mania, but vigilance is required for adverse effects. Steady-state levels are usually achieved 5 days after a dose adjustment.

As treatment continues lithium estimations should be carried out every 3–6 months or whenever the clinical status of the patient changes. Thyroid and renal function tests should be checked every 12 months. It is important to have a way of reminding the doctor about the times for the next repeat investigation. If two consecutive thyroid function tests a month apart show hypothyroidism, lithium should be stopped or L-thyroxine prescribed. Mild but troublesome polyuria is a reason for attempting a reduction in dose, whereas severe persistent polyuria is an indication for specialist renal investigation. A persistent leucocytosis is not uncommon and is apparently harmless; it reverses soon after the drug is stopped.

While lithium is continued, the doctor must keep in mind the possibility of interactions if new drugs are required by the patient.

Sodium valproate

Pharmacology. Like carbamazepine, sodium valproate was introduced as an anticonvulsant. Later it was found to control acute mania. It is probably less effective than lithium in preventing recurrence of bipolar disorder, but it is increasingly used and, in the USA, is now used more commonly than lithium. There are several formulations of valproate which vary in terms of pharmacokinetics. Most trials have investigated valproate semisodium, but this is currently more expensive than other formulations.

Dosage and plasma concentration. The doses depend on the formulation. Here we refer to valproate semisodium—the equivalent doses for other formulations may need to be 30 per cent higher. For most outpatients valproate should be started at 250–500 mg in divided doses or as a single dose at night. The dose can be titrated upward by 250–500 mg per day every few days, depending on adverse effects. The usual maintenance dose is between 750 and 1250 mg per day.

Adverse effects. Common adverse effects include sedation, tiredness, tremor, and gastrointestinal disturbance. Reversible hair loss may occur in 10 per cent of patients. Sodium valproate may cause thrombocytopenia and has other unwanted effects that should be studied in a reference source before a patient is treated.

Drug interactions. Valproate displaces highly protein-bound drugs such as other antiepileptic drugs from their protein-binding sites and may therefore increase plasma levels. Valproate inhibits the metabolism of lamotrigine, which must be used at about 50 per cent of the usual dose when prescribed in combination.

Teratogenesis. Valproate is teratogenetic and so must be avoided if possible in pregnant women and used with caution in women of childbearing potential.

Lamotrigine

Pharmacology. Lamotrigine also is primarily an anticonvulsant. It may be effective in bipolar depression—possibly without inducing mania—and it also prevents depressive (but not manic) relapse in bipolar disorder.

Dosage and plasma concentration. Lamotrigine must be initiated very gradually, initially 25 mg daily for 2 weeks, then 50 mg daily for 2 weeks, and then further gradual increase. The usual dose in bipolar disorder is 100–300 mg daily.

Adverse effects. A rash may occur in 3–5 per cent of patients—the risk can be reduced by using gradual dosing (see above). Other side effects include nausea, headache, tremor, and dizziness.

Drug interactions. Lamotrigine levels are increased by valproate. The combination of lamotrigine and carbamazepine may cause neurotoxicity.

Teratogenesis. Lamotrigine has been found to increase rates of cleft palate.

Carbamazepine

Pharmacology. Carbamazepine was introduced as an anticonvulsant. Later it was found to prevent the recurrence of affective disorder. It is effective in some patients who are unresponsive to lithium, and for some with rapidly recurring bipolar disorder. Both the effect in acute mania and the long-term efficacy of carbamazepine are less certain than those of lithium, but it is used successfully both as monotherapy and in combination with lithium in some patients.

Dosage and plasma concentration. Carbamazepine is usually started at 400 mg daily in outpatients but may be increased up to 800–1000 mg or higher in inpatients. The doses used for long-term treatment depend on tolerability and can range from 200–1600 mg daily. Monitoring of blood levels is less important than continued clinical vigilance for the emergence of adverse effects.

Adverse effects. Adverse effects may be troublesome if plasma levels are high, and include drowsiness, dizziness, nausea, double vision, and skin rash. A rare but serious side effect is agranulocytosis. A full blood count and liver function tests should be done before commencing treatment.

Drug interactions. Carbamazepine can accelerate the metabolism of some other drugs and of the hormones in the contraceptive pill, reducing its effectiveness. It is advisable therefore to consider another form of contraception. Drug interactions should be checked in a reference source before prescribing other drugs to a patient taking carbamazepine.

Teratogenesis. Carbamazepine seems to be one of the safest mood stabilizers.

Cognition-enhancing drugs

Anticholinesterase inhibitors

These drugs, including donepezil, rivastigmine, and galantamine, increase the function of acetylcholine, which can improve cognitive functioning, and they are used in the treatment of Alzheimer's disease. On average, they have a modest beneficial effect that might persist for a number of months but they do not halt or reverse the disorder. These drugs are used following assessment in a specialist clinic, including tests of cognitive, global, and behavioural functioning and assessment of activities of daily living.

Adverse effects. The main adverse effects of anticholinesterase inhibitors include anorexia, nausea, vomiting, and diarrhoea.

■ Other physical treatments

Electroconvulsive therapy (ECT)

ECT is a specialist treatment and the reader requires only a general knowledge of its use; those requiring further information should consult the *Shorter Oxford Textbook of Psychiatry* or another specialist text.

In ECT, an electric current is applied to the skull of an anaesthetized patient to produce seizure activity while the consequent motor effects are prevented with a muscle relaxant. The electrodes which deliver the current can be placed with one on each side of the head (**bilateral ECT**) or with both on the same side (**unilateral ECT**).

Unilateral placement on the *non-dominant side* results in less memory impairment but may be less effective than bilateral ECT. Bilateral placement is therefore preferred when a rapid response is essential, or when unilateral ECT has not been effective.

The beneficial effect, which depends on the cerebral seizure, not on the motor component, is thought to result from neurotransmitter changes, probably involving 5-HT and noradrenaline transmission. ECT acts more quickly than antidepressant drugs, although the outcome after 3 months is similar.

Indications

The main indications for ECT are:

1 **The need for an urgent response:**

   (i) when life is threatened in a severe depressive disorder by refusal to drink or eat or very intense suicidal ideation;

   (ii) in puerperal psychiatric disorders when it is important that the mother should resume the care of her baby as quickly as possible.

2 **For a resistant depressive disorder,** following failure to respond to thorough treatment with antidepressant medication.

3 **For two uncommon syndromes:**

   (i) catatonic schizophrenia (see p. 249);

   (ii) depressive stupor (see p. 226).

Adverse effects of ECT

ECT has a number of adverse effects. Patients often have a brief period of headache after the treatment.

A degree of cognitive impairment after treatment is relatively common although this clears rapidly in most patients. The more effective forms of ECT (e.g. higher dose, bilateral) appear to be more likely to cause cognitive problems. Some patients report a persistent loss of autobiographical memories but this has been difficult to show objectively in research studies. Depressive disorder can also lead to cognitive impairment, including memory problems, and it is therefore possible that the disorder itself is responsible. It is probably best to inform the patient that they may experience some short-term problems and that some patients report longer-term problems but that these appear to be uncommon. There are occasional effects from the anaesthetic procedure: the teeth, tongue, or lips may be injured while the airway is introduced and, rarely, muscle relaxants cause prolonged apnoea.

Mortality of ECT

The death rate from ECT is about 4 per 100 000 treatments, closely similar to that of an anaesthetic given for any minor procedure to a similar group of patients. Mortality is greater in patients with cardiovascular disease, and due usually to ventricular fibrillation or myocardial infarction.

Contraindications

The contraindications are those for any anaesthetic procedure and any condition made worse by the changes in blood pressure and cardiac rhythm which occur even in a well-modified fit: serious heart disease, cerebral aneurysm, and raised intracranial pressure. Extra care is required with diabetic patients who take insulin and for patients with sickle cell trait. Although risks rise somewhat in old age, so do the risks of untreated depressive disorder and of drug treatment.

Consent to ECT

Before ECT, a full explanation is given of the procedure and its risks and benefits, before asking for consent. If a patient refuses consent or is unable to give it, for example because he is in a stupor, and if the procedure is essential, the psychiatrist seeks a second opinion and discusses the situation with relatives (although they cannot consent on behalf of the patient). In the UK and many other countries, there are procedures for authorizing ECT when the patient refuses but it is essential (these are set out in the Mental Health Act or corresponding legislation). Patients treated under these provisions seldom question the need for treatment once they have recovered.

The technique

ECT is administered by a psychiatrist, who applies the current, and an anaesthetist and a nurse. The procedure is described in specialist textbooks. ECT is usually given twice a week with a total of 6–12 treatments, according to progress. Response begins usually after two or three treatments; if there has been no response after six to eight treatments, it is unlikely that more ECT will produce useful change.

As some patients relapse after ECT, antidepressants are usually started towards the end of the course to reduce the risk of relapse.

Treatment with bright light

There is some evidence that bright light treatment is effective in seasonal affective disorder (SAD) (see p. 227). When a therapeutic effect appears it is rapid, but relapse is common. Light is administered usually at 6–8 am using a commercially available light box. The intensity of the light is usually about that of a bright spring day. The mode of action is uncertain; the light may correct circadian rhythms, which seem to be phase-delayed in seasonal affective disorder.

Psychosurgery

Psychosurgery refers to the use of neurological procedures to modify the symptoms of psychiatric illness by operating either on the nuclei of the brain or on the white matter. The treatment had a period of wide use after its introduction in 1936 and until the development of effective psychotropic drugs in the 1960s. Nowadays, it is used rarely and then only in a few special centres, mainly for a very small minority of patients with obsessional or prolonged depressive disorders which have failed to respond to vigorous and prolonged pharmacological and behavioural treatment.

Modern surgery involves small lesions placed by stereotaxic methods, usually to interrupt the frontolimbic connections. With these restricted lesions, side effects are unusual; when they occur they include apathy, weight gain, disinhibition, and epilepsy. There have been no randomized controlled trials to test the value of the operation, and its use is diminishing even further as pharmacological and behavioural treatments continue to improve.

■ Prescribing for special groups

Children

Most childhood psychiatric disorders are treated without medication. Many drugs that are licensed for use in adults have not been adequately studied in children. The indications for drug treatment are considered in Chapter 32. When drugs are required, care must be taken in selecting the appropriate dose. Usually, medication will have been started by a specialist who will advise about continuing treatment.

Elderly patients

These patients are often sensitive to drug side effects and may have impaired renal or hepatic function, so it is important to start with low doses and increase to about half the adult dose in appropriate cases.

Pregnant women

Psychotropic drugs should be avoided if possible during the first trimester of pregnancy because of the risk of teratogenesis. If medication is needed for a woman who could become pregnant, advice is given about contraception. If the patient is already pregnant and medication is essential the manufacturer's advice should be followed and the risks discussed with the patient. If the patient becomes pregnant while taking a psychotropic drug the risk of relapse should be weighed against the reported teratogenic risk of the drug. In general, it is safer to use long-established drugs for which there has been ample time to accumulate experience about safety. The following points concern the classes of psychotropic drugs.

- **Anxiolytics** are seldom essential in early pregnancy since psychological treatment is usually an effective alternative.

- **If antidepressants are required,** amitriptyline and imipramine have been in long use, without convincing evidence of teratogenic effects.

- **Antipsychotic drugs.** It is important to discuss contraception with schizophrenic women, and to re-evaluate the need for antipsychotics if the patient becomes pregnant.

- **Lithium carbonate** should not be started in pregnancy because its use is associated with an increased rate of cardiac abnormality in the fetus. Contraception is especially important for women who may become manic, and it is prudent to leave a month between the last dose of lithium and the ending of contraceptive measures. If a patient conceives when taking lithium, there is no absolute indication for termination but the risks should be explained, specialist advice obtained, and the fetus examined by ultrasound. Mothers who are taking lithium at term should, if possible, stop gradually well before delivery. The drug should not be taken during labour. Serum lithium concentration should be measured frequently during labour and the use of diuretics avoided.

- **Valproate** should be used cautiously in women of childbearing potential, and should not be started in pregnancy, because of its teratogenic potential.

Mothers who are breast-feeding

Psychotropic drugs should be prescribed cautiously to women who are breast-feeding because these pass into breast milk and the possibility is not ruled out that they may affect brain development. Some authorities recommend that women receiving psychotropic medication should not breast-feed. Others continue treatment cautiously with careful monitoring of the baby. Benzodiazepines pass readily into breast milk, causing sedation. Most neuroleptics and antidepressants pass rather less readily into the milk; sulpiride, doxepin, and dothiepin are secreted in larger amounts and should be avoided. Lithium carbonate enters milk freely and breast-feeding should be avoided. The advice of a specialist should be obtained.

Patients with concurrent medical illness

Special care is needed in prescribing for patients with medical illness, especially liver and kidney disorders, which may interfere with metabolism and excretion of drugs. Conversely, medical disorders may be exacerbated by the side effects of some psychotropic drugs. For example, cardiac disorder and epilepsy may be affected adversely by some antidepressant drugs (see p. 125), while drugs with anticholinergic side effects exacerbate glaucoma and may provoke retention of urine.

 Further reading

Stahl, S.M. (2008). *Essential Psychopharmacology*, 3rd edn. Cambridge University Press. A comprehensive and very well illustrated review of psychopharmacology.

Psychological treatment

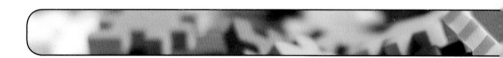

■ Core psychological techniques

Psychological treatment is ubiquitous in medical practice; all doctors use psychological treatment techniques every day, with every patient. This is because the words that we use when we speak (or write) to patients have the power to heal and to harm. This is the essence of the psychological treatments—they are treatments that use the power of words to improve the physical and emotional status of patients.

Carefully chosen words can improve your patient's morale, engage them with self-care, encourage them to adhere to medicines and to attend appointments, and reassure them that the resumption of normal daily activities is permissible and indeed desirable. Ill-chosen words can increase dependency, disability, and distress. All doctors therefore need to be able to employ **core psychological techniques** in their everyday practice. These core psychological techniques (Table 14.1) are involved in every therapeutic relationship, whether in psychiatry or other branches of medicine. They are also involved in most formal psychological treatments.

Develop a therapeutic relationship. This can improve the patient's adherence to more specific psychological methods, sustain them through periods of distress, and instil hope. In an appropriate therapeutic relationship, patients should feel that the professional is concerned about them and takes time for them, but also understand that the relationship is distinct from friendship, and is one that the professional has also with other patients. Occasionally, a patient–professional relationship can become too intense so that it impedes progress—see 'Independence versus dependence' below.

Table 14.1 Core psychological techniques

- Develop a therapeutic relationship
- Actively listen to your patient's concerns
- Provide information, explanation, and advice (psychoeducation)
- Allow the expression of emotion
- Improve morale
- Review and develop personal strengths
- Actively endorse, encourage, and facilitate self-help
- Involve, educate, and support carers

Actively listen to your patient's concerns. Patients feel helped when they describe their problems to a sympathetic person, and many complain that doctors (whether in primary care, general hospitals, or mental health settings) do not listen for long enough before they offer advice. To be effective, listening requires adequate time, and patients should feel that they have the doctor's undivided attention and have been understood. Non-verbal signs of attention and occasional summarizing/checking out understanding of what has been said can help, as can summarizing the patient's perspective in clinical letters which are copied to patients.

Allow the release of emotion. It is a common experience that the expression of strong emotion is followed by a sense of relief. Some patients feel ashamed to reveal their feelings to others and need to be assured that to do this is not a sign of weakness. If a patient or relative cries, offer support by looking concerned, by acknowledging verbally that they are upset (e.g. 'I'm sorry you're upset, it's clearly a difficult time for you'), and by offering a tissue (have some handy on your desk). After an appropriate period of time, aim to improve morale by saying something about the way forward, such as 'Perhaps now would be a good time to start to think about how things can be better for you—how does that sound?'.

Improve morale. Patients who have prolonged or recurrent medical or social problems may give up hope of improvement. Low morale, caused in this or other ways, undermines further treatment and rehabilitation. Even if there is no hope of recovery, such as in terminal cancer, it is usually possible to improve morale, for example by describing how pain and distress can be minimized, and who will be there to help near the end.

Review and develop personal strengths. Medical diagnosis focuses on what is wrong, rather than what is right. However, an effective treatment plan should take into account what abilities and social supports are intact, and help patients to bolster them, in order to overcome the current episode of illness, and to reduce risk of relapse in the future.

Provide information, explanation, and advice. In mental health settings, this is termed **psychoeducation**. It is an important part of every patient's management. What is said (or written) needs to be accurate, clear, free from jargon, and relevant to the patient's physical and mental condition. It should attempt to correct any misunderstandings about the nature of the condition or the likely outcome. Further details of psychoeducation are given below. In the general hospital, explanations of the cause of physical symptoms should be positive; it is not enough to say that no physical disease has been found. Rather, a convincing model of the genesis of the physical symptoms via physiological processes, and psychological and social factors, should be described.

Actively endorse, encourage, and facilitate self-help. Patients should be helped to achieve an appropriate balance between collaboration with medical treatment and a determination to be self-sufficient. It is usually possible to achieve this important aim even with the most handicapped patients, provided a dependent relationship on the professional is not allowed to develop. It is the patient's illness, and it may be lifelong. It is, therefore, very much in the patient's interest for them to develop the knowledge about their illness, skills in self-management, and day-to-day behaviours that will help to get them well and to keep them well. As patients recover and their confidence grows, self-management can and should play an increasing role in their daily care, progressively replacing the input of healthcare professionals.

Involve, educate, and support carers. Carers are partners in the care of the patient, and may play a crucial role in supporting patients through and out of illness. They may also play a crucial role in perpetuating illness, if their attitudes to and beliefs about the illness are unhelpful. For these reasons, involving the carer in some aspects of psychological treatment, with the consent of the patient, can be beneficial. Written materials used during psychological treatment can be shared with carers, for example, or carers can be invited into meetings with patients at which diagnosis and treatment plans are discussed.

■ Psychoeducation

Psychoeducation is, simply, the education of patients (and their carers, if appropriate) about their illness. It is usual to inform the patient of:

1 the name and nature of their illness;

2 the likely causes of the illness, in their particular case;

3 what health services can do to help them;

4 what they can do to help themselves (i.e. self-help).

It is closely related to several core psychological techniques, including the provision of information, explanation and advice, active endorsement, encouragement and facilitation of self-help, and the involvement, education, and support of carers (see above). It often involves bibliotherapy (see below), and is often considered to be the first level of stepped care (see below).

■ Provision of psychological support

For most people facing adverse events (e.g. death of a close relative, or diagnosis of a life-threatening condition) or coping with adverse circumstances (e.g. coping with a handicapped child), psychological support is provided informally by their social network, including their close and extended family. In other circumstances, it can be provided by statutory bodies (such as social work services) or non-statutory bodies (such as charities and voluntary organizations). Occasionally, however, it will be provided by health services, and it can be an effective and valuable use of healthcare professionals' time.

Psychological support involves the use of the core psychological techniques described above to:

- reduce distress during a short episode of self-limiting illness or personal misfortune;
- support the patient and instil hope until a specific treatment has a beneficial effect (e.g. while waiting for the therapeutic effects of an antidepressant drug);
- sustain patients whose medical or psychiatric condition cannot be treated, or whose stressful life problems cannot be resolved (e.g. the problems of caring for a handicapped child).

Before choosing supportive treatment, the vital question is whether a more structured and active form of psychological or other treatment could bring about change. Supportive sessions generally last for about 15 minutes, though the first session of treatment is often longer. Sessions are often weekly at first but may become less frequent. The length, frequency, and number of sessions should be agreed with the patient at the start, to avoid the development of dependency.

■ Stepped care in psychological treatment

Psychological treatments may be time-consuming, and often need to be delivered by specially trained staff. As a result, there are often waiting lists with significant delays before starting treatment. A 'one size fits all' approach to treatment is now seen as inappropriate and, instead, a 'stepped care approach' is desirable. This means that most patients with a particular disorder will start with 'level one' treatment, which is simple, quick to provide, and usually inexpensive. If level one treatment fails, the patient moves to the level two treatment and, again, if this fails, to level three. Treatment algorithms may dictate that a patient misses out one or more levels if there is a clear clinical need.

In psychological treatments, **level one** of this stepped care approach often involves basic information about the disorder and self-help approaches, delivered by booklet, book, or the Internet. At this level, there is minimal input by professionals. **Level two** may involve group treatment (see below) or supported computerized delivery of a psychological treatment. **Level three** may involve individual treatment, that is face to face and one to one. Finally, there may be a further level, for the very few treatment-resistant patients who need specialist or particularly intensive treatments.

Bibliotherapy is the use as a treatment by patients of books or similar reading. It often comprises the first level of psychological treatment. A healthcare practitioner should recommend, in almost every case, appropriate reading material for the particular patient and, potentially, also their carer(s). Their recommendation should bear in mind the patient's existing level of knowledge, their motivation, and the nature of their clinical problem. As with any treatment, adherence to bibliotherapy is sometimes poor. Adherence can be increased by the professional in the following ways.

1 **Providing a clear rationale for the self-help approach.** The professional might say:

   'You need to become the expert in managing this problem. I can be here to help and support from time to time, but I can't be there when you most need me.'

2 **Actively endorsing a particular resource:**

   'Lots of people with problems like yours find this book useful (show patient the book, from your bookshelf). It's easy to read, and is available in most public libraries and bookstores. I'll give you the details . . .'

3 **Suggesting reading particular chapters or sections.** In larger texts, some sections may be much more relevant than others:

   'Chapters X and Y are particularly relevant to your problems. Chapter X describes anxiety symptoms and their causes, and Chapter Y describes the beginnings of a self-help approach to managing anxiety.'

4 **Making a follow-up appointment,** to review the patient's progress with the self-help approach:

   'I'd like to see you again in 2 weeks' time, when we can review how you've got on with those chapters. Do you have any questions?'

■ Independence versus dependence

The aim of doctors, other healthcare professionals, and treatments including psychological treatments, is to maximize the patient's functioning and to enhance their independence, wherever possible. This is why modern management always incorporates elements of self-management, and why psychoeducation is an essential part of every management plan. However, those aspects of the doctor–patient interaction that can be therapeutic and supportive can also be difficult to give up for some patients, who can become excessively dependent on healthcare professionals.

Dependence is most likely to arise during psychological treatment but it can occur in the course of any treatment. Signs that the relationship is becoming too dependent include (i) asking questions about the doctor's personal life, (ii) efforts to prolong interviews beyond the agreed time, (iii) attempts to contact the doctor for unwarranted reasons, (iv) presentation of new or increased problems when reduction in or termination of contact is discussed, and (v) repeatedly bringing or offering gifts.

Dependent patients do not make appropriate efforts to help themselves. They request or demand increased attention and, if the therapist does not respond, they may become anxious or angry, or make increasingly unreasonable demands. In these circumstances, the following approaches can be helpful.

● Remember how important the relationship is to the patient. Make and keep appointments in a reliable manner, letting the patient know when you will be unavailable, for example due to leave.

● Maintain usual professional boundaries, and behave as a professional rather than as a friend. For example, make sure that you have a 'buffer' between you and the patient, by giving only your secretary's or ward administrator's phone number, rather than your office number, mobile, or email address. Do not fit in additional appointments at the request of the patient, unless there is a definite clinical need. Maintain the usual rules about touching patients; expressing sympathy and offering a tissue to a sobbing patient is desirable, but hugging them is not. Do not agree to meet the patient 'outside work'. Treat the patient as you would any other. Keep accurate and contemporaneous notes of all interactions with the patient, whether in person, in phone, by email, or in writing. Seek advice from another doctor or healthcare professional and, perhaps, ongoing support and supervision—sharing such problems with another professional can be very helpful.

● Discuss the perceived difficulties with the patient, alongside a discussion of the way forward, towards independence, when the patient will have the confidence to deal with their life's problems alone. Recognize that this transition can be frightening for the patient, but encourage them to believe that it is possible.

Transference

In the practice of psychotherapy, an intense relationship between the patient and doctor is called transference. The term originates from Freud's theory that, in such a relationship, the patient transfers to the doctor feelings and thoughts that originated in a close relationship during childhood—usually with one or other parent. When the current feelings are positive, there is said to be **positive transference**; when the current feelings are negative, there is said to be **negative transference**.

Countertransference

Not only may patients transfer to their therapists feelings that properly belong elsewhere, but therapists may also do the same with their patients. Thus therapists may develop strong positive or negative feelings because a particular patient reminds them, consciously or unconsciously, of a parent or another close figure in their life. Such feelings toward the patient are called countertransference. If countertransference is not recognized in its early stages and corrected, it may impair the doctor's ability to maintain an appropriate professional relationship and to provide impartial advice.

■ Formal psychological treatments

In contrast to the core psychological techniques, which every doctor should employ every day, only a few of the **formal psychological treatments** are of direct concern to non-mental-health specialists. These treatments are discrete psychological interventions which are separate to routine clinical care, and for which patients would usually be referred to another healthcare professional, such as a clinical psychologist or specialist nurse.

In this chapter, the formal psychological treatments are described under the following headings:

1 **problem-solving treatment,** which is useful for patients with adjustment disorders, depression, and deliberate-self-harm;

2 **behavioural and cognitive therapies,** which are used to alter patterns of behaviour (**behaviour therapy**) and

thinking (**cognitive therapy**) that predispose to certain psychiatric disorders, which can prevent recovery from those disorders, and which can be combined to form a common psychological treatment, known as **cognitive behaviour therapy** or **CBT**;

3 **dynamic psychotherapy,** which enables patients to recognize unconscious determinants of their behaviour and thereby gain more control over it;

4 **group treatments,** which are used either as a first step in psychological treatment, when efficiency of delivery is as important as effectiveness, or when the group nature of the intervention may be particularly helpful, such as in the treatment of personality disorders;

5 **couple and family treatments,** which are used when the core problem appears to be related to the couple's relationship or family interactions.

Terminology

Some terms may cause confusion because they are used with more than one meaning.

- The term **psychotherapy** is sometimes used to mean *all* forms of psychological treatment, often with an additional qualifying term, such as behavioural psychotherapy. Alternatively, the term can be used to refer solely to dynamic psychotherapy. In addition, the term **therapy** is sometimes used as an abbreviation of psychotherapy. We prefer the term **psychological treatment** to psychotherapy. However, the term **cognitive behaviour therapy** is used almost universally, rather than cognitive behavioural treatment, and so we have stuck with the commonly used term.

- The term **counselling** refers to a wide range of the less technically complicated psychological treatments ranging from the giving of advice, through sympathetic listening, to structured ways of encouraging problem solving. By itself, the term does not have a precise meaning and it should be qualified to indicate either the procedures that are employed (e.g. problem-solving counselling) or the problem that is being addressed (e.g. relationship counselling, bereavement counselling).

■ Problem-solving treatment

The problem-solving approach

The aim of problem-solving treatment is to help patients to solve stressful problems and to make changes in their lives. Problem solving is used as the main treatment for acute reactions to stress and for adjustment disorders, and as an addition to other treatments for psychiatric

disorders in which associated life problems need to be resolved.

Problem solving is used for problems requiring:

- **a decision**—for example, whether a pregnancy is to be terminated, or an unhappy marriage brought to an end;

- **adjustment** to new circumstances, such as bereavement or the discovery of terminal illness, or a move to an unfamiliar environment (e.g. by a student starting university);

- **change** from an unsatisfactory way of life to a healthier one—for example, as part of treatment for dependence on alcohol or drugs.

Problem-solving treatment includes the basic supportive processes described above together with the techniques summarized in Table 14.2. Throughout treatment, patients are encouraged to take the lead in identifying problems and solutions so that they learn not only a way of resolving the present difficulties but also a strategy for dealing with future problems. Sessions of treatment last

Table 14.2 Basic problem-solving techniques

1 **Define and list current problems.** A *list of problems* is drawn up by the patient with help from the therapist, who helps to define and separate the various aspects of a complex set of problems.

2 **Choose a problem.** The patient *chooses one of the problems* to work on.

3 **List alternative solutions for this problem.** The therapist helps the patient to *list alternative solutions* that could solve or reduce the problem. A written list of problems and possible actions helps the patient to identify a plan of action that is specific, practical, and likely to succeed. The listed problems and actions are considered one by one to determine what should be done, and how success will be judged.

4 **Evaluate the alternative solutions and choose the best.** The patient *considers the pros and cons* of each plan of action and *chooses the most promising one.*

5 **Try the chosen course of action.** The patient *attempts the chosen course of action* for the first problem.

6 **Evaluate the results.** The *results are evaluated.* If successful, the next problem is acted upon. If the plan for the first has not succeeded, the attempt is reviewed constructively by the patient and therapist to decide how to increase the chance of success on the next occasion. Lack of success is not viewed as a personal failure but as an opportunity to learn more about the person's situation.

7 **Repeat until all the important problems have been resolved.** The *sequence is repeated* until all the selected problems have been resolved.

for about 30 minutes. Four to eight sessions are usual according to the complexity of the problems.

Problem solving and crisis intervention

When patients are overwhelmed by stressful events or adverse circumstances they are said to be in crisis, and help for them is called crisis intervention. People in crisis include those who have harmed themselves, victims of physical or sexual assault, and people involved in man-made or natural disasters. Such patients are highly aroused and usually require some additional help to reduce this arousal before they can concentrate effectively on problem solving.

Crisis intervention is prompt, brief, and goal directed. It uses the techniques of problem solving, applied to a crisis situation and its early aftermath. The risk of suicide and self-harm should be assessed at each meeting. The therapist encourages the patient to express their distress, within a supportive setting. The patient is also encouraged to seek support from appropriate non-professionals, that is, friends and family. Coping mechanisms are discussed, adaptive mechanisms encouraged (e.g. phased return to work and leisure activities, use of distraction), and maladaptive coping mechanisms discouraged (e.g. avoidance of thinking about the traumatic event and its consequences, use of alcohol or illicit drugs to numb feelings, use of self-harm to numb feelings). Advice about improving sleep may well be needed. When distress is severe, an anxiolytic or hypnotic drug (usually a benzodiazepine) may be needed for a few days to calm the patient and assist sleep.

■ Behavioural and cognitive treatments

Behaviour therapy

This is used to treat symptoms and abnormal behaviours that persist because of certain actions of *the patient* or *other people* that produce immediate relief of distress but nevertheless prolong the disorder.

1 **Maintaining actions by the patient.** For example, patients *avoid* situations that provoke anxiety, such as flying phobics avoiding plane travel, or agoraphobics avoiding rush-hour buses or busy supermarkets. While in the short term the patient gains, due to the prevention or alleviation of distress, in the long term they lose, due to inability to fly, and inability to shop when they choose.

2 **Maintaining actions by other people.** For example, parents, teachers, or friends may pay more attention to children when they behave badly than when they behave well.

Commonly used techniques in behaviour therapy

1 **Distraction.** This can reduce the impact of worrying thoughts and preoccupations. One approach is to encourage the patient to focus *attention* on some external object (e.g. they may count blue cars in the street or look intently at an object in the room), or to use *mental exercises*, such as mental arithmetic, that require full attention. Another is to build activities into the patient's life that are inherently distracting. If a patient is alone, at home, and under-occupied, worrying thoughts can gain the upper hand. If, however, they are cooking, or cleaning, or with friends, or at work, their activities will help to distract them.

2 **Relaxation training.** This treatment is used to reduce anxiety by lowering muscle tone and autonomic arousal. Used alone relaxation is not effective for severe anxiety disorders, but it is a component of anxiety management training (see below), which is often effective in these conditions. Relaxation training is useful in the treatment of some physical conditions that are made worse by stressful events (e.g. some cases of mild hypertension). The essential procedures are (i) relaxing muscle groups one by one, (ii) breathing slowly as in sleep, and (iii) clearing the mind of worrying thoughts by concentrating on a calming image, such as a tranquil scene.

These techniques can be combined in a variety of ways but the results of all methods appear to be similar. One typical form of relaxation training has the following steps.

- Distinguish between tension and relaxation by first tensing a group of muscles and then letting go.
- Breathe slowly and regularly.
- Imagine a restful scene such as a quiet beach on a warm cloudless day.
- Relax one muscle group (e.g. the muscles of the left forearm). Follow this by relaxing other groups one by one, for example the left upper arm, right forearm, right upper arm, neck and shoulders, face, abdomen, back, left thigh, left calf, right thigh, and right calf.
- Relax larger muscle groups (e.g. all the muscles of a limb together) so that complete relaxation is achieved more rapidly.
- Resume activity gradually as in waking from sleep.

The first relaxation session usually lasts for about 30 minutes and each subsequent session usually lasts about 15 minutes. Throughout the sessions the person continues to breathe slowly and imagine restful scenes. After about six sessions, most people can relax rapidly. This is a time-consuming and therefore poorly available and expensive intervention for healthcare professionals to deliver. However, there are various audio-recorded relaxation programmes available to purchase which patients can use at home, in quiet surroundings at a time when disturbance is unlikely. There are three steps: (i) the full intervention should be used regularly, with the audio-recording, so that the patient develops confidence and skill; (ii) the patient can practise the full intervention without the recording; (iii) finally, the patient can shorten the intervention, so that it is a brief, easy-to-use intervention that can be used whenever they feel stressed.

3 **Graded exposure.** Exposure is used mainly for phobic disorders. The basic procedure is to persuade patients to enter, repeatedly, situations that they have avoided previously. This is usually achieved in real life (*in vivo*), but, if this is not practicable, there is good evidence for the effectiveness of exposure in the patient's imagination (*in imagino*). This exposure is usually achieved in a graded way—graded exposure or **desensitization**. Patients should practise graded exposure for about an hour every day. To ensure this it is often helpful to enlist a relative or friend who can encourage practice, praise success, and sustain motivation. When the re-entry to feared situations is rapid, the term **flooding** is used.

The stages of graded exposure are as follows.

(i)   Determine in detail which *situations* are *avoided*, and rate the degree of anxiety experienced (out of 10) for each.

(ii) Arrange these situations in order of the amount of anxiety that each provokes (the resulting list is called a **hierarchy**), where 0 is no anxiety and 10 is the worst anxiety possible. Check whether the difference in the amount of anxiety induced by each item in the hierarchy and the next is about the same throughout the list. If it is not, add or remove items until this aim has been achieved. A hierarchy for a supermarket (agora-)phobic might include items such as the local shop when there are no other customers (3/10), the local shop when it is crowded (5/10), a supermarket when there are no queues at the checkouts (7/10), and a supermarket at a busy time, with long queues impairing escape (10/10).

(iii) *Teach relaxation training* (see above) so that it can be used subsequently to reduce anxiety during exposure.

(iv) Persuade the patient *to enter a situation* at the bottom of the hierarchy, monitor their anxiety regularly, and stay until anxiety has gone (e.g. from 3/10 to 0/10). It is important that anxiety should have subsided significantly before the patient leaves the situation, otherwise no benefit will follow. The procedure is repeated until the situation at the bottom of the hierarchy can be experienced without anxiety.

(v)   Repeat with the next situation up the hierarchy, whose predicted anxiety level is likely to have reduced a little following this early success, e.g. rating for the local shop when it is crowded might have reduced from 5/10 to 3/10. Then repeat until the top of the hierarchy is reached.

4 **Response prevention** is used to treat obsessional rituals. It is based on the observation that rituals become less frequent and intense when patients make prolonged and repeated efforts to suppress them. To be effective, the ritual must be suppressed until the associated anxiety has waned, and this may take up to an hour. Since the immediate effect of response prevention is to increase anxiety, patients require much support if they are to suppress the rituals for the required time. When this stage has been achieved, the procedure is repeated in the presence of any factors that tend to provoke the rituals. For example, a patient with a fear of contamination and associated ritualistic cleaning and washing would (i) clean a dirty smelly bin, using a small brush and no gloves, in order to get their hands smelly and dirty, (ii) experience intense anxiety and an associated impulse to reduce that anxiety with rituals including washing and disinfecting, but (iii) resist the impulse until the anxiety has subsided and the dirt on their hands is less meaningful ('it's just dirt'). Usually, any associated obsessional thoughts decline as the rituals improve.

5 **Thought stopping** is used to treat obsessional thoughts occurring without obsessional rituals (and therefore not treatable by response prevention). A sudden, intrusive stimulus is used to interrupt the thoughts; for example, the mildly painful effect of snapping an elastic band worn around the wrist. When treatment is successful, patients become able to interrupt the thoughts without the aid of the distracting stimulus.

6 **Assertiveness training.** This method is for people who are abnormally shy or socially awkward. Socially acceptable expression of thoughts and feelings is encouraged as follows:

(i)   *analyse the problem* in terms of facial expression, eye contact, posture, and tone of voice, and what is said;

(ii) *exchange roles* to help the patient understand the viewpoint of the other person in the situation;

(iii) *demonstrate* appropriate social behaviour;

(iv) *practise* appropriate behaviour within the sessions;

(v)   *practise* appropriate social behaviour in everyday life;

(vi) *record* the outcome of this practice.

7 **Self-control techniques** are used to increase control over behaviours such as excessive eating or smoking. The treatment may be used alone or as part of a wider treatment,

such as in CBT for bulimia nervosa. The treatment has two stages. During the first stage, **self-monitoring** is the keeping of daily records of the problem behaviour and of the circumstances in which it occurs. For example, a patient who overeats would record what is eaten, when it is eaten, and any associations between eating and stressful events or moods. The keeping of such records is itself a powerful aid to self-control, because many patients have previously avoided facing the true extent of their problems. The second stage, **self-reinforcement**, is the rewarding of oneself when a goal has been achieved successfully. For example, a woman who has reached a target might have a weekend away with her partner. Rewards of this kind help to maintain motivation.

8 **Contingency management** is used to control abnormal behaviour that is being reinforced unwittingly by other people; for example, by parents who attend more to a child during temper tantrums than at other times. The treatment has two aims: first, to identify and reduce the reinforcers of the abnormal behaviour; and, second, to find ways of rewarding desirable behaviour. Praise and encouragement are the usual rewards, but they may be added to with material rewards such as points or stars that will earn a child a desired toy or treat. The approach may seem mechanistic, but in practice the procedures can be carried out in a caring way. Contingency management has several components.

(i) **The behaviour to be changed is recorded** by the patient or another person (e.g. a parent might count the frequency of a child's temper tantrums).

(ii) **Triggers are identified.** These are events that immediately precede the behaviour. For example, the child's temper tantrums may occur after the mother pays attention to a younger sibling.

(iii) **Reinforcers are identified.** These are events that immediately follow the behaviour; usually these events involve extra attention being given to the child when behaving badly.

(iv) **The undesirable behaviour is ignored** as far as this is practicable.

(v) **Appropriate behaviour is rewarded** (e.g. the parent would attend to the child when behaving well).

(vi) **Parents or others monitor progress** by continuing to record the frequency of the relevant behaviour.

Cognitive therapy

This is used to treat symptoms and abnormal behaviours that persist because of the way that patients think about them. For example, an agoraphobic experiencing intense anxiety as they approach a busy supermarket may believe that their palpitations, occurring as part of the anxiety response, are evidence of an impending heart attack. Their beliefs are therefore important **maintaining factors** in their disorder.

Outline of cognitive therapy

Cognitive therapy proceeds through four stages.

1 **Identify maladaptive thinking** by asking patients to keep a daily record of the thoughts that precede and accompany their symptoms or abnormal behaviour. The thoughts are recorded as soon as possible after they have occurred. This record is often called a **dysfunctional thought record**.

2 **Challenge the maladaptive thinking** by correcting misunderstandings with accurate information, and pointing out illogical ways of reasoning.

3 **Devise more realistic alternatives** to the maladaptive ways of thinking. 'More realistic' is a better term to use than 'more positive'.

4 **Test out these alternatives.**

Until maladaptive thinking has changed, *distraction* (a behavioural technique) can be used to control the thoughts.

Cognitive behaviour therapy (CBT)

CBT merges aspects of behaviour and cognitive therapies to form a treatment which may be more than the sum of its parts. An agoraphobic may be *exposed* to their feared stimulus (e.g. busy supermarket). This might be beneficial alone, by reducing avoidance, but it will also trigger physical symptoms (palpitations) and associated **negative automatic thoughts** (e.g. 'I'm having a heart attack'). These can be used as the basis for simple cognitive interventions, using a dysfunctional thought record (e.g. Table 14.3), which can help the patient to regain control over their anxious thoughts. This increase in self-perception of control makes further exposure easier. **Behavioural experiments** can be prescribed that test out the beliefs that patients have about how their body and the world around them work (e.g. running up and down stairs to increase heart rate and give 'palpitations', and to thereby demonstrate a benign cause of 'palpitations'). CBT therapists can help the patient to analyse the varied forms of avoidance in their life, which are maintained by their beliefs about their vulnerabilities (in this case cardiac). Avoidance includes overt avoidance, such as avoiding busy shops, and also covert avoidance, which includes **safety behaviours.** These are personal ways of reducing the sense of threat, such as always carrying a mobile phone in case of the need to summon assistance, or hanging on very tightly to a supermarket trolley to avoid the risk of collapse.

Table 14.3 Examples of CBT symptom diaries

A. A diary to record anxiety

Date/time	The situation in which you felt anxious	Symptoms	Rating of anxiety (0–10)	What you were thinking	What you did
12/6/98 4 pm	In a queue at the supermarket	Palpitations and dizziness	8	I am going to die	Ran away from the queue
13/6/98 10 am	In town centre	Palpitations and sweating	5	I must relax	Stood still Tried to relax

B. A diary to record an eating disorder

Date/time	The problem	The situation at the time	What you were thinking before	What you did
18/7/98 7 pm	Ate a whole loaf of bread with butter and jam	Feeling despondent after being criticized at work	Everything I do goes wrong	Made myself vomit
19/7/98 1 pm	Bought 3 bars of chocolate and a cake	Angry with my friend	No one respects me	Sat alone and ate it all

CBT requires special training, and generalists need know only the principles of the treatments and the main reasons for referral. There are, however, some simpler procedures that can be used by non-specialists, such as *relaxation*, *graded exposure*, and *anxiety management*.

Principles of cognitive behaviour therapy

- The general approach to CBT is that the therapist helps patients first to become aware of, and then to modify, their maladaptive thinking and behaviour.

- The treatment is *collaborative*, and the patient is treated as an active and expert partner in care.

- Patients practise new ways of thinking and behaving between the sessions of treatment; this is called *homework*.

- Written instructions are often used to supplement the explanations given by the therapist during treatment sessions, because it is important that they understand the procedures clearly and are well motivated to carry them out.

- Symptoms, cognitions, and associated behaviours are monitored by recording them in a *diary* or *dysfunctional thought record*, in which are noted the occurrence of (i) symptoms, (ii) thoughts and events that precede and possibly provoke the symptoms, and (iii) thoughts and events that follow and possibly reinforce the symptoms (Table 14.3).

- Treatment takes the form of a *graded* series of tasks and activities such that patients gain confidence in dealing with less severe problems before attempting more severe ones.

- Tasks and activities are presented as *experiments* in which the achievement of a goal is a success, while non-achievement is not a failure but an opportunity to learn more by analysing constructively what went wrong. This format helps to avoid discouragement and maintain motivation.

- *Behavioural experiments* can be used to test out a patient's predictions (invariably negative, due to active *cognitive biases*) of what will happen in a particular circumstance

CBT for common problems

CBT for anxiety management. The components of anxiety management are (i) assessment of the problem, (ii) relaxation, (iii) techniques for changing anxiety-provoking cognitions, and (iv) exposure (see Box 14.1).

Anxiety management is a time-limited, focused intervention. However, when delivered face to face, one to one, it still demands a significant amount of a healthcare professional's time, with a resulting impact on feasibility and cost. In many cases, it will be delivered within a *stepped care model*. The first step, applicable to most patients, is *bibliotherapy*, with the recommendation or provision of self-help materials including a booklet or book and relaxation tape or CD. Examples are listed at the end of this chapter. The second step, applicable to some patients, might be group anxiety management. The final step, for a few patients who have not been helped by steps one and/or two, is individual anxiety management. In this way, the most intensive intervention is restricted to those patients who need it most.

CBT for panic disorder. Patients with panic disorder are convinced that some of the physical symptoms are not caused by anxiety but are the first indications of a serious physical illness (often that palpitations signal an impending

BOX 14.1 Anxiety management

- Organize *a diary record* (see Table 14.3) to assess the nature and severity of symptoms, situations in which anxiety occurs, and avoidance.
- Give *information* to correct misunderstanding about the cause of symptoms (e.g. palpitations, chest pain, and lightheadedness are due to normal 'fight or flight' anxiety response/hyperventilation, rather than heart attack or stroke) and the consequences of symptoms (they are harmless).
- *Discuss the patient's specific concerns* about their symptom(s); for example, that dizziness will lead to fainting.
- *Explain the vicious circle of anxiety* ('*fear of fear*'), including the importance of fearful concerns about the symptoms.
- *Explain the maintaining effects of avoidance.*
- Teach *relaxation* (see p. 135).
- Teach *graded exposure* (see p. 136).
- Teach *distraction* (see p. 135) to reduce the anxiety-producing effect of any remaining thoughts.

heart attack). This conviction causes further anxiety so that a cycle of mounting anxiety is set up. The treatment includes the general components listed above under anxiety management, with the following additional features.

- **The therapist explains** that physical symptoms are part of the normal response to stress, and that fear of these symptoms sets up a vicious circle of anxiety.
- **Patients record** the fearful thoughts that precede and accompany their panic attacks. Patients who cannot identify their thoughts during naturally occurring panic attacks

can often do so if panic-like symptoms are induced by voluntary hyperventilation.

- **The therapist demonstrates** that fearful cognitions can induce anxiety, by asking patients to remember and dwell on these cognitions and observe the effect.
- **Patients attempt to think in the new way** when they experience symptoms, and they observe the effect of this change on the severity of the panic attacks. By repeating this sequence many times they gradually gain control of the panic attacks.

CBT for depressive disorder. As in the treatment of anxiety, cognitive and behavioural techniques are used alongside each other. The three kinds of cognitive abnormality in depressive disorder (see p. 225) are dealt with as follows.

1. **Intrusive thoughts**, usually of a self-depreciating kind (e.g. 'I am a failure'). When they are weak such thoughts can be counteracted by *distraction*, using the methods described above, but when they are strong they are difficult to control.
2. **Logical errors** distort the way in which experiences are interpreted, and maintain the intrusive thoughts (Box 14.2). The therapist helps the patient to recognize these irrational ways of thinking and change them into more *realistic* thoughts.
3. **Maladaptive assumptions** are often about social acceptability; for example, the assumption that only good-looking and successful people are liked by others. The patient is helped to examine how ideas of this kind influence the ways in which they think about themselves and other people.

Depressed patients tend to withdraw from or avoid their usual social and occupational activities, and to lead unstructured, inactive lives. The therapist therefore uses a behavioural intervention, **activity scheduling**, to help the patient to increase their activity levels, by building satisfying or enjoyable activities into their life.

BOX 14.2 Logical errors/cognitive distortions in depressive disorders

- **Exaggeration:** magnifying small mistakes or problems and thinking of them as major failures or issues, i.e. 'making a mountain out of a molehill'. At its worst, this is termed catastrophizing.
- **Catastrophizing:** expecting serious consequences of minor problems (e.g. thinking that a relative who is late home has been involved in an accident).
- **Minimization:** minimizing or ignoring successes or personal positive qualities.
- **Overgeneralizing:** thinking that the bad outcome of one event will be repeated in every similar event in the future (e.g. that having lost one partner, the person will never find a lasting relationship).
- **Mental filter:** dwelling on personal shortcomings or on the unfavourable aspects of a situation while overlooking the favourable aspects.

The cognitive-behavioural approach in everyday clinical practice

Although formal CBT is a complex procedure that requires special training, three features of the cognitive-behavioural approach are useful in everyday clinical practice.

1 **Recording thoughts** that occur when symptoms are experienced, via a diary. There is no fixed design for a diary/dysfunctional thought record—the professional and patient can design one together that will work for that patient's particular circumstances. However, standard templates are widely available.

2 **Recording abnormal behaviours and events** that precede and follow them (the ABC approach—**A**ntecedents, **B**ehaviours, **C**onsequences).

3 **Asking patients to monitor and record their progress**, both as a way of judging the success of treatment and as a way of increasing their collaboration with treatment.

■ Dynamic psychotherapy

In this treatment, patients are helped to obtain a greater understanding of aspects of their problems and of themselves, with the expectation that this will help them to overcome these problems. The focus of treatment is on aspects of the problems and of the self of which the person was previously unaware (unconscious aspects). The treatment may be brief and focused on a small number of specific problems (**brief focal dynamic psychotherapy**) or long term and dealing with a broader range of problems (**long-term dynamic psychotherapy**). Dynamic psychotherapy is a specialist treatment requiring training. Those who are not specialists need to understand the indications for referral and broad principles of treatment.

Brief focal psychodynamic therapy

The main *indications* for brief dynamic therapy are problems of low self-esteem and difficulties in forming relationships, either of which may be accompanied by emotional disorders, eating disorders, or sexual disorders. Patients referred for dynamic psychotherapy need to be insightful and willing to consider links between their present difficulties and events at earlier stages of their life. Because treatment is so much concerned with self-concept and relationships, which involve judgements about the kind of change that is desirable, it highlights some ethical problems concerned with values (Box 14.3).

The principal steps of treatment are as follows.

1 The patient and therapist *agree on the problems* that will be the focus of treatment.

2 Patients *discuss recent and past experiences* of the problem. To encourage the necessary self-revelation, the therapist speaks infrequently and responds more to the emotional than the factual content of what is said. For example, instead of asking for more factual detail he may say 'You seemed angry when you spoke about that experience.'

3 Patients are encouraged to *review their own part in problems* that they ascribe to other people.

4 Patients are helped to *identify common themes* in what they are describing; for example, fear of being rejected by other people.

5 Patients are helped to *recall similar problems* at an earlier stage of life. They are encouraged to consider whether the present maladaptive behaviour may have originated as a way of coping that was adaptive at that time but is now self-defeating; for example, failure to trust others following the experience of sexual abuse in childhood.

6 The *therapist makes interpretations* to help patients discover connections between past and present behaviour, or between different aspects of their present behaviour. Interpretations should be presented as hypotheses to be considered by the patient, rather than truths to be accepted.

7 The patient is encouraged to *consider alternative ways of thinking and relating* and to try these out first with the therapist and then in everyday life.

 BOX 14.3 Ethical issues of imposing values in dynamic psychotherapy

Therapists should always respect their patients' values and never impose their own. This rule applies to all therapeutic situations—for example, when counselling about a possible termination of pregnancy. It is especially important in dynamic psychotherapy in which value judgements are often involved—for example, in deciding what relationship changes would be desirable. Therapists may impose their own values:

- directly by expressing their values or challenging those of the patient;

- indirectly—for example, by giving more attention to arguments against a course of action than to arguments for it.

The problem arises also in couple therapy and family therapy in which therapists should not support, directly or indirectly, the values and approach of one member of the couple or family against those of the others.

Dynamic psychotherapy tends to give rise to intense emotional relationships between the patient and therapist (*transference*). In some forms of brief psychotherapy, the transference is examined to throw light on the patient's relationship with his parents, as in long-term therapy. Whether or not transference is used in this way, it is important to reduce its intensity before the planned end of treatment, otherwise patients are left in a dependent state, which makes it difficult to end the therapy.

Long-term dynamic psychotherapy

This treatment, which originates from Freud's original methods of psychoanalysis, aims to change long-standing patterns of thinking and behaviour that contribute to personal and relationship problems and may be associated with psychiatric disorder. Patients are seen three or more times a week, for at least a year. The problems of dependency, noted above under brief dynamic therapy, are even greater with long-term therapy, and the end of treatment (termination) should be anticipated and discussed very early.

No randomized controlled trials have demonstrated that this long and intensive form of psychotherapy is more effective than brief dynamic treatment or cognitive behaviour therapies. For this reason, these methods are seldom used in everyday practice.

As well as the basic procedures of psychotherapy, the following special techniques are used.

1 **Free association.** In this technique, the patient is encouraged to allow their thoughts to wander freely, and potentially illogically, from a starting point of relevance to the problem. This technique and the next are used to encourage the recall of previously repressed memories.

2 **Recall of dreams** and discussion of their meaning.

3 **Interpretation of transference.** Intense transference develops readily in this form of treatment because the therapist sees the patient frequently and over a long period but reveals little of himself. Transference is used as a tool of treatment on the assumption that it reflects patients' relationships with their parents in earlier life; in psychodynamic theory these early relationships are important in aetiology. The therapist comments on the significance of the transference reactions (he makes transference interpretations), and helps the patient to practise controlling the strong emotions that are part of the transference, and which are likely to be similar to emotions experienced outside the therapy sessions.

4 **Control of countertransference.** The factors that encourage transference in the patient also provoke *counter-transference* on the part of the therapist. It is for this reason that therapists are required to understand their emotional reactions better by undergoing dynamic psychotherapy themselves before using these intensive methods with patients.

■ Treatment in groups

Rationale

Some psychological treatment takes place in groups. There are two main reasons for this.

1 **Cost-effectiveness and availability.** Psychological treatments often need to be delivered by highly trained staff, who may be expensive and scarce. Providing individual, one-to-one treatment may therefore lead to expensive services and long waits for treatment. It is often possible to provide basic, first-level psychological treatment, such as CBT, in a group environment. Any disadvantage of the reduction in personalized care may be balanced out by additional therapeutic processes that may arise in groups.

2 **Additional therapeutic processes in groups.** These processes are useful both in psychiatric treatment and in the general practice of medicine where groups can be used to support patients or their relatives. They include:

(i) **Understanding you are not alone.** This is sometimes called normalization—meeting other people with similar problems to your own can be reassuring.

(ii) **Support from others,** which can help the members through difficult periods in their treatment or in their lives.

(iii) **Learning from others**—for example, how others in the group have overcome problems similar to the patient's own.

(iv) **Pressure from others in the group to modify behaviour within the group.** For example, disruptive outbursts, dominating the group, or excessively criticizing other members may trigger feedback from one or more members of the group.

(v) **Testing beliefs, opinions, and attitudes** against those of other people. This experience is often more effective in bringing about change than is advice from a professional.

(vi) **Practising adaptive social behaviour,** especially by those who are shy or socially awkward.

Specific issues

In group therapy, close relationships develop between patients as well as between each patient and the therapist. The therapist should ensure that these relationships do not become too intense. Depending on the form of therapy, relationships may be discouraged between members of the group outside the actual meetings, although in others, such as group CBT for anxiety disorders, there is no reason why this should not happen.

In individual psychotherapy, patients have a confidential relationship with the therapist. Members of a group reveal their personal problems not only to the therapist but also to each other. Due to this, patients need to agree some group rules, which usually include (i) that they will speak about personal matters in the group, so that they can play an active role and (ii) that they will treat as confidential anything that other group members say. In addition, therapists need to ensure that anything that they have learned in a one-to-one interview (e.g. as part of an assessment for group therapy) is not revealed to the group. If such information is important for the group process, the therapist must wait until the patient reveals it, or have the agreement of the patient to reveal it on their behalf.

Small group treatment

A small group usually has about eight patients. Group therapy can be used for any of the purposes for which individual therapy is used, that is, for *support*, *problem solving*, *behavioural treatment*, *cognitive behavioural therapy*, and *dynamic psychotherapy*. The length of treatment, its intensity, and the techniques vary according to the purpose, as they do with individual therapy.

Large group treatment

In some psychiatric wards, patients meet regularly in a group containing 20 or more people. The usual purpose is supportive, enabling patients to talk about the problems of living together in the ward, and thereby to reduce these problems whenever possible.

A **therapeutic community** uses group methods not just for support but also to modify personality. Patients reside in the community for many months, living and working together, and attending small and large groups in which they discuss problems in relationships and try to help each other to recognize and resolve their problems. This kind of treatment has been used mainly for patients with personality disorders characterized by antisocial or aggressive behaviour. The value of the methods is uncertain and the approach is available in only a few special centres.

Self-help groups

These groups are organized by people who have a problem in common — for example, obesity, alcoholism, postnatal depression, or the rearing of a child with a congenital disorder. The group is often led by a person who has coped successfully with the problem. The members usually meet without a professional therapist, although the leader may have a professional adviser. *Alcoholics Anonymous*, *Depression Alliance* and *MDF: The Bipolar Organization* are prominent examples of such groups. They are important sources of support and advice, and many can and should be recommended to patients.

■ Treatment for couples and families

Couple therapy

Couple therapy (or **marital therapy**) is used to help couples who have problems in their relationships. In medical practice this therapy is used when relationship problems are maintaining a psychiatric disorder (e.g. a depressive disorder) in one or both partners. Treatment focuses on the ways in which the couple interact rather than on their individual problems. The aim is to promote concern by each partner for the welfare of the other, tolerance of differences, and an agreed balance of decision making and dominance. To avoid imposing the therapist's own values, the couple first identify the difficulties that they wish to put right. The therapist does not take sides with either partner but helps the couple understand each other's point of view. Problems of communication are pointed out. Common problems of this kind include failure to express wishes directly, failure to listen to the other's point of view, 'mind reading' (A knows better than B what is in B's mind), and following positive comments with criticism (the 'sting in the tail').

Marital therapy can be carried out in several ways using a number of approaches:

1 **problem-solving methods** like those described earlier;

2 **behavioural approaches** that focus on the ways that each person reinforces, or fails to reinforce, the behaviour of the other;

3 **transactional methods** in which attention is given to the private rules that govern the couple's behaviour towards each other, and to the question of who makes these rules (e.g. whose work takes priority and who decides this);

4 **dynamic methods** intended to uncover hitherto unconscious aspects of the couple's interaction—for example, the possibility that a husband repeatedly criticizes his wife because she fails to show the self-reliance that he lacks himself.

Depending on the nature of the marital problem, and on the couple's capacity for psychological insight, each approach can be of value. There is, however, insufficient evidence available from clinical trials on which to evaluate the effectiveness of these treatments.

Family therapy

Family therapy is usually employed when a child or adolescent has an emotional or conduct disorder. In addition to the young person, the parents are involved together with any other family members (such as siblings or grandparents) who are involved closely with the young person. The aim of treatment is to reduce the problem(s) rather than to produce some ideal state of family life.

Problem-solving methods, transactional methods, and dynamic approaches can be used, as in marital therapy. Specific forms of family therapy have been devised to deal with factors thought to lead to relapse in eating disorders and schizophrenia.

Further reading

Butler, G. & Hope, T. (2007). *Manage Your Mind: The Mental Fitness Guide*. Oxford University Press, Oxford.

Gelder, M., Andreasen, N., Lopez-Ibor, J., & Geddes, J. (eds) (2009). *New Oxford Textbook of Psychiatry*, 2nd edn. Section 6.3 Psychological treatments. Oxford University Press, Oxford.

Resources suitable for patients

Butler, G. & Hope, T. (2007). *Manage Your Mind: The Mental Fitness Guide*. Oxford University Press, Oxford. This comprehensive self-help book makes extensive use of cognitive and behavioural techniques and insights, and includes chapters on, among other topics, anxiety, panic, depression, alcohol, smoking, sleep, and relationships. It is useful reading for all healthcare professionals, both to help inform their patients, and for the maintenance of their own emotional well-being.

The Oxford Cognitive Therapy Centre publishes a variety of booklets and books which are based on cognitive behavioural approaches and are ideal for patients wanting to know more about their illness and how to manage it. Their website is at www.octc.co.uk Examples include:

Kennerley, H. *Managing Anxiety: A User's Manual*. An eight-part self-help programme for managing anxiety, which also includes a relaxation tape.

Westbrook, D. *Managing Depression*. Information and self-help advice for people who are depressed.

Sanders, D. *Overcoming Phobias*. Deals with specific phobias such as insects, animals, blood and needles, loud noises, and enclosed spaces.

Close, H., Rouf, K., & Rosen, K. *Managing Psychosis*. Explains how people suffering from psychosis can understand and manage psychotic symptoms using CBT.

Whitehead, L. *Overcoming Eating Disorders*. A CBT approach to overcoming eating disorders, focusing on getting ready to change, providing suggestions for how to manage key eating disorder features, and how family and friends can help.

Social treatments

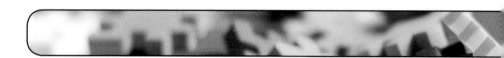

The most common approach to providing comprehensive treatment for patients with mental health problems is the biopsychosocial model. This chapter will focus on social interventions.

■ Rehabilitation

For patients with severe, enduring mental health problems, social treatments are known as **rehabilitation**. The aim of rehabilitation is to reintegrate the individual back into their community and ensure their ongoing wellbeing. Ideally, rehabilitation aims to change the natural course of a psychiatric disorder, but more frequently it just assists the patient in making life changes that allow them to manage more satisfactorily in their environment. The patients who most commonly benefit from rehabilitation are those with the following features:

- persistent psychopathology (e.g. ongoing hallucinations in schizophrenia);
- frequent relapses (e.g. mania or depression in bipolar disorder);
- social maladaption (e.g. isolation, chaotic antisocial behaviour).

The key benefits of rehabilitation have been shown to be as follows:

- the patient moves away from the 'sick role' and starts to see him- or herself as a well individual again;
- quality of life improves;

- reduction in relapses of bipolar disorder and psychotic illnesses;
- reduction in social stigma surrounding mental health disorders.

In the UK and many other countries, social workers are key players in arranging social interventions for patients. In order for an appropriate care package to be put together, it is essential that the multidisciplinary team (psychiatrist, GP, community psychiatric nurse (CPN), and social worker) all work together. The usual areas that a social worker can help with include:

- help with claiming and managing benefits;
- applying for funding for social or supported accommodation;
- assisting with child protection or vulnerability issues;
- role in Mental Health Act proceedings—social workers can train to be approved mental health practitioners (AMHPs);
- helping patients to stay within the limits of their community treatment order;
- advising for families on available services for their particular situation.

A rehabilitation programme will usually include help with housing, employment/education, finances, daily activities, medication management, social skills training, and family interventions. There is usually some overlap between psychological and social treatments. The rest of this chapter will briefly consider each of these areas in turn. However, it should be remembered that many individuals with less severe mental health problems may benefit from an intervention focused on a specific problem; for example, lack of housing, anxiety leading to problems getting to the benefit office or job centre, or lack of transport for getting to the supermarket. Many social interventions are also very specific to the particular country or region a patient is living in; as a clinician you should find out what your local options are.

The voluntary sector plays a huge role in the provision of social treatments. In other chapters in this book specific voluntary organizations have been mentioned—for example, MIND, Alcoholics Anonymous—but there are thousands of local charities providing invaluable support in their community.

Housing

Since the Second World War there has been huge change in the way people with mental health problems are housed. Previously, many lived in long-term institutions whereas now the emphasis is on providing appropriate accommodation in the community. The majority of people who have a mental health disorder will live independently, but those with more severe debilitating illnesses may need extra support. There is good evidence that patients living in the community in a supported environment are much less likely to be re-hospitalized than those who go straight from inpatient care to independent living. In most countries there is a hierarchy of accommodation available, depending on the individual's needs.

- **Twenty-four-hour staffed sheltered accommodation.** These houses or 'group homes' have staff available at all times to provide meals, manage medications, and sort out problems. The staff are usually trained in mental health and provide basic behavioural therapy to help patients adapt to living more independently over time. Some group homes are diagnosis specific—for example, specializing in schizophrenia or learning disabilities—and others only provide accommodation for young people or the elderly. Usually people will live there for a long period, but sometimes just as a step-down between hospital and more independent living.
- **Sheltered accommodation staffed in the daytime.** This is the most commonly available type of supported accommodation in the UK, and provides less intensive assistance to the people living there. Sometimes help with medication management is available, and the staff frequently encourage and help the inhabitants to organize cooking meals, cleaning, and finding daytime activities.
- **Warden-controlled apartments.** These are similar to those that many elderly people choose to live in; the person has their own apartment and manages life almost independently, but the warden is available to help with problems and check up on them. There are some larger organizations which provide staffed sheltered accommodation, but with the option for patients to move into apartments once they are able to manage.
- **Independent living.** Patients living in rented or owned accommodation can live completely independently, but occasionally a little support is required. A social worker or community support worker can be invaluable in helping them to remember to pay the rent, sort out utility bills, or keep the house clean.

In the UK, some supported accommodation is funded through the social housing budget but much needs to be privately funded. The voluntary sector also provides some accommodation, but usually with very specific referral criteria.

Employment and education

In the majority of societies, education and/or employment take up the majority of our time and play a large part in defining us 'as a person'. Mental health problems frequently disrupt education in the adolescent and early adult years, and often people with severe psychiatric conditions are not able to continue with their chosen career. It is extremely important to provide individuals with help to re-establish themselves in the world of work. Return to employment has been shown to have many benefits. It:

- provides a daily routine and structure;
- improves social contact;
- increases quality of life;
- improves self-esteem: people develop a sense of 'mastery';
- reduces the likelihood of living in poverty.

Employment should be carefully chosen to minimize stress and the risk of relapses. The best approach uses graded steps to return to work.

1 Patients frequently have not been in employment for prolonged periods and usually need help in learning the process of looking for, applying for, and maintaining employment. In the UK, some trusts have specific mental health employment advisers who meet with patients to help them with this, but often this is provided by the job centre. Practical assistance includes, for example, putting together a curriculum vitae or writing covering letters to potential employers.

2 Learning new skills—sheltered workshops or college classes are invaluable in helping people with few transferable skills to improve their chances of finding work. A common example is learning how to use a computer, but specific skills relating to a trade (e.g. welding, decorating, etc.) are widely taught.

3 Temporary, part-time, sheltered employment that helps patients get used to the work environment greatly increases the chance that, in the long term, mainstream employment will work out. These jobs might include volunteering in a charity shop, serving lunch at a local mental health day centre, or working with a supportive employment. This is another opportunity for learning new skills.

4 Supported employment—there are a surprising number of employers who are sympathetic to those with mental health problems and will support them in maintaining employment. Social workers, CPNs, and community support workers provide assistance to help the patient get used to going to work and to managing their wages sensibly.

5 Mainstream independent employment.

For young people who have been out of education due to illness, finding an appropriate educational environment can be a challenge. Many adolescents can return to their previous school (e.g. after an acute episode of depression or anorexia nervosa) but some may need more specialist environments. There are schools that cater for specific conditions (e.g. autism, schizophrenia, learning disabilities) but the trickiest situations concern those with substance misuse problems, conduct disorder, or other ongoing risky behaviours.

In the UK, a scheme called 'Building Bridges' has become used widely within mental health services. The course runs as a series of group sessions over 6–9 weeks, and may take place in a hospital, day centre, or the community. The aim is to help patients think about making a new start in their life, and point them in the right direction for achieving this. The focus is on learning social and communication skills and improving confidence and self-belief. Patients can also learn about what opportunities are available for education, employment, and housing, and start to investigate them. Building Bridges is extremely popular amongst patients and carers.

Benefits and finances

Unfortunately many patients with mental health problems find themselves reliant on state benefits and may be living on very restricted incomes. This may well be due to an objective low income, but frequently habits such as smoking and alcohol and substance abuse eat into what little there is. Sometimes patients with mania or disorganized behaviour find managing their money very difficult, and will go out on spending sprees for unnecessary items. Whilst patients are in hospital, it is common for limits to be put on the money they can withdraw daily/weekly, to help with budgeting. Where possible, this should be continued in the community—often sheltered accommodation staff or family can assist with this. Social workers or community support workers can help with setting up direct debits for utilities, or working out a budget.

Most countries have state benefits available for those with long-term illnesses. As an example, some UK benefits which those with mental health problems may be eligible for are listed below.

- **Incapacity benefit.** If one is unable to work (and is under state retirement age) due to illness or disability then incapacity benefit is available to help with everyday costs.

- **Disability living allowance.** This benefit is specifically aimed at people who need assistance with activities of daily living (cooking, dressing, washing) due to illness. The money is supposed to be used to pay/assist the person who cares for them.

- **Carer's allowance.** This a benefit to help people who look after someone who is disabled.

- **Income support.** This is extra money to help those who are working but are on a low income.

- **Housing benefit.** This is a monthly payment to help with rent payments for those on low incomes.

- **Council tax benefits.** Those on a low income—whether they are working or not—can be eligible for a reduction in their council tax payments.
- **Job seeker's allowance.** This is the 'dole' payment that those currently unemployed but actively looking for work are entitled to.

A social worker is the best person to advise on appropriate benefits and to help patients fill out the application forms, although this is often done by family or carers.

Social interaction and activities

An integral part of many mental health disorders is the tendency for isolation. Many patients cut themselves off from friends or family, and if they are unable to work then they become very isolated and sometimes house-bound. A very important aspect of rehabilitation is encouraging the patient to engage with activity scheduling—to build a structure back into their days and to interact with other people. This may be as simple as visiting the local swimming pool twice a week or meeting a friend regularly for coffee. CPNs are particularly well placed to help develop an activity schedule and encourage the patient to stick to it.

There are many options available in the community, including the following.

- **Specialist community or day centres.** These are open on most weekdays for at least half a day and often provide lunch. Some will provide transport to and from the day centre free of charge. During the day there may be scheduled activities—for example, art or creative writing, help with daily problems, an opportunity to mingle with others, or a therapeutic group.
- **Voluntary sector organizations.** Many charities provide a range of services, including day centres as above. In the UK, the largest charity is MIND, who provide daily drop-in sessions for socialization, a rota of activities, and specialist advice (on legal problems, medication, benefits, housing) free of charge. MIND also has supported housing in the community and runs therapeutic groups covering areas such as anxiety management and problem solving.
- **Classes and courses.** These may be evening classes, run at a local college, or be part of mental health services. Not only can patients learn new skills but they can also engage in exercise (e.g. dance classes) or other hobbies (e.g. fishing club or painting).
- **Structured projects.** One example is the Root and Branch project in the UK. This provides therapeutic gardening and training in rural crafts for people experiencing mental health difficulties. The benefits of this scheme include meeting new people, learning new skills, and becoming more physically active. Some patients go on to gain employment with their new skills.

Social skills training

Social skills training is a behavioural therapy-based programme which helps patients improve their interpersonal skills and coping skills, learn workplace essentials, and improve their self-care. It is delivered as a structured course and in the UK is available from the NHS, voluntary organizations, or the private sector. There are various adaptations for specific diagnoses or age groups. Social skills training has been shown to be particularly useful for the following groups:

- adults and adolescents with schizophrenia (especially with predominantly negative symptoms and/or chaotic, disorganized behaviour);
- adults and adolescents with severe bipolar disorder;
- adults with personality disorders;
- adolescents with autism spectrum disorders, ADHD, or conduct disorders;
- children with ADHD.

Family interventions

Formal family therapy is an essential part of the management of many major psychiatric conditions—for example, most childhood disorders, eating disorders, schizophrenia, bipolar disorder, severe depression, and personality disorders. It addresses problems within the family—for example, interpersonal communication difficulties and unrealistic expectations—and provides education. Skilled family therapists or clinical psychologists usually facilitate the sessions.

There is also a role for less formal psychoeducation and involvement of the family, especially if the patient is continuing to live with them. Frequently a CPN is in a good position to deliver this, but it may also be done by allied health professionals. The prognosis of a patient can be highly dependent upon the environment in which they are living and the support within it. There is good evidence that a reduction in highly expressed emotions in the home reduces the chance of relapse in schizophrenia and bipolar disorder. CPNs use basic CBT techniques to educate and change the behaviours of the family to reduce the emotional load within the household. Working with the family can have a range of other benefits:

- they can be taught to encourage the patient to stick to their activity schedule and to help them to engage in work or hobbies;
- helping with managing medications, belongings, and money;
- learning to be more tolerant of abnormal behaviours;

- monitoring for signs of relapse and taking responsibility for informing the patient's care team immediately;
- encouraging the family to talk to their friends and advocate a reduction in social stigma surrounding mental illness.

Medication

Compliance with medications is one of the greatest challenges in psychiatry. Studies estimate that only about 40–60% of patients take medications regularly, and only about 30% take them according to the doctor's instructions. Teaching patients and their carers the importance of taking medications and helping them to do so is therefore essential. Whilst medications may be initially given in hospital, most patients are treated entirely in the community. Psychiatrists and GPs provide prescriptions and encourage patients to take their medications, but it falls to family, carers, community support workers, CPNs, and other health professionals to try and enforce this. It can be a difficult situation if the patient has limited insight into their condition but is not subject to a community treatment order. There are a variety of simple ways of helping patients with medication compliance.

1 Doctors should use the best available evidence to choose effective drugs with positive side-effect profiles. They should enquire about side effects regularly and treat them aggressively or change the medication.

2 Avoid prescribing complex regimes (e.g. take four times daily *versus* take once daily). This may mean using slow-release formulations or choosing a different medication.

3 Offer a depot injection.

4 Arrange for prescriptions to be produced in advance and sent to the pharmacy automatically. Many pharmacies offer a free home delivery service if it would be helpful for the patient.

5 Use medication aids such as prefilled trays for each day of the week.

6 CPNs can remind patients about the importance of taking their medication, and help to educate their family/carers to support the patient with this.

7 In limited areas, SMS text messaging is being used to deliver automatic reminders to patients when their medication is due. Special applications for smart phones are now available that sound an alarm at a set time and remind the patient exactly which tablets to take.

■ Allied health professionals

Whilst the provision of specific services for psychiatric disorders lies with the mental health services, there are various allied professions based in the community which patients can benefit from. Frequently the physical health of patients is poor and they may be overweight, lacking in regular exercise, and living in poverty. Maximizing overall health—including mobility and pain reduction—is an essential part of a rehabilitation programme. Some helpful professionals include the following.

- **Occupational therapists (OTs).** Within the UK, OTs provide a limited community service within the NHS and are also available through voluntary organizations and privately. They are experts in providing equipment to increase safety at home and to assist with activities of daily living. Specifically targeting mental health, OTs can reinforce behavioural modifications to daily activities at home and in the community (e.g. shopping, swimming) and help patients to develop coping skills.

- **Physiotherapists.** Physiotherapists work to maintain maximum function and mobility of the body. Patients may have co-morbid musculoskeletal disorders, have been bed-bound due to severe psychiatric disturbance, or had a restricted environment in which to exercise whilst in hospital. Most people benefit from the individual input the physiotherapist can give in strengthening the body and preventing further injury.

- **Podiatrists.** Many individuals with self neglect secondary to their mental disorder can benefit from some treatments on their feet.

- **Dietitians.** There is a strong association between severe mental health problems and obesity, partly related to medications. A community-based dietitian can give practical advice on weight loss or avoiding further weight gain, especially whilst on a restricted budget. For patients with eating disorders, advice on a healthy balanced diet should be given alongside psychological therapy.

- **Sports/personal fitness instructors.** Exercise promotes both a healthy body and a healthy mind. For patients with anxious or depressive disorders, a structured exercise programme (3×45 minutes per week) has been shown to reduce symptoms and the risk of relapse. Sports are also a good way to meet people and engage in a structured activity. Some gyms and sports centres offer discounted rates for patients referred in from health services, and local clubs (e.g. badminton in a school hall) are usually very cheap.

■ Legal support

Whilst the majority of individuals who experience mental health disorders will never have the need for any legal support, a minority may find themselves having committed an offence or needing advice on treatment under the Mental Health Act. Each country has individual structures for providing this support, but it is widely available.

In the UK, voluntary organizations provide the majority of legal support to those with limited resources or a disability. The mental health charity MIND (www.mind.org.uk) has a legal unit which offers general advice regarding the Mental Health Act, mental capacity, community care, human rights, and discrimination/equality related to mental health. Community Legal Advice is a charity that provides free, confidential, and independent legal advice to any member of the public (www.communitylegaladvice.org.uk). This includes advice on family issues, finances, employment, benefits, crimes, and healthcare. They also have specific advisors trained in dealing with criminal acts undertaken during an acute psychiatric illness.

There is more information about the safeguarding and rights of patients being treated under the Mental Health Act in Chapter 12.

■ Cultural considerations

When designing a rehabilitation programme for a patient, it is important to take into consideration the cultural background from which they come. This may mean having to ask for assistance from colleagues or specialists who know more about a specific religion, culture, or community than you do. Appropriate interpreters should always be provided for patients if the interviewer does not speak the same language as them; these should be independent interpreters rather than family members wherever possible. It is not acceptable to leave the patient out of discussions regarding their care because of a language barrier. There are various specific points to consider.

- Cultural beliefs may be very different from those of the clinician's culture. Certain events or experiences may be interpreted differently and this needs to be handled sensitively; for example, a woman who has been raped may find it hard to attract a husband now that she is no longer 'clean' or a virgin.

- Roles within the family and community may differ. It may be difficult for women to leave the home and attend medical services; more of their care should therefore be provided in the home. Activity scheduling and engaging with others can be a particular problem in this situation. It may not be possible for a patient to live in supported housing if this would ostracize them from their community.

- Patients may present with very different symptoms to those usual for a specific diagnosis; for example, 'total body pain' is a common manifestation of depression in Afro-Caribbeans. Early warning signs, and relapse plans must take this into account.

- Expectations and acceptance of treatments may be different. Some cultures do not believe in mental health problems and it may be very difficult to persuade a patient or carer of the need for treatment. Medication compliance can be challenging. One key factor is to make sure the patient is able to leave the house and visit the pharmacy and there are no ingredients in the tablets that are forbidden in their religion.

 ## Further reading

Gelder, M. G., Lopez-Ibor, J. J., Andreasen, N. C. & Geddes, J. R. (2009). *New Oxford Textbook of Psychiatry*, 2nd edn. Section 7: Social psychiatry and service provision, pp. 1425–1493. Oxford University Press, Oxford.

CHAPTER 16

Managing acute behavioural disturbance

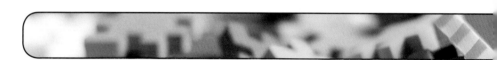

Chapter contents

The safe management of episodes of acute behavioural disturbance is a basic skill that all doctors need to possess because it may occur in all settings.

Acute behavioural disturbances may develop in people suffering from mental disorders at any time during the course of the illness, and may also be a manifestation of systemic organic illness (e.g. sepsis). During an acute exacerbation, a patient with schizophrenia or bipolar disorder may be agitated, aggressive, or violent towards others. This may be directly due to psychotic symptoms (e.g. paranoid or grandiose delusions, or hallucinations) or non-psychotic symptoms (e.g. high levels of arousal or anxiety).

In the UK, the National Institute for Health and Clinical Excellence (NICE) published detailed guidance on the management of acute behavioural disturbance in 2005, but most hospitals will also have local guidelines that doctors should follow where possible.

A useful framework for thinking about managing behaviour disturbance is as follows:

1 **prediction** of the risk of behavioural disturbance;

2 **prevention** of behaviour escalating once a patient starts to become disturbed;

3 **intervention** to prioritize safety of staff and patients;

4 **review** of events and planning for future risk reduction.

Many mental health trusts now have psychiatric intensive care units (PICUs), which specialize in providing a safer and more secure environment for patients at high risk of acute behavioural disturbance. These wards are locked, have a higher ratio of staff to patients, and have facilities for physical restraint and seclusion. As a rule, patients are transferred to the PICU for the shortest time possible, before being 'stepped down' on to the open wards as soon as it is safe to do so.

■ Prediction

Predicting the likelihood of behavioural disturbance in any given patient should be part of the overall risk assessment done when a patient is first seen or admitted to hospital. This is frequently undertaken in mental health services, but rarely done in the general hospital. It is helpful to think of both the common causes of disturbed behaviour and the personal or situational variables relating to the individual patient (Tables 16.1 and 16.2). Simple measures such as searching the patient's belongings and person for potential weapons and making sure that basic needs (e.g. warmth, hunger) are considered can reduce risks considerably.

■ Prevention

In some cases (e.g. acute confusional state secondary to sepsis) it may be very difficult to predict or prevent

Table 16.1 Causes of acute behavioural disturbance

Organic disorders
Acute confusional state (delirium), see p. 315
Dementia
Intracranial pathology (e.g. tumours, chronic degenerative conditions, epilepsy)
Endocrine conditions (e.g. thyroid disorders)
Infections (e.g. sepsis, HIV, syphilis)
Autoimmune disorders (e.g. SLE)
Psychiatric disorders
Schizophrenia, bipolar disorder, personality disorders (the following features increase risk):
Acute psychosis
Delusions or hallucinations focused on one individual
Command hallucinations
Delusions of control
Preoccupation with violent fantasy
Paranoia and overt hostility
Antisocial or impulsive personality traits
Co-morbid organic disorders
Learning disabilities
Substances
Intoxication or withdrawal from alcohol
Intoxication or withdrawal from illicit substances
Difficult drug adverse effects (e.g. akathasia, dyskinesias)

Table 16.2 Personal and social risk factors for acute behavioural disturbance

Personal history
Previous violent behaviour
Previous use of substances
Use of weapons
History of impulsivity
Lack of insight
Known personal triggers for violence
Verbal threats
Recent severe stress or loss
As a child: cruelty to animals, bed wetting, fire setting
Reckless driving
Social circumstances
Lack of social support
Availability of weapons
Relationship difficulties
Access to potential victims
Difficulty complying with rules and limit setting

behavioural disturbance, but within mental health services it is much easier. All staff should undergo mandatory training covering risk assessment, warning signs of violence, de-escalation techniques, and breakaway. If a patient does start to become aggressive, the first stage is to recognize this and to take steps to de-escalate the situation immediately. All mental health facilities should have an inbuilt alarm system within the building, and many staff carry individual alarms which they can activate to summon immediate support. Some common warning signs of impending aggression are shown in Table 16.3.

Table 16.3 Warning signs of violent behaviour

- Angry facial expression
- Restlessness or pacing
- Shouting
- Prolonged, direct eye contact
- Refusal to communicate or cooperate
- Evidence of delusions or hallucinations with violent content
- Verbal threats or reporting thoughts of violence
- Blocking escape routes
- Evidence of arousal (sympathetic nervous system activation)

De-escalation techniques

The aim is to anticipate possible violence and to *de-escalate* the situation as quickly as possible. Many situations will respond to such measures, and physical restraint or seclusion should only be used when appropriate psychological and behavioural approaches have failed or are inappropriate. One member of staff should be in charge of the situation and should carry out the following steps.

- Encourage the patient to go into a room or area designated for reducing agitation, which is away from other patients and visitors.

- Speak confidently, using clear, slow speech and avoiding changes in volume or tone.

- Adopt a non-threatening body posture—reduce direct eye contact, keep both hands visible, and make slow movements (or pre-warn 'I am going to get up now').

- Explain clearly to the patient what is happening, why, and what will happen next.

- Ask the patient to explain any problems, how they are feeling, and why the situation has arisen. Try and develop a rapport with the patient, show empathy and concern, and offer realistic solutions to any problems.

- If weapons are involved, make sure the minimum number of people are in the room and ask the patient to put the weapon down in a neutral position.

- Use non-threatening verbal and non-verbal communication.

■ Intervention

Whilst non-pharmacological de-escalation techniques are the first line of management, pharmacological treatments ('rapid tranquillization'), physical restraint, or seclusion may need to be used if the risk is not reduced. The aim of drug treatment in such circumstances is to calm the person and reduce the risk of violence and harm, rather than treat the underlying psychiatric condition. One disadvantage of using sedation is that the patient is then unable to participate in further assessment and treatment at that time.

Rapid tranquillization should only be carried out by well-trained teams of professionals (including doctors and nurses) who are able to assess the situation and manage the risks of using medications. The equipment and expertise to do cardiopulmonary resuscitation should be available, as should antidotes to commonly used sedatives (e.g. flumazenil, a benzodiazepine antagonist).

Ideally, a drug would be used that has a rapid onset, short half-life, minimal side effects, and is easily reversible. However, the realistic situation is that all medications have disadvantages and there are a number of risks of rapid tranquillization whatever treatment option you choose (Box 16.1). It is important that after administration of a medication, the appropriate observation and care is carried out.

Figure 16.1 gives a frequently used rapid tranquillization algorithm and some safety considerations that go along with it. Even if the rapid tranquillization medications are prescribed on the 'as needed' part of a medication chart and given at nursing discretion, a doctor should be called to examine the patient as soon as possible. In the UK, the maximum daily doses specified in the *British National Formulary (BNF)* should not be exceeded.

Physical interventions and seclusion

Physical restraint of a patient should be avoided wherever possible, and only used for the shortest amount of time possible. It should only be carried out by trained members of staff according to a specific protocol. Some examples of when it may be appropriate to use physical restraint include the following:

- to administer essential intramuscular medications;

- to allow a doctor to perform an essential physical examination or conduct investigations (e.g. a blood test or vital signs monitoring);

- in order to move a patient to a place of safety so as to reduce the risk to others;

- to prevent continued serious self-harm.

Throughout the restraint, you should continue to use de-escalation techniques and to keep the patient as calm as possible. It is essential that the patient's head and neck are supported and vital signs are monitored. After the

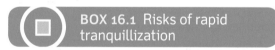

BOX 16.1 Risks of rapid tranquillization

- Over-sedation and loss of consciousness
- Loss of airway
- Cardiovascular or respiratory collapse
- Interactions with other medications
- Arrhythmias (check admission ECG for pre-existing abnormalities)
- Hypo- or hyperthermia
- Neuroleptic malignant syndrome (antipsychotics)
- Seizures (antipsychotics, benzodiazepines)
- Involuntary movements (antipsychotics)
- **Damage to the therapeutic relationship**

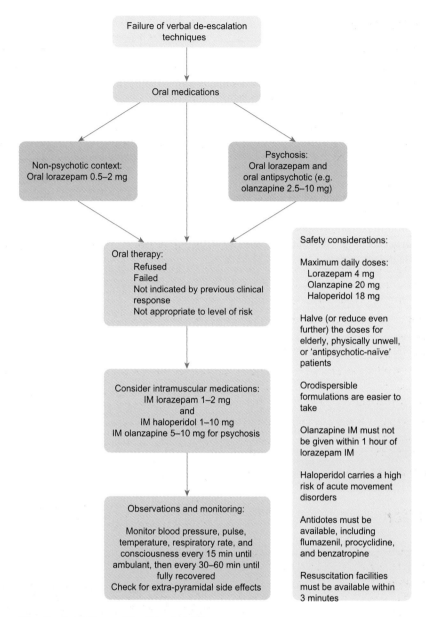

Fig. 16.1 Rapid tranquillization algorithm.

event, it is important to explain to the patient why restraint was needed and help them to understand how to avoid it happening again.

Seclusion is the last resort in managing behavioural disturbance with high risk to others, and should only be carried out on units with a designated seclusion room and highly trained staff. It should not be used as a punishment or because there are staff shortages on the open ward. In most places in the UK, seclusion only occurs on the PICUs. The seclusion room must:

- have clear facilities for staff observation (within eyesight);
- have a comfortable area for the patient to lie down and sleep (e.g. a mattress);

- be well insulated and ventilated;
- have a private toilet and washing facilities;
- be able to withstand attacks/damage.

Patients should only be put into seclusion if verbal de-escalation has failed and rapid tranquillization is not possible or has not had the desired effect. The law states that patients in seclusion must be reviewed by staff every 2 hours, and by a doctor every 4 hours. They must be offered adequate food and drink. It is not appropriate to use seclusion if this may increase the risk of suicide. If rapid tranquillization starts to take effect while the patient is in seclusion, they should be moved back into their usual environment.

■ Review

If a patient has required rapid tranquillization, physical restraint, or seclusion, a post-incident review should take place within 24–72 hours. This will usually be done by the nursing staff on the ward with the involvement of the patient's usual medical team. It is important to review what happened, the triggers, what was successful/unsuccessful in management, and the ongoing impact upon the patient and staff. This helps to provide a more realistic risk management plan for the patient in the future.

 Further reading

National Institute of Health and Clinical Excellence (2005). *CG25 Violence: The short-term management of disturbed/violent behaviour in in-patient psychiatric settings and emergency departments.* http://guidance.nice.org.uk/CG25/QuickRefGuide/pdf/English

Management of specific groups

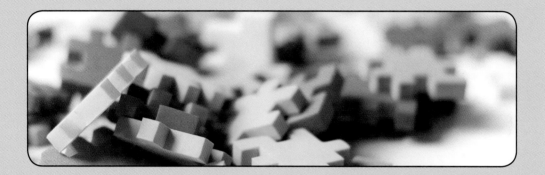

Child and adolescent psychiatry: general aspects of care

CHAPTER 17

Introduction

Child and adolescent psychiatry is relevant to all clinicians who treat either young people or their family members. Emotional, behavioural, and developmental problems are common among children of all ages, and doctors in many specialties are often asked for advice about them by parents. A recent UK prevalence study reported 10 per cent of children aged 5 to 15 years reached diagnostic criteria for a psychiatric disorder. Many of these children are successfully managed in primary care, with about half needing input from specialist child and adolescent psychiatric services. To help these children and their families effectively requires knowledge of normal child development and of the behavioural disorders of this time of life, together with the skills needed to interview the child, assess the problem, and use basic forms of management. This book aims to cover the essential points on each of these topics in enough detail for undergraduates and generalists; however, more detailed texts can be found in the Further Reading section. This chapter covers general aspects of epidemiology, aetiology, assessment, and treatment that are relevant to all of child and adolescent psychiatry, while Chapter 32 deals with common and/or important psychiatric disorders that are specific to childhood. An overview of the differences between child and adult psychiatry is shown in Box 17.1.

Normal child development

Detailed accounts of child development can be found in textbooks of paediatrics (see Further Reading). The

Chapter contents

BOX 17.1 Child and adolescent psychiatry versus adult psychiatry

- Development is a dynamic process; children's behaviour and emotions change with age and psychiatrists' assessment and treatment need to reflect this.

- A child is not an isolated individual; they come in the midst of a family unit and social situation. It may not always be the child who has the greatest need for psychiatric attention.

- It is usually the parents who present with concern that there is a problem with their child, rather than the patient themselves identifying a difficulty.

- Children are smaller than and have different physiology from adults; therefore appropriate medications must be prescribed.

- Children are dependent on others for all of their needs.

- Young people tend to have less choice about their home environment, school, activities, and friends than adults do.

- Children are highly receptive to changes in their environment. Therefore many forms of treatment (behaviour, art, play therapy) that use this have much greater importance.

- There are some conditions (e.g. enuresis) that the majority of children will 'grow out of.

- Those less than 18 years of age are minors in the eyes of the law, and therefore others can make decisions for them.

following account summarizes points that are particularly relevant to the study of childhood emotional and behavioural disorders. It is important to remember that there are wide variations in the speed of development of healthy children.

First year

The child learns about the basic attributes of common objects, spatial relationships, and simple links between cause and effect. By 3 months, they have developed a preference for humans over inanimate objects, and in the next 4 months start to distinguish between people and form specific attachments. From about 7 months most children can sit without support, and by about 12–14 months most can take a few steps unaided. At a year, the child will cooperate with dressing, wave good-bye, and understand simple commands. They should also have a regular pattern of feeding and sleeping. The child forms a strong, secure emotional bond with their regular carers. By about 8 months the child shows signs of distress when separated from the mother, and in the presence of strangers.

Second year

The child begins to walk, explores the environment, and learns that this exploration will be limited at times by the parents (e.g. to avoid danger). The parents demand more of the child as they encourage bowel and bladder training. From 18 months, the child will show some interest in peers, and by 2 years will play alongside (but not with) them. They will be able to recognize themselves in a mirror, and start to understand symbols and make-believe play. By the age of 20 months most children have learnt the words 'dada', 'mama', and three others. As speech and language comprehension increase, it becomes easier for the parents to understand their child's wishes and feelings and to respond to them appropriately.

Age 2–5 years

The child can run, and learns to draw circles, crosses, and then triangles. In this period there is rapid development of language and intellectual functions and children ask many questions. Attention span increases, motor skills are refined, and continence is achieved. Children become less self-centred and more sociable and they learn to share in the life of the family. Gender roles become established, the parents' values are absorbed, and a sense of conscience develops. During this period children are capable of vivid fantasy, expressed in imaginative games. Play helps children to learn how to relate to other children and adults, explore objects, and increase their motor skills.

Later childhood

By 6 years, the child should be able to skip and hop, draw simple shapes, and know left from right. Speech is usually fluent, and they are able to dress themselves alone. Upon starting school, children learn about social relationships with other children and with adults other than the parents. Skills and knowledge increase. Ideas of right and wrong develop further at this age as the influence of school is added to that of the family. Children develop a feeling of self-worth, while learning that they are less successful in some activities than their peers are.

Adolescence

Considerable changes—physical, psychosexual, and social—take place in adolescence and they are usually accompanied by some emotional turmoil. The individual has to come to terms with a new physical self, develop a sense of personal identity and a value system, meet school demands, establish vocational skills, adapt to emotional independence from their parents, and develop peer relationships. In most this occurs relatively smoothly, but it can be a difficult time, and is frequently when psychiatric problems develop. Among older adolescents rebellious behaviour is common, especially during the last years of compulsory attendance at school. Other common problems include relationships, sexual difficulties, delinquent behaviour, excessive drinking of alcohol, and abuse of drugs and solvents. These behaviours and the associated emotional turmoil may be difficult to distinguish from psychiatric disorder.

■ Classification

As in adult psychiatry, diagnosis of psychiatric disorders often relies on the clinician being able to recognize variants of and the limits of normal behaviour and emotions. In children, problems should be classified as either a delay in, or a deviation from, the usual pattern of development. Sometimes problems are due to an excess of what is an inherently normal characteristic in young people (e.g. dieting in anorexia nervosa, anger in oppositional defiance disorder), rather than a new phenomenon (e.g. hallucinations or self-harm) as is frequently seen in adults.

There are four types of symptoms that typically present to child and adolescent psychiatry services:

1 **emotional symptoms** (e.g. anxiety, fears, obsessions, mood, sleep, appetite, somatization);

2 **behavioural disorders** (e.g. defiant behaviour, aggression, antisocial behaviour, eating disorders);

3 **developmental delays** (e.g. motor, speech, play, attention, bladder/bowels, reading, writing and maths);

4 **relationship difficulties** with other children or adults.

There will also be other presenting complaints which fit the usual presentation of an adult disorder (e.g. mania, psychosis), and these are classified as they would be in an adult. Occasionally, there will also be a situation where the child is healthy, but the problem is either a parental illness, or abuse of the child by an adult. Learning disorders are covered in Chapter 19.

Formal classification systems

The DSM-IV and ICD-10 cover all psychiatric conditions, and therefore are just as relevant to children as to adults unless they include a specific age limit. In both classifications there is a section on 'disorders with onset usually in childhood and adolescence' which contains the conditions primarily seen in under-18s. Table 17.1 outlines the conditions diagnosed at less than 18 years, and Table 17.2 lists general psychiatric conditions that are also commonly found in children.

■ Epidemiology

Epidemiological studies carried out in the UK and the USA consistently report that the prevalence of any psychiatric disorder in children and adolescents is approximately 10 per cent. Whilst 1 in 5 children may have a mental health problem, only 1 in 10 need specialist treatment by psychiatrists. Boys are more likely than girls to receive a psychiatric diagnosis, and those aged 11–15 years have a higher prevalence (11 per cent) than children under 11 years (8 per cent). Girls are more likely to have an emotional disorder whilst boys tend to have behavioural disorders. It is important to remember that research in adults has shown half of all patients' problems started in childhood. By 24 years, 75 per cent of individuals who are going to develop a psychiatric disorder at some point will have been diagnosed. The prevalence and 1-year incidence of some of the major conditions found in young people are shown in Table 17.3.

■ Aetiology

Although there are causes specific to each disorder, many others are general. As in adult psychiatry, causes are multiple and fall into four interacting groups: **genetics, physical disease, family, and social or cultural factors** (Table 17.4). Of these, family factors are particularly important.

Genetics

Genetic factors in child psychiatry are mostly polygenic and, as in the disorders of adult life, they interact with environmental factors. Estimates of heritability for most of the common psychiatric disorders are between 50 and 80 per cent, meaning they are the principal determinant of whether or not a child develops the condition. A good example is attention deficit hyperactivity disorder (ADHD), for which the heritability is estimated to be 65 to 75 per cent. First-degree relatives of children with

Table 17.1 ICD-10 and DSM-IV classification of childhood psychiatric disorders

Category of disorder	DSM-IV	ICD-10 (if different from DSM-IV)
PDD	Autistic disorder	Childhood autism
	Rett's disorder	
	Asperger's disorder	
	PDD NOS	Atypical autism
Attention deficit and disruptive behaviour disorders	Attention deficit hyperactivity disorder (ADHD)	Attention deficit disorder with hyperactivity
	ADHD NOS	Hyperkinetic disorder, unspecified
	Conduct disorder	Conduct disorder (confined to the family, unsocialized or socialized)
	Oppositional defiance disorder	Mixed disorder of conduct and emotions
Feeding and eating disorders (anorexia and bulimia nervosa are categorized as in adults)	Pica	
	Rumination disorder	
	Feeding disorder of infancy or childhood	
Tic disorders	Tourette's disorder	
	Chronic motor or vocal tic disorder	
	Transient tic disorder	
	Tic disorder NOS	
Elimination disorders	Encopresis	Non-organic encopresis
	Enuresis	Non-organic enuresis
Other disorders	Separation anxiety disorder	
	Selective mutism	
	Reactive attachment disorder	
	Stereotypic movement disorder	

NOS, not otherwise specified; PDD, pervasive developmental disorder.

ADHD have a three- to fivefold increased risk of also having the disorder, and monozygotic twin studies show 60 per cent concordance.

Physical disease

In childhood, any serious physical disease can lead to psychological problems, but brain disorders (e.g. injury at birth) are particularly likely to have this effect. It has been suggested that minor damage to the brain may be a cause of some otherwise unexplained psychiatric disorders such as conduct disorder. However, evidence for this latter idea is not convincing.

Family factors

To progress successfully from complete parental dependence to independence, children need a stable and secure family environment in which they are loved, accepted, and provided with consistent discipline. Lack of any of these elements can predispose to psychiatric disorder. Examples include the following.

Poor parenting. Parenting skills are predominantly learnt behaviours and, whilst perfection is not needed to successfully raise a child, lack of a stable, organized, attentive relationship can lead to problems. Neglect, abuse, poor boundary setting, and humiliation are particular risk factors.

Family conflict. Arguments within the family—especially between parents—predispose to emotional disorders.

Prolonged absence or loss of a parent can predispose to both emotional and conduct disorders in the child.

Parental illness, whether physical or mental health related, can be a worrying time for a child, especially if they are not included in the discussions and decisions surrounding it.

Care provided outside of the family home. There is a very high rate of psychiatric morbidity in children who have been

Table 17.2 Psychiatric disorders found in all ages, including children and adolescents

- Schizophrenia and other psychotic disorders
- Bipolar disorder
- Depression
- Suicide and deliberate self-harm
- Anxiety disorders and obsessive-compulsive disorder
- Post-traumatic stress disorder
- Eating disorders
- Substance abuse
- Somatoform disorders
- Sleep disorders

Table 17.3 Epidemiology of psychiatric conditions in adolescents. Reproduced (with alterations) with permission from Roberts, R. E., Roberts, C. R., Chan, W. (2009). One-year incidence of psychiatric disorders and associated risk factors among adolescents in the community. *Child Psychology and Psychiatry* **50**: 405–15.

Diagnosis	Prevalence (%)	1-year incidence (%)
Anxiety disorder	6.9	2.9
Mood disorder	2.9	1.9
ADHD	2.0	1.2
Conduct disorder or ODD	5.2	2.6
Substance misuse	5.3	3.8
Anorexia nervosa	0.7	0.01
One or more DSM-IV diagnoses	17.0	7.5
Two or more DSM-IV diagnoses	5.9	3.0

brought up under social services supervision, be it in an institution or a foster home. It is currently unclear how much of the cause is due to experiences prior to going 'into care' and how much is due to being raised in an abnormal family environment.

Social and cultural factors

Wider social influences become increasingly significant as the child grows older, spends more time outside the family, and is influenced by the attitudes and behaviour of other children, teachers, and older people in the neighbourhood. The importance of social factors is reflected in the finding that rates of childhood psychiatric disorder are higher in areas of social disadvantage.

Table 17.4 Causes of childhood psychiatric disorder

Genetics

Physical disease

Family factors

Poor parenting

Separation or divorce of parents

Losses and bereavements

Illness of a parent (physical or mental)

Parental discord

Personality deviance of parent

Large family size

Child abuse and neglect

Care provided by social services

Social and cultural factors

Large changes in lifestyle (new school, new house)

Influences at school

Bullying

Peer group behaviours

Racism or discrimination

Poor social amenities and overcrowding

Lack of community involvement

Break-up of peer relationships (teenagers)

■ The structure of child and adolescent mental health services (CAMHS)

In the UK, and many other countries, child and adolescent mental health services work via a tiered system. The idea is the child enters at the lowest tier that is appropriate for their current problems, and can move up or down as the requirement for treatment changes.

Tier 1: Non-specialists who work with children, e.g. primary care, social work, education, and the voluntary sector.

Tier 2: CAMHS specialists working in the community and primary care.

Tier 3: Multidisciplinary service working in a specialist child psychiatry outpatient service. It is for children with more severe, persistent, or complex disorders. The team will include psychiatrists, psychologists, occupational therapy, social workers, family therapists, dietitians, and play therapists.

Tier 4: Comprehensive tertiary level services such as day-patient and inpatient units, and highly specialized outpatient teams.

■ Assessment of a psychiatric problem in childhood

The aims of assessing a child or adolescent are fourfold;

to obtain a clear account of the presenting problems and detect psychopathology; this includes understanding the parents' attitudes, state of health, and family problems;

5 to relate the problems to the child's temperament, development, and physical condition;

6 to produce a treatment plan;

7 to identify factors inherent to the child, home, or school that may influence the effectiveness of treatment, and work out how to manage these.

Differences between the assessment of children and adults

Although the psychiatric assessment of children resembles that of adults, there are three important differences.

1 When the child is young, the *parents supply most of the verbal information*. Despite this, the child should usually be seen without the parents at some stage.

2 When interviewing a child it is often difficult to follow a set routine, and *a flexible approach is required*.

3 The child should be assessed by *at least two members of the multidisciplinary team,* including a psychiatrist.

An assessment may be done in an outpatient clinic, at school, or at the child's home.

History taking

A full psychiatric, general health, developmental, and family history should be taken. The majority of the information typically comes from the child's parents, but it is also important to get permission to talk to relevant teachers, social workers, childcare providers, significant other family (e.g. grandparents), siblings, other involved clinicians, and the primary care doctor.

Interviewing the parents

The parents are usually seen together, with siblings and any other relevant family members. They should feel that they are part of the solution to the child's difficulties rather than part of the problem. While interviewing the family it is important to note the patterns of interaction between family members (alliances, scapegoating, avoidance), and how easily they communicate with one

another. The important areas to cover in the interview are shown in Table 17.5.

Table 17.5 History taking in child psychiatry

The presenting problem

Who initiated the referral and why

Nature, severity, and frequency

Situations in which it occurs

Factors that make it better or worse

Stresses at home, school, or elsewhere that might be important

Other current problems

Mood and energy level: sadness, depression, suicidal feelings

Anxiety level and specific fears

Activity level, attention, concentration

Eating, sleeping, elimination

Relationship with parents and siblings

Relationships with other children, special friends

Antisocial behaviour

School performance and attendance

Sexual interest and behaviours

Physical symptoms, hearing and vision

Previous psychiatric history

Previous problems and diagnoses

Treatments (including efficacy)

Family history

Family structure—draw a family tree

Current emotional state of parents and children

Separations from and illness of parents

Siblings: age, temperament, health problems

Home circumstances, sleeping arrangements

Psychiatric problems in the wider family

Personal and developmental history

Problems in pregnancy, type of delivery, birth weight, and gestation

Early life—need for special care, early feeding and sleeping patterns, maternal postpartum depression, mother–child relationship

Developmental history, age key milestones reached

Current level of development (language, motor skills)

Past illness and injury, hospital stays

Schooling history: difficulties, abilities, and attainments

Interests, hobbies, talents, and strengths of the child

Interviewing and observing the child

Starting the interview. It is important to (i) establish a friendly atmosphere and win the child's confidence before asking about the problems, and (ii) explain how the psychiatrist and other team members may be able to help. With younger children an indirect and gradual approach is needed, starting with general topics that may engage the child's interest such as pets, games, or birthdays, before asking about the problems. With older children and adolescents it may be possible to follow an approach similar to that for adults.

Continuing the interview. Older children can usually talk about their problems and their circumstances directly but young children need to be helped, for example by asking what they would ask for if given three wishes. Children who have difficulty in expressing their problems and feelings in words may be able to show them in other ways, for example in imaginative play or creative writing.

Observing behaviour. While trying to engage a child in these ways, the interviewer should observe how the child interacts with clinicians and with the parents when they are present. Specific items of the child's behaviour and mental state should be recorded (Table 17.6).

Interviewing other informants

The most important additional informants, other than members of the family, are the child's *teachers*. They can describe classroom behaviour, educational achievements, and relationships with other children. They may also have useful information about the family and their circumstances. In some situations it may be necessary to arrange a school visit to observe classroom behaviour.

Psychological tests

Sometimes questionnaires or other psychological tests can provide information to supplement the clinical assessment, or be used as a quantitative measure of symptoms over time. Some examples are listed below.

- Assessment of IQ can help compare academic performance with potential. The Weschler Intelligence Scale for Children is a commonly used tool.

- Conner's Rating Scales are a screening tool used in the diagnosis and monitoring of ADHD.

- The Eating Disorders Examination (child version) and Eating Disorders Inventory for Children are commonly used to screen for and assess children with suspected eating disorders.

- The Beck Youth Depression Scale or the Mood and Feelings Questionnaire are used in assessment of depression.

Physical examination

A full general examination of the child should be undertaken, especially in those presenting with eating disorders (pp. 341–342). Emphasis should be on a thorough neurological screening, to exclude organic pathology in the CNS. The examination should include:

- height, weight, BMI, head circumference plotted on standard charts;

- standard paediatric cardiovascular, respiratory, ENT, and abdominal examinations;

- any evidence of congenital disorders, dysmorphism features, neglect, or abuse;

- detailed neurological examination.

Investigations

The majority of children presenting with mental health problems will need no investigations. Be guided by the presenting problems and examination results. Some examples include CT/MRI for neurological deficits, genetic testing for dysmorphic features, and thyroid function tests in mood disorders. A full list of the investigations that should be undertaken in eating disorders can be found on p. 342.

Table 17.6 Principal observations of a child's behaviour and emotional state

Rapport with the interviewers, eye contact, spontaneous talk, disinhibition
Relationship with parents
Appearance (dysmorphism, nutrition state, cleanliness, evidence of neglect or abuse)
Stage of development
Activity level and concentration
Mood (sadness, irritability, anxiety, tension)
Involuntary movements
Habits and mannerisms
Presence of delusions, hallucinations, thought disorder
Intellectual abilities, memory
Judgement and insight into problems

■ General aspects of treatment

Although treatment differs in important ways according to the type of disorder, there are many common features (Table 17.7).

Table 17.7 Treatment of child and adolescent mental health problems

Assessment

Diagnosis of psychiatric disorders, co-morbidities, and complications

Risk assessment

Decide upon appropriate level of care:

    Primary care team (Tier 1)

    Specialist mental health workers based in primary care (Tier 2)

    Multidisciplinary specialist CAMHS team (Tier 3)

    Specialist outpatient team (Tier 4)

    Day-patient or inpatient programme (Tier 4)

    Admission to general hospital for medical stabilization

General measures for all patients

Agree a clear treatment plan and assign a care coordinator

Psychoeducation for parents and for the child

Self-help resources for parents and for the child

Reduce any stressors: problem-solving and relaxation techniques

Recommendation of appropriate generic or specific parenting programmes

Regular monitoring of physical health and mental state

Psychological treatments

Behavioural therapy or cognitive behavioural therapy (CBT)

Interpersonal therapy

Group therapy

Family therapy

Play and art therapy

Pharmacological treatments

Stimulants

Antidepressants

Mood stabilizers

Antipsychotics

Social interventions

Assistance with school placements (or work if over 16 years)

Placements with social services for child protection or other issues

Choosing an appropriate setting of care

In most cases, the primary care team can treat the child initially using the general measures in Table 17.7, but a proportion will need specialist treatment. The vast majority of children will be treated as outpatients, with day or inpatient care used only in the following situations:

1 *to treat a severe behaviour disorder* that cannot be managed in another way (e.g. unstable emaciated patients with anorexia nervosa);

2 if the child is deemed to be at *high risk of suicide or deliberate self-harm*;

3 *for observation* when the diagnosis is uncertain;

4 *to separate the child* temporarily from home to assess behaviour in a different environment.

Inpatient admissions are kept as short as possible and used only as a last resort.

Psychoeducation and self-help

An opportunity should be provided for the child and their parents to discuss the diagnosis, and to learn about the nature of the disorder. It is important to cover any preconceptions the parents have surrounding a diagnosis and discuss all available treatment options.

Stressors in the family, at home, at school, or elsewhere often exacerbate the child's psychiatric symptoms, and it is important to help the family to realize this, and to put in place strategies to reduce stressors in the child's life.

There are a wide range of self-help materials available for adults, children, adolescents, and those with special needs. Young people often prefer computer-based programmes. Self-help can be used to impart information, advise on lifestyle choices, teach CBT approaches to problem solving, or provide strategies for parents managing a child with a specific condition.

Parenting programmes

Parenting programmes are now commonly used in child psychiatry, and aim to teach parents techniques to appropriately reward and encourage good behaviour, whilst ignoring and discouraging bad behaviours. Parenting programmes are very good at reducing oppositional behaviour in young children, but are not effective for adolescents. Some commonly used programmes are the Incredible Years Programme and Triple P, but there are also specialized programmes for some specific disorders—for example, the Early Bird Programme for autism run by the National Autistic Society.

Psychological treatments

Behaviour therapy. Behavioural principles are used in the management of many kinds of childhood psychiatric problem. It is based on the idea that behaviour can be changed by altering the consequence of the behaviour, or whatever environmental stimulus triggers it. It may be used alone or as part of cognitive behavioural therapy. Behavioural therapy is based on the principles of conditioning theory, and can be used either to increase desirable behaviours or decrease undesirable behaviours. It is frequently used in ADHD, oppositional defiance disorder (ODD), and autistic spectrum disorder (ASD). Activity scheduling can also be very valuable in those with low mood.

Cognitive behavioural therapy (CBT). CBT in children uses the same principles as in adults (p. 135). As CBT requires the child to be able to identify and label thoughts and feelings and consider the impacts of their behaviour, it is only suitable for children at least 7–8 years old, with behavioural therapy more suitable for those less than 7 years. Cognitive therapy is best in disorders where there is some cognitive distortion as part of the psychopathology or when a purely behavioural approach has only been partly effective. Homework is an important part of CBT, and parents can often be involved with this. Disorders in which CBT is commonly used include depression, anxiety disorders, eating disorders, and conduct disorder. Occasionally, adolescents will be unwilling to engage with a therapist, as they are not yet ready to change their behaviours—in this case it is often helpful to use motivational interviewing as a step prior to starting CBT.

Interpersonal therapy (IPT). IPT works to identify, challenge, and change dysfunctional interpersonal relationships that are having a negative effect upon the child's well-being. It is used frequently in depression, as interpersonal problems are a common precipitating and maintaining factor in depressed patients.

Psychodynamic psychotherapy is usually employed after simpler measures have been tried. Its aim is to identify thought processes that underlie behaviour. The principle is that past events influence current emotions and behaviour. The therapy helps the child to explore issues surrounding past events, and so reduce the effect they have on current behaviour.

Family therapy. Families are always involved in some way in the treatment of children. Family therapy refers to a specific psychological treatment in which the child's symptoms are considered as an expression of difficulties in the functioning of the family. Members of the family meet to discuss their difficulties that appear related to the child's disorder, while the therapist helps them to find ways of overcoming the problems. It is commonly used in mood disorders, OCD, psychosis, eating disorders, and somatization disorders.

Group therapy. Group therapies are used extensively in child and adult day-patient and inpatient programmes for almost every psychiatric condition, and are usually based on CBT principles. They are a cost-effective way of providing therapy, but also help to make the child feel less isolated, learn social skills, and have the chance to explore common issues with peers.

Play and art therapies. For young children, often the best method of making them feel at ease and expressing their true emotions and behaviour is to engage them in an activity they enjoy. It allows the child to communicate with a therapist without speech. Play can be used to show how the child is feeling at that moment, and to recreate past experiences and try to make sense of them. Play therapy is particularly useful for issues surrounding neglect, abuse, loss, bereavement, or separation.

Pharmacological treatments

Medication is considered last because it has only a limited place in the treatment of childhood psychiatric disorders. Medication is first-line treatment for very few conditions, and should only be prescribed in a more severe disorder when psychological and social interventions have failed. Table 17.8 gives an overview of which drugs are used in children, and for which conditions. Benzodiazepines are not recommended for use in those less than 18 years of age.

■ Ethical and legal issues

Consent for treatment

In English legal terms, a 'child' is anyone under the age of 18 years. Children develop psychologically at different speeds, but the law has to decide on set age-related guidelines for obtaining consent, below which the parents typically provide proxy consent. The only caveat is that adolescents may have the right to consent to or refuse treatment if deemed to have capacity to make the specific decision (Gillick competence). Even below the age of consent, the child's agreement should be obtained whenever possible since without it treatment will be more difficult. Parents may refuse treatment for a child, though only when this does not conflict with their duty to protect the child. If the parents' refusal seems not to be in the interests of the child, most countries provide for a decision by a court of law. The Mental Health Act may be used at any age and can be very useful in older children who are disengaging with essential inpatient treatment.

Table 17.8 Use of medications in child and adolescent psychiatry

Class of medication	Indications
Stimulants	ADHD
	ADHD with co-morbid ODD or conduct disorder
	ASD
Antidepressants (SSRIs unless otherwise stated)	Depression
	Anxiety disorders and OCD
	Enuresis (tricyclics)
	Tics with co-morbid anxiety
	Bulimia nervosa
Antipsychotics	Schizophrenia
	Other psychoses
	ASD
	Tics and Tourette's syndrome
	Bipolar disorder
Mood stabilizers	Bipolar disorder
	ASD
Alpha-agonists (e.g. clonidine)	Tics and Tourette's syndrome

ADHD, attention deficit hyperactivity disorder; ASD, autism spectrum disorder; ODD, oppositional defiance disorder; OCD, obsessive-compulsive disorder.

Consent for psychiatric research follows the rules above. Parents may find it difficult to balance the risks to their child against the benefits for others in the future; adequate explanation and discussion are therefore essential.

Conflicts of interest

Usually, the interests of the child are the same as those of the parents. When they are not, those of the child generally take precedence—for example, in suspected abuse. Occasionally, the decision is less obvious—for example, when a depressed mother is neglecting her child but is likely to become more depressed if substitute care is arranged. If the problems are anticipated, they can usually be resolved by discussion with the parents and between the professionals caring for the mother and child.

Confidentiality

Patients of any age have the right to expect that information about them will be held in confidence by their doctor. The care of children often involves the sharing of information with non-medical agencies that do not have identical policies about the confidentiality of records.

Careful thought should be given to the information that it is essential to share, and the need should be discussed with the parents and, if they are old enough, with the children concerned.

■ Child protection issues and child abuse (Table 17.9)

Breakdown of the normal caring relationship between adults in the parental role and children can lead to abuse.

Both the United Nations *Convention on the Rights of the Child* and the World Health Organization have produced a basic set of rights and standards relating to a child's health and living circumstances. Child abuse or neglect may not necessarily occur in the home; it includes child labour, sexual exploitation, and children involved in conflict. Abuse, neglect, or exploitation of a child affects their development in every domain, and is never acceptable.

In the UK, unlike many other countries, there is no legal obligation for anyone except social workers and the police to report suspicions of child abuse. However, the General Medical Council recommends to all doctors that they report to authorities whenever they have reasonable concern about a child's safety. Investigation of a child protection case usually involves social workers, the police, paediatricians (physical investigations), and child psychiatrists. Each hospital trust will have a designated team to deal with these situations, and all doctors should be aware of how to contact them.

Prevalence

It is extremely difficult to obtain accurate figures regarding the epidemiology of child abuse, because most cases never come to the attention of health services. Official incidence statistics report maltreatment of 2–12 per 1000 children in the UK, the USA, and Australia. Of these,

Table 17.9 Forms of child abuse

Child abuse
Physical abuse
Sexual abuse
Emotional abuse
Neglect
Fetal abuse: behaviour detrimental to the fetus (e.g. physical assault on the mother, taking of substances toxic to the fetus by the mother)
Munchausen syndrome by proxy

neglect is the most common (30–50 per cent of cases), followed by physical abuse (15–30 per cent), sexual abuse (10–20 per cent), and then emotional abuse. The sex ratio is equal, except for sexual abuse, which is more commonly against girls. Physically disabled children are three times more likely to be abused. The most vulnerable age group is 0–3 years.

Physical abuse (non-accidental injury)

These terms refer to deliberate infliction of injury on a child by any person having custody, care, or charge of that child. Each year about 1 per 1000 children receive injuries of such severity as to cause a fracture or cerebral haemorrhage. Less severe injury is more frequent, but rarely comes to professional attention. Failure to prevent injury is considered neglect rather than abuse. Discipline through smacking or hitting is common in some countries; there is a blurred line between acceptable and non-acceptable acts.

Detecting abuse

Physical abuse is usually detected when a child presents with injuries for which no other explanation can be found. The problem may become apparent when the parents bring a child to the doctor with an injury said to have been caused accidentally. Alternatively, relatives, neighbours, teachers, or other people may become concerned and report the problem to the police, social workers, or voluntary agencies. Rarely a child or witness may come forward directly. Suspicion of physical abuse should be aroused by:

- the nature of the injuries (Table 17.10);
- previous suspicious injury;
- unconvincing explanations of the way in which the injury was sustained;
- delay in seeking help;
- incongruous reactions to the injury by the carers;

Table 17.10 Injuries caused by physical abuse

- Multiple bruising
- Abrasions
- Bites
- Burns
- Torn lips
- Fractures
- Retinal haemorrhage
- Subdural haemorrhage

- fearful responses of the child to the carers ('frozen watchfulness')
- evidence of distress, such as social withdrawal, regression, low self-esteem, or aggressive behaviour.

Aetiology

There are three sets of aetiological factors relating to the parents, the child, and the social circumstances (Table 17.11). The common factor is a failure of the normal emotional bonding between the parent or other carer and the infant. Knowledge of these risk factors assists in the detection of child abuse.

Management

Assessment of the injuries. When abuse is suspected a specialist assessment should be arranged, giving a full account of the reasons for suspicion. Usually, the child will be admitted to a paediatric ward for assessment, which includes taking photographs of the injuries and a radiological examination, which may show evidence of previous fractures. Occasionally, an organic cause of the injuries will be found—for example, osteogenesis imperfecta. All findings should be clearly and fully documented since evidence may be needed at subsequent legal proceedings.

Subsequent action. Each area has a child protection team who will take over the case and follow the local protocols. If it appears that non-accidental injury is probable, an experienced senior doctor and social worker should *talk to the parents* and arrange to examine other children in their care.

Table 17.11 Risk factors for physical abuse

In the parents	Young age
	Single parent
	Poverty and/or unemployment
	Social isolation
	Mental health or personality disorder
	Personal experience of abuse
	Criminal record
In the child	Premature and/or needing special neonatal care
	Age 0–12 months
	Congenital malformations or disability
	Difficult temperament
In the environment	Poor housing
	Family violence
	Lack of community support

Returning the child. Sometimes the abused child can return home if support and close supervision are provided for the parents. Others need temporary foster care or a permanent alternative home. These very difficult decisions are usually made by a paediatrician or child psychiatrist and a social worker, both experienced in such problems, after discussion with the family doctor.

Prognosis

Children who have been subjected to physical abuse are at high risk of delayed development, learning difficulties, and emotional and behavioural disorders extending into adult life. As adults, former victims of abuse may have difficulties in rearing their own children, and some abuse them. Abuse in childhood is a risk factor for almost every psychiatric condition, and there is a strong association with suicide and deliberate self-harm.

Sexual abuse

The term sexual abuse refers to the involvement of children in sexual activities to which they cannot give legally

---

Science box 17.1 Are retinal haemorrhages a good indicator of non-accidental injury in young children?

Head injuries caused by child abuse are the most common cause of traumatic death in children less than 1 year old. Being able to spot which children presenting with injuries are likely to have been victims of non-accidental injury (NAI) is a frequent diagnostic dilemma, and one which can have grave consequences if missed. In 1974, a radiologist named John Caffey first described the association between retinal haemorrhages (RHs) and 'shaken baby syndrome'.[1] The presence of RH is highly suggestive of intracranial bleeding, and carries a high risk of long-term brain damage. Subsequently, RHs have been widely taught to be a good indicator of NAI, and much research on the topic has been conducted. So, with the hindsight of 40 years' experience and an extensive evidence base, is it still the case that RHs are a sensitive and specific marker of NAI?

At the time of writing, Maguire and colleagues had carried out the largest systematic review on this topic.[2] They included studies primarily comparing the clinical characteristics of children up to 18 years presenting with accidental injury (AI) versus NAI. Unfortunately, this did exclude papers only describing characteristics of children with either NAI or AI. In total, 1655 children were included, 779 with NAI and the rest with AI. They report that in a child with an intracranial injury, apnoea and RH were the features most predictive of NAI, with odds ratios of 17.0 (positive predictive value (PPV) 93%) and 3.5 (PPV 71%), respectively.

A large proportion of severe head injuries caused by abuse occur in less mobile infants and toddlers, primarily those under 2 years. In 2004, Keenan *et al.* reviewed the presenting physical findings of all children under 2 years with intracranial injuries who were admitted to paediatric intensive care units in North Carolina.[3] They included 152 children, half with NAI and half with AI. Children who had suffered NAI were significantly more likely to have RH on admission. Bechtel and colleagues published a smaller prospective study of infants presenting with head injuries.[4] They also report RH to be significantly more frequent in children with NAIs ($P < 0.01$).

There is a good evidence base backing the association between RH and NAI. One important point made in many publications is unless NAI is strongly suspected on first contact with medical services, fundoscopy is often not performed. With the added knowledge that non-ophthalmologists conducting fundoscopy miss up to 15 per cent of RHs, it is imperative that all children should be thoroughly assessed when attending the emergency room with head injuries, including slit-lamp examination by an ophthalmologist.[5]

1 Caffey, J. (1974). The whiplash shaken infant syndrome: manual shaking by the extremities with whiplash-induced intracranial and intraocular bleedings, linked with residual permanent brain damage and mental retardation. *Pediatrics* **54**: 396–403.

2 Maguire, S., Pickerd, N., Farewell, D., *et al.* (2009). Which clinical features distinguish inflicted from non-inflicted brain injury? A systematic review. *Archives of Diseases of Childhood* **94**: 860–7.

3 Keenan, H. T., Runyan, D. K., Marshall, S. W., *et al.* (2004). A population-based comparison of clinical and outcome characteristics of young children with serious inflicted and noninflicted traumatic brain injury. *Pediatrics* **114**: 633–9.

4 Bechtel, K., Stoessel, K., Leventhal, J. M., *et al.* (2004). Characteristics that distinguish accidental from abusive injury in hospitalized young children with head trauma. *Pediatrics* **114**: 165–8.

5 Morad, Y., Kim, Y. M., Mian, M., *et al.* (2003). Nonophthalmologist accuracy in diagnosing retinal hemorrhages in the shaken baby syndrome. *Journal of Pediatrics* **142**: 431–4.

informed consent, or which violate generally accepted cultural rules, and which they may not fully comprehend. The term covers penetrative sexual contact, touching of genitalia, exhibitionism, pornographic photography, and inciting children to engage in sexual practices together. The abuser is usually known to the child and is often a member of the family.

Prevalence

The prevalence of sexual abuse is difficult to determine; UK figures currently suggest approximately 6 per cent of children experience sexual abuse. Half of these cases involved penetration or orogenital contact.

Clinical features

The children are more often female and the offenders usually male. Sexual abuse may be reported directly by the child or by a relative or other person. Children are more likely to report abuse when the offender is a stranger than when he is a family member. Sometimes, sexual abuse is discovered during the investigation of other conditions; for example, symptoms in the urogenital or anal area, behavioural or emotional disturbance, inappropriate sexual behaviour, or pregnancy.

The *immediate consequences* of sexual abuse include anxiety, depression, and anger, inappropriate sexual behaviour, and unwanted pregnancy. *Long-term effects* include low self-esteem, mood disorder, self-harm, difficulties in relationships, and sexual maladjustment.

Assessment

It is important to be alert to the possibility of sexual abuse, and to give serious attention to any complaint made by a child of being abused in this way. It is also important not to make the diagnosis without adequate evidence from a thorough social investigation of the family, and from physical and psychological examinations of the child.

It is essential that information from children is obtained carefully. The child should be encouraged sympathetically to describe what has happened. Drawings or toys may help younger children to give a description, but great care should be taken not to suggest answers to the child. When the circumstances make it appropriate a physical examination is carried out by a paediatrician, including inspection of the genitalia and anal region. If intercourse may have taken place in the past 72 hours, specimens should be collected from the genital and any other relevant regions.

Management

The initial management and the measures to protect the child are similar to those for physical abuse. In families where sexual abuse has occurred, the members may deny the seriousness of the abuse and the existence of other family problems. The discovery of abuse may lead to family conflict that adds to the child's distress. Decisions about treatment and removal from home are taken only after the most careful consideration of all the implications. The sexual development of the abused child is often abnormal, requiring help long after the event. A variety of forms of therapeutic work are used with victims of sexual abuse—the exact type of therapy depends largely upon the needs of the individual child. There is some evidence that group and individual CBT-based programmes reduce the longer-term effects of sexual abuse.

Emotional abuse

The term emotional abuse usually refers to severe and persistent emotional neglect, verbal abuse, or rejection sufficient to impair a child's physical or psychological development. Emotional abuse often accompanies other forms of child abuse but may occur alone. Management resembles that for cases of physical abuse. The parents require help for their own emotional problems, and the child needs counselling, and, in severe cases, a period of separation from the parents.

Neglect

Child neglect includes neglect of the child's physical or emotional needs, upbringing, safety, or medical care, all of which may lead to physical or psychological harm. It may occur within the family home, or within institutions such as children's homes or schools. Neglect may begin prenatally (e.g. maternal substance abuse) and continue through to 18 years old. There are four types of neglect:

1 **physical neglect:** inadequate provision of food, shelter, and clothing;

2 **supervisory neglect:** inadequate parental supervision or interest in the child—this includes failing to provide an education, healthcare needs, and using unsafe care situations;

3 **emotional neglect:** insufficient parental attention to the child's need for affection;

4 **cognitive neglect:** insufficient attention to the child's intellectual, speech, and neurological development, including the provision of adequate schooling.

Neglect of a child's emotional needs and nutrition may lead to **failure to thrive** physically in the absence of a detectable organic cause; height and weight are reduced and development is delayed. The aetiological factors associated with neglect are shown in Table 17.12.

Neglected children soon recover their physical health when provided with adequate nutrition and healthcare. However, they often show significant developmental

Table 17.12 Risk factors for child neglect

Parental characteristics

Living in poverty

Personality difficulties: immaturity, impulsivity, chaotic lifestyle

Low self-esteem

Unrealistic expectations of the child

Psychiatric illness (mood disorders, schizophrenia, substance misuse)

Family characteristics

Lack of affection between family members

Household disorganization

Lack of cognitive stimulation

Poor intrafamilial relationships

delays, especially in speech, language, attention, and school achievements. Many children remain attention-seeking, passive, and helpless.

Munchausen syndrome by proxy

This rare disorder is where a parent or carer repeatedly fabricates an illness or disability in a child they are looking after, for the benefit of themselves. The adult involved is most frequently the child's mother, but not always. There are several important aspects to this condition:

- the physical harm caused to the child through falsification of illness;
- the impact upon the child's physical and emotional development;
- the psychological status of the adult involved.

The clinical presentation may be with any symptom or sign. Fabrication may be at the level of the history of presenting complaint given, an inaccurate past medical history, interference with hospital notes/blood specimens/equipment readings or induction of an illness (e.g. by poisoning or hurting the child). The diagnosis is usually made by an alert paediatrician, for whom the story does not quite add up. The majority of children involved are under 5 years, and over 80 per cent of fabricators are females. Half of these fit diagnostic criteria for a personality disorder. Once the diagnosis is made, the child usually recovers quickly from any physical consequences, but remains at high risk of developing genuine psychiatric conditions in later years. Treatment of the fabricator is paramount.

 Further reading

Gelder, M., Andreasen, N., Lopez-Ibor, J, & Geddes, J. (eds) (2009). *New Oxford Textbook of Psychiatry*, 2nd edn. Child and adolescent psychiatry, pp. 1587–816. Oxford University Press, Oxford.

National Institute of Health and Clinical Excellence (2009). *When to Suspect Child Maltreatment*. http://guidance.nice.org.uk/CG89.

Lissauer, T. & Clayden, G. (2007). *Illustrated Textbook of Paediatrics*, 3rd edn. Mosby Elsevier, London.

CHAPTER 18

Psychiatry of older adults

■ Epidemiology and principles of management

The provision of mental health services for older adults faces two main challenges. Our ageing population is leading to an ever increasing number of patients (Figure 18.1), and those patients often present with multiple, complex co-morbidities, which must be manageing alongside acute psychiatric problems. As many illnesses, including most of the dementias, occur more frequently with increasing age, the proportion with cognitive impairment will double in the UK in the next 50 years and will increase even more dramatically in less developed countries.

People with mental health problems are often physically and mentally frail and services must be designed with this in mind. Physical illness may cause the patient to present in different ways, and often has poor prognostic implications. The practice and organization of services must take psychological, physical, and social needs into account; for example, the use of day patient programmes is a common strategy. The multidisciplinary team is key to providing effective treatment.

Normal ageing

A huge number of physical, psychological, and social changes occur within the normal process of ageing. A basic understanding of these is necessary in order to identify those individuals in whom there is pathology.

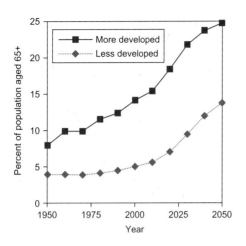

Fig. 18.1 The percentage of the population aged 65 and over for more developed and less developed countries. (Data from 1996 United Nations population estimates and projections from Jorm, A. F. (2000).) Fratiglioni, L. & Henderson, S. (2009). The ageing population and epidemiology of mental disorders among the elderly. In *New Oxford Textbook of Psychiatry*, 2nd edn. Eds Gelder, M., Andreasen, N., Lopez-Ibor, J, & Geddes, J. Oxford University Press, Oxford.

Biological theories

Ageing is defined as *'the accumulation of changes in an organism or object over time'*, and is known as senescence in biology. There are two main theories of ageing.

The genomic theory states that ageing is primarily due to changes in the genetic constitution of the organism. It was originally suggested from the observation that most species have characteristic lifespans. As lifespan increases, there are increased numbers of errors in DNA replication, reduced efficiency of DSN repair genes, increased epigenetic errors, and a decline in mitochondrial function. All of these lead to abnormal or ineffectual proteins, which cause cell malfunction or death. A popular idea within this theory is that of telomere loss—within cells the telomerase is down-regulated with increasing age and so telomeres (which are essential for DNA stability and maintenance) are gradually lost. It is known that 25–30 per cent of life expectancy is genetically determined.

The stochastic theory suggests that an accumulation of random adverse events at the cellular level leads to a gradual functional decline. This could be via an accumulation of waste products, free radical formulation, or gradual cross-linkage between macromolecules. The theory is mainly based on evidence showing that basal metabolic rate is inversely proportional to life expectancy, and that calorie restriction (with adequate nutrients) leads to an increase in lifespan.

Physical changes

The following changes are seen in the brain in normal ageing.

- The weight of the brain decreases by 5–20 per cent between age 70 and 90 years. There is a compensatory increase in ventricular size.
- There is neuron loss, especially in the hippocampus, cortex, substantia nigra, and cerebellum.
- Senile plaques are found in the neocortex, amygdala, and hippocampus.
- Tau proteins form neurofibrillary tangles, which are usually only in the hippocampus.
- Lewy bodies are seen in the substantia nigra.
- Ischaemic lesions (reduced blood flow, lacunar infarcts) are seen in 50 per cent of normal people over 65 years.

Psychological changes

From mid life there is a decline in intellectual functions, as measured with standard intelligence tests, together with deterioration of short-term memory and slowness. IQ peaks at 25 years, remains stable until 60–70 years and then declines. Problem solving reduces after about age 60. Also, there may be alterations in personality and attitudes, such as increasing cautiousness, rigidity, and 'disengagement' from the outside world.

Social changes

Later life presents a series of major changes. Many individuals retire, lose partners, lose their physical health, and are forced to live on much lower incomes and in poorer-quality housing than younger people. These are difficult transitions which may predispose to mental illness. The majority of older people remain living at home—half with a partner, and 10 per cent with other family members. Those who live alone may be isolated and lonely.

Use of medical services

Older people consult their family doctors more often than younger people and they occupy two-thirds of all general hospital beds. These demands are particularly great in those aged over 75. Treatment is often made difficult by the presence of more than one disorder and by increased sensitivity to drug side effects.

Epidemiology

It is estimated that there will be over 1 billion people aged over 65 years by 2030, of whom 70 per cent are found in developed countries. Psychiatric disorders, like physical illness, are especially prevalent in older adults

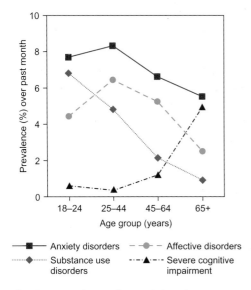

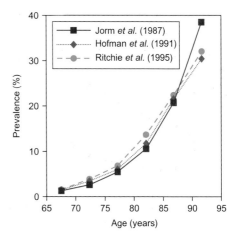

Fig. 18.2 The prevalence of mental disorders across age groups. (Data from 1-month prevalence rates from the Epidemiologic Catchment Area Study using DSM-III criteria; from Jorm, A. F. (2000).) Fratiglioni, L. & Henderson, S. (2009). The ageing population and epidemiology of mental disorders among the elderly. In *New Oxford Textbook of Psychiatry*, 2nd edn. Eds Gelder, M., Andreasen, N., Lopez-Ibor, J, & Geddes, J. Oxford University Press, Oxford.

Fig. 18.3 Prevalence rates for dementia across age groups: data from three meta-analyses. (From Jorm, A. F. (2000).) Fratiglioni, L. & Henderson, S. (2009). The ageing population and epidemiology of mental disorders among the elderly. In *New Oxford Textbook of Psychiatry*, 2nd edn. Eds Gelder, M., Andreasen, N., Lopez-Ibor, J, & Geddes, J. Oxford University Press, Oxford.

(Figure 18.2). Although psychiatric disorders in old age have some special features, they do not differ greatly from the psychiatric disorders of younger adults. Table 18.1 compares the prevalence of some common psychiatric conditions in the older and general adult populations. The greatest burden of disease is in two areas: mood and anxiety disorders, and cognitive impairment. Dementia

makes up a large proportion of an old age psychiatrist's caseload, and its prevalence is highly correlated to increasing age (Figure 18.3).

What types of mental disorder are seen in older patients?

Many of the same disorders affect older people as affect younger people. They can be subdivided into three types:

1 pre-existing problems that continue into older age;

2 new diagnoses after the age of 65;

3 mental health disorders associated with ageing.

Management and prognosis may depend on which of these subgroups are relevant, information which is usually gained from a comprehensive history. Common diagnoses include:

Table 18.1 Prevalence of common psychiatric conditions in older adults. From the UK Office for National Statistics 2010, www.statistics.gov.uk.

Diagnosis	Prevalence in adults aged 18–64	Prevalence in adults over 65
Depression	5.8%	10%
Psychosis	0.5%	< 1%
Bipolar disorder	1.5%	1%
Generalized anxiety disorder	5–6%	10%
Alzheimer's disease	< 1% before 65 years	1% aged 60
		5% aged 70
		40% aged 85
Completed suicides per year	11/100 000	14/100 000

- dementia;
- delirium;
- mood disorders: depression and bipolar disorder;
- anxiety disorders;
- psychoses: schizophrenia and delusional disorder;
- suicide and deliberate self-harm;
- alcohol and substance misuse.

As in child and adolescent psychiatry, much of the assessment, management, and service provision are standardized via a multidisciplinary assessment, no matter what the diagnosis.

Assessment of mental health disorders in older patients

The assessment of older people presenting with a psychiatric problem is fundamentally the same as in the younger population, but extra consideration must be given to several areas.

1 Is this an episode of a recurrent problem, or a completely new diagnosis?

2 Are the symptoms being caused by mental illness, or could it be an organic pathology (e.g. brain tumour, dementia)?

3 What physical illnesses does the patient have, and how do these complicate the situation?

4 What is the patient's social situation, and what is their level of function in activities of daily living?

The general practitioner usually refers to psychiatric services, but it may be a social worker, clinician in any specialty, residential home staff, or someone else in contact with the patient. The referral should clearly state the problem and its context. Once a referral has been received, an assessment will be arranged. In the UK, this is usually by the old age psychiatry team, who look after a specific geographical area. A place to assess the patient must be chosen, taking account of their cognitive state, sensory losses, and preferences. It is always best to assess someone in their home environment if possible, as this maximizes the chance of them performing at their best, and reduces the difficulties in arranging transport. However, it is less convenient for the medical team.

A full assessment of an older adult should be undertaken by a multidisciplinary team including a psychiatrist, psychologist, occupational therapist, physiotherapist, and social worker. A patient advocate (an independent party representing the patient) may also be needed if there is pronounced cognitive impairment. The full assessment will include:

- full history from the patient, family, carers, GP, and other clinicians;
- full physical and neurological examination;
- full cognitive assessment, including a Mini Mental State Examination (MMSE);
- functional assessment (activities of daily living and mobilization);
- social assessment (housing, finances, activities);
- assessment of carers' needs.

History

Most older adults are able to give a full, accurate account of their symptoms and situation themselves, but sometimes they are unable to do so, and it is necessary to speak to family, friends, carers, GP, and other relevant clinicians/professionals to obtain information. The general history in terms of presenting symptoms is no different to that in younger patients. The specific information to be gathered is shown in Box 18.1.

The Mental State Examination

This is fundamentally the same as in other age groups. One important point is to try to distinguish between depression and dementia.

Appearance and behaviour. Observation of the patient's clothing, personal cleanliness, and home environment often provides valuable information. They may point to mental illness, or to neglect. Look for signs that suggest these are chronic problems rather than caused by an acute illness (e.g. delirium). Agitation or psychomotor retardation may be obvious. Wandering, incontinence, and disorientation may point to dementia.

Speech. Dysphasia is frequently seen in moderate to advanced dementia, or after a stroke. In delirium, dementia, or alcohol excess, speech may be inappropriate. Lack of speech may suggest depression, and excessive quantities of rapid speech may suggest mania.

BOX 18.1 Taking a psychiatric history in an older adult

The following specific information should be obtained during the assessment:

- timing of onset of symptoms and their subsequent course;
- any previous similar episodes;
- a description of behaviour over a typical 24 hours;
- previous medical and psychiatric history (including previous intellectual ability and personality characteristics);
- accurate drug history;
- family history of psychiatric problems;
- living conditions;
- financial position;
- ability for self-care, shopping, cooking, laundry;
- ability to manage finances and deal with hazards such as fire;
- any behaviour that may cause difficulties for carers or neighbours;
- the ability of family and friends to help;
- other services already involved in the patient's care.

Mood. Older people may not admit to low mood, sadness, or depression. Anhedonia, fatigue, weight loss, anorexia, and insomnia are common. Suicidal ideation and passive death wish are more common in older than in younger adults. Florid mania is rare, but presents as in younger patients.

Thoughts. There are no specific differences in older people. Anxiety is very common. Delusions are seen in depression, delusional disorder, delirium, and dementia.

Perceptual disturbances. Hallucinations are common in dementia and delirium, but also in pre-existing or late-onset psychoses. Visual hallucinations are particularly associated with delirium and alcohol withdrawal.

Cognition. The MMSE (see below) is the best tool to assess cognition. A 10-point abbreviated mini mental test score may also be helpful.

Insight. This is typically poor. Good insight into low mood suggests depression rather than dementia.

Examination and investigation

Physical examination. A detailed physical examination should be carried out on all patients, as there are likely to be physical co-morbidities. This should include a neurological examination, and an assessment of vision and hearing.

Physical investigations. It is wise to carry out a number of screening investigations, to exclude an organic cause for the symptoms. Those in italics are needed for patients presenting with relatively acute symptoms, primarily to exclude delirium:

- blood for full blood count, urea and electrolytes, liver function tests, thyroid function tests (FBC, U + Es, LFTs, TFTs,) calcium, phosphate, magnesium, glucose, lactate, troponin, albumin, haematinics, syphilis serology;
- chest X-ray;
- imageing, e.g. computed tomography of the head;
- *blood and urine cultures;*
- *arterial blood gas;*
- *electrocardiogram (ECG);*
- *urinalysis.*

Psychological and cognitive assessment

Tests should be used within the wider context of obtaining information from the history and clinical examination. They should be regularly repeated, especially after any acute illness or stressor. The Geriatric Depression Scale or Beck Depression Index may be used to screen for depression. Complex cognitive investigations are usually not needed, but the following are useful simple tests to quantify the level of impairment.

- **Abbreviated Mental Test Score (AMTS)** out of 10 points, score of 6 or less taken as delirium (http://en.wikipedia.org/wiki/Abbreviated_mental_test_score).

- **Mini Mental State Examination (MMSE)** out of 30 points, with more than or equal to 25 taken as normal, mild dementia 21–24, moderate 10–20 and severe <10 points. It tests the domains of orientation, attention, calculation, memory and language.

The AMTS is often used sequentially to monitor for improvement or decline in functioning. The MMSE is primarily used for dementia, but may be helpful in delirium. In severe depression, the phenomenon of 'psuedodementia' may occur, in which the patient complains of poor memory. However, on formal memory testing they show no deficit.

Provision of psychiatric services for older adults

In the UK, the National Framework for Older People (2001) sets out standards to ensure older adults receive person-centred care in appropriate settings, without suffering age discrimination. It is similar to the World Health Organization's (WHO) CARITAS consensus, which is a set of values agreed by many countries as to which mental health services should be available for older people. As in the rest of psychiatry, there is a basic separation of services into outpatient, day-patient, and inpatient facilities, with some additional settings of care. These are outlined in Table 18.2. There is also a large number of voluntary sector provided services, mostly in the form of day centres or home visiting schemes, which are accessible free of charge. They are helpful in providing help or advice on

Table 18.2 Types of psychiatric services available for the older patient

Type of service	Setting	Characteristics and treatments provided
Psychiatric inpatient units	Hospital	24-hour specialist care
		MDT assessment
		Treatment with drugs, ECT, specialist nursing, talking therapies
		Rehabilitation
		Case management
		Usually short admissions
		Can accept patients under section
Acute medical wards	Hospital	Treatment of acute physical illness
		Basic assessment of mental health state
		Usually as a temporary or emergency measure

Table 18.2 Types of psychiatric services available for the older patient (*Continued*)

Type of service	Setting	Characteristics and treatments provided
Consultation and liaison services	Hospital	Psychiatrist visits patients in the general hospital
		Support for acute medical services
		Direct referrals to appropriate follow-up on discharge
Day hospitals	Hospital	Often cater for specialist groups (e.g. advanced dementia)
		Hospital-level treatment whilst remaining at home
		Respite for carers
Community outpatient services	Community	MDT assessment at home
		Case management
		Drug treatments and talking therapies
Specialist residential care	Community	May be private, state funded, or run by a voluntary agency
		For those unable to live independently
		24-hour personal and nursing care
		Often specialize in particular diagnoses
		Psychiatrists may visit the home to see patients
Respite care	Hospital or community	Brief admissions to a residential home or hospital
		Gives carers some time off
		Financially difficult to support
Primary care	Community	Consistent support and treatment
		Basic assessment
		Treatments
		Integrating treatment for mental and physical health problems

MDT, multidisciplinary team.

social and financial aspects, and are complementary to traditional medical services. Admission to an inpatient facility should only occur when less intensive treatment options have not been successful, or when life is at risk.

Principles of treatment

Although treatment differs in important ways according to the type of disorder, there are many common features. Specific treatments for particular conditions are covered in the latter half of this chapter, or in Chapter 26 for cognitive disorders. Table 18.3 outlines the major options for treatment in old age psychiatry, but for any given patient, only a few of these will be relevant.

Table 18.3 Treatment options in old age psychiatry

Assessment

Physical, psychological, cognitive, and social

Decide on an appropriate level of care

Primary care team

Specialist mental health workers based in primary care

Specialist outpatient, day patient, or inpatient care

Admission to general hospital for acute medical treatment

General measures

Treat any physical disorders

Psychoeducation of patient, family, and carers

Promote and maintain independence with a written care plan

Make decisions regarding capacity

Provide and assist with the use of self-help materials

Offer physiotherapy and occupational therapy

Provide training courses, support groups, and respite care for carers

Pharmacological

Antidepressants

Antipsychotics

Acetylcholinesterase inhibitors

Benzodiazepines

Psychological

CBT, individual or group

Group therapy

Psychological support for carers

Social

Arrange suitable living environment and personal care if required

Financial advice and assistance

Arrange appropriate social activities

In most situations, the treatment of psychiatric disorders in older adults resembles that of the same conditions in younger adults, although there are some differences in emphasis:

- it is more often necessary to treat concurrent physical disorders;
- maintaining function and independence is paramount;
- special caution is needed in drug dosages;
- social measures and services are even more important;
- families need to be involved and supported, even more than with younger patients;
- capacity and other ethical issues are important (Box 18.2).

Ethical issues

Ethical issues are similar to those in younger people but problems relating to impaired capacity are much more common (Box 18.2). It may be necessary to consider practical matters as well as the ability to consent to treatment. In the UK, the Mental Capacity Act 2005 sets out to protect those individuals who do not have the capacity to make decisions for themselves, and provides the principles by which decisions of capacity may be made. A summary of the guidance it gives is shown in Box 18.3.

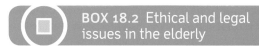

BOX 18.2 Ethical and legal issues in the elderly

- Confidentiality in relation to information from carers
- Confidentiality of information about financial circumstances
- Consent to treatment:
  - capacity to consent to physical and psychological treatment
  - advance directives
  - decisions 'not to treat'
- Management of financial affairs:
  - nominating another to take responsibility (Power of Attorney)
  - procedures to enable others to take responsibility
- Entitlement to drive a car

Deciding on an appropriate level of care

Decisions upon the setting in which to treat an older patient are fundamentally the same as for younger patients. The indications for admission to hospital for depression, psychoses, etc. are as outlined in the chapters covering these conditions. Patients may be treated

BOX 18.3 The Mental Capacity Act 2005

Mental capacity is the ability to make decisions for ourselves. The Mental Capacity Act provides the means to assess whether or not an individual has capacity, and, if not, how those caring for them can make decisions in their best interests. There are various elements contained within the act:

Assessing capacity. The act sets out a clear test for assessing whether a person lacks capacity to make a particular decision at a particular time. To make a decision a person must:

- have a general un derstanding of the decision and why they need to make it;
- have a general understanding of the likely consequences of making, or not making, the decision;
- be able to understand, retain, use, and weigh up the information presented to them;
- be able to communicate their decision to others.

Best interests. The act contains a checklist of factors that must be worked through to decide what is in a person's best interests.

Acts in connection with care or treatment. The Act offers statutory protection from prosecution where a person is performing an act in connection with care or treatment of someone who lacks capacity. For example, providing medical treatment in the patient's best interests.

Lasting Powers of Attorney (LPA). This allows a person to appoint an attorney to act on their behalf if they should lose capacity in the future. There is a formal legal protocol to register an attorney.

Advance decisions to refuse treatment. The act makes it possible to make an advance decision to refuse treatment should a person lack capacity in the future.

Safeguards. A number of safeguards have been put in place to ensure that individuals lacking capacity are treated in the rightful manner. These include a court of protection, a public guardian (who is responsible for creating all LPA), and independent mental capacity advocates (IMCAs). The latter are individuals appointed to speak for a person who lacks capacity and has no one to speak for them.

Office of the Public Guardian and Ministry for Justice. *Mental Capacity Act 2005*, www.justice.gov.uk/about/mental-capacity.htm

involuntarily (under 'section' or 'commitment') in the usual way. One specific consideration is safety at home—they may be unable to provide adequately for their own physical needs (such as warmth, food, and personal hygiene), or lack a physically safe environment (trip-free floors, risk-free heating, and cooking facilities).

General measures

Physical conditions. The first issue to address is the treatment of any physical disorder causing organic mental disorder. A good example of this is the correction of electrolyte abnormalities in delirium (which may be hiding an underlying dementia) or hypothyroidism in depression. The treatment of other physical disorders may benefit the mental state in a non-specific way. The latter is especially true for cardiorespiratory disorders. Mobility should be encouraged, and is often helped by physiotherapy and occupational therapy. A nutritional assessment by a dietitian is essential.

Psychoeducation should begin at the time a diagnosis of mental illness is made and continue throughout the illness. The patient, their relatives, and carers should all be actively informed of the following: symptoms of the condition, course and prognosis, treatments, support groups, financial and legal considerations (e.g. capacity and driving), and where to look for further information.

A written care plan is the recommended way of ensuring consistent, high-quality treatment tailored to the individual's needs. This can be drawn up soon after the diagnosis is made, and includes important decisions such as views on residential accommodation, end-of-life care, and resuscitation. The majority of patients will want to remain living independently for as long as possible, and this should be supported and respected.

Support for carers is as important as treatment of the patients themselves. There are many training courses and support groups for carers available, many of which are run by the voluntary sector and are free of charge. Information and help in making capacity decision—for instance, setting up a Lasting Power of Attorney—should be offered. Having respite care available for short-term use is invaluable to carers, especially in the later stages of dementia. Frequently, carers may suffer distress themselves during the illness; psychological interventions such as cognitive behavioural therapy (CBT) or counselling should be offered where appropriate.

Memory aids. Patients with memory disorder may be helped by simple measures such as the use of notebooks and alarm clocks to aid memory. In residential accommodation, aids such as colour coding of furniture can help recall.

Pharmacological treatment

Drug-induced morbidity is common among older adults who may develop side effects at lower doses than younger people, and may not be in a position to communicate these easily to others. It is therefore essential to consider very carefully before starting any new medications. However, patients should not be denied effective drug treatment, especially for depressive disorders. Some drugs may cause psychiatric symptoms as side effects; most often these are drugs that are:

- used to treat cardiovascular disorders (antihypertensives, diuretics, and digoxin);
- acting on the central nervous system (antidepressants, hypnotics, anxiolytics, antipsychotics, and antiparkinsonian drugs);
- acting on the endocrine system (steroids, thyroxine, hormones).

It is prudent to start treatment with small doses and increase these gradually to find the minimal effective dose. With increasing age, liver metabolism is slowed and renal function may become impaired. Lower doses of drugs may therefore be needed, and the threshold for toxicity is lower. Older people are more prone to extrapyramidal and anticholinergic side effects. Response to the medication should be reviewed regularly.

It is worth remembering that patients may not take drugs as prescribed, especially when they are living alone, have poor vision, or are confused. For this reason, the drug regimen should be as simple as possible, medicine bottles should be labelled clearly and easy to open, and the patient should be provided with memory aids (e.g. by containers with separate compartments for the drugs to be taken at each time of day). If possible, drug taking should be supervised by one of the carers or by a community nurse, both of whom need to be adequately informed of the drug regimen.

Many older people sleep poorly, and some take hypnotics regularly. Such drugs should be avoided as they may cause daytime drowsiness, confusion, falls, incontinence, and hypothermia. If a hypnotic is essential, the minimum effective dose should be used, the side effects monitored carefully, and the course of treatment made as short as possible. Z-drugs (e.g. zopiclone) and medium- or short-acting benzodiazepines are the safer hypnotics.

Psychological treatment

It is sometimes thought that older people do not want to engage in, or respond to, psychological treatments. This is not true. Many older people prefer talking treatments to medicines and they are just as effective as in younger adults. The UK NICE guidelines for depression and anxiety recommend that the same psychological options should be offered to all ages. Those with mild to moderate cognitive impairment can benefit from adapted therapeutic programmes.

- **Discussion and problem solving** are often helpful, especially when important life decisions such as possible changes in living arrangements need to be made.
- **Group supportive psychotherapy** can be helpful and also provides some social interaction. This may be carried out at a day-patient programme or day centre.
- **Individual cognitive behavioural therapy** should be offered to those with mood or anxiety disorders.
- **Interpretative psychotherapy** is seldom appropriate.

Social measures

Organizing a suitable living environment is essential to manageing both physical and mental health. Eighty per cent remain in their own home, and many patients can be helped to remain independent by attendance at a day centre. These provide activities, social contact, a cooked meal, and access to medical and social services. More severely impaired patients may benefit from moving to a residential or nursing home, provided that their individual needs and dignity are respected. Table 18.4 summarizes social considerations.

■ Specific psychiatric disorders

Cognitive impairment: delirium and dementia

These common disorders are covered in Chapter 26 (pp. 312–329).

Depressive disorders

Older people experience profound changes—loss of a partner, reduction in income, physical illness—which influence their mood and predispose to depression. Clinicians are poor at identifying depression in older adults, but it worsens the prognosis of most physical conditions and is treatable, and so it should always be considered.

Clinical features

There are no fundamental differences in the management of depressive disorders in older and younger people, but some symptoms are more common. Anxiety, somatic, and hypochondriacal symptoms are frequent. Depressive delusions of poverty, nihilism, and physical illness are more common among severely depressed patients, as are hallucinations of an accusing or obscene kind. Deliberate self-harm is rare, and should be taken seriously. Occasionally, behavioural changes can be an indicator of depression; for instance, new-onset incontinence, poor oral intake, or alcohol misuse.

Some depressed patients have conspicuous difficulty in concentrating and remembering but there is no corresponding defect in clinical tests of memory function (**pseudodementia**). The differences between dementia and pseudodementia are shown in Table 18.5. Psychomotor agitation or retardation occurs in 30 per cent of depressed older patients. The possibility of a depressive disorder should be considered whenever a patient develops apparent cognitive impairment, anxiety, or hypochondriacal symptoms.

The diagnostic criteria are the same as for younger adults, and are described on p. 223.

Prevalence

The prevalence of clinically significant depressive disorders in older people living at home is 10–15 per cent.

Table 18.4 Social considerations in treating older adults

Psychosocial treatments
Encourage self-care
Social contacts
Legal and financial advice
Financial
Driving
Determining mental capacity
Social services
Domiciliary
Day care
Residential and nursing care
Voluntary services

Table 18.5 Distinguishing the pseudodementia of depression from dementia

Dementia	Depression ('pseudodementia')
Insidious onset over months	Quicker onset, days to weeks
Mood and behaviour fluctuate	Mood and behaviour consistent
Biological symptoms absent	Biological symptoms present
Denies (or attempts to hide) poor memory	Admits to poor memory
Impaired orientation	Normal orientation
Reduced MMSE on testing	Normal MMSE on testing
Less often a personal history of depression	Often a personal history of depression
No response to antidepressants	Responds to antidepressants

MMSE, Mini Mental State Examination.

In residential care or general medical wards the prevalence is higher, at 20–40 per cent. Many of these disorders are found in people who have had a depressive disorder at an earlier age; first depressive illnesses decline in incidence after the age of 60, and are rare after the age of 80. Unlike in younger adults, the numbers of cases in males and females are approximately equal. The incidence of **suicide** increases steadily with age and is usually associated with depressive disorder.

Differential diagnosis

- **Dementia.** The most difficult differential diagnosis is between depressive pseudodementia and dementia, and a specialist opinion is often required. The distinction depends on a detailed history from other informants, and careful observation of the mental state and behaviour of the patient (Table 18.5). The diagnostic problem is made more difficult because dementia and depressive disorder sometimes coexist.

- **Paranoid disorder.** In a depressive disorder, the patient usually believes that the supposed persecution is justified by his own wickedness; in a paranoid disorder he usually resents it as unjustified. Depressive symptoms usually follow the onset of paranoid disorder, but it is often difficult to be certain of the sequence.

- **Anxiety disorder.** A depressive disorder with symptoms of agitation may be mistaken at first for an anxiety disorder. Look for low mood, anhedonia, and fatigue.

- **Stroke.** It may be difficult to distinguish between mood symptoms caused by cerebral damage (especially of left frontal lobe) and depression secondary to an adverse situation caused by the stroke. Practically, treatment should be as for any depressive episode.

- **Parkinson's disease.** Mood symptoms may be an intrinsic part of Parkinson's disease itself, or be side effects of antiparkinsonian medications.

- **Organic mood disorders.** The most common are hypothyroidism, cancer, chronic infection, and medication side effects.

Aetiology

In general, the aetiology of depressive disorders in late life resembles that of similar disorders occurring in earlier life (see Chapter 21), except that genetic factors may be less important. As in other groups, a depressive episode tends to present when a precipitating event (usually an adverse life event) occurs in a vulnerable individual. The most important risk factors are neurological or other chronic physical illnesses, and loss of a partner. Common stressors include:

- retirement;
- loss of mobility leading to social isolation;
- poverty;
- lack of support from family or friends;
- moving from own home into a residential or nursing home;
- hospital admission.

Course

Untreated depressive disorders often have a prolonged course, some lasting for years. With treatment, most patients improve considerably within a few months, but about 15 per cent do not recover completely even after vigorous treatment. Long-term follow-up of recovered patients shows that relapse is frequent. Suicide is more likely than in younger people.

The factors predicting a better prognosis are:

- onset before the age of 70;
- short duration of illness;
- good previous adjustment;
- no concurrent disabling physical illness;
- good recovery from previous episodes.

There is some evidence that depression is a risk factor for later developing dementia. This is not yet well characterized, but may be due to chronic depression precipitating hippocampal atrophy, or it may be that the depressive episode is actually one early way that dementia may present.

Assessment

A full assessment should be carried out as outlined in the section above. The best clinical screening tool is the **Geriatric Depression Score**, a questionnaire of 30 (or 15 in the condensed version) yes/no statements, which has reasonable sensitivity and specificity. A score of more than or equal to 11 (or 5 in the condensed version) is suggestive of depression. A full set of blood tests is usually all that is needed in terms of investigations.

Management

In the UK, management of depressive disorders is as outlined in the National Institute for Health and Clinical Excellence (NICE) guidelines, last updated in 2005. These are relevant to all ages. Full details can be found in Chapter 21, so what follows are specific points relating to treatment in older adults. Table 18.6 contains a summary of the various options.

Antidepressant drugs are effective, but should be used cautiously and adjusted according to side effects and response. A Cochrane systematic review of patients over 55 years has found no difference in the efficacy of SSRIs compared with tricyclic antidepressants (TCAs). However,

Table 18.6 Treatment of depression in older people

General measures
Optimize treatment of physical conditions
Psychoeducation
Offer advice about social and financial support
Evaluate need for community treatment, for example community mental health nurse or social worker
Mild depression
Antidepressants are not recommended
Choices include guided self-help, supervised exercise programmes or computerized cognitive behavioural therapy (CBT)
Moderate depression
SSRI antidepressant
Individual CBT
Offer a social group activity
Severe depression
Antidepressants: SSRIs or TCAs
Consider lithium augmentation
Consider ECT
Individual CBT
Group therapy or activities

NICE recommends the use of SSRIs as the first-line treatment, as they have fewer anticholinergic side effects and are safer in overdose. TCAs should be avoided in those at risk of cardiac arrhythmias. They also have a high risk of postural hypotension. The starting dose should be half the usual dose for younger adults (to avoid side effects), but often a full therapeutic dose will be needed. After recovery, antidepressant medication should be reduced slowly and then continued in reduced dose for at least 2 years. As in younger patients, recurrent depression requires long-term continuation treatment and mirtazapine or lithium are suitable augmentation choices for resistant depression.

Electroconvulsive therapy (ECT) is useful for the small minority of patients with severe and distressing agitation, life-threatening stupor, or failure to respond to drugs. Special care is needed with the anaesthesia. It may be necessary to space out treatments at longer intervals than in younger patients to reduce post-treatment memory impairment.

Psychological treatments. Cognitive behavioural therapy (CBT) and interpersonal therapy (IPT) are proven to be efficacious, in either individual or group format. As anxiety is often a large part of mood disorders, specific anxiety-reduction and relaxation techniques may be helpful.

Bipolar disorder

The natural course of bipolar disorder is such that most patients who are diagnosed as young adults will continue to have episodes throughout life. The diagnostic criteria are outlined in Chapter 21. For those patients who develop bipolar disorder after the age of 50, the prognosis is significantly worse. Depressive episodes in the context of bipolar disorder present and are treated as in younger adults.

Clinical features

There are few differences between the clinical presentation of a manic episode in older versus younger adults, but they are more likely to be confused or disorientated, whilst euphoria and grandiosity are less frequently seen. Typical presenting symptoms include:

- labile mood;
- rapid speech and flight of ideas;
- reduced or disturbed sleep;
- psychomotor agitation or aggression;
- distractibility;
- acute confusion;
- reckless behaviour;
- paranoid delusions;
- new focal neurology (which resolves with treatment).

There is a greater propensity for sudden switching between mania and depression. Mixed episodes are also common, and may lead to misdiagnosis as delirium or dementia.

Prevalence

The prevalence of bipolar disorder in the general population is 1.5 per cent, reducing to 1 per cent in the over-65s. Only about 10 per cent of new diagnoses of bipolar disorder occur in patients over 50 years, and in retrospect it is usually possible to see that the patient has had episodes earlier in their life. Males and females are equally represented.

Differential diagnosis

The differential depends upon whether the presenting episode is mania or depression. For the latter, the list in the section above is relevant. The main differentials of a manic episode are as follows

- **Schizophrenia or schizoaffective disorder.** As manic episodes frequently include psychotic elements, distinguishing between schizophrenia and mania can be difficult. Search carefully for the characteristic features of

Science box 18.1 Cognitive behavioural therapy for depression in older adults

There is good evidence that CBT is an effective treatment for moderate to severe depression and it is now included in most treatment guidelines used across the world.[1] Depression in older people is often resistant to treatment, but only 5 per cent of patients currently receive psychological therapies. There appears to be a general belief that therapies such as CBT are less effective with increasing age, but this has not been evidence based.[2] So is CBT as effective in the older population as in younger patients?

In 2008, the Cochrane Collaboration published a meta-analysis of randomized controlled trials (RCTs) comparing various psychotherapies with 'waiting list' or active control interventions.[3] The latter included advice and a non-therapeutic bibliography. Nine RCTs were identified, including trials of both CBT and psychodynamic therapy. The mean duration of the trials was 12 weeks, delivering 16–20 sessions of individual therapy. The patients who received CBT showed a significantly greater reduction in symptoms compared with waiting list controls. CBT was directly compared with psychodynamic therapy in three small trials, but despite limited data they appeared to be equally efficacious.

It was widely recognized that the study above (and several similar reviews) involved relatively small groups of patients with heterogeneous 'control' groups. In 2009, Sertafy *et al.* conducted a larger primary care-based trial

of 204 patients, mean age 74 years, who were randomized to treatment as usual (TAU), TAU plus a talking control, or TAU plus CBT.[4] The CBT arm improved significantly when compared with either of the other groups, based on response to standard mood disorder questionnaires. Many other similar trials are currently under way.

As it stands, the evidence does confirm that CBT is an effective treatment for older people with depression. It should be routinely available to patients presenting with mood disorders, irrespective of their age.

1 National Institute of Clinical Excellence. *Depression: Management of Depression in Primary and Secondary Care: NICE guidance reference CG23*. www.nice.org.uk/CG23.

2 Pinquart, M., Duberstein, P. R., & Lyness, J. M. (2006). Treatments for later-life depressive conditions: a meta-analytic comparison of pharmacotherapy and psychotherapy. *American Journal of Psychiatry* **163**: 1493–501.

3 Wilson, K. C. M., Mottram, P. G., & Vassilas, C. A. (2008). Psychotherapeutic treatments for older depressed people. *Cochrane Database Systematic Review* **1**(1): CD004853.

4 Serfaty, M.A., Haworth, D., Blanchard, M., *et al.* (2009). Clinical effectiveness of individual cognitive behavioral therapy for depressed older people in primary care. *Archives of General Psychiatry* **66**: 1332–40.

---

schizophrenia. Delusions are typically mood congruent in a mood disorder, and not in schizophrenia. In mania the content of delusions or hallucinations often changes rapidly, and usually ceases with a reduction in the overactive state.

- **Delirium.** A sudden-onset, acute confusional state with disorientation in a patient with no history of a mood disorder is highly suggestive of delirium. Look for a precipitating cause (infection, electrolyte abnormality, etc.).

- **Dementia.** It is rare for dementia to present suddenly; symptoms have usually taken months to develop, whereas a mood disorder is relatively quick in onset. Always consider dementia when patients with no history of mood disorders present with altered behaviour.

- **Organic causes.** Endocrine disorders (hyperthyroidism, Cushing's) may present exactly as a manic episode. Neurological conditions such as space-occupying lesions, epilepsy, stroke, head injuries, multiple sclerosis, HIV, or systemic lupus erythematosus may also present with mood symptoms. Extreme social disinhibition is characteristic of frontal lobe lesions.

- **Abuse of stimulant drugs.** Amphetamines, hallucinogens, and opiates can all cause a mania-like state.

- **Medications.** Virtually any drug affecting the central nervous system can cause mania. Other culprits include antituberculosis drugs, antihypertensives, respiratory drugs, steroids, analgesics, and antacid preparations.

Aetiology

For late-onset bipolar disorder, heritability is somewhat reduced, but is still important. It is thought that organic cerebral factors may be related to the onset of late-life mania. Many of these patients have mild cognitive impairment, and MRI scans have shown an increased number of white matter lesions, especially in those with soft neurological signs.

Course and prognosis

In those presenting with a first episode of mania in late life, 80 to 90 per cent recover fully with treatment. About half of these will go on to have recurrent episodes. In patients with a long history of bipolar disorder there is a reduced rate of full response, and the chance of further (and often more severe) episodes is higher.

Management

Assessment of the patient should be carried out as in the Assessment section at the beginning of this chapter. Treatment of bipolar disorder is covered by the NICE guideline for the management of bipolar disorder, and is discussed in detail in Chapter 21. A summary of its guidance is shown in Table 18.7.

Drug treatments

As in a manic episode at any age, the basic treatment is with an antipsychotic (usually an atypical) and a mood stabilizer. The usual choices for the latter are lithium or sodium valproate. Older people tend to metabolize drugs more slowly than younger patients, and may need lower doses. The advised therapeutic level of lithium in

Table 18.7 Management of bipolar disorder in older adults

General measures

Optimize treatment of physical conditions

Psychoeducation

Organize calming activities, structured supported routine

Offer psychological and social support

Manic episodes (not already on antimanic drugs)

Stop antidepressants

Atypical antipsychotic

Mood stabilizer: lithium or valproate

Short-term use of benzodiazepines

Consider ECT for resistant cases

Manic episodes (already on antimanic drugs)

Stop antidepressants

Check doses and compliance with antipsychotic medications

Increase dose of antipsychotic

Add (or increase dose of) mood stabilizer: lithium or valproate

Check blood levels of lithium regularly

Depressive episode

Antidepressant: SSRI

Add lithium

Consider a second mood stabilizer: valproate or carbamazepine

Consider an atypical antipsychotic

Consider ECT for severe resistant cases

Psychological and social measures as usual

adults is 0.5–1.0 mmol/l for maintenance, which can be raised slightly in an acute episode. Older patients may become toxic at these levels, and many old age psychiatrists work to a lower range. There is an increased risk of falls on sedating medications, which needs to be carefully monitored.

Schizophrenia and paranoid disorders

Patients with psychosis in later life can be divided into three groups:

1 those with pre-existing schizophrenia;

2 new diagnoses of schizophrenia ('late-life schizophrenia', also known as 'late paraphrenia');

3 other conditions producing hallucinations or delusions (dementia, delirium, mood disorders, delusional disorder, paranoid personality disorders).

As the population ages and treatments improve, the first group is getting significantly larger and making up a greater proportion of mental illness.

Clinical features

The classical clinical features and diagnostic criteria of schizophrenia are described in Chapter 22. Generally, older patients have less severe positive symptoms than younger adults, and may have fewer negative symptoms. Persecutory delusions are the most common symptom (over 90 per cent of late-life schizophrenic patients), followed by auditory hallucinations. Hallucinations in other senses (visual, tactile, olfactory) are more common. Some degree of cognitive impairment is typical, and may precede the onset of positive symptoms, making the diagnosis more difficult.

Prevalence

The prevalence of all psychotic disorders over 65 years of age is 4 to 6 per cent, rising to 10 per cent over 85 years. However, a large proportion of these cases are related to dementia. True schizophrenia or delusional disorder in the over-65s has a prevalence of 0.5–1.0 per cent. There is a female preponderance, with a ratio of female to males of 5:1, which is partly because the onset of schizophrenia tends to be later in females. Sixty per cent of cases are paranoid schizophrenia, 30 per cent delusional disorder, and only 10 per cent all other forms of psychosis.

Differential diagnosis

- **Dementia.** This is the main differential for psychosis in the older patient. Memory testing is paramount; those with schizophrenia usually have a good memory. Persecutory delusions are common in dementia, but other forms of delusion are not. The time scale of symptom development will also be useful, as dementia usually has an insidious onset.

- **Delirium.** An acute confusional state with disorientation and florid visual hallucinations is typical of delirium.

- **Bipolar disorder with psychosis.**

- **Severe depression with psychosis.**

- **Paranoid personality disorder.** In paranoid personality disorder there is lifelong suspiciousness and distrust, with sensitive ideas but no delusions.

- **Organic cerebral disease.** Stroke, tumours, temporal lobe epilepsy, vCJD, HIV, syphilis, multiple sclerosis, and any other diffuse brain disease should all be excluded.

- **Drug-induced states.** Amphetamines, cannabis, cocaine, and ecstasy all cause psychosis. Prescribed medications—especially steroids, antiparkinsonian drugs, and psychoactive drugs—may be the primary cause, or exacerbate symptoms.

- **Hallucinations of sensory deprivation (Charles–Bonnet syndrome).** Complex visual hallucinations may occur in older people with low vision, especially in the context of significant hearing loss. Usually, there are no other psychotic symptoms, and the patient has more insight than in schizophrenia.

Aetiology

See Chapter 22. The significant social changes of old age may well trigger the onset of the condition, or precipitate another episode.

Course and prognosis

There is little evidence currently on the prognosis of late-life schizophrenia.

Treatment

In general, the treatment of these disorders in older people is similar to that for younger people (see Chapter 22). This is summarized in Table 18.8. Outpatient treatment may be possible, but admission to hospital is often required for adequate assessment and treatment. Hospital admission is essential if there is risk of suicide or violence, severe psychosis or catatonia, lack of capacity or willingness to comply with treatments, no social supports, or complex co-morbidities. Day hospitals are often very useful in this patient group, and a short inpatient admission can be followed by tapering attendance at the day programme. This aims to avoid social isolation, ensure adequate supervision, and prevent relapse. Any sensory deficit, such as deafness or cataract, should be assessed and, if possible, treated.

Most patients require antipsychotic medication but the dosage is usually less than that needed for younger adults. There is a higher risk of extrapyramidal symptoms and

Table 18.8 Treatment of late-life schizophrenia

- Refer urgently to mental health services and early intervention team
- Choose appropriate setting of care
- Allocate a CPN and a social worker
- Offer an antipsychotic to all patients (first-line, atypical antipsychotic)
- Consider clozapine after trials of two other antipsychotics
- Short-term low-dose benzodiazepines for agitation or poor sleep
- Offer a course of 16–20 sessions of individual CBT
- Consider group therapeutic sessions
- Social interventions: appropriate housing, activities, financial assistance

tardive dyskinesia than in younger people, so the older typical antipsychotics should be avoided. Medications should be introduced at the lowest dose and the patient carefully monitored for physical side effects. The most common side effects are postural hypotension (and therefore falls), urinary retention, and constipation. As with younger patients a depot preparation should be considered. It is recommended that medications be continued for at least 2 years after full recovery (see Case study 18.1).

Stress-related and anxiety disorders

These 'minor' psychiatric disorders are the mostly common mental health problems of old age, and are frequently encountered by all clinicians. Ten per cent of the population fit diagnostic criteria for an anxiety disorder, and the majority of these are new diagnoses in old age. They are common reasons for admission to the general hospital, are highly associated with physical illness, and are very costly to health services in time and money. The main features of all of the separate conditions are described in detail in the relevant chapters; what follows is a summary of the differences seen in older patients.

Clinical features

In an older population, there is much less distinction between different types of stress-related and anxiety disorder. Generalized anxiety disorder is by far the most common condition. Symptoms frequently encountered are shown in Table 18.9.

Differential diagnosis

Patients usually present to the GP or general hospital with physical symptoms; it is therefore important (but

Case study 18.1 Paranoid symptoms

The son of an 82-year-old widow comes to your surgery to say that he is concerned about his mother. He has noticed, over a period of months, that his mother has complained of increasingly numerous events in which neighbours and other people have apparently shouted abuse from outside her house and persecuted her. She believes that they have stolen objects and that they have moved her furniture around. She thinks that there is a complex conspiracy that involves a number of her neighbours and which is intended to drive her out of her own home. The son has realized that many of the allegations are a fantasy and unbelievable and has tried to persuade his mother to seek help. However, she has maintained that she is perfectly well and that the problem lies with her neighbours' behaviour.

You have known the patient for many years and have occasionally visited her to treat minor ailments. You say that you will visit her home and say that you are making one of your regular visits to the older patients in your practice. When you arrive, the patient is initially somewhat suspicious but lets you in and tells you about her beliefs that she is being persecuted. When you express some doubt, it is clear that she will not be dissuaded from these beliefs.

You feel that it is unlikely that she would agree to a visit from a psychiatrist and that you should try and establish the diagnosis. While your patient is upset about what has been happening, it is also apparent that when she discusses her own family and other issues she is cheerful and retains her usual sense of humour. You conclude she is not suffering from a depressive illness. At the same time, it is apparent that her memory of past events and of previous discussions with you is excellent and that she has a good knowledge of current events. It is clear that she is not suffering from dementia. She is not deaf. You conclude that she is almost certainly suffering from primary paranoid disorder.

You conclude that medication would be appropriate and you are eventually able to persuade your patient that she should try some new tablets to treat the very considerable distress that she reports in association with the persecutory symptoms. You prescribe olanzapine 2.5 mg per day and arrange to visit her again. When you return to your surgery, you consult the local psychiatrist for older adults and agree that the present plan is appropriate and that, if necessary and the patient consents, a psychiatric consultation could be arranged at a later stage.

Two weeks later you are pleased to find that the patient is no longer describing the persecutory symptoms, which she says stopped several days previously (although she apparently still believes that they were genuine). She agrees that the medication has been helpful for her distress and is willing to continue for the time being. You suggest that you will check on the medication when you see her for her usual blood pressure review.

---

sometimes impossible) to distinguish them from symptoms caused by organic pathology. It is frequently the case that symptoms may be an exaggeration of those caused by an underlying pathology—for example, shortness of breath in chronic obstructive pulmonary disorder—which are extremely difficult to treat. It is helpful to distinguish between the following:

- **Depression.** Anxiety and stress-related disorders often coexist with depression, but this does not mean depression should be ignored. In depression the physical symptoms are more stereotyped—sleep disturbance, anorexia, weight loss, fatigue—and are usually in the context of low mood.

- **Dementia.** Early dementia often presents with anxiety or obsessions. It may not be possible to make a definite diagnosis until more characteristic symptoms of dementia develop.

- **Delirium.** This is characterized by a relatively sudden onset of disorientation and other features of confusion, and is usually associated with common physical problems in the elderly such as chest infection, urinary tract infection, constipation, or electrolyte disturbance.

- **Paranoid delusional disorder or schizophrenia.** The presence of hallucinations or delusions is usually relatively obvious.

- **Physical illness.** There is a high correlation between the diagnosis of a physical illness and the onset of anxiety symptoms. Frequently, it is best to treat both concurrently, if only to try and maximize symptom relief.

Aetiology

The likelihood of developing an anxiety disorder in later life is primarily related to prior vulnerability, personality, and life experiences. It is rare for a clinically significant disorder (especially if unrelated to physical illness) to develop *de novo* in a patient with no previous history of any anxiety or mental health disturbance. The genetic predisposition to anxiety continues into later life. Psychosocial factors that may predispose to or precipitate an episode are similar to those for depression (p. 228).

Table 18.9 Symptoms of stress-related and anxiety disorders in older adults

Psychological	Physical (somatic)	Behavioural
Fearful anticipation	Abdominal pain	Phobic avoidance
Irritability	Diarrhoea	Fear of mobilizing
Hyperacusis	Dry mouth	Social isolation
Restlessness	Dysphagia	Use of alcohol or drugs
Poor concentration	Tight chest	Frequent attendance at the GP or hospital admissions
Worrying thoughts	Shortness of breath	
	Palpitations	
Fear of losing control	Chest pain	
Depersonalization	Sweating	
Panic attacks	Urinary frequency and urgency	
	Tremor	
	Headache	
	Fatigue	
	Pain	
	Insomnia	
	Nightmares	

Course and prognosis

Anxiety disorders tend to become chronic and are very difficult to treat. Those illnesses that develop with an obvious precipitating factor have a poorer prognosis.

Treatment

There is a little evidence on the treatment of anxiety and stress disorders in older people. Treatment should follow the recommendations for younger people. Most patients are treated in primary care and do not need to be referred to a psychiatrist. A typical management plan would include:

- a clear explanation of the diagnosis, the cause of the symptoms, and what the treatment will be;
- psychoeducation;
- provision of self-help materials and exercises;
- psychological treatment;
- medications;
- regular review.

There is some evidence that CBT is effective in this group of patients. Frequently, the techniques need to be altered for those with sensory losses, physical disability, or cognitive impairment. Individual treatment is usually more appropriate than group therapy, but there is a role for group social activities. Antidepressants are the first-line choice for generalized anxiety, and an SSRI is the safest option. They should be used as described in the depression section above. Benzodiazepines are frequently used in older adults, but they carry a high risk of sedation, falls, tolerance, and dependence and therefore should be avoided wherever possible.

Suicide and deliberate self-harm

Suicide and deliberate self-harm are relatively common in older adults, with the highest rates of suicide being amongst men over 75. In the USA, the overall population rate of completed suicide in 2002 was 17.9/100 000, but in older men was 40.7/100 000. With an increasing proportion of society reaching old age, suicide in this group is likely to become a more prominent problem. In younger people there is a spectrum of self-harm, from suicidal thoughts to acts of deliberate self-harm to suicide attempts and completed suicide. This is also seen in the older population, but they are also more prone to passive methods of self-harm: refusing to eat and drink, non-compliance with medical treatments, or complete withdrawal from the world. Fifteen per cent of older people living in the community admit to fleeting suicidal ideation from time to time, although very few have more severe symptoms than that.

Deliberate self-harm (DSH)

There are many fewer cases of active deliberate self-harm in the old compared with the young. It is therefore important to consider every act as a failed suicide, and act accordingly. Unlike completed suicide, DSH is more common in females, although there is less preponderance than seen in young adults. Deliberate overdose of prescribed medications (typically benzodiazepines, analgesics, or antidepressants) is the most common presentation, with few cases of over-the-counter paracetamol or aspirin-based attempts. Self-cutting is seen, but only occasionally. A psychiatric disorder is present in at least 90 per cent of patients, most of whom will be depressed. Two-thirds have severe physical illness of some type, and most have a psychiatric history. Risk factors for DSH (and suicide) are shown in Box 18.4. Those who are the most likely to go on to complete suicide are males with a prior psychiatric history under current treatment for a depressive illness.

BOX 18.4 Risk factors for DSH and suicide in the elderly

- Age
- Physical illness
- Widowed, divorced, or separated
- Social isolation
- Loneliness
- Grief
- Threat of moving to a residential home
- Alcohol abuse
- Depression, past or present
- Recent contact with a psychiatrist

Completed suicide

Completed suicide is a natural progression from DSH, but in many patients it is the first and final act. Only one-third have had a previous attempt at DSH or suicide. The method of suicide is highly dependent on geographical location; for instance, in the USA shooting is the most common, whereas in the UK (which has very tight fire-arms laws) drug overdose, suffocation, and hanging are frequently used. More so than in younger patients, older people plan their suicide carefully, leaving an explanatory note and their affairs in order. Surprisingly, fewer patients who kill themselves appear to have been suffering from a psychiatric illness prior to their death than those who commit DSH. The figure is thought to be around 70 per cent, with almost all of these having depression.

Risk assessment

As mentioned above, all acts of DSH should be taken seriously. Clinicians also need to be alert to the chance of depressed patients having suicidal thoughts, even with no previous history. Careful prescriptions—for instance only prescribed 1–2 weeks' medication at a time—and/or monitoring the taking of medications may be necessary. In some cases it may be appropriate to move a patient temporarily into accommodation where they are not alone for long periods, and involve family and friends in the care plan.

Abuse of alcohol

Alcohol use disorders are common in older adults, and are under-recognized and undertreated. One-third of those who develop a problem with alcohol only do so after the age of 65, and most have no prior psychiatric history. As liver metabolism slows and reduces in efficiency

with increasing age, lower levels of alcohol are needed to provoke the characteristic symptoms and alcohol dependence syndrome. In the UK, the national recommendations for alcohol are not more than 14 units per week for women, and 21 units per week for men. There are no separate guidelines for the over-65s, for whom this is probably too much. Community-based prevalence studies have reported alcohol dependence to be around 2–4 per cent of older patients, but for those in institutional care or hospitals the figure is 15–20 per cent. It is not known how accurate these figures are. The clinical features are similar to those in younger patients, described in Chapter 29. Alcohol can cause a range of neuropsychiatric symptoms including cognitive impairment, depression, Wernicke–Korsakoff syndrome, cerebellar atropy, psychosis, or a withdrawal syndrome.

The aetiology of alcohol use disorders in older patients is as complex as in younger ones. There remains a genetic risk, but social factors are probably more important. Retirement, bereavement or divorce, reduced socioeconomic status, and physical ill health are common precipitating events. Those patients who exhibited antisocial personality traits, hyperactivity, or impulsivity in former years are at higher risk.

Patients should be assessed as outlined at the start of this chapter, with an emphasis on determining the type, amount, and pattern of drinking. Extensive physical investigations should be carried out to determine the secondary effects of alcohol excess (Box 18.5).

Treatment is similar to that in younger adults. Any underlying psychiatric or physical illness should be treated along normal guidelines. If a reducing benzodiazepine regimen is used, the doses should be significantly lower than in standard guidelines as there is a high risk of sedation and falls. Chlordiazepoxide or lorazepam are the safest choices. Concurrently, either oral or parenteral thiamine should be given to avoid Wernicke–Korsakoff syndrome. Evidence suggests that oral thiamine is as effective as IV thiamine complexes (Pabrinex®). Newer therapies for alcohol abuse, such as disulfiram, acamprosate, and naltrexone, are licensed for use in all ages, but there is no real evidence on safety or efficacy over 65 years.

Abuse of older adults

The mistreatment of older people is often known as elder abuse, and is much more commonplace than the general public realize. Abuse may occur in any setting, not just in institutions or residential care. Epidemiological studies report a prevalence of 5 per cent in the community, rising to 10 per cent in residential care. As in children and other

BOX 18.5 Physical investigations into harmful use of alcohol

Physical examination: look for signs of hepatic damage, malnutrition, focal neurological deficits, and cognitive decline.

Blood tests:

- Blood alcohol concentration (via either a breathalyser or laboratory assay)
- Full blood count: MCV is raised in 60% of people with drinking problems; anaemia may occur in cases of malnutrition
- Liver function tests: hepatocellular damage is indicated by raised AST and ALT

- Gamma-glutamyltranspeptidase (GGT) is raised in 80% of people with chronic drinking problems
- Serum urate may be raised in some people with high alcohol intakes
- Renal function: always worth checking in older people, especially before starting any new medications

Imageing:

- Abdominal ultrasound may be useful to identify hepatomegaly ± cirrhosis
- Chest X-ray: if patients present acutely unwell, excluding a chest infection is important

---

vulnerable groups, there are a variety of different forms that abuse may take:

- **neglect:** refusal or failure to provide basic rights, or other obligations;
- **physical abuse:** the infliction of pain or injury, physical or drug-induced restraint;
- **emotional abuse:** the infliction of mental anguish;
- **sexual abuse:** any non-consensual sexual contact;
- **financial or material exploitation:** illegal or improper use of financial or other resources belonging to the elderly person.

Risk factors for elder abuse tend to depend strongly upon the context, but the most vulnerable people are those with cognitive and/or physical impairments, or those who are socially isolated. The consequences of abuse may be great, as older people are weaker physically, and bones or other wounds may not heal in the same way as in younger victims. They often live in financially tighter circumstances, where the loss of relatively small amounts of money may push them into poverty. One devastating result of abuse is the loss of confidence; this sets up a spiral of social isolation and increasing vulnerability to further abuse.

Clinicians need to be aware of the possibility of abuse and be prepared to intervene in whatever way will prevent continuing abuse and to deal with underlying problems. If there is any concern, a social worker and senior clinicians with experience in such cases should be contacted, and a thorough history, physical examination, and investigations undertaken. A similar process should be gone through as for child abuse, which is discussed in Chapter 17. Alternative accommodation and care may need to be found for the patient, if only in the short term. Many developed countries now have mechanisms in place to prevent elder abuse, but there is still a lack of education amongst the general population.

Further reading

Jacoby, R., Oppenheimer, C., Dening, T., &Thomas, A. (2008). *Oxford Textbook of Old Age Psychiatry.* Oxford University Press, Oxford.

Gelder, M., Andreasen, N., Lopez-Ibor, J, & Geddes, J. (eds) (2009). *New Oxford Textbook of Psychiatry*, 2nd edn. Section 8: The psychiatry of old age, pp. 1505–86. Oxford University Press, Oxford.

National Institute of Clinical Excellence (2006). *Dementia: Supporting people with dementia and their carers in health and social care.* http://guidance.nice.org.uk/CG42.

Alexopoulos, G.S. (2005). Depression in the elderly. *Lancet* **365**: 1961–70.

Kirmizioglu, Y., Doğan, O., Kuğu, N., *et al.* (2009). Prevalence of anxiety disorders amongst elderly people. *International Journal of Geriatric Psychiatry* **14**: 1026–33.

Learning disability

The term **learning disability (LD)** and the alternative phrase **mental retardation** denote an irreversible impairment of intelligence originating early in life which is associated with limitations of social functioning. A distinction is to be made between learning disability and dementia, the former originating in childhood and the latter after 18 years of age. Although not reversible, much can be done to enable people with learning disabilities to live as normally as possible. To achieve this, the main interventions are educational and social rather than medical: special schooling, sheltered work and housing, and support for the affected person and for the family. Nevertheless, general practitioners are involved in important aspects of the care of people with learning disability; they may be the first to identify the problem, they help the family to come to terms with the condition, and they provide general medical services throughout the person's life. And whatever their specialty, all doctors will see people with learning disability who are seeking help for a medical or surgical condition. Therefore, all doctors need to be able to interview people with learning disability and understand their special needs. They need to know something of its causes and have a broad understanding of the range of services available for these patients and when to refer to a psychiatrist. This chapter is divided into three parts: firstly, an overview of the epidemiology, aetiology, and clinical features of learning disabilities; then an approach to assessment and management of the individual patient; and finally a brief description of some of the more common and/or important clinical syndromes.

Chapter contents

■ Overview of aetiology and clinical features

Classification and terminology

Several terms are used to describe people with intellectual impairment originating early in life. In the UK, the term **learning disability (LD)** is generally used, and this chapter will reflect this. In many other countries, the term is **mental retardation** and this is the one used in the diagnostic classification systems. In the past, the condition has been known at various times as mental deficiency, mental subnormality, and mental handicap.

The term learning disability implies more than intellectual impairment. The word disability draws attention to what the DSM definition refers to as 'concurrent deficits and impairments in adaptive behaviour, taking into account the person's age'. It therefore separates those who cannot lead a near normal life from people of the same IQ level who can. Despite this emphasis on disability, the degree of intellectual impairment is still important and LD is divided into subgroups based on IQ. These are shown in Table 19.1, and the full diagnostic criteria in Box 19.1.

LD is not a clinical diagnosis in its own right, just a way of describing a particular clinical syndrome of impairments with disability and handicaps. The underlying diagnosis is the cause of these impairments, which may or may not have been identified. The terms impairment, disability, and handicap are not interchangeable. The value of their use is in describing an individual's specific needs, irrespective of their aetiological diagnosis.

- **Impairment** is any loss or abnormality of psychological, physical, or anatomical structure or function. It is not dependent upon aetiology.
- **Disability** is any restriction in the ability to perform an activity within the range considered normal for a human at a corresponding level of development.
- **A handicap** is a disadvantage for a person, due to their impairment or disability, that prevents them from fulfilling a role that is normal for that individual.

Epidemiology

The definition of LD as an IQ < 70 is based upon the assumption that IQ is normally distributed with a mean of 100 and standard deviation of 15. Two standard deviations below the mean is 70, representing 2.5 per cent of the population. However, reported rates of LD are actually 2–3 per cent. This is because average IQ varies with a number of factors:

- **Country.** Learning disabilities are more common in developing than developed countries. This is primarily due to preventable causes (e.g. iodine deficiency).
- **Genetics.** Different ethnic groups show variable intellectual abilities.
- **Age.** Prevalence of LD is higher in child than adult cohorts, with a peak at 10 years. This is partly due to the reduced life expectancy of some individuals with LD, but also due to diagnostic bias.
- **Method of data collection.** Ascertaining the true level of LD is difficult. Data collected from education registers of

Table 19.1 Classification and epidemiology of learning disability

Learning disability	IQ level	Proportion of patients (%)	Prevalence in general population (%)
Mild	50–69	80	2.5
Moderate	35–49	12	0.4
Severe	20–34	7	0.1
Profound	< 20	1	

BOX 19.1 dSM-IV diagnostic criteria for mental retardation (learning disability)

1 Significantly subaverage intellectual functioning (IQ < 70).
2 Concurrent deficits or impairments in present adaptive functioning in at least two of the following areas: communication, self-care, home living, social skills, use of community resources, self-direction, academic skills, work, leisure, health and safety.
3 The onset is before 18 years.

The ICD-10 definition of mental retardation is:

A condition of arrested or incomplete development of the mind, which is especially characterized by impairment of skills manifested during the developmental period, skills which contribute to the overall level of intelligence, i.e. cognitive, language, motor, and social abilities. Retardation can occur with or without any other mental or physical condition.

special needs or specialist health services underestimate the general population figures.

Not all individuals with an IQ < 70 have LD; they must also have impairment of functioning. Table 19.1 outlines the relative prevalence of differing levels of LD in the UK population. The rate of moderate or severe LD is three to four per 1000 of the population aged 15–19 years, or six to eight people in a general practitioner's average list of 2000 patients. This **prevalence** has changed little since the 1930s even though the **incidence** of severe mental retardation has fallen by one-third to one-half in the same period, partly as a result of improved antenatal and neonatal care. The reason that the prevalence has not changed despite the lower incidence is that people with LD are living longer.

Causes of learning disability

There are a myriad of different causes of LD, representing a heterogeneous group of individuals. A specific cause can be identified in 80 per cent of severe cases, but only in 50 per cent overall. There are three main reasons for making an aetiological diagnosis for a given patient.

1 A diagnosis may guide treatment options.

2 It allows prediction of likely disabilities and prognosis, allowing for planning of services, education, finances, and family life.

3 It may provide information relating to the likely risk of recurrence in future pregnancies.

Mild LD is usually due to a combination of genetic and adverse environmental factors, such as extreme prematurity and damage to the brain during birth. **Severe and profound LD** is usually due to specific pathological conditions, most of which can be diagnosed in life and about two-thirds of which can be diagnosed before birth. The causes of **moderate LD** are varied. An overview is shown in Table 19.2.

Genetic causes

The heritability of IQ is estimated to be 50 per cent, but we do not currently know which (combination of) genes are responsible for this. Many specific causes of LD have been identified, many of which are abnormalities of chromosomes or genes, and some associated with specific biochemical abnormalities. There are five main genetic aetiological groups.

1 **Single gene disorders: autosomal dominant conditions.** Neurofibromatosis, myotonic dystrophy, and tuberose sclerosis are examples of these rare conditions.

2 **Single gene disorders: recessive conditions.** This is the largest group of specific genetic disorders. It includes

Table 19.2 Aetiology of learning disability

Aetiology	Subgroup	Examples
Genetics	Dominant genes	Neurofibromatosis
		Tuberose sclerosis
	Recessive genes (mostly errors of metabolism)	Phenylketonuria
		Homocystinuria
		Urea cycle abnormalities
		Tay–Sach's, Gaucher's
	Chromosomal abnormalities	Down's syndrome
		Kleinfelter's syndrome
		Turner's syndrome
	X-linked disorders	Lesch–Nyhan syndrome
		Fragile X syndrome
		Hydrocephaly
	Genomic imprinting	Prader–Willi syndrome
		Angelman's syndrome
Antenatal	Infections	Rubella, CMV, syphilis
	Intoxification	Alcohol, cocaine, lead
	Physical damage	Injury, radiation, hypoxia
	Endocrine disorders	Hypothyroidism
		Hypoparathyroidism
Perinatal		Birth asphyxia
		Kernicterus
		Intraventricular haemorrhage
		Neonatal infections
Postnatal	Injury	Accidental or non-accidental
	Infections	Meningoencephalitis
	Intoxification	Lead, drugs
Malnutrition		Protein–energy malnutrition Iodine deficiency

most of the inherited metabolic conditions, such as phenylketonuria, homocystinuria, and galactosaemia.

3 **Chromosome abnormalities.** The most common chromosome abnormality is Down's syndrome (trisomy 21). Abnormalities in the number of sex chromosomes, as in Klinefelter's syndrome (XXY) and Turner's syndrome (XO), sometimes lead to LD as well as to physical abnormalities.

4 **X-linked conditions.** Specific genes on the X chromosome cause rare syndromes including the Lesch–Nyhan syndrome and Duchenne's muscular dystrophy.

5 **Genomic imprinting** is gene expression dependent on the parent of origin. Prader–Willi and Angelman's syndromes are both due to an abnormality in the 15q11-13 region. Altered paternal expression of genes in this region causes the Prader–Willi syndrome with hypotonia, hyperphagia, obesity, and daytime sleepiness. Altered maternal expression of a gene in this region leads to Angelman's syndrome with characteristic abnormal movements and a sociable disposition.

Antenatal damage is caused by **intrauterine infection** (such as rubella, HIV, toxoplasmosis, CMV, syphilis) or toxic substances (such as *lead poisoning* or *excessive alcohol* use by the mother). In some developing countries, **hypothyroidism** due to iodine deficiency is important. Maternal diabetes, pre-eclampsia, and placental insufficiency can also be damaging.

Perinatal damage. Birth injuries, hypoxia, or intraventricular haemorrhage may all occur around the delivery. Newborn complications such as kernicterus, hypoglycaemia, respiratory distress or infections (meningitis, sepsis, pneumonia or congenital) can have long-lasting effects.

Postnatal damage is due to injury or resulting from infections (encephalitis and meningitis), brain tumours, hypoxia, vascular events, or child abuse. Historically, lead poisoning has been a common cause of LD.

Social factors include associations with lower social class, poverty, poor housing, and an unstable family environment.

Malnutrition is a common cause of LD in developing countries. It includes hypothyroidism secondary to iodine deficiency, and all kinds of protein–energy malnutrition (e.g. marasmus and/or kwashiorkor).

Prevention and early detection

Primary prevention depends mainly on genetic screening and counselling, together with good antenatal and obstetric care (Table 19.3). In some developing countries, correction of iodine deficiency and malnutrition is important.

Secondary prevention aims to reduce the effect of the primary disorder; for example, by providing 'enriching' education.

Genetic screening and counselling. Most parents seek advice only after the birth of a first child with LD. Those asking for advice before or during the first pregnancy usually do so because there is a person with LD in the extended family. Specialist advice is usually needed to assess the risk that an abnormal child will be born, and to explain this risk to the parents so that they can make their own decision whether to start or continue the pregnancy.

Table 19.3 Prevention and early detection of learning disability

Prevention
Before pregnancy:
Rubella immunization
Folic acid supplementation (5 mg daily from conception to 12 weeks)
Genetic counselling and preimplantation diagnosis
During pregnancy:
Avoid excess alcohol, drugs, and toxic substances
Protection against sexually transmitted diseases
During and after delivery:
Care of premature infants
Early detection
During pregnancy:
Ultrasound screening, amniocentesis, fetoscopy
After delivery:
Screening for phenylketonuria, hypothyroidism, galactosaemia (heel-prick)
Aggressive treatment of neonatal complications in special care
Good nutrition

Early detection

Prenatal care. Ultrasound scanning of the fetus, **amniocentesis**, and **fetoscopy** can reveal disorders due to chromosomal abnormalities, most open neural tube defects, and about half of inborn errors of metabolism. Because amniocentesis carries a small but definite risk, it is usually offered only to women who have carried a previous abnormal fetus, women with a family history of congenital disorder, and those over 35 years of age.

Postnatal care. Phenylketonuria, hypothyroidism, medium-chain acyl-coenzyme A dehydrogenase deficiency and galactosaemia can be detected by routine heel-prick testing of infants.

Clinical features

The clinical features of each specific diagnosis are obviously different, but some general points that may assist with management can be made. People with LD perform badly on all kinds of intellectual task including learning, short-term memory, the use of concepts, and problem solving. Sometimes, one specific function is impaired more than the rest, for example the use of language. The clinical features are described best by reference to the subgroups of mild, moderate, severe, and profound disability (Table 19.4).

Table 19.4 Levels of learning disability

Mild (IQ 50–70)

Specific causes uncommon

Many need practical help and special education

Few need special psychiatric or social services

Moderate (IQ 35–49)

Most can manage some independent activities

Require special education, sheltered occupation, and supervision

Severe (IQ 20–34)

Specific causes usual

Many physical impairments

Social skills and communication severely limited

Require close supervision and much practical help

Profound (IQ below 20)

Specific causes usual

Little or no language and communication skills

Multiple complex physical problems

Require help with basic self-care

Mild learning disability (IQ 50–70)

About 80 per cent of people with LD fall into this group. Their appearance is usually normal and any sensory or motor deficits are slight. Most develop more or less normal language abilities and social behaviour during the preschool years, so that in the least severe cases the LD may not be identified until the child starts school. In adult life most can live independently, although some need help with housing and employment, and support when they are experiencing stress.

Moderate learning disability (IQ 35–49)

Individuals in this group account for about 12 per cent of those with LD. Most have enough language development to communicate, and most can learn to care for themselves, albeit with supervision. As adults, most continue to do this and are able to undertake simple routine work.

Severe learning disability (IQ 20–34)

About 7 per cent of the people with LD are in this group. In the preschool years their development is greatly slowed, and so is their learning when they go to school. With special training, many can eventually look after themselves under supervision and they can communicate, albeit in simple ways. As adults, most are able to undertake simple tasks and limited social activities. Many have associated physical disorders. A small number of these people have a single, highly developed cognitive ability of a kind normally associated with superior intelligence, such as the ability to carry out feats of mental arithmetic or memory. Such people were historically called **idiots savants.**

Profound learning disability (IQ below 20)

About 1 per cent of those with LD are in this group. Few learn to care for themselves completely. A few achieve some simple speech and social behaviour. Physical disorders are very frequent.

General problems in people with learning disability

From a medical perspective, the problems that patients with an LD (and/or their families) present with can be divided into four categories: emotional and behavioural problems; physical disorders; effects of the LD upon the family; and psychiatric disorders.

Emotional and behavioural problems

Behavioural disorders, at any given age, are more common in individuals with learning disabilities than in the general population. As well as the direct effects of intellectual impairment, children with LD may show any of the common behavioural problems of childhood (see Chapter 32). These problems tend to occur at a later age than in a child of normal intelligence, and to last longer, although they usually improve slowly with time. A minority show severely disordered behaviour that threatens the well-being of the patient or the carers. Such behaviour is referred to as **challenging behaviour.** There are a variety of common behaviours which can be difficult to manage.

- Aggression and/or antisocial behaviour: this may be shouting and screaming, faecal smearing, and self-induced vomiting in youngsters. Aggressive outbursts towards people or property are common in adolescence, but dangerous physical violence is not. These behaviours usually reduce in early adulthood.

- Self-injury: biting, cutting, burning, and head banging. These are inversely proportionate to IQ in frequency. Overall, 40 per cent of children and 20 per cent of adults with LD self-injure.

- Stereotyped behaviours such as rocking, mannerisms, and flapping usually seen in autistic spectrum disorders. The presence of these does not necessarily mean the child is autistic.

- Hyperactivity is common, and needs to be distinguished from the triad of impairments seen in ADHD.

- Anxiety.

- Social withdrawal.

Behavioural problems are usually multifactorial in origin, combining genetics, characteristics inherent to the specific cause of the LD, and environmental factors. Frequent causes are shown in Table 19.5. It is important to recognize the cause of the problem if possible, for this may aid management.

Sexual problems. Some people with LD show a child-like curiosity about other people's bodies, which can be misunderstood as sexual. Many need sympathetic help in understanding sexual feelings at and after puberty. Concern is sometimes expressed that people with LD may give birth to children with LD. However, many of the causes of LD are not inherited, and most of those that are inherited are associated with infertility. A more important concern is that people with severe LD are unlikely to be able to function well as parents. If termination of pregnancy or sterilization is considered, difficult ethical and legal problems can arise relating to consent, and specialist advice is usually necessary.

Physical disorders among people with learning disability

Physical disorders are most frequent among those with severe and profound LD, many of whom have motor disabilities (20–30 per cent) or epilepsy (40 per cent). Impaired hearing or vision may add an important additional obstacle to normal cognitive development, and is found in 10–20 per cent of those with an IQ < 35. Motor disabilities, which are frequent, include spasticity, ataxia, and athetosis, and are often due to cerebral palsy. Only a third of such people are continent and ambulant, and a quarter are highly dependent on other people. The majority of genetic phenotypes (e.g. Down's syndrome, fragile X) produce physical and cognitive impairments. It is important to recognize these, but also to look for non-associated conditions in every individual.

Epilepsy is frequent in LD and may present at any age. It needs to be carefully distinguished from stereotypies or mannerisms (e.g. rolling eyes) and from episodes of complete social withdrawal. All forms of epilepsy may occur, and the seizure pattern may change over time. Increased frequency of seizures may indicate physical illness, stress, or non-epileptic seizures. Whilst 40 per cent of individuals with severe or profound LD have epilepsy, it is also seen in 10 per cent of mild cases. Severe epilepsy can cause permanent loss of intellectual ability in anyone, and this is more frequent in those with LD to begin with. Epilepsy can usually be controlled effectively with anti-epileptic drugs.

Effects of learning disability on the family

The effects of a child with LD upon their family should not be underestimated. Prenatal diagnosis now means that parents can be put in a situation of having to make choices about an unborn child. This is extremely stressful, and the couple will need advice and counselling from professionals to make the choice that is best for them. When a newborn child is found to have LD, the parents are distressed and some reject the child at first, although this rejection seldom lasts long. More often the diagnosis is not made until after the first year of life. When this happens, the parents have to abandon their earlier hopes and expectations, and many experience a period of bereavement, depression, guilt, shame, or anger. Most parents eventually achieve a satisfactory adjustment but, however well they adjust psychologically, they are faced with the prospect of prolonged hard work and significant social problems. If the child also

Table 19.5 Causes of behavioural problems in learning disability

Causal factor	Description and examples
Stressful events	When people with LD react to stress, they often display their distress through behaviour rather than words; for example in agitation, fearfulness, irritability, and dramatic behaviours
Over- or under-stimulation	An over-stimulating environment may cause problems such as agitation or aggression, while an under-stimulating environment may lead to withdrawal, self-stimulation, or self-injury
Undiagnosed physical illness	Gastrointestinal disorders, epilepsy, otitis media, migraine, and pain are common examples
Psychiatric illness	For example schizophrenia, depression, anxiety disorders
Brain damage	The underlying damage causing the LD may also cause behavioural problems
Epilepsy	The first sign of epilepsy may be the onset of challenging behaviour
Behavioural phenotypes	Some genetic causes of LD also cause a specific pattern of behaviour problems, e.g. individuals with:
	• Prader–Willi syndrome have voracious appetite, pick and scratch their skin, and show outbursts of unprovoked rage
	• Lesch–Nyhan syndrome injure themselves seriously by biting their lips and fingers
	• Fragile X are shy, anxious, and avoidant
Frustration	With lack of communication, sensory deprivation, etc.
Iatrogenic	Medication side effects are commonplace

has a physical handicap, these problems are greater. Depression is very common, especially amongst those parents who cannot work or socialize due to having to care for their child. Siblings may also be affected, either by the stress and anxiety caused by family life, or from reduced parental attention. For these reasons, the whole family of a child with learning disability needs long-term support. Specific problems may arise when the parents of a severely LD child become too old or unwell to take care of their dependent child.

Psychiatric disorder in people with learning disability

Psychiatric disorders are more common in individuals with LD than in those within the normal range of intelligence and add an additional burden to the patient, their carers, and the community. All types of mental disorder may occur at any degree of LD, but at the severe level the most frequent are autism, hyperkinetic syndrome, stereotyped movements, pica, and self-mutilation. Those patients with epilepsy have a higher risk of serious psychiatric disorders. The assessment and management of all psychiatric diagnoses are as for any patient presenting with the corresponding symptoms.

Diagnosis

There are several reasons why psychiatric diagnosis is difficult in people with LD.

1 Patients may have *insufficient verbal ability* to describe abnormal experiences accurately (the level of ability corresponds to an IQ level of about 50).

2 Some people with LD are *suggestible* and may answer positively to a question about a symptom when they have not in fact experienced it.

For the above reasons, diagnosis often has to be *based on reports by others* of changes in the patient's behaviour. These informants may know little about the patient's past history, may not have spent much time with them recently, or may not be observant.

3 *Some causes of LD also cause abnormal behaviour.* Behaviour problems due to psychiatric disorder may be wrongly ascribed to this other cause, or vice versa.

4 LD is *associated with autism*, and some of the symptoms of autism can be mistaken for those of another psychiatric disorder, for example obsessive-compulsive disorder. Psychiatric disorder should be diagnosed only after deciding whether a pervasive developmental disorder is present (see p. 430).

5 *Physical illness* or *stressful events* can cause changes in behaviour, and both should be considered before the diagnosis of mental disorder is made.

The diagnostic criteria in the DSM-IV and ICD-10 classification systems apply to all individuals, and can be used for those with LD. However, the reliability and validity of these criteria are poorly characterized, especially for children. The criteria that include judgements based on whether or not a symptom is consistent with developmental level are particularly difficult. There are diagnostic guidelines being developed for those with LD; the Royal College of Psychiatrists have produced a set for adults with LD and there is also a modified form of the DSM-IV-TR. However, these are not yet widely used.

Specific psychiatric disorders

Attention deficit hyperactivity disorder (ADHD). ADHD is seen in up to 20 per cent of children with LD. It should be diagnosed using the usual criteria and observation of the patient. Attention and concentration should be judged against those of a child of a comparable developmental, not chronological, age. Hyperactivity is typically the most prominent symptom, and usually responds well to stimulants.

Autistic spectrum disorders (ASD). ASD are more common in people with LD than in the rest of the population, with a prevalence of about 1–2 per cent in all children with LD, and about 5 per cent in people with severe LD. Looked at in another way, about two-thirds of children with ASD also have some degree of LD. There is a particular association with tuberous sclerosis, congenital rubella, severe epilepsy, and phenylketonuria. It can be quite difficult to tell between those children with LD who have stereotypies and a limited range of interest, and those with autism. Most children with LD will try to communicate, use gestures/facial expressions, and display emotions, whilst these are reduced or absent in ASD.

Mood disorder. When people with LD develop a **depressive disorder** they are less likely than people of normal intelligence to complain of low mood or to express depressive ideas. Diagnosis has to be made mainly on observable features such as an appearance of sadness, reduction of appetite, disturbance of sleep, retardation, or agitation. Atypical features such as a regression to child-like behaviours, incontinence, and loss of social skills are more common. A severely depressed patient with adequate verbal abilities may describe depressive ideas, delusions, or hallucinations. Any change in behaviour in someone with a LD should lead to the exclusion of a mood disorder as the cause. A few of these patients make attempts at suicide, although these are usually poorly planned. Classical bipolar disorder I is occasionally seen in LD, with rapid cycling being a prominent feature. Mania has to be diagnosed mainly on overactivity and behavioural signs indicating excitement and irritability.

Anxiety disorders. The most commonly reported anxiety disorders are simple phobia, social phobia, and generalized anxiety disorder (GAD). Behaviour problems, irritability, withdrawal, insomnia, and somatic complaints are the usual symptoms seen. In GAD, conversion and dissociative symptoms are more conspicuous than in the corresponding disorders of people of normal intelligence. Anxiety disorders occasionally improve with stress reduction strategies, but are much harder to treat than in the general population. SSRIs are frequently used, but there is less good evidence of their efficacy. Similarly, stress-related and adjustment disorders occur commonly among people with mild and moderate LD, especially when they are facing changes in the routine of their lives.

Psychosis. In individuals with mild LD, the classical symptoms of schizophrenia (or other psychoses) are present, and diagnosis is relatively simple. However, delusions are less elaborate than they are among schizophrenics of normal intelligence, and hallucinations have a simple and repetitive content. Delusions frequently contain ideas gathered from the person's immediate environment, for example television shows. 'First rank' and other typical symptoms of schizophrenia are uncommon, and often the main features are a further impoverishment of a person's already limited thinking, and an increased disturbance of behaviour and social functioning. Catatonic symptoms are much more common. The negative symptoms of schizophrenia appear early, and are relatively treatment resistant. When the IQ is below 45, it is difficult to make a definite diagnosis of schizophrenia. When the diagnosis of schizophrenia is probable but not certain, a trial of treatment with antipsychotic drugs may be carried out.

Delirium and dementia. As at the extremes of age, the threshold for delirium is lower in those with LD. Disturbed behaviour resulting from delirium may be the first indication of physical illness. Dementia causes a progressive global decline in intellectual and social functioning from the previous level. It presents at a younger age, and may progress more quickly, in those with severe or profound LD. The typical symptoms are present, but may be difficult to identify. Nocturnal confusion ('sun downing'), forgetting the usual domestic routine, and late-onset epilepsy are sensitive markers of dementia. All forms of dementia may occur, but Alzheimer's disease is especially common in Down's syndrome.

Personality disorder. There is some debate as to whether or not personality disorders are a valid concept in those with moderate to profound LD. Epidemiological data suggests that personality disorders are common amongst people with mild LD and sometimes lead to greater problems in management than the learning problems. Because psychological development is delayed, the diagnosis is not generally made until the age of 20 years. There is no specific treatment, and management has to be directed at finding an environment as suitable as possible for the patient's temperament.

■ An approach to assessment and management

Assessment

Severe LD is usually diagnosed in infancy, as it is often associated with physical abnormalities or with delayed motor development. It is more difficult to diagnose less severe LD, which has to be done on the basis of delays in psychological development. Patients may therefore present at any age, including in adulthood, although this is fairly uncommon. In the UK, a structured method of assessment is used throughout psychiatry and paediatrics, the Care Plan Approach. This includes a multidisciplinary assessment, with a view to producing a full needs assessment, including the physical, psychological, and social needs of the patient and their carers. The specific aims of assessing a patient presenting with LD are:

- to make a diagnosis of LD;
- to search for the specific cause of the LD;
- to diagnose co-morbid physical and psychiatric disorders;
- to identify the specific needs of the patient and their family;
- to put together a coherent, long-term management plan.

The multidisciplinary team will vary depending upon the setting and age of the patient, but usually includes the family GP, psychiatrist, developmental paediatrician, psychologist, social workers, community psychiatric nurse, occupational therapist, physiotherapist, speech and language therapist, audiologist, and play specialist.

A full assessment includes history taking, interviewing, behavioural assessments, mental state examination, physical examination, psychological testing, and physical investigations.

Suggestibility among people with learning disability

When interviewing people with LD, the interviewer should remember that some are unusually suggestible. There are several reasons for this increased suggestibility:

- a strong wish to please others, especially people in authority;
- reliance on cues from the interviewer when deciding what answer to give, rather than reliance on factual information;
- a tendency to reply 'yes' rather than 'no' to yes/no questions, regardless of the appropriateness of this response.

Interviewing people with learning disability

The procedure is generally similar to those described in Chapter 5 for interviewing people of normal intelligence, but some special points should be noted.

1 **Ask simple questions.** avoiding subordinate clauses, passive verb constructions, figures of speech, and other complexities of grammar.

2 **Allow adequate time** for the patient to respond, and do not appear impatient.

3 **Check answers to closed questions** (e.g. 'Do you feel sad?'), which may have to be used because the patient cannot volunteer information. A positive answer can be checked by asking the opposite (e.g. 'Do you feel happy?').

4 **Avoid leading questions and check responses.** Because some people with LD are suggestible (see above), it is especially important to avoid leading questions. Some people with LD repeat the interviewer's last words. For example, interviewer: 'Do you feel sad?'; patient: 'Sad'.

5 **Check with an informant.** People with learning disabilities often have difficulty in timing the onset or describing the sequence of symptoms. Whenever possible, these and other important points should be checked with an informant.

History taking

The aim of the history is to understand what has brought the patient to the attention of medical services, and to gather information which can help with specific diagnosis. The parents or another informant should be interviewed in every case; patients who have reasonable language ability should be interviewed as well. It is usually helpful to talk to teachers, childminders, the GP, and members of the extended family. Particular points which should be covered include the following (see also Table 17.5, Chapter 17).

- presenting symptoms (e.g. aggressive behaviour, social withdrawal, failure to learn at school);
- previous medical and psychiatric history; current medications;
- the pregnancy, maternal infections/complications (e.g. pre-eclampsia); use of alcohol or drugs in pregnancy; labour and birth; neonatal complications, early feeding and weight gain;
- developmental history, including dates of passing key developmental milestones, review of growth charts;
- behaviour and physical disorders in the early years; head injuries;
- school/nursery attendance, attainment, and behaviour; for older patients, exam performance;
- family history; age of parents, consanguinity, family history of LD/congenital abnormalities/psychiatric disorders; current family structure and set-up.

Interviewing and observation

In younger children or those with limited communication, interviewing is not possible. A behavioural assessment will therefore need to be based on the account given by the parents or other informants and on observations of: (i) the child's *ability to communicate*; (ii) *sensorimotor skills*; (iii) any *unusual behaviour*; (iv) ability to *self-care*. The child may need to be visited at home or school to build a full picture of the behavioural problems. In older patients, a Mental State Examination should be carried out in the usual way, making adaptations as necessary.

Developmental and psychological testing

This is a complex procedure, which is performed usually in a specialist unit. IQ testing is important, usually using the Wechsler Intelligence Scales. Developmental delay and adaptive skills can be measured using the Griffiths or Bailey Developmental Scales, and the Vineland Adaptive Behaviour Scales. These quantify the problems the patient has, and can be useful aids when planning appropriate interventions and applying for social benefits. Conner's scales for ADHD can be used as for any child, but are not usually necessary.

Physical examination

The physical examination is best carried out by a paediatrician with knowledge of developmental and neurological disorders. It should include the recording of *head circumference*, *height*, and *weight*. Look carefully for dysmorphic features and congenital abnormalities. It may be helpful to examine close relatives to determine if any abnormalities are present in them too. A full neurological examination is essential, including speech and language, hearing, and vision assessments.

Investigations

In some cases, the clinical phenotype will clearly point to a cause for the LD (e.g. Down's syndrome) and little further investigation will be necessary. However, in cases of moderate to profound LD without obvious causation, a series of investigations should be carried out. Some examples of these include:

- blood tests for FBC, U&Es, liver function, renal function, clotting, thyroid function, glucose, and lipids;
- infection screening or serology (blood, urine, occasionally CSF) for rubella, toxoplasmosis, HIV, CMV, EBV, HSV, and syphilis;

- metabolic screening of blood for inborn errors of metabolism;

- genetics: karyotyping, single gene disorder testing (e.g. fragile X DNA testing);

- imaging of dysmorphia or abnormalities seen on physical examination, e.g. X-rays, CT/MRI (especially cranial);

- ECG, echocardiography;

- EEG, visual evoked potentials, muscle biopsy.

Overall assessment

At the end of the assessment, the clinician should have an idea of the cause of the LD and a clear view of the current behavioural, psychiatric, and social problems the patient has. These should be carefully documented, with specific individuals assigned to managing particular problems (e.g. ADHD—psychiatrist; schooling—social worker and educational psychologist).

Management approaches

The management of a patient with LD should be as for any other complex patient, with special attention to the psychological and social needs of the family (Table 19.6).

Few people with mild LD need specialist services. Most live with their families, cared for when necessary by the family doctor. When specialist treatment is needed it is

Table 19.6 Goals of service provision for a person with learning disability

'Normalize' the person's life
Recognize individual needs
Develop abilities
Offer choice and involve the patient in management decisions
Provide the best possible care for physical and psychiatric problems
Support the family or carers

usually for associated physical disability or illness, emotional disorder, or psychiatric illness. When placement away from home is needed it is usually because of difficulties in the family, or physical problems. Sometimes help may be needed by providing day care or respite care, for example parental illness. In these cases fostering or boarding school placement for children or residential care for adults is arranged. Adults with mild LD may need extra support when they are facing problems with housing and employment or with the problems of growing old (Table 19.7).

The remaining one-third of children with severe LD need residential care, often because of physical disability,

 Case study 19.1 The value of collateral information in learning disability

Philip, a 43-year-old forklift truck driver, presented to the emergency room with abdominal pain. He was unable to give much history, saying that his mum told him to come to hospital after work because he was ill. On examination, he was distended, diffusely tender, had tinkling bowel sounds, and had had a right orchidectomy. Philip seemed surprised to hear he was missing a testicle, and couldn't remember why it had been removed. He was admitted under the suspicion of bowel obstruction. During the night, Philip became agitated and aggressive towards staff. He was hyperactive, running around the ward and disturbing other patients. A doctor was called, who gave him IM sedation. In the morning, the surgeons called the on-call psychiatrist for help with his management. A psychiatrist came, who immediately called Philip's mother, his GP, his social worker, and his employer to gather the history of presenting complaint and background. This revealed that Philip had moderate LD, and had had testicular cancer for which he had received a radical right orchidectomy and radiotherapy 25 years earlier. He also tended to become anxious at night without his mum, and usually took stimulants (for hyperactivity) and low-dose zopiclone to help him sleep.

That night, Philip's mum was invited to stay in hospital with him, and his usual medications were given. There were no behavioural problems. Philip underwent a laparoscopy, revealing small bowel obstruction secondary to adhesions, probably secondary to radiotherapy. He did well post-operatively, and was discharged on day 3. His community psychiatric nurse was contacted, and she arranged for the district nurses to help his mum with dressing the wounds, and also visited more regularly for the next 3 weeks.

Learning points

- Always gather as much collateral history and information as possible; this may not be possible from the patient.

- Remember changes in routine can upset those with LD, who may show distress as challenging behaviour.

- Check regular medications with the patient, family, GP, and other involved professionals.

- Consider carefully if the patient has capacity, and, if not, how to make a medical decision ethically.

Table 19.7 Components of a service for people with learning disability

Social and psychological

Support for family at home; respite admissions

Education, training, and occupation

Social activities

Accommodation

Help with financial and other problems

Medical

Treatment of physical disorders

Management of challenging behaviour

Behavioural therapy

Cognitive behavioural therapy

Treatment of psychiatric disorders

Psychological treatments

Pharmacological treatments

behavioural problems, or autism too great for the parents to manage.

As people with LD live longer, provision is needed increasingly for the later years of their lives. At this stage, parents are no longer able to provide care and physical illness or dementia may add to the person's disability. It is important to recognize these problems when planning services.

Social interventions

Help for families. Parents need help as soon as the diagnosis of LD is made. It is seldom enough to explain the problem once; most parents need to hear the information several times before they can take in all its implications. Adequate time is needed to explain the prognosis, indicate what help can be provided, and discuss the part the parents can play in helping their child achieve his full potential. As explained above, parents need continuing psychological support and help with practical matters such as day care during school holidays, babysitting, or arrangements for family vacations. These provisions are needed in particular at times of change for the patient, especially leaving school, and at times when there are additional problems in the family such as the illness of another child. The rise of self-help and support groups for parents has been useful, and volunteers can play a valuable part in the arrangements. The Internet is now providing a huge support base for parents with children suffering from rare conditions.

Education. Education and training should begin early. Extra education and training before school age (**compensatory education**) helps children with LD to realize their

potential. When the normal school age is reached, the least disabled children can be educated in a special class in an ordinary school. More disabled children benefit more from attendance at a school for children with learning difficulties. For intermediate levels of disability, a choice has to be made between education in an ordinary school or a special school. The former offers the advantages of more normal social surroundings and greater expectations of progress; it has the disadvantages of lack of special teaching skills and the risk that the child may not be accepted by more able children. Since learning is slow, education may need to extend into adult life.

The period after leaving school is difficult for people with LD and they need a lot of help from their general practitioner and the specialist services. It is important to review the prospects for employment, suitability for further training, and requirements for day care. At this stage of life, it may be difficult for the parents to look after a young person with severe LD and residential care may be required. Wherever the person is living, there is a need for sheltered work or other occupation after leaving school.

Training and work. Most people with mild learning difficulties are capable of work and benefit from appropriate training. However, except at times of full employment, suitable work may not be available and sheltered occupation is needed. Most school-leavers with moderately severe LD need sheltered work or further training when they leave school. Most need these special provisions throughout their lives, although some do progress to normal employment.

Social activities. People with LD need to develop leisure activities appropriate to their age, ability, and interests. Whenever possible this should be achieved by joining activities arranged for able people, but clubs and day centres for the disabled are also needed. For the most disabled, leisure activities need to be arranged as part of the programme of the training centres that provide sheltered work.

Accommodation. Many people with LD live with their families. For the rest, a variety of accommodation is required ranging from ordinary housing to staffed hostels. A useful intermediate level of supervision is provided in a 'core and cluster' system in which several group homes are sited near to a central staffed unit. When parents grow old and can no longer care for their disabled son or daughter, special accommodation is required. In most places, the supply of such accommodation has not kept pace with the increasing life expectancy of people with LD.

Help with financial and other practical problems. People with LD may need help in managing their money, dealing with forms, regulations, and other problems of daily life. In most developed countries there are various social benefits available for people with special needs; patients and their families may need help and advice in order to access these. Special equipment for the home is also available and occupational and physiotherapists can be very helpful in arranging this.

Medical and psychological interventions

General medical services. People with LD sometimes receive substandard medical care because doctors do not detect their needs or do not provide the extra support needed to enable these patients to cooperate with treatment. It is good practice to keep a register of these patients and arrange regular health checks. Basic physical problems (e.g. toothache, hay fever) are a great source of behavioural disturbance, and should be actively sought and aggressively managed.

Treatment of challenging behaviour. The most important step in treating challenging behaviour is to identify the cause; if possible, this is then removed/treated. If the behaviour persists, behavioural treatment may be tried, directed to changing any factors that appear to be reinforcing the behaviour.

- **Behavioural therapy.** Behavioural techniques are very helpful in teaching basic self-care skills and establishing normal patterns of behaviour. Eating, sleep, and disobedience problems respond well to simple parenting skills such as ignoring poor and rewarding good behaviour. Phobias and anxiety disorders can be treated in the standard way. It can be used in people without verbal skills, which is a benefit over most other treatments.

- **Cognitive behavioural therapy.** CBT can be successfully used in people with mild to moderate LD. Anger management, aggression, interpersonal skills, low self-esteem, and problem-solving skills can all be treated with CBT in LD. There has been particular success in the treatment of sex offenders. It has been found that CBT for LD actually works best when delivered in a group format.

Psychodynamic therapy and counselling. As in the rest of psychiatry, the emphasis on psychodynamic therapy has reduced significantly in the field of LD. However, the principles of a comprehensive analysis can be very useful in treating patients with a LD who have suffered emotional abuse and severe psychological disturbance at an early age. Family members and carers may also benefit from counselling, or a CBT course for mood disorders.

Treatment of psychiatric disorder. Treatment of mental disorder among people with LD is similar to that of the same disorder in a patient of normal intelligence. There is typically a lower threshold for admission to hospital, which is usually related to the family/carer's ability to cope at home, rather than the patient being a risk to themselves or society.

Psychopharmacological treatments are widely used in LD, partly because the patients frequently have physical disorders (e.g. epilepsy) which are independent indications for them. Whilst medications do have a role to play in relieving specific symptoms and behaviours, they should not be used without a good indication. Because patients are less likely to report the side effects of drugs, particular care is needed in adjusting dosage. They are also more prone to atypical or idiosyncratic reactions.

- **Antipsychotics.** Antipsychotic drugs are used for psychosis, challenging behaviour (especially in autism, self-injury, and social withdrawal), tic disorders, and in severe mood disorders. Patients with LD are more prone to the metabolic side effects of atypical antipsychotics (weight gain, metabolic syndrome) and should be carefully monitored. There is good randomized controlled evidence for the use of risperidone in challenging behaviour.

- **Antidepressants.** Depression, OCD, anxiety disorders, and self-injury all respond well to standard antidepressant therapy.

- **Mood stabilizers** are used in the treatment of bipolar disorder and severe depression, and are a particularly good choice in patients with co-morbid epilepsy.

- **Stimulants** are now widely used to tackle hyperactivity and ADHD, and there is some evidence that they can improve behaviour more globally (improving eating, sleep, and mood).

- **Opiate antagonists.** There is a hypothesis that opioid excess may underlie autism and self-injury, and naltrexone has been used to treat both these conditions. There is little evidence that it improves symptoms in autism, but it does reduce the frequency and severity of self-injury.

Ethical problems in the care of people with learning disability

Most of the ethical problems encountered in the care of people with LD are similar in kind to those in the care of other patients. Two problems will be mentioned further.

Normalization, autonomy, and conflicts of interest

If people with LD are to live as normally as possible, they require support. Often this support comes from their family and arrangements that were entered into willingly at one time may become unduly burdensome if the needs of the disabled person increase, other children have additional needs, or the carers grow older. The problem can usually be resolved by discussion between the disabled person, the carers and other members of the family, and professionals with a duty of care for the various people involved. Comparable conflicts of interest may arise also when deciding whether a disabled child should be educated in an ordinary school or a special school for handicapped children.

Consent to treatment and research

Most learning disabled people can give informed consent provided that explanations are in clear and simple language, and adequate time is set aside for discussion. In the UK, when an adult with (usually severe) LD cannot give informed consent, no one can consent for him and the doctor has to decide what is in his best interests. The new Mental Capacity Act (see Box 18.3, p. 177) has made the process of making these decisions clearer. If there is time and the problem is particularly difficult—for example, termination of pregnancy—it may be appropriate to seek a ruling from the courts. If the condition is urgent and life-threatening it may be possible to proceed under common law, although expert medicolegal advice should be obtained first.

■ Specific clinical syndromes

Whilst the majority of people with mild LD do not have a unifying diagnosis for their problems, one can be identified in 50–80 per cent of those with moderate to profound LD. In many cases, the diagnosis is of a 'clinical syndrome'. *A syndrome is a characteristic pattern of clinical features, including both signs and symptoms.* It may include physical, genetic, cognitive, and emotional features. A syndrome may not necessarily have only one aetiological basis. Whilst some diagnoses will inevitably produce certain characteristics (e.g. LD in Angelman's syndrome), others are more variable in their phenotype (e.g. cardiac abnormalities in Down's syndrome). In these latter cases, the syndrome is said to be associated with the abnormality,

Science box 19.1 What is the evidence for the use of antipsychotic drugs in the treatment of challenging behaviour in patients with learning disability?

Challenging behaviour is difficult for patients, carers, and clinicians to manage. Given the availability of cheap antipsychotic medications (especially the 'safer' atypicals), there has been a rise in the use of drugs to manage this behaviour. However, evidence to support this usage has been lacking.

One of the first studies to describe the use of antipsychotics in the LD population was published by Bair and Herold in 1955.[1] They concluded that chlorpromazine (in high dosage) was an effective method of treatment. Over the next 30 years, the use of antipsychotics, especially amongst patients hospitalized or living in institutions, rose dramatically. Since the millennium, it has been realized that this usage may not have an evidence base to support it, and further work has been carried out.

In 2000, Robertson *et al.* carried out a study of 500 UK residents with LD living in the community (family home or sheltered accommodation), hospitals, or other institutions.[2] They found 20–50 per cent of patients were taking an antipsychotic, with the highest rates in hospitalized individuals. The study reports that mental illness was not the greatest predictor of being on an antipsychotic; associations were strongest with challenging behaviour, normal mobility, and living away from the family. The authors suggest that antipsychotics are being used to manage difficult behaviour in mobile patients, rather than mental illness.

A series of randomized controlled trials (RCTs) have been conducted to establish if antipsychotics are efficacious in managing challenging behaviour. Tyrer and colleagues published an RCT comparing risperidone, haloperidol, and placebo for up to 26 weeks in 86

non-psychotic patients with LD.[3] They report that aggression reduced significantly by 4 weeks in all three groups, with the placebo group showing the greatest change. A follow-up publication at the end of the 6 months confirmed these results, concluding that there is currently no indication for using antipsychotics for challenging behaviour in the absence of a mental disorder that would usually benefit from one.[4] Importantly, they did not find an increase in the quality of life of carers with antipsychotic use.

Currently, it seems that antipsychotics should not be thrown at all patients with challenging behaviour. It is not ethically sound to use them at extremely low dosage for 'the placebo effect', due to the potential for harmful side effects. More work is needed, especially in exploring the use of psychological treatments to tackle challenging behaviour.

1 Bair, H. V. & Herold, W. (1955). Efficacy of chlorpromazine in hyperactive mentally retarded children. *Archives of Neurology and Psychiatry* **74**: 363–4.

2 Robertson, J., Emerson, E., Gregory, N., *et al.* (2000). Receipt of psychotropic medication by people with intellectual disability in residential settings. *Journal of Intellectual Disability Research* **44**: 666–76.

3 Tyrer, P., Oliver-Africano, P. C., Ahmed, Z., *et al.* (2008). Risperidone, haloperidol and placebo in the treatment of aggressive challenging behaviour in patients with intellectual disability: a randomised controlled trial. *Lancet* **371**: 57–63.

4 Tyrer, P., Oliver-Africano, P., Romeo, R., *et al.* (2009). Neuroleptics in the treatment of aggressive challenging behaviour for people with intellectual disabilities: a randomised controlled trial (NACHBID). *Health Technology Assessment* **13**: 1–54.

or it is said that the patients will have vulnerability towards it. One of the advantages of recognizing a syndrome is that it allows clinicians to look for associated anomalies and treat them early; it also helps parents to plan for the future and families to access specialist support and services.

There are a large number of clinical syndromes that include or are associated with LD, but by far the most common are Down's, fragile X, and Kleinfelter's syndrome. These three examples will be explored in some detail, and Table 19.8 outlines the features of some rare conditions.

Down's syndrome

Down's syndrome was described by John Langdon Down in 1887, but it was not until 1959 when it was discovered to be (in the majority of cases) caused by the chromosomal abnormality trisomy 21. Down's syndrome is the most common autosomal trisomy, and the most prevalent cause of moderate to profound learning disability. The natural prevalence of Down's syndrome is 1 in 600 live births, but this has been significantly reduced by prenatal screening, and in the UK is now 1 in 1000 live births. The rate of Down's syndrome increases with increasing maternal age, such that the risk is 1 in 37 births once the mother is age 44.

There are three different ways in which trisomy 21 may come about:

1 **Non-disjunction (94% of cases).** One pair of chromosome 21 fail to separate at meiosis, such that one gamete has two chromosome 21s, rising to three after fertilization.

2 **Translocation (5%).** An extra chromosome 21 is joined on to another chromosome (usually 14, 15, or 22), so that whilst the child has 46 chromosomes, there are three copies of the chromosome 21 material.

3 **Mosaicism (1%).** This is due to non-disjunction at mitosis. Some of the cells in the body have three chromosome 21s and others have two. The clinical phenotype is often less severe.

Clinical features

The characteristic clinical features are shown in Table 19.9. The syndrome can usually be accurately diagnosed soon after birth, but nowadays most parents have had prenatal testing, and know in advance that their child has trisomy 21. For further information about the physical abnormalities typical of Down's syndrome, see the Further Reading section on p. 206.

Learning disability. In Down's syndrome the degree of LD varies considerably from person to person; usually the IQ is between 20 and 50, but in 15 per cent it is greater than 50. Many people are able to self-care (with prompting) by adolescence, and the majority to live with their families.

Temperament. The temperament of children with Down's syndrome is usually affectionate and easygoing, and many show an interest in music. Most have some obsessional characteristics and behaviours, and may be very stubborn about their daily routine, but these are usually subclinical problems.

Behaviour problems are less frequent than in most other forms of LD; nevertheless about a quarter of children with Down's syndrome are chaotic and difficult to engage. They relish attention and do very well with behavioural therapy approaches.

Ageing. In the past, many people with Down's syndrome died in infancy, but with improved medical care about half now live beyond the age of 50. Signs of ageing appear prematurely and **Alzheimer-like neuropathological changes** are found in the brain of most of those dying at the age of 40 years or more. However, for unknown reasons, survivors do not show signs of dementia until later, with a mean age of onset of about 50 years.

Co-morbidities. The most common psychiatric co-morbidities are ADHD, depression, OCD, and schizophrenia.

Fragile X syndrome

The condition is so called because a break is seen in an X chromosome of a proportion of cells when cultured in a medium deficient in folate. Fragile X is a trinucleotide repeat expansion mutation, similar in mechanism to those seen in Huntington's or Friedrich's ataxia. The basis of the abnormality is a region of CGG repeats in the gene *FMR1*. The repeats accumulate with successive copying, and affect the function of the gene when their number exceeds 200. Men and women with 50–200 repeats are carriers, though men are unlikely to pass on the condition as *FMR*, which is found active mainly in the brain and testis, probably modifies the activity of other genes. Testing can identify heterozygous females who are clinically normal, and males who are carriers. As the condition is inherited as an X-linked recessive disorder, all mothers of affected males are carriers, but there are some affected women, and unaffected males can pass the condition on to their grandsons via a daughter.

The disorder occurs in about 1 in 4000 males and in a milder form in 1 in 8000 females. The condition is the second most frequent cause of mental retardation (Down's syndrome is the first), accounting for about 7 per cent of moderate and about 4 per cent of mild LD among males, and about 3 per cent of moderate and mild mental retardation among females.

Clinical features

Affected children have *characteristic features*, none of which is diagnostic, and the clinical picture varies greatly from one affected person to another.

Table 19.8 Notes on some causes of learning disability

Syndrome	Aetiology	Clinical features	Comments
Chromosome abnormalities			
Down's, fragile X, and Kleinfelter's syndrome are described in the text			
Triple X	Trisomy X	Tall and thin	1 in 1000 female births
		Mild LD	
Cri du chat	Deletion in chromosome 5	Microcephaly, hypertelorism, typical cat-like cry, failure to thrive	1 in 35 000 births
		Hyperactivity	
		Language problems	
Angelman's syndrome	Deletion of 15q11q13 from maternal chromosome	Excessive laughter	Genomic imprinting condition
		Epilepsy and ataxia	
		Blond hair, blue eyes	
		Severe to profound LD	
		Fewer than 6 words by adulthood	
Prader–Willi syndrome	Deletion of 15q11q13 from paternal chromosome	Hypotonia	Genomic imprinting condition; complement of Angelman's syndrome
		Short stature	
		Hypogenitalism	
		Overeating	
		DSH	
		Mild to moderate LD	
Inborn errors of metabolism			
Phenylketonuria	Autosomal recessive causing lack of liver phenylalanine hydroxylase	Lack of pigment (fair hair, blue eyes)	Detectable by postnatal screening of blood or urine
		Retarded growth	
	Commonest inborn error of metabolism (1 in 10 000)	Epilepsy, microcephaly, eczema, hyperactivity, autism and self-injury	Treated by exclusion of phenylalanine from the diet during early years of life
		Untreated leads to severe LD	
Homocystinuria	Autosomal recessive causing lack of cystathione synthetase	Ectopia lentis, fine fair hair, joint enlargement, skeletal abnormalities similar to Marfan's syndrome	Sometimes treatable by methionine restriction
		Associated with thromboembolic episodes	
		Variable severity of LD	
Galactosaemia	Autosomal recessive causing lack of galactose-1-phosphate uridyltransferase	Presents after the introduction of milk into the diet	Detectable by postnatal screening for the enzymic defect
		Failure to thrive, hepatosplenomegaly, cataracts	Treatable by galactose-free diet
			Toluidine blue test on urine
Tay–Sachs disease	Autosomal recessive resulting in increased lipid storage (the earliest form of cerebromacular degeneration)	Progressive loss of vision and hearing	Death at 2–4 years
		Spastic paralysis	
		Cherry red spot at macula of retina	
		Epilepsy	
Hurler's syndrome (gargoylism)	Autosomal recessive affecting mucopolysaccharide storage	Grotesque features	Death before adolescence
		Protuberant abdomen	
		Hepatosplenomegaly. Associated cardiac abnormalities	
		Severe LD	

continued

Table 19.8 Notes on some causes of learning disability (*Continued*)

Syndrome	Aetiology	Clinical features	Comments
Lesch–Nyhan syndrome	X-linked recessive leading to enzyme defect affecting purine metabolism Excessive uric acid production and excretion	Normal at birth Development of choreoathetoid movements, scissoring position of legs, and self-mutilation (finger and lip biting) IQ 40–80 Death in second or third decade from renal failure	Can be diagnosed prenatally by culture of amniotic fluid and estimation of relevant enzyme Postnatal diagnosis by enzyme estimation in a single hair root Self-mutilation may be reduced by treatment with hydroxytryptophan
Other inherited disorders			
Neurofibromatosis (Von Recklinghausen's syndrome)	Autosomal dominant inheritance, mutation in neurofibromin gene	Neurofibromata, café au lait spots, vitiligo Associated with symptoms determined by the site of neurofibromata Astrocytomas, meningioma LD in a minority Speech defects	1 in 3000 births High spontaneous mutation rate, 50% have no family history
Tuberose sclerosis (epiloia)	Autosomal dominant (very variable penetrance) Up to 80% arise from spontaneous mutations	Epilepsy, adenoma sebaceum on face, white skin patches, shagreen skin, retinal phakoma, periungual fibromata Associated multiple tumours in kidney, spleen, and lungs LD in about 70% High rates of autism, OCD, ADHD, and self-injury	1 in 7000 in UK
Lawrence–Moon–Biedl syndrome	Autosomal recessive	Retinitis pigmentosa, polydactyly, obesity, infertility, diabetes Mild to moderate LD	Common in Kuwait and Canada
De Lange syndrome	Mutation in *NIPBL* gene on chromosome 5	Growth retardation Distinct facial features Feeding problems Self-injury Autism Severe to profound LD	1 in 60 000 births
Rett's syndrome	Mutation of *MeCP* gene on X chromosome, affects females only	Normal to 1 year, then loss of motor skills Scoliosis, spasticity, leg deformities Epilepsy Sleep disturbance Profound LD	Few girls survive beyond mid-adolescence
Infection			
Rubella	Viral infection of mother in first trimester	Cataract, microphthalmia, deafness, microcephaly, congenital heart disease	If mother infected in first trimester, 10–15% of infants are affected (infection may be subclinical)
Toxoplasmosis	Protozoal infection of mother	Hydrocephaly, microcephaly, intracerebral calcification, retinal damage, hepatosplenomegaly, jaundice, epilepsy	Wide variation in severity

Table 19.8 Notes on some causes of learning disability (*Continued*)

Syndrome	Aetiology	Clinical features	Comments
Cytomegalovirus	Virus infection of mother	Brain damage	
		Only severe cases are apparent at birth	
Congenital syphilis	Syphilitic infection of mother	Many die at birth	Uncommon since routine testing of pregnant women
		Variable neurological signs	
		'Stigmata' (Hutchinson teeth and rhagades often absent)	
Cranial malformations			
Hydrocephalus	Sex-linked recessive	Rapid enlargement of head in early infancy, symptoms of raised CSF pressure	Mild cases may arrest spontaneously
	Inherited developmental abnormality (e.g. atresia of aqueduct, Arnold–Chiari malformation, meningitis, spina bifida)		May be symptomatically treated by CSF shunt
		Other features depend on aetiology	Intelligence can be normal
Microcephaly	Recessive inheritance, irradiation in pregnancy, maternal infections	Features depend on aetiology	Evident in up to 20% of institutionalized patients with LD
Miscellaneous			
Spina bifida	Aetiology multiple and complex	Failure of vertebral fusion	Hydrocephalus in 80% of those with myelomeningocole
		Spina bifida cystica is associated with meningocole or, in 15–20%, myelomeningocole	LD frequent in this group
		Latter causes spinal cord damage, with lower limb paralysis, incontinence, etc.	
Cerebral palsy	Perinatal brain damage	Spastic (commonest), athetoid, and ataxic types	Majority are below average intelligence
	Strong association with prematurity	Variable in severity	Athetoid are more likely to be of normal IQ
Congenital hypothyroidism	Iodine deficiency or (rarely) atrophic thyroid	Appearance normal at birth Abnormalities appear at 6 months	Now rare in the UK
		Growth failure, puffy skin, large tongue, lethargy, constipation	Responds to early replacement treatment
		Moderate LD	
Hyperbilirubinaemia	Haemolysis, rhesus incompatibility, and prematurity	Kernicterus	Prevention by antirhesus globulin
		Choreoathetosis, opisthotonus, spasticity, convulsions	Neonatal treatment by exchange transfusion
Fetal alcohol syndrome	Exposure to alcohol during development	Mild to moderate LD	0.3 per 1000 live births
		Hyperactivity	
		Facial dysmorphia	
		Stunted growth	
		Skeletal, heart, and urological abnormalities	

Table 19.9 Abnormalities found in Down's syndrome

External abnormalities at birth

Flat occiput

Oblique palpebral fissures

Epicanthic folds

Small mouth, high-arched palate

Macroglossia

Short, broad hands

Single transverse palmar crease

Curved fifth finger

Hypotonia and extensive joints

Brushfield spots in the iris

Congenital heart disease (40%)

Deafness (and recurrent otitis media)

Duodenal atresia or Hirschsprung's disease

Later physical problems

Delayed motor milestones

Short stature and obesity

Immunocompromise—high risk of bronchopneumonia

Visual problems

Leukaemia

Atlantoaxial instability

Hypothyroidism (25%)

Epilepsy

Behavioural and psychiatric characteristics

Moderate to severe LD

Speech and language delay

Early-onset Alzheimer's disease

Obsessional and stubborn behaviours

Physical characteristics

The most specific physical feature is that 95 per cent of postpubertal men have large testes (macro-orchidism). Other typical features include a high forehead, prominent supraorbital ridges, and large everted ears. Connective tissues are often abnormal, leading to mitral valve prolapse (and other cardiac anomalies), hyperflexibility, cataracts, flat feet, and ear infections. Approximately 30 per cent of affected men have epilepsy. Since absence of these physical characteristics does not exclude the diagnosis, it is appropriate to test for the disorder in all unexplained cases of mental retardation.

Behavioural and psychiatric characteristics

People with fragile X almost inevitably have LD, varying from IQ 20–80. They have increased rates of abnormalities of speech and language, with speech that is rapid and disorganized with frequent repetition of words and phrases (a disorder known as **cluttering**). There are behaviours similar to those seen in autism: hand flapping, gaze avoidance, repetitive movements, and social anxiety. However, they can usually self-care and are more socially responsive than autistic children. Poor attention and concentration, and hyperactivity, are almost universal.

Kleinfelter's syndrome (47, XXY)

Kleinfelter's syndrome is a trisomy of the sex chromosomes, resulting in the karyotype 47, XXY. Prevalence at birth is 1–2 per 1000 live males, although this again is being reduced by prenatal diagnosis. The majority of males with Kleinfelter's do not present until young adulthood, when they are found to be infertile. They are tall, on average the 75th centile, and have no distinctive facial features. The testes and penis are small in childhood, and whilst the penis grows normally at puberty, the testes do not. Most men have gynaecomastia (60 per cent) and little bodily hair, which is another method of presentation.

The majority of boys with Kleinfelter's have an IQ of 50–90, and whilst they attend normal schools, do poorly. Many have speech and language problems, which do improve with therapy. From adolescence there is a high level of aggression, antisocial behaviour, and violence towards themselves and others. Data have shown a high proportion of UK prison inmates are found to have XXY (or XYY) on karyotyping. Behavioural therapy can help to an extent, but is not very successful.

Further reading

Gelder, M., Andreasen, N., Lopez-Ibor, J, & Geddes, J. (2009). *New Oxford Textbook of Psychiatry*, 2nd edn, pp. 1819–1887. Oxford University Press, Oxford.

Fraser, W. & Kerr, M. (eds) (2003). *The Psychiatry of Learning Disability*, 2nd edn. Gaskell, London.

Royal College of Psychiatrists. *Learning Disabilities*. www.rcpsych.ac.uk/mentalhealthinfoforall/problems/learningdisabilities.aspx

Royal College of Psychiatry (2001). *DC-LD: Diagnostic Criteria for Psychiatric Disorders for Use with Adults with Learning Disabilities/Mental Retardation*, 1st edn. RCPsych Publications.

Hagerman, R., Berry-Kravis, E., Kaufmann, W. E., *et al.* (2009). Advances in the treatment of fragile X syndrome. *Pediatrics* **123**: 378–90.

Lissauer, T. & Clayden, G. (2007). *Illustrated Textbook of Paediatrics*, 3rd edn. Mosby, St Louis.

People presenting with physical disorder

It is vital that all healthcare professionals dealing primarily with people presenting with physical disorder have a working knowledge of relevant psychological factors and psychiatric disorders in this population. Despite the geographical and, often, cultural separation of most 'general' (i.e. physical) and psychiatric hospitals in the developed world, there are close links between physical and psychological disorders, and between physical and psychological factors in the aetiology, presentation, and management of illness. This chapter aims to stimulate you to think about some of these issues when you are studying in primary care or the general hospital and, of course, aims to equip you with some of the knowledge required to think in a more integrated way about your patients' problems.

The links between physical and psychological factors are multiple. They include:

- psychiatric and physical disorders occurring together by chance, as they are both common;

- psychiatric disorders causing physical symptoms; for example, depression is associated with low physical energy (anergia), amenorrhoea, and constipation;

- psychiatric disorder adversely affecting the outcome of physical disorder; for example, a depressive disorder might make a patient less able to manage longstanding diabetes mellitus, because low motivation is a common symptom of depression, and may reduce adherence to self-monitoring of glucose;

- psychological factors increasing disability associated with physical disorder; for example, if a patient recovering from a myocardial infarction believes that it has led to a permanent reduction in their cardiac function, they are less likely to return to work, less likely to take regular exercise, and less likely to have a normal sex life;

- untreated psychological problems leading to the inappropriate use of medical resources and to poor compliance with medical advice; for example, people with panic disorder are more likely to attend Accident and Emergency departments with acute chest pain;

- physical symptoms and disorders having psychological consequences, which include psychiatric disorder; for example, hypothyroidism and cerebrovascular disease may lead to depression;

- physical disorder exacerbating unrelated psychiatric symptoms; for example, a viral infection could delay recovery from a depressive disorder by impeding the person's usual activities, at work and at home, which would otherwise provide therapeutic distraction and stimulation.

■ Epidemiology

In the *general population* psychiatric disorder is two to three times more likely when physical ill health is present (Figure 20.1). Also, disabling functional symptoms (see Chapter 25) are frequent.

In *primary care*, psychological issues are important in the management of many patients with serious acute or chronic physical illness. Functional physical symptoms are among the commonest reasons for seeking treatment and are often due to psychiatric disorder.

In *secondary care*, psychological problems are especially frequent in Accident and Emergency departments, gynaecological and medical outpatient clinics, and elderly patients, including those on specialist units such as stroke units.

About a quarter of patients in medical wards have a psychiatric disorder of some kind. **Mood disorders** are commonly seen in younger women, **organic mental disorders** such as dementia and delirium in the elderly, and **drinking problems** in young men and women. In outpatient clinics, about 15 per cent of patients with a definite medical diagnosis have an associated psychiatric disorder, and about 40 per cent of those with no medical diagnosis have a psychiatric disorder.

■ Psychological factors as causes of physical disorders

It used to be thought that certain 'psychosomatic' diseases, such as asthma and ulcerative colitis, were caused mainly by psychological factors. Research evidence has not supported this view, but has certainly supported the contribution of psychological factors to the aetiology, presentation, and outcome of physical illness. Psychological factors may, for example:

- **lead to unhealthy habits** such as overeating, smoking, and excessive use of alcohol, which are risk factors for physical disease;

- **result in hormonal, immunological, or neurophysiological changes**, which contribute to the onset or affect the course of the physicopathological process. It has been suggested, for example, that increased mortality among patients depressed after myocardial infarction is caused in this way;

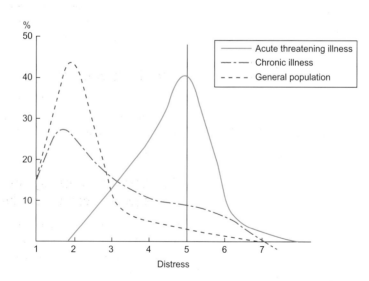

Fig. 20.1 The distribution of emotional distress in the general population and in those with physical illness. Level 5 and over indicates a diagnostic psychiatric disorder.

- **affect symptom perception**, such as people experiencing more physical pain when they are depressed;
- **affect medical help seeking;** for example, a person who would not seek help for backache when in a normal mood may do so when depressed;
- **affect treatment adherence;** for example, a depressed patient may neglect his part in the treatment of diabetes.

■ Psychological complications of physical disorders

Delirium (acute global impairment of cognitive functioning) is frequent in those who are severely ill, and is often not diagnosed (see Chapter 26). Most anxiety and depression associated with physical illness are part of the psychological reaction to that illness, but several medical disorders also cause anxiety and depressive symptoms directly, through physiological mechanisms (Table 20.1). Finally, some drugs used in the management of physical disorders have psychiatric side effects, and it is important to be aware of the possibility of iatrogenic psychiatric disorder (Table 20.2).

Most people are remarkably resilient when ill and are able to carry on without undue distress. However, all physical illness has some psychological impact, including:

- disturbances of mental state, of which about a quarter are severe enough to be classified as a psychiatric disorder;
- heightened perception of physical symptoms and disability;
- impaired quality of everyday life;
- unnecessarily poor physical outcome;
- adverse effects on family and others;

Table 20.1 Psychiatric symptoms and some physical causes

Depression
Neurological disorder, including cerebrovascular disease
Endocrine disorder, including hypothyroidism
Carcinoma, including lung and pancreatic cancer
Infections
Anxiety
Hyperthyroidism
Hyperventilation
Hypoglycaemia
Withdrawal from psychoactive drugs, including cannabis, benzodiazepines

Table 20.2 Some medications reported to cause depression

- Antihypertensives, e.g. beta-blockers, calcium channel blockers, reserpine, alpha-methyl-DOPA
- Gastrointestinal drugs, including cimetidine, ranitidine
- Interferon
- NSAIDs
- Corticosteroids, e.g. dexamethasone, prednisolone (although mood elevation is much more common)
- Combined oral contraceptive pill
- Roaccutane
- L-DOPA

- inappropriate or excessive consultation with doctors or other healthcare professionals;
- poor adherence to treatment plans.

Psychological reactions to illness

The usual reaction to **acute illness** is anxiety, which may be followed by depression. In up to a quarter of patients these reactions reach the diagnostic threshold for anxiety, depressive, or adjustment disorder. These responses are similar to those to other types of stress (see Chapter 23). Other reactions are also common, for example anger and the complete or partial denial of a life-threatening diagnosis. Both these responses can lead to poor collaboration with treatment.

In **chronic illness**, anxiety and depressive disorders are up to twice as common as in the general population, and psychological and social variables are strong determinants of outcome, such as employment status. The special problems of **terminal illness** are discussed in Chapter 23.

Psychiatric disorder

Although adjustment disorder, anxiety, and depression are the commonest psychiatric complications of physical illness, other psychiatric disorders may also be precipitated by physical illness (Table 20.3).

Determinants of the psychological consequences of physical illness

Some illnesses and treatments are particularly threatening (Table 20.4). However, the psychological reactions depend more upon a patient's perception of the illness than its objective nature (Table 20.5). If patients see their illness as particularly unpleasant or if their ability to cope with stress is poor, then severe distress is more likely. The

Table 20.3 Common psychiatric disorders in the physically ill

More common

- Adjustment disorder
- Depressive disorder
- Anxiety disorders
- Delirium

Less common

- Somatoform disorders
- Dementia
- Post-traumatic stress disorder
- Mania
- Schizophrenia and delusional disorder

Table 20.5 Determinants of the psychological impact of physical illness

Illness factors

- Pain
- Threat to life
- Duration
- Disability
- Conspicuousness to others

Treatment factors

- Side effects of medication
- Uncertainty of outcome
- Self-care demands

Patient factors

- Psychological vulnerability
- Social circumstances
- Beliefs about illness and treatment

Reactions of others

- Family
- Employers
- Doctors and others involved in care

reactions of others may also affect patients' perceptions and their ability to cope.

Patients at high risk are especially likely to be encountered in hospital emergency departments and in specialized units, such as those responsible for terminal care, cancer, severe neurological problems, and pain.

Psychiatric assessment of a physically ill patient

Among severely ill patients distress is often seen as understandable and inevitable and no help is offered. This is incorrect. Most people cope remarkably well with even the most severe medical problems, and, by implication, marked distress is abnormal and requires assessment and treatment.

The psychiatric assessment of a physically ill patient is similar to that of a patient presenting solely with

Table 20.4 Factors associated with a high risk of psychiatric problems

Physical factors

- Severe illness: unpleasant, threatening, relapsing, progressive or terminal
- Unpleasant treatment: e.g. major surgery, chemo- or radiotherapy
- Very demanding self-care

Psychological factors

- Previous psychiatric disorder

Social factors

- Poor social support, social isolation
- Other adverse social circumstances

psychiatric symptoms (see Chapter 5), except that it requires knowledge of the nature and prognosis of the physical illness. Box 20.1 lists some screening questions. It is best if these questions do not come out of the blue but, rather, that there is a clear introductory rationale; for example, 'It's clear that your illness has been tough on you, and we do find that some people with illnesses like yours have trouble coping. Has that been the case with you? ... I'd like to ask you some questions about that.'

It is important to:

- speak to relatives who can provide extra information, and also because families frequently require help themselves;
- review medical notes and referral letters as they often contain useful medical history and other information;
- be aware that some symptoms, such as mental and physical fatigue, and poor sleep, may occur in both physical and psychiatric disorder.

Management

Treatment of **acute reactions** to illness is discussed in Chapter 23. Some emotional distress is an almost inevitable accompaniment of the stress of physical illness and its treatment, although it can often be reduced by appropriate management. An important part of good psychological care is effective patient education, which should

BOX 20.1 Recognition of emotional disorder in the physically ill

Psychiatric symptoms

- How have you been feeling in yourself?
- Have you been very worried about your health?
- How have you been sleeping?
- Are you taking any tablets for your nerves or for your sleep?
- Have you ever suffered from tension or nerves?

Social factors

- Have you had any problems recently that have upset you?

- Do you have any problems at home or at work?
- How is your relationship with your husband/wife/partner/children?

Beliefs and concerns

- What do you think is the cause of your symptoms?
- What effects do you think they will have on your life?
- How will things turn out?
- How hopeful are you?

---

comprise an explanation of (i) the nature of the illness, (ii) the likely causes of the illness, (iii) the proposed treatment plan, and (iv) advice about the ways the patient can help himself. In addition, simple questions to elicit the patient's queries or concerns are helpful, and involving the patient's primary carer can be useful. Give written information to back up verbal messages, copy patients in to GP letters that are written appropriately, and inform patients of available support organizations such as, in the field of cancer in the UK, Maggie's Cancer Caring Centres and Macmillan Cancer Support.

As well as systematic assessment and alertness to verbal and non-verbal cues of distress, good care depends on the ability to provide and discuss information and advice with patients and their relatives. Basic psychological skills are important, including:

- knowledge of the recognition and treatment of depression;
- basic anxiety management skills (see p. 138);
- knowledge of basic cognitive behavioural principles (see pp. 135–140);
- an ability to encourage self-care.

Management of the psychological problems of **chronic illness** is best organized as a process of 'stepped' care. At **step one**, psychosocially informed medical care is provided for everyone, and includes:

- information about and encouragement of self-care, including symptom management;
- discussion of how the patient and their family will be involved in care;
- explanation of who will be providing treatment, and routine and emergency contact arrangements, including a named key worker where possible;

- practical support with occupational, financial, and accommodation problems, perhaps with the assistance of a social worker or benefits expert;
- systematic monitoring of progress;
- the identification of those needing step two care.

Step two care is provided by the patient's GP or by the team providing the patient's physical care, and comprises initial treatment of common psychiatric disorder such as depression, perhaps following telephone advice from mental health specialists. If the problem persists despite step two care, or there are specific concerns, such as significant suicidality, **step three** care is provided by mental health professionals, based either within the physical setting (as a liaison psychiatry service) or within community mental health teams.

Psychiatric disorder

The treatment of any specific psychiatric disorder among the physically ill is similar to that of the same condition in a physically healthy person, with one proviso—particular attention should be paid to adverse consequences of the side effects of antidepressant and other drugs, and to drug interactions.

Adjustment disorder. Patients need opportunities for discussion, explanation, and problem solving. Simple advice about the disadvantages of using alcohol and other substances to manage distress may be appropriate.

Anxiety disorder. Advice, and self-help via cognitive-behaviourally informed books, is important. Formal psychological treatment or pharmacological treatment (usually an SSRI) may be required, if the anxiety is severe or persistent.

Depressive disorder. Mild depression can often be helped by illness support, advice or problem solving, and encouragement of re-engagement with aspects of the patient's occupational, home, and social life that they have given up following diagnosis. These are simple approaches which can be delivered by a member of the team treating the physical disorder. Moderate or severe disorders require antidepressant medication or formal psychological treatments such as CBT. The choice of antidepressant may be affected by side effects, cautions, and contraindications, so it is vital to consult the *British National Formulary* or a similar reference. Tricyclic antidepressants, for example, are contraindicated in the immediate days after myocardial infarction, and cautioned in cardiovascular disease more generally.

Effects on families

Close relatives may suffer as much, or even more, distress than patients. It is important to include relatives in discussions about the patient's treatment, involve them in the programme of self-care, and consider ways of helping with their own distress and any practical problems caused by the patient's illness.

■ Some practical problems

Acutely distressed patients

Distress, anxiety, or anger often reflects patients' uncertainties and fears about what is happening to them. It is important to try to understand the cause, to show sympathy, and to correct misunderstandings. It is always important to remain calm and to take time to understand the patient's concerns and to avoid unintentional exacerbation of problems. When anxiety remains severe, small amounts of anxiolytic medication may be helpful.

Patients who refuse consent to medical treatment

Occasionally, patients are unwilling to accept their doctor's advice about treatment that seems essential for a serious medical condition. There are many reasons for such refusal. Commonly, this is because the patient is frightened or angry, does not understand fully what is happening, has had aversive previous experience of medical care, or knows someone who has. Remember that your views and experiences, as a member of the healthcare team, may be very different to many members of the public, who may have good reason to hold different views to you. Frequently, taking time to explain and to discuss the patient's situation, perhaps involving a close relative, and steadily building trust over a series of meetings, will result in informed consent. Occasionally, the cause of refusal is a mental illness that interferes with the patient's ability to make an informed decision and, if this is the case, the illness should be treated, if appropriate under the Mental Health Act. It is important to note that the Mental Health Act does not give the right to treat physical disorder, except in the unusual case when physical disorder is thought to be the direct cause of the mental disorder.

It has to be accepted that some mentally healthy patients will continue to refuse treatment even after a full and rational discussion of the reasons for carrying it out. It is the absolute right of a conscious, mentally competent adult to refuse treatment (see Chapter 12). In the UK, the Mental Capacity Act provides important guidance in this area.

Psychiatric emergencies in general hospital practice

However urgent the problem, the successful management of a psychiatric emergency, like any other medical emergency, depends greatly on a thorough clinical assessment. The aims are to:

- establish a satisfactory relationship with the patient;
- take a brief history, from the patient and a key healthcare professional;
- assess the mental state, including observation of behaviour.

When the patient's behaviour is very disturbed, the history may have to be obtained from other people, such as relatives or nurses. Although in managing emergencies there may not be the time or opportunity to follow the usual systematic scheme of history taking and examination, mistakes will be avoided and time saved if the assessment is as complete as the circumstances permit. Several common problems are discussed elsewhere in this book, including deliberate self-harm (see Chapter 9), substance intoxication (see Chapter 29), acute stress reactions to trauma (see Chapter 23), and delirium (see Chapter 26).

Acute disturbed behaviour and violence

The conditions most often leading to disturbed behaviour requiring immediate action in a general hospital or in primary care are delirium (i.e. physical disorder), schizophrenia, mania, agitated depression, and alcohol- and drug-related problems. Among inpatients, delirium is the most common.

■ Psychiatric services for a general hospital

General practitioners are responsible for all aspects of their patients' care: physical, psychological, and social. Similarly, in a general hospital, psychological aspects of illness are part of the consultant team's responsibilities, as are social aspects such as arranging an appropriate discharge route and social support. Step one psychological care (assessment, advice about self-care, simple cognitive-behavioural strategies, first-line medication) should be within the domain of the physical healthcare team. Sometimes, specialist psychiatric advice is needed. In larger hospitals, this advice may be from a special **liaison** (also known as **consultation liaison**) **service**. This service is staffed by psychiatrists, nurses, and psychologists, usually with a social worker. The consultation liaison service may provide (i) an emergency service for patients admitted after deliberate self-harm, (ii) emergency consultation for other Accident and Emergency department attenders, (iii) a consultation service, to provide advice on the management of inpatients, (iv) outpatient care for patients referred with psychiatric complications of physical illness or functional somatic symptoms, and (v) regular visits to selected medical and surgical units in which psychiatric problems are especially common (e.g. neurology, renal dialysis, terminal care), to develop knowledge and skills among the physical healthcare team.

Because specialist psychiatric care is provided by a multidisciplinary team, referral is usually made to that team rather than to a specific doctor. The team will decide (i) which of its members is best placed to respond (availability, skill set) and (ii) how they will respond (phone call, visit, or phone call followed by visit; emergency, urgent, or routine). Referral to a mental health team should provide basic information about:

- the medical problem(s);
- the reason(s) for the referral;
- the specific question to be asked, or specific nature of the help required;
- the urgency of the referral.

■ Some examples of psychiatric aspects of physical disorders

Cancer

As the most frightening of diseases, cancer causes considerable distress to many patients and their families. Psychological and social problems include family worries, financial and work difficulties, and worries about appearance. Patients may be angry. Sexual difficulties are common, sometimes due to direct effects of the illness or its treatment, but often due to cancer's impact on self-esteem, self-confidence, and personal relationships. Only a minority develop a psychiatric disorder, such as adjustment disorder (on diagnosis or recurrence), anxiety, depression, or rarer psychiatric syndromes due to metastases or paraneoplastic syndromes. Cancer and its treatment vary considerably in the nature, intensity, and duration of their physical impact on an individual and, by implication, in the nature of their psychological impact. Distress is particularly likely to occur at particular points during the patient's experience of cancer, including at diagnosis, during treatment (surgery, radiotherapy, or chemotherapy), and at the point (or points) of recurrence.

Care should be planned to involve patients and families to prevent or minimize psychological and social problems. Almost all psychological care is provided in primary care or in specialist cancer services in secondary care, which are increasingly well equipped to think in an integrated, biopsychosocial way about the management of cancer. This includes information and explanation, provided in a staged manner as patients and families require it. It is accompanied by practical and social support and willingness to encourage patients to talk about their worries. Specific psychiatric treatments (pharmacological and psychological) are effective for anxiety and depression and in helping patients to cope with physical symptoms.

Surgical treatment

Most patients are anxious before major surgery; those who are most anxious before surgery are also most likely to be distressed afterwards. Anxiety can be reduced by a clear explanation of the operation, its likely consequences, and the plan for post-operative care, including the effective treatment of pain. In addition, a written handout is helpful since anxious people do not remember all that they have been told. Delirium is common after major surgery, especially in the elderly.

When surgery leads to changes in the body's appearance (e.g. mastectomy) or function (e.g. colostomy) there may be additional psychological problems. These patients benefit from psychological support, which may be given by a specially trained nurse.

Screening for physical disorder or risk

Screening procedures for physical disorders, such as hypertension or early cancer, or for major risk factors, such as high blood lipid levels, are used increasingly. Screening usually causes little distress if it is properly explained. However, a few recipients are made anxious by the screening, whatever the result, 'positive' or 'negative' and, for these people, extra help is needed. Screening programmes should incorporate the routine provision of background information, the opportunity for the discussion of anxieties, and additional help for the small proportion of people who become anxious.

Genetic counselling

Counselling about the risk of hereditary disease is mainly given to couples planning or expecting a child. It includes providing information about risks, help with worry about increased risk, help in taking well-informed decisions about family planning (including sterilization), and treatment. Genetic counselling is usually provided in obstetric and genetic clinics, but there is also a need for advice and support by family doctors. There are important ethical issues to consider (Box 20.2).

Genetic counselling is often undertaken in the context of specific tests or test results. The following guidelines are helpful.

- The written protocol for the testing programme should detail how the laboratory tests will be conducted and how communications with patients will be managed.
- Before they decide whether to undergo a test, clear and simple information should be presented to those eligible for testing. This should include the advantages and disadvantages of testing, as well as the meaning of each possible test result.
- The initial offer of a test should be separated by at least a day from the collection of the biological sample, to allow time for reflection and 'cooling off'.
- Test results should be explained and support offered to all those tested and, where appropriate, their relatives.

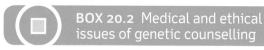

BOX 20.2 Medical and ethical issues of genetic counselling

- Confidentiality
- Informed consent
- Storage and use of genetic information
- Testing children: it is probably wise to delay testing until an age at which individuals have the capacity to make their own decisions
- Implications for life insurance

■ Psychiatric aspects of obstetrics and gynaecology

Pregnancy

Psychiatric disorder is more common in the first and third trimesters of pregnancy than in the second (Box 20.3). In the first trimester, unwanted pregnancies are associated with anxiety and depression, and the news of the pregnancy, even when welcomed by both partners, brings the prospect of uncertainty and significant lifestyle change. In the third trimester, there may be fears about the impending delivery, or doubts about the

 BOX 20.3 Some psychological problems of pregnancy

Unwanted pregnancy (common)

Most medical decisions about termination are made by the family doctor or gynaecologist. In a small proportion of patients with psychiatric disorder, a specialist opinion should be obtained.

Hyperemesis gravidarum (unusual)

Severe and repeated vomiting, much worse than the usual 'morning sickness', appears to have primary physiological causes but the psychological reaction may exacerbate the severity and duration of the symptoms and result in greater difficulty in management.

Pseudocyesis (rare)

A condition in which a woman believes she is pregnant when she is not and develops amenorrhoea, abdominal distension, and other changes resembling early pregnancy. It usually resolves quickly following diagnosis. It may be recurrent.

Couvade syndrome (rare)

A condition in which the husband or partner of a pregnant woman experiences some of the symptoms of pregnancy, including minor weight gain, morning nausea, and disturbed sleep.

normality of the fetus. Psychiatric symptoms in pregnancy are more common in women with a history of previous psychiatric disorder, although some women with chronic psychiatric disorders may improve during pregnancy. Women with chronic psychiatric problems often attend irregularly for antenatal care, and are at increased risk of obstetric problems.

Treatment of psychiatric disorder during pregnancy

During pregnancy great care must be taken in the use of psychotropic drugs because of the possible risk of fetal malformations, impaired growth, and perinatal problems (Box 20.4). The current *British National Formulary* provides up-to-date guidance.

Abuse of *alcohol* and *street drugs* may affect the fetus and should be strongly discouraged, especially in the first trimester when the risk to the fetus is greatest. Current advice about alcohol consumption is that, when trying to conceive and during the first trimester, alcohol should be avoided entirely. In the second and third trimester, small amounts of alcohol may be drunk on 1 or 2 days a week.

Loss of a fetus and stillbirth

Loss of a fetus during pregnancy or at delivery (stillbirth) has substantial and immediate psychological impact for the mother and also for the father. The loss leads to significant depression, which may continue for several weeks. **Spontaneous abortion** at any stage of pregnancy causes distress and depression is frequent. **Stillbirth** is associated with even greater distress than loss of the pregnancy at an earlier stage. The distress is likely to be greatest when the pregnancy was particularly wanted, for example when there have been previous miscarriages or stillbirths. **Termination of pregnancy for medical reasons** is especially likely to cause distress, depression, and feelings of guilt, which usually improve over a period of 2–3 months. After abortion, termination, or stillbirth, mothers and fathers should be encouraged to grieve the loss as they would the death of an infant.

Postpartum mental disorders

There are three kinds of postpartum psychiatric disorder:

- maternity 'blues';
- puerperal psychosis;
- other depressive disorders of moderate severity.

 BOX 20.4 Use of psychiatric medicines during pregnancy and breast-feeding

Pregnancy

Avoid all medication *if possible*, especially during the first trimester. Use only if the expected benefit to the mother is greater than the possibility of risk to the fetus. Clearly there will be circumstances, such as perceived high risk of relapse of a challenging mental disorder, when continued prescription is considered appropriate, despite theoretical risks to the fetus.

Antidepressants. There is no evidence that tricyclics or SSRIs cause fetal abnormality, but use only where there are very clear indications and in minimal dosage. There is a possibility of SSRI withdrawal in neonates.

Lithium. There is a small risk of teratogenicity in the first trimester, and of toxic effects on the fetus in late pregnancy. Risks are reduced by careful monitoring of levels. Ideally, lithium should be avoided in the period of conception and early pregnancy, but careful represcription is possible in the final trimester. In an unplanned pregnancy during long-term therapy, discuss with the parents, consider termination, and also careful screening

for malformations. The dose may need to be increased during the second and third trimesters, but take care—pharmacokinetics return rapidly to normal at delivery.

Antipsychotics. Continue in minimal dose if there are major clinical indications. Occasional extrapyramidal side effects are seen in neonates.

Breast-feeding

Take care with all medications. This advice is motivated by a relative absence of evidence.

Antidepressants. Although there is no convincing evidence of possible harm, most manufacturers advise avoiding these during breast-feeding. Avoid if possible, but if risks to the woman's mood are considered high, carefully consider the risks and benefits with the parents.

Lithium. Present in breast milk, with possible risk of toxicity. Breast-feeding cannot be recommended with confidence.

Antipsychotic drugs. The risk is probably very small, but there is a theoretical risk to nervous system development, so avoid if possible.

The management of depressive disorder is more fully described in Chapter 21. Abuse and neglect, which also occasionally occur in infancy, are discussed in Chapter 17.

Maternity 'blues'

Between one-half and two-thirds of women delivered of a normal child experience a brief episode of irritability, muddled thinking, tearfulness, and lability of mood, which is particularly characteristic. All these symptoms reach their peak on the third or fourth postpartum day. The patient and her partner should be reassured that the condition is common and short lived. No other treatment is needed.

Puerperal psychosis

Puerperal psychosis begins, typically, 2–3 days after delivery and nearly always in the first 1–2 postpartum weeks. There are three types of psychosis. **Affective** syndromes are the most common in high-income nations, followed by **schizophreniform** syndromes and, finally, **delirium,** which was common before antibiotics were introduced to treat puerperal sepsis, but is now rare in high-income nations. The clinical features of each of these syndromes are similar to those of the corresponding syndromes occurring outside the puerperium.

Puerperal psychosis occurs in about 1 in 500 births. It is more frequent among primiparous women, those who have suffered previous serious psychiatric disorder, and those with a family history of psychiatric disorder. Puerperal psychosis is not more common after complicated deliveries.

Assessment. As well as taking a *history* and examining the *mental state* in the usual way, *it is essential to ascertain the mother's ideas concerning the baby.* Severely depressed patients may have delusional ideas that the child is malformed or otherwise imperfect and some patients may attempt to kill the child to spare it from future suffering. Assessment of *suicidal intent* is also important.

Treatment is as described for affective disorder and schizophrenia occurring outside pregnancy. For depressive disorders of marked or moderate severity, *ECT* is often the best treatment because its rapid effect enables the mother to resume the care of her baby quickly. When the disorder is not severe and the mother has no ideas of harming herself or the baby, treatment can be at home with appropriate help to ensure the safe care of the baby. When the disorder is more severe, or there are ideas of harm to self or baby, the mother should usually be admitted to hospital, if possible to a specialist mother and baby unit. If psychiatric medicines have to be prescribed, the safety of breast-feeding must be assessed.

Prognosis. Most patients recover fully from a puerperal psychosis but a few (mostly those with a schizophrenic psychosis) remain chronically ill. At a subsequent birth, the recurrence rate for puerperal affective disorder is much higher than in those without previous puerperal affective disorder.

Treatment during subsequent pregnancies. Women who have had a puerperal psychosis should be referred to a psychiatrist and monitored very closely in the hours and days after delivery. Patients who have a history of bipolar disorder may require lithium prophylaxis, avoiding the first trimester and stopping for a short period at delivery.

Other puerperal depressive disorders

Postnatal depression of mild or moderate severity is much more common than puerperal psychosis, occurring in 10–15 per cent of recently delivered women. However, this prevalence is little different to that in the general population of young women. Tiredness, irritability, and anxiety are often more prominent than depressive mood and there may be prominent phobic symptoms.

Clinical observation suggests these disorders are caused mainly by the psychological adjustments required after childbirth, by loss of sleep, and by the hard work involved in the care of the baby. Some of these women have a history of psychiatric illness and some have experienced stressful events near the time of onset of the disorder.

There is evidence that postnatal depression adversely affects the mother–infant relationship and the cognitive and emotional development of the infant. It is not clear whether these adverse effects persist into early and later childhood.

Early detection is important and those providing care to the mother and baby need to be alert to the possibility of depression. In the UK, the Edinburgh Postnatal Depression Scale is commonly used as a screening tool by community midwives and health visitors. Management may include advice about childcare, help with childcare, advice on sexual relationships, and more general marital guidance. Otherwise, management of postnatal depression is similar to that of depression in general.

Menstrual disorders

Premenstrual syndrome

This term denotes psychological and physical symptoms starting a few days before, and ending shortly after, the onset of a menstrual period. The psychological symptoms include anxiety, irritability, and depression, and the physical symptoms include breast tenderness, abdominal discomfort, and a feeling of distension.

Estimates of the frequency of the premenstrual syndrome in the general population vary widely from 30 to 80 per cent of women of reproductive age, depending on the diagnostic criteria used. The cause is uncertain. Psychological factors may exacerbate distress and disability originating from physiological changes around menstruation.

Many pharmacological treatments have been tried, including serotonin-reuptake-inhibiting drugs such as the tricyclic clomipramine and the SSRIs. To determine whether this approach is effective in a particular patient, a daily symptom diary can be helpful, in which the main emotional and physical symptoms are rated, day by day. Cognitive behavioural therapy can be helpful in enabling women to cope with symptoms and their consequences in a positive way that enables them to feel more in control of their everyday life. There is some randomized evidence to support the effectiveness of both SSRIs and CBT.

Menopause

Some menopausal women complain of physical symptoms of flushing, sweating, vaginal dryness, headache, and dizziness, and psychological symptoms such as depression and anxiety. Although there is a widespread belief that emotional problems are an inevitable part of the menopause, it is not certain whether psychological symptoms are more common in menopausal women than in other women of similar age. Depressive and anxiety-related symptoms around the time of the menopause could be related to hormonal changes but this has not been proved. Alternatively, or additionally, the symptoms could result from changes in the woman's role as her children leave home, her relationship with her partner alters, and her own parents become ill or die.

Hormone replacement therapy (HRT) should not be seen as a treatment of depressive illness in those of menopausal age. Psychiatric disorders around the menopause should be treated as at other times of life.

Further reading

Gelder, M. G., Andreasen, N. C., Lopez-Ibor, J. J., & Geddes, J. R. (eds) (2009). *New Oxford Textbook of Psychiatry*, 2nd edn. Section 5: Psychiatry and medicine. Oxford University Press, Oxford.

The specific disorders

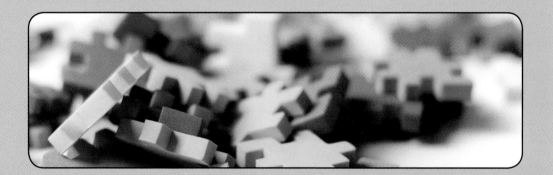

Mood disorders

Changes of mood are common in all psychiatric disorders and also frequently accompany physical illness. In mood disorders, the mood—either low mood or elation—is more intense and persistent than normal variation and leads to problems in occupational and social functioning. There may be associated symptoms, such as disturbances of thinking and sleeping.

■ Classification of mood disorders

As with all psychiatric disorders, classification is descriptive and based on clinical characteristics. The most useful current approach to classification is based on the clinical course. As well as classifying an illness as a single episode, recurrent, or persistent, there is an important distinction between people who only have depressed mood (unipolar) and those who also have elated mood. Episodes of illness are also classified according to severity—depressive episodes may be mild, moderate, or severe, and abnormally elated mood may be hypomanic or manic.

Mood disorders have also been classified according to presumed aetiology. Illnesses apparently caused by factors within the individual person such as genes were called **endogenous** and those apparently related to external stressors, **reactive**. In fact, mood disorders are probably multifactorial in aetiology, involving gene–environment interaction, and this is not a very clinically useful basis for classification. Nonetheless, in the individual case, it is always worth considering predisposing, precipitating, and maintaining factors as these may have implications for treatment and prognosis.

Depressive disorders may also be classified according to the nature and intensity of symptoms (neurotic and psychotic). In both depressive and manic illnesses, the presence of psychotic symptoms probably reflects the severity of the disorder, although they may be important for clinical management. The distribution of mood variation in the general population is probably continuous, producing a spectrum of severity (Figure 21.1).

For clinical purposes, diagnostic criteria are used to define specific mood disorders and episodes. The categories used for classification in ICD-10 and DSM-IV are broadly similar, although the terms are not quite the same (Table 21.1).

As well as classifying disorders by severity, it can be useful to subtype depression, for example disorders that have a seasonal pattern and those in which general medical conditions or substance dependence appear to be aetiological factors. The classification includes two categories for less severe and more chronic illnesses:

1 **dysthymia**, with chronic, constant, or fluctuating mild depressive symptoms;

2 **cyclothymia**, with chronic instability of mood with mild depressive and manic symptoms.

Table 21.1 The classification of affective disorders in ICD-10 and DSM-IV

ICD-10	DSM-IV
Manic episode	Manic episode
Depressive episode	Major depressive episode
Mild	
Moderate	
Severe	
Bipolar affective disorder	Bipolar disorders
Persistent mood (affective) states	
Cyclothymia	Cyclothymia
Dysthymia	Dysthymia

■ Unipolar depressive disorder

Epidemiology

The lifetime risk of depressive disorder is around 20% in both developed and developing countries and it is one of the most important causes of disability. It is more common in women than in men: the sex ratio is about 2 to 1. In the UK, it is common in patients attending primary care (up to 40% of attenders) and the general hospital.

Depressive disorders are more common in urban than rural populations and, in general, the prevalence is

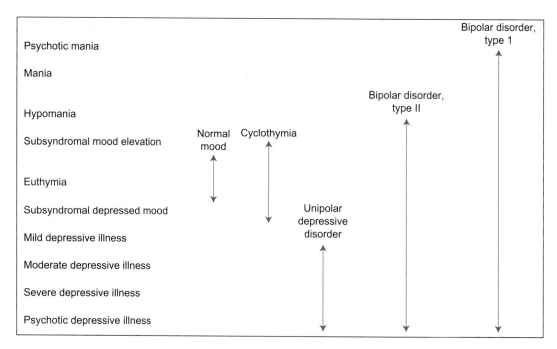

Fig. 21.1 Spectrum of mood disorders.

higher in groups with adverse socio-economic factors (for example in homeless people). The high prevalence means that depressive disorders are one of the most important causes of disability in all countries. Depressive disorders cause both direct costs to health services, and much greater indirect costs due to inability to work.

Depression may be undetected, especially when there are accompanying physical symptoms. Unrecognized depressive disorder may slow recovery and worsen prognosis in physical illness. It is important, therefore, that all clinicians should be able to recognize the condition, treat the less severe cases, and identify those requiring specialist care because of suicidal risk or for other reasons.

General clinical features

Pathological low mood is the central symptom of depressive disorder and needs to be distinguished from normal sadness commonly experienced by healthy people in response to misfortunes, especially loss, including grief. Low mood can be viewed as a spectrum from normal mood variability through to profound and severe depressive disorder (Figure 21.1). In depressive disorder, the low mood is persistent and is often accompanied by anxiety, loss of pleasure (**anhedonia**), lack of energy, general malaise, and poor sleep. As the low mood becomes more severe, the patient's ability to function in normal daily activities, for example employment or childcare, is increasingly impaired. Low mood may be hidden because the patient smiles and denies feeling miserable. Diagnosing depressive disorder therefore requires a careful search for the whole range of symptoms described below, especially anhedonia, sleep disturbance, diurnal mood variation, and a pessimistic view of the future. Diagnostic criteria for a depressive episode are shown below.

BOX 21.1 DSM-IV-TR diagnostic criteria for major depressive disorder

A Five (or more) of the following symptoms have been present during the same 2-week period and represent a change from previous functioning; at least one of the symptoms is either (1) depressed mood or (2) loss of interest or pleasure.

Note: do not include symptoms that are clearly due to a general medical condition, or mood-incongruent delusions or hallucinations.

1 Depressed mood most of the day, nearly every day, as indicated by either subjective report (e.g. feels sad or empty) or observation made by others (e.g. appears tearful). Note: in children and adolescents, can be irritable mood.

2 Markedly diminished interest in pleasure in all, or almost all, activities most of the day, nearly every day (as indicated by either subjective account or observation made by others).

3 Significant weight loss when not dieting or weight gain (e.g. a change of more than 5% body weight in a month), or decrease or increase in appetite nearly every day. Note: in children, consider failure to make expected weight gains.

4 Insomnia or hypersomnia nearly every day.

5 Psychomotor agitation or retardation nearly every day (observable by others, not merely subjective feelings of restlessness or being slowed down).

6 Fatigue or loss of energy nearly every day.

7 Feelings of worthlessness or excessive or inappropriate guilt (which may be delusional) nearly every day (not merely self-reproach or guilt about being sick).

8 Diminished ability to think or concentrate, or indecisiveness, nearly every day (either by subjective account or as observed by others).

9 Thoughts of death (not just a fear of dying), recurrent suicidal ideation without a specific plan, or a suicide attempt, or a specific plan for committing suicide.

B The symptoms do not meet criteria for a mixed episode.

C The symptoms cause clinically significant distress or impairment in social, occupational, or other important areas of functioning.

D The symptoms are not due to the direct physiological effects of a substance (e.g. a drug of abuse, a medication) or a general medical condition (e.g. hypothyroidism).

The symptoms are not better accounted for by bereavement, i.e. after the loss of a loved one, the symptoms persist for longer than 2 months or are characterized by marked functional impairment, morbid preoccupation with worthlessness, suicidal ideation, psychotic symptoms, or psychomotor retardation.

Q2

Table 21.2 Clinical characteristics of depressive disorder

Mild depressive disorder

- Low mood
- Seen by others as different to normal character and behaviour
- Lack of energy or enjoyment
- Anxiety symptoms
- Poor sleep
- Mood often worse in the evenings
- Pessimism, but not suicidal ideation

Moderately severe depressive disorder

Appearance

- Sad appearance
- Psychomotor retardation

Low mood

- Misery and unhappiness
- Diurnal variation—worse in morning
- Anxiety, irritability, agitation
- Lack of interest and enjoyment
- Reduced energy
- Poor concentration
- Subjective poor memory

Depressive thinking

- Pessimistic and guilty thoughts
- Ideas of personal failure
- Hopelessness
- Suicidal ideas
- Self-blame
- Hypochondriacal ideas

Biological symptoms

- Early wakening and other sleep disturbance
- Weight loss
- Reduced appetite
- Reduced sexual drive

Other symptoms

- Obsessional symptoms
- Depersonalization, etc.

Severe depressive disorder

Delusions of worthlessness

- Guilt
- Ill health
- Poverty
- Nihilism

Table 21.2 Clinical characteristics of depressive disorder (*Continued*)

- Persecution

Hallucinations

- Auditory
- Rarely visual

Within the range of depression that meets diagnostic criteria for depressive disorder there are, of course, varying degrees of severity. Depressive episodes can be divided into mild, moderate, or severe; the characteristic clinical features of these subtypes (although there is a large range of overlap) are shown in Table 21.2.

Minor depressive episode and disorders

In primary care, the most frequent presentation of mild depressive disorder is a mixture of anxiety and depression. This term covers a range of disorders in which the symptoms may not be sufficiently severe to meet diagnostic criteria for depressive disorder, but may still be disabling for the patient. Such conditions are common in general practice. Looked at in another way, minor mood disorders probably make up about two-thirds of the psychiatric disorders seen in general practice. The most frequent symptoms are:

- anxiety and worrying thoughts;
- sadness and depressive thoughts;
- irritability;
- poor concentration;
- insomnia;
- fatigue;
- somatic symptoms, including abdominal discomfort, indigestion, flatulence, and poor appetite, palpitations, precordial discomfort, and concerns about heart disease, headache, and pain in the neck, back, and shoulders;
- excessive concern about bodily function.

About half of patients with minor mood disorders improve within 3 months and a further quarter within 6 months. The rest persist as minor mood disorders, or become more severe so that they are diagnosed as anxiety disorders, depressive disorders, or somatoform syndromes (p. 306).

Moderate depressive disorder

In depressive disorders of moderate severity (Table 21.2), the central features are again low mood, lack of enjoyment, reduced energy, and pessimistic thinking but the functional impairment is likely to be more profound and the patient might find it difficult to work, for example.

Appearance

The patient's appearance is often characteristic. Psycho-motor retardation, which is a slowing of mental and motor activity, is frequent. There may be agitation, a feeling of rest-lessness, which may manifest itself as an inability to relax accompanied by restless activity. When agitation is severe the patient cannot sit for long and may pace up and down.

Mood

The patient is usually miserable. The low mood is usually experienced as having a different quality to ordinary sadness. There is diurnal variation of mood, which is characteristically worse in the morning than in the later part of the day (see biological symptoms, below).

Anxiety and irritability are frequent.

Lack of interest and loss of enjoyment (anhedonia) are frequent and important symptoms, though not always complained of spontaneously. Patients show no enthusi-asm for activities and hobbies that they would normally enjoy, and describe a loss of zest for living and for the pleasure from everyday things. They often withdraw from social encounters.

Reduced energy is characteristic (although when accompanied by physical restlessness it can be over-looked). The patient feels lethargic, finds everything an effort, and leaves tasks unfinished. For example, a nor-mally house-proud woman may leave beds unmade and dirty plates on the table. Understandably, many patients attribute this lack of energy to physical illness and seek help for this rather than for depression.

Poor concentration and complaints of poor memory are common. However, if the patient is encouraged to make a special effort, retention and recall can usually be shown to be normal. Sometimes, however, apparent impairment of memory is so severe that the clinical pres-entation resembles that of dementia. This presentation, which is particularly common in the elderly, is some-times called depressive pseudodementia (see p. 179).

Complaints about physical symptoms are common in depressive disorders. They take many forms, but com-plaints of constipation and of aching discomfort in any part of the body are particularly common. Complaints about any pre-existing physical disorders usually increase, and hypochondriacal preoccupations are common.

Depressive thinking

- **Pessimistic thinking ('depressive cognitions').** Low mood is associated with gloomy thoughts about the present, future, and the past.

- **Thoughts concerned with the present.** Patients see the unhappy side of every event, think that they are failing in everything they do and that other people see them as a failure, and they lose confidence and discount any success as a chance happening for which they can take no credit.

- **Thoughts concerned with the future.** Patients expect the worst. They may foresee failure in their work, the ruin of their finances, misfortune for their families, and an inevitable deterioration in their physical health. These ideas of hopelessness are often accompanied by the thought that life is no longer worth living and that death would come as a welcome release. These gloomy pre-occupations may progress to thoughts of, and plans for, suicide. It is important to ask about suicide in every case of depressive disorder. (The assessment of suicidal risk is considered further in Chapter 9.)

- **Thoughts concerned with the past.** These thoughts often take the form of unreasonable guilt and self-blame about minor matters; for example, patients may feel guilty about some trivial act of dishonesty in the past or about letting someone down. Usually, the patient has not thought about these events for years, but as the depres-sion developed they have flooded back into memory accompanied by intense feelings of guilt. Gloomy pre-occupations of this kind strongly suggest depressive disor-der. Some patients have similar feelings of guilt but do not attach them to any particular event. Other memories are focused on unhappy events; patients remember occasions when they were sad, when they failed, or when their for-tunes were at a low ebb. These gloomy memories become more frequent as the depression deepens.

Biological symptoms

This term is used to denote sleep disturbance, diurnal variation of mood, loss of appetite, loss of weight, consti-pation, loss of libido, and, in women, amenorrhoea. These symptoms are more common in severe depression than in cases of moderate severity (see below).

1 Sleep disturbance is of several kinds:

   (i) Early morning waking is the most characteristic form of sleep disturbance. The patient wakes 2 or 3 hours before their usual time. Patients do not fall asleep again, but lie awake feeling unrefreshed and often restless and agitated. They think about the coming day with pessimism, brood about past failures, and ponder gloomily about the more distant future. This combination of early waking with depressive think-ing is important in diagnosis.

   (ii) Delay in falling asleep, and waking during the night.

   (iii) Excessive sleep. The patient wakes late feeling unrefreshed.

2   Variation of appetite and weight. The characteristic pattern is for loss of appetite and weight loss, which often seems greater than can be explained by the loss of appetite alone. Instead of eating too little and losing weight, some patients eat more and gain weight. Sometimes they do this because eating brings them temporary relief from their distressing feelings. In other cases it is a side effect of medication.

3   Loss of libido with decreased interest in sex is common.

Other psychiatric symptoms

Many other symptoms may occur as part of a depressive disorder, including depersonalization, obsessional symptoms, phobias, and conversion symptoms such as fugue or loss of function of a limb (Chapter 1). Occasionally, one of these dominates the clinical picture and it is always important to consider the possibility of a depressive disorder.

Severe depressive disorder

As depressive disorders become more severe, all the features described under moderate depressive disorder occur with greater intensity (Table 21.2). There may also be additional symptoms not seen in moderate depressive disorder, namely delusions and hallucinations ('psychotic' symptoms; a disorder with these symptoms is called psychotic depression). The delusions of severe depressive disorders are concerned with the same themes as the non-delusional thinking of moderate depressive disorders, namely worthlessness, guilt, ill health, and, more rarely, poverty. When delusions with this kind of content occur in depressive disorder, they are termed mood-congruent. Such delusions have been described in Chapter 4, and include the following.

- A patient with a delusion of guilt may believe that some dishonest act, such as a minor concealment in making a tax return, will be discovered and that he will be punished severely and humiliated. He is likely to believe that such punishment is deserved.

- A patient with hypochondriacal delusions may be convinced that he has cancer or a sexually transmitted disease.

- A patient with a delusion of impoverishment may wrongly believe that he has lost all his money in a business venture.

- A patient with nihilistic delusions may believe that he has no future, or that some part of him has ceased to exist or function (e.g. that his bowels are wholly blocked—sometimes called **Cotard's syndrome**).

- A patient with persecutory delusions may believe that other people are discussing him in a derogatory way, or are about to take revenge on him. When persecutory delusions are part of a depressive syndrome, typically the patient accepts the supposed persecution as something he deserves.

Mood-incongruent delusions may also occur: when they do, the course of the illness may be more like schizophrenia.

Perceptual disturbances may also be found in severe depressive disorder. When hallucinations occur, these are usually auditory in the form of voices addressing repetitive words and phrases to the patient. The voices may seem to confirm their ideas of worthlessness (e.g. 'You are evil; you should die'), or to make derisive comments, or urge suicide. Visual hallucinations may also occur, sometimes in the form of scenes of death and destruction.

Suicidal ideas should be enquired about carefully in any patient with a severe depressive disorder. Rarely, there are homicidal ideas and when these occur, they may concern family members, including children. This possibility needs to be considered in the assessment of postnatal depressive disorder (see below).

Variants of moderate and severe depressive disorder

The clinical picture of severe depressive disorders is varied and several terms are sometimes used to describe common patterns.

- Agitated depression is a condition in which agitation is particularly severe. Agitated depression occurs more commonly among older patients.

- Retarded depression is a condition in which psychomotor retardation is prominent.

- Depressive stupor is a rare variant of severe depressive disorder in which retardation is so extreme that the patient is motionless, mute, and refuses to eat and drink. On recovering, patients can recall the events taking place at the time they were in stupor.

- Atypical depression is characterized by **reversed biological symptoms,** such as *increased* sleep, *increased* appetite, severe anxiety, and interpersonal sensitivity.

Mood disorder following childbirth

Following childbirth, women may experience several forms of mood disturbance.

Mild depression (baby blues) occurring in the first few days following childbirth. This is a normal phenomenon occurring in about 70 per cent of mothers and is self-limiting, usually disappearing within a few days. The main symptoms are irritability, lability of mood, muddled thinking, and tearfulness. Of these symptoms, lability of mood is particularly characteristic. All these symptoms reach their peak on the third or fourth postpartum day. Both the frequency of the emotional changes and their timing suggest that maternity 'blues' may be related to readjustment in hormones after delivery, but there is no direct evidence to support this idea.

Postnatal depressive disorder. Depressive disorder occurring in the first 3 months after childbirth occurs in about 10 per cent of mothers and the symptoms are similar to depressive disorder occurring at any other time although tiredness, irritability, and anxiety may be more prominent than depressive mood and there may be prominent phobic symptoms. Several factors are thought to be involved in the aetiology of postnatal depressive disorder, including history of psychiatric illness, experience of stressful events around pregnancy and childbirth, the psychological adjustments required after childbirth, loss of sleep, and fatigue secondary to caring for the baby. Some of these women have a history of psychiatric illness and some have experienced stressful events near the time of onset of the disorder. Depressive disorder can have a negative effect on bonding between mother and baby and this can delay the infant's development. Screening tests such as the Edinburgh Postnatal Depression Scale are often used.

Puerperal psychosis (see also Chapter 22). Puerperal psychosis usually begins in the first or second week after delivery and occurs in about 1 in 500 births. It is more frequent among primiparous women, those who have suffered previous serious major psychiatric disorder, and those with a family history of psychiatric disorder. Delirium used to be common before antibiotics were introduced to treat puerperal sepsis. Nowadays, the usual clinical picture is of a severe psychotic mood disorder or schizoaffective disorder although varying levels of confusion and disorientation lend an organic 'flavour' to the clinical picture.

Seasonal affective disorder (SAD)

Some people repeatedly develop a depressive disorder at the same time of year. In some cases, this timing reflects extra demands on the person at a particular time of year; in other cases there is no such extra demand, and it has been suggested that the cause is related to changes in the season, for example in the length of daylight. Although these affective disorders are characterized mainly by the season in which they occur, they are also said to be characterized by some symptoms that are less common in other affective disorders, for example hypersomnia and increased appetite with cravings for carbohydrates.

The most common pattern is onset in the autumn or winter, and recovery in the spring or summer. This pattern has led to the suggestion that shortening of daylight is important. Some patients improve after exposure to artificial light, given usually in the early morning. It is uncertain for which patients the treatment is effective, or how lasting are its effects.

Differential diagnosis

Depressive disorders should be distinguished from:

- **Normal sadness.** As explained on p. 223, the distinction from normal sadness depends on the presence of other symptoms of the syndrome of depressive disorder.

- **Grief.** Although depressive disorder resembles uncomplicated grief in many ways, severe pessimism, suicidal thoughts, profound guilt, and psychotic symptoms are all rare in grief. Severe symptoms persisting more than 2 months after bereavement suggest a depressive disorder.

- **Bipolar disorder.** It is important always to enquire about a history of elevated mood because this will indicate bipolar, rather than unipolar, disorder and the treatment is different. In particular, antidepressant medicines must be used cautiously in bipolar disorder because of the risk of inducing mood instability or mania.

- **Anxiety disorder.** Mild depressive disorders are sometimes difficult to distinguish from anxiety disorders. Accurate diagnosis depends on assessment of the relative severity of anxiety and depressive symptoms, and on the order in which they appeared. Similar problems arise when there are prominent phobic or obsessional symptoms. (These points are discussed further in Chapter 24).

- **Functional physical symptoms.** (See p. 306.) It is not uncommon for depressive disorder to present with concern about non-specific and medically unexplained physical symptoms, without a direct complaint of the psychological symptoms. Careful enquiry will elicit these additional symptoms.

- **Schizophrenia.** The differential diagnosis of depressive disorder from schizophrenia depends on a careful search for the characteristic features of schizophrenia (see Chapter 22). Diagnosis may be difficult when a patient has both depressive symptoms and persecutory delusions, but the distinction can usually be made by examining the mental state carefully and by establishing whether the delusions followed, and are consistent with, the depressive symptoms (mood-congruent—depressive disorder) or the delusions came first or are not congruent with the mood disorder (schizophrenia). For example, in depressive disorder, persecution is usually accepted as the deserved consequence of the patient's own failings; in schizophrenia it is strongly rejected. Some patients have symptoms of both depressive disorder and schizophrenia; these schizoaffective disorders are discussed in Chapter 22. A depressive syndrome may also occur following treatment of the psychotic symptoms of schizophrenia. It is called post-psychotic depression.

- **Dementia.** In middle and late life, depressive disorders may be difficult to distinguish from dementia because some patients with depressive disorder complain of considerable difficulty in remembering, and some demented patients are depressed. In depressive disorders, difficulty in remembering occurs because poor concentration leads to inadequate registration. The distinction between the two conditions can often be made by careful memory testing; standard psychological tests are required in doubtful cases, but even these may not decide the issue. If memory disorder does not improve with recovery of normal mood, dementia is probable.

- **Substance abuse.** Depressive symptoms are common in substance abuse, and some patients with depressive disorder abuse alcohol or non-prescribed drugs to relieve their distress. The sequence of the depressive symptoms and substance abuse should be determined, as well as the presence of the features of depressive disorder other than low mood.

Aetiology of depressive disorders

In broad terms, mood disorders are caused by an interaction between (i) stressful events and (ii) constitutional factors resulting from genetic endowment and childhood experience. These aetiological factors act through biochemical and psychological processes, which have been partly identified by research. More is known about the aetiology of depressive than of manic disorders. For this reason, and because it illustrates the multifactorial approach to aetiology in psychiatry, here we focus on depressive disorders.

Genetic causes

Genetic factors have been studied mainly in moderate to severe cases of mood disorder, rather than in milder cases. Parents, siblings, and children of severely depressed patients have a higher lifetime risk for mood disorder (10–15%) than the general population (1–2%). Twin studies indicate that these high rates among families are due to genetic factors. Thus the concordance of bipolar disorder is the same (about 70%) among monozygotic twins reared together and monozygotic twins reared apart, and higher than the concordance between dizygotic twins (23%). Studies of adopted children confirm the importance of genetic causes of depressive disorder because the risk of

developing the disorder is higher in a child who was born to a parent with a history of serious depressive disorder but raised by adoptive parents with no such history, than in a child who was born to parents with no history of serious depressive disorder. Although the circumstantial evidence for genetic factors is therefore strong, no single gene, or combination of genes, causing depression has yet been consistently identified. The intriguing possibility of an interaction between a polymorphism in the serotonin transporter gene and the environment has been raised but awaits confirmation (see Science box 21.1).

Personality

It has been suggested that genetic factors might predispose to affective disorder through an effect on personality, or alternatively that variations in personality (e.g. cyclothymic personality, p. 422) reflect the same genetic factors that cause illness. Unipolar depressive disorders have not been found to be associated with a single personality type.

Predisposing environmental factors

Depressive disorders often seem to begin after prolonged adversity, such as difficulties in marriage or at work. These adverse circumstances seem to prepare the ground for a final acute stressor, which precipitates the disorder. For example, there is evidence that having the care of several young children, poor economic circumstances, and an unsupportive marriage increase vulnerability to depression.

Looked at another way, certain factors protect against the action of stressors and people who lack them are more vulnerable. Thus, some women appear to be more vulnerable to depressive disorder when they have nobody in whom they can confide. Clearly, there is some overlap between the concepts of vulnerability and protective factors.

Precipitating environmental factors

Clinically, depressive disorders often seem to follow stressful life events. This association is not necessarily causal; instead it might be coincidental or the stressful event itself might be a consequence of the early, but unrecognized, stages of the illness (e.g. losing a job because of deteriorating performance) rather than a cause in its own right (e.g. losing a job when a whole factory closes). Epidemiological research has shown that there is an excess of life events independent of the illness in the week preceding a depressive disorder, but this association is non-specific since life events also occur in excess in the weeks before the onset of schizophrenia, and before acts of deliberate self-harm. The effect is substantial; the risk of developing a depressive disorder is increased about sixfold in the 6 months after experiencing moderately severe life events (the

Science box 21.1 The serotonin transporter gene, gene–environment interaction, and depression

Despite strong evidence from family and twin studies for an important genetic predisposition to many mental disorders, the identification of specific genes has been slow and frustrating. Finally, some genes are being identified but these tend to be of small effect and not specific—in other words, the same genes seem to predispose to several disorders. It looks as if the cause of most mental disorders will be multiple genes and environmental factors acting together.

A report of a study published in *Science* in 2003 (Caspi *et al.* 2003) attracted a great deal of interest. In this study, people with a serotonin transporter gene (5-HTT) promoter polymorphism exhibited more depressive symptoms than people without the polymorphism when they had experienced stressful life events. These findings suggested that there is an *interaction* between having the gene and experiencing stressful life events—the risk of developing a depressive disorder following a stressful life event is *much* higher in people with the polymorphism, rather than simply being the additive effect of two risk factors.

This would be an example of **gene–environment interaction** and, should it be confirmed, could be very important because a gene of small overall effect may prove to

have a more substantial effect in the presence of a specific environmental risk factor. This could provide important clues to the neurobiology of mental disorders, and Caspi *et al.* became the most highly cited paper of the decade in the field of mood disorders.[1]

In 2009, however, a meta-analysis (Risch *et al.* 2009) found evidence for an increased risk of depression in people with stressful life events but no association with the 5-HTT polymorphism and, crucially, no evidence of an interaction.[2]

So what should we conclude? First, the possibility of an interaction with the 5-HTT polymorphism remains unconfirmed. Second, it is certainly possible to get a little carried away when a new, exciting finding is reported, and, lastly, systematic review and meta-analysis is one of the most sobering research methods we have!

1 Caspi, A., Sugden, K., Moffitt, T. E., *et al.* (2003). Influence of life stress on depression: moderation by a polymorphism in the 5-HTT gene. *Science* **301**: 386–9.

2 Risch, N., Herrell, R., Lehner, T., *et al.* (2009). Interaction between the serotonin transporter gene (5-HTTLPR), stressful life events, and risk of depression: a meta-analysis. *JAMA* **301**: 2462–71.

corresponding figure for schizophrenia is about threefold). Loss events, such as bereavement, are particularly likely to lead to depressive disorder.

Physical conditions as predisposing or precipitating factors

Most physical conditions are non-specific stressors but a few appear to precipitate depressive disorder by direct biological mechanisms. They include influenza and some other viral infections, childbirth (see p. 226), and Parkinson's disease.

Mediating processes

Two kinds of complementary mediating processes have been studied: psychological and biochemical.

Psychological mediating processes. Depressed patients may process information in a way that causes and then prolongs the initial change of mood (cognitive biases). Several abnormalities have been proposed.

1 Abnormalities of emotional processing; for example, people who are susceptible to depression may be more likely to interpret facial expression as negative.

2 Tendency to remember unhappy events more easily than happy ones.

3 Unrealistic beliefs; for example, 'I cannot be happy unless I am liked by everyone I know'.

4 Cognitive distortions in drawing a general conclusion from a single event; for example, 'I have failed in this relationship, so I will never be loved by anyone'. These illogical ways of thinking allow the intrusive gloomy thoughts and the unrealistic expectations to persist despite evidence to the contrary.

Biochemical mediating processes. There is increasing evidence of biochemical abnormalities, at least in the more severe depressive disorders, but their nature is uncertain. Also, it is not known whether there is a single abnormality present in every patient with depressive disorder, or different abnormalities leading to the same clinical picture. The strongest evidence is for an abnormality of 5-HT (serotonin) function. There are three main strands of evidence.

1 Concentrations of the main 5-HT metabolite (5-HIAA) are reduced in the cerebrospinal fluid (CSF) of patients with severe depressive disorders. This is very indirect evidence since concentrations of 5-HT in the brain could be very different from those in CSF.

2 5-HT concentrations are reduced in the brains of depressed patients who have died by suicide. This reduction could,

however, be caused by drugs used to commit suicide or by post-mortem changes.

3 Neuroendocrine functions that involve 5-HT transmission are reduced in depressed patients. However, the finding of an abnormality in neurons controlling endocrine function is not necessarily evidence for the same abnormality in neurons controlling mood.

4 Tryptophan (amino acid precursor of 5-HT) depletion via diet can lead to increased depressive mood in people who have recovered.

If low 5-HT function is important in causing depressive disorder, then increasing this function should be therapeutic and this is a common effect of most antidepressant drugs.

Noradrenergic (NA) function also seems to be reduced in depressive disorders, and antidepressant agents that affect both 5-HT and NA may be moderately more effective than agents that work on one neurotransmitter.

Endocrine abnormalities

A causal role for endocrine abnormalities is suggested by the association of mood disorder with Cushing's syndrome, Addison's disease, and hyperparathyroidism (Cushing's syndrome is sometimes associated with elation rather than depression of mood). It has also been suggested that depressive disorders occurring after childbirth or at the menopause are related to endocrine changes at these times, but there is no strong evidence for this.

Plasma cortisol is increased in about half of patients with depressive disorder. However, this increase in cortisol is not specific to depressive disorder; it occurs also in mania and schizophrenia. The change does not seem to be just a reaction to the stress of being ill, for it involves a change in the diurnal pattern of secretion of cortisol (being high in the afternoon and early evening after which time it normally decreases), a change not seen after exposure to stressors. It has been suggested that the elevation of cortisol may arise after a prolonged life stress and may predispose to depression by interfering with brain 5-HT function.

Course and prognosis of depressive disorders

Unipolar depressive disorders may start at any time from childhood to late life, the most common age of onset being in the late twenties. Untreated illnesses last 6 months or more, with a significant minority lasting for years. With treatment, each episode lasts 2 to 3 months on average. Most patients eventually recover from the episode, although recurrences are common. At least half of those who have a single episode followed by complete recovery will eventually have another episode.

Suicide is substantially more frequent among patients with affective disorder than among the general population. Among patients with severe depressive disorder about 1 in 10 eventually commit suicide.

Management of depressive disorders

Most patients with depressive disorders are treated in primary care. However, not all those needing treatment are recognized. This is partly due to a lack of understanding of the recognition and treatment of the condition.

Detection of depressive disorders

It is important that all doctors remain aware of the high prevalence of depression in all settings. The detection of depression can be improved if the doctor always remembers to ask two simple screening questions:

1 During the last month, have you often been bothered by feeling down, depressed, or hopeless?

2 During the last month, have you often been bothered by little interest or pleasure in doing things?

Doctors with good interviewing skills are also more likely to detect depression and also to lead to better outcomes, possibly because good interviewing provides non-specific benefits as well as leading to improved diagnosis and the provision of effective treatment.

Assessment

A patient who is suspected of having a depressive disorder needs a comprehensive assessment, which includes a consideration of medical, psychological, and social needs and an assessment of the risk (Table 21.3).

Diagnosis depends on thorough history taking and examination of the physical and mental state. Differential diagnosis has been discussed earlier in this chapter (p. 227). Particular care should be taken:

- not to overlook a depressive disorder in a patient who complains of the physical symptoms of depression such as fatigue or poor sleep rather than depressed mood ('masked depression');

- not to diagnose a depressive disorder simply on the grounds of prominent depressive symptoms; the latter could be part of another disorder, for example an organic psychiatric syndrome caused by cerebral neoplasm;

- to remember that certain drugs can induce depression (see p. 209);

- to determine if the patient has suffered from a previous episode of mania, in which case the diagnosis would be bipolar depression and the treatment would be as described below (p. 243).

Table 21.3 Assessment of depressive disorder

Diagnosis

- History
- Mental state
- Relevant physical examination
- Relevant physical investigation
- Informants' accounts

Severity

- Biological symptoms
- Psychotic symptoms
- Suicide risk, risk to others
- Effect on social functioning

Aetiology

- Psychological
- Social
- Physical illness
- Drug therapy
- Constitutional

Social consequences

- Patient's everyday life
- Partner and family
- Dangers at work

Social resources

- Family support
- Housing
- Work

Severity. The severity of the disorder is judged from the symptoms, behaviour, and level of functional impairment. Whenever possible, an informant should be interviewed as well as the patient. The risk of suicide must be assessed in every case (the methods of assessment are described in Chapter 9). It is also important to assess how far the depressive disorder has reduced the patient's capacity to work or to engage in family life and social activities. In this assessment, the duration and course of the condition should be taken into account as well as the severity of the present symptoms and disability. The length of history not only affects prognosis, it also gives an indication of the patient's capacity to tolerate further distress. A long-continued disorder, even if not severe, can bring the patient to the point of desperation.

Aetiological factors. Possible aetiological factors may include both known medical and psychiatric causes and precipitating, predisposing, maintaining, and pathoplastic factors. Precipitating causes may be psychological and social

(the 'life events' discussed earlier in the chapter) or they may be physical illness or its treatment. In assessing such causes, enquiries should be made into the patient's work, finances, family life, social activities, general living conditions, and physical health. Problems in these areas may be recent and acute, or chronic background difficulties such as prolonged marital tension, problems with children, and financial hardship. In planning treatment, maintaining factors are usually of most relevance.

Social consequences. The impact on the patient's everyday life should be considered by asking about ability to work, effects on leisure interests, and particularly consequences for family life. Such information is not only an indication of the severity of the disorder, but may bring up issues that require advice and discussion with the patient and family.

The effect of the disorder on other people should be considered. It is important to consider whether the patient could endanger other people by remaining at work (e.g. as a bus driver). Effects on the family are important, especially on young children. A severely depressed mother may, for example, neglect her children. Danger may also arise when there are depressive delusions that could lead to action. Severely depressed mothers may sometimes kill their children because of the belief that they are doomed to suffer if they remain alive. Severely depressed patients occasionally kill their partner. In the longer term, depressive disorder in either parent is associated with the development of emotional disorder in the children.

Social resources. The patient's social resources are considered next. Enquiries should cover family, friends, and work. Supportive families and friends can help patients through periods of depressive disorder by providing company, encouraging them when confidence is lost, and guiding them into suitable activities. For some patients, work is a valuable social resource, providing distraction and comradeship. For others it is a source of stress. A careful assessment is needed in each case.

Treatment of the acute phase of depression

Treatment of depressive disorder can be divided into three main stages:

1 an acute phase to relieve symptoms of depression and achieve recovery;

2 continuation therapy to preserve the improvement;

3 a maintenance phase to protect vulnerable patients from further episodes (see also Figure 21.2).

There are several effective treatments for depressive disorders and the choice of treatment for each individual patient will depend on several factors, including the

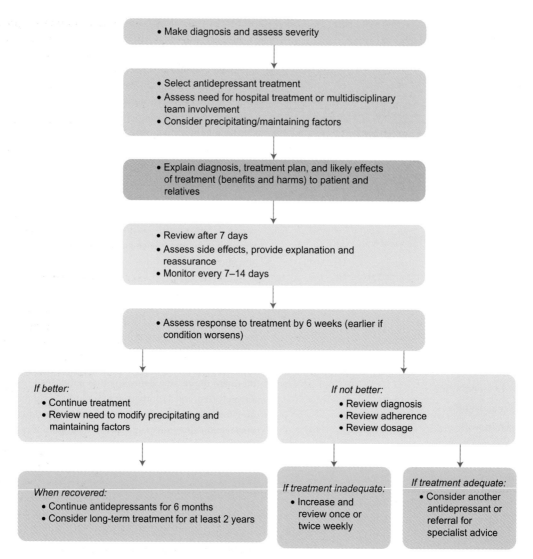

• Make diagnosis and assess severity

• Select antidepressant treatment
• Assess need for hospital treatment or multidisciplinary team involvement
• Consider precipitating/maintaining factors

• Explain diagnosis, treatment plan, and likely effects of treatment (benefits and harms) to patient and relatives

• Review after 7 days
• Assess side effects, provide explanation and reassurance
• Monitor every 7–14 days

• Assess response to treatment by 6 weeks (earlier if condition worsens)

If better:
• Continue treatment
• Review need to modify precipitating and maintaining factors

If not better:
• Review diagnosis
• Review adherence
• Review dosage

When recovered:
• Continue antidepressants for 6 months
• Consider long-term treatment for at least 2 years

If treatment inadequate:
• Increase and review once or twice weekly

If treatment adequate:
• Consider another antidepressant or referral for specialist advice

Fig. 21.2 Treatment of depressive disorders.

severity of the disorder, the patient's own preferences, and the availability of the treatments.

General aspects of the treatment of the acute phase

As well as the specific treatments outlined above, non-specific and supportive measures are very important. The patient may have an unclear view of the nature of depressive disorder and its treatment. The doctor should therefore provide a clear outline of the nature of the disorder and the available treatments, including both likely benefits and possible adverse effects, should discuss the patient's preferences, and agree a treatment plan. Active follow-up with early identification of any problems leads to better adherence to the prescribed therapy and improved outcomes. During the initial weeks of treatment, patients should be seen and supported; those with severe disorders may need to be seen

every 2 or 3 days, others usually weekly. The possibility of the emergence of a manic episode should be kept in mind when depression is being treated, because the first manic episode follows treatment for a depressive disorder in some patients with bipolar disorder.

It is important to advise the patient that there are a number of things that they can do themselves to promote recovery from depression:

Activity. The level of activity should be considered for every patient. Depressed patients give up activities and withdraw from other people. In this way, they become deprived of social stimulation and rewarding experiences, and their original feelings of depression increase. It is important to make sure that patients are occupied adequately, but also that they are not pushed into activities in which they may fail because of slowness or poor concentration. Hence, the range of activity appropriate for a depressed patient is narrow and changes as the illness runs its course. If the patient is treated at home, it may be helpful to discuss with relatives how much the patient should do each day.

Diet. Appetite may be diminished in depression and the patient should be encouraged to eat regularly and healthily.

Sleep. Simple advice should be given on how to deal with any insomnia that accompanies the depression (see p. 361).

It can be helpful to involve the patient's relatives in the treatment plan. In particular, they should be helped to understand the disorder as an illness, to avoid criticizing the patient, and to encourage appropriate activity.

Psychological help. Even when not being treated with a specific psychological treatment, all depressed patients require support, encouragement, and repeated explanation that they are suffering from illness, not moral failure. When the depressive disorder appears to have been precipitated by life problems, discussion and problem-solving counselling may be required. However, when the depressive disorder is severe, discussion of problems may increase hopelessness. The more depressed the patient, the more the doctor and others should take over problems in the early days of treatment. When mood improves, the problems can be reconsidered.

Specific treatments for depressive disorder

Antidepressant drug treatment

Antidepressant drugs remain the most widely available, effective treatments for depressive disorder and are prescribed widely in both primary and secondary care. They are not without adverse effects and so their use should generally be restricted to patients with at least a moderate level of symptom severity in whom depressive symptoms are causing impaired functioning.

There are five main groups of antidepressant drugs (see p. 119).

1 Specific serotonin reuptake inhibitors (SSRIs). SSRIs (including fluoxetine, paroxetine, sertraline, citalopram, and escitalopram) have specific 5-HT uptake blocking effects (see p. 119) and have been shown to be effective in randomized trials. SSRIs are generally well tolerated although they may cause nausea, agitation, insomnia, and sexual dysfunction. They are relatively safe in overdose. While there does not seem to be evidence of large differences in efficacy between SSRIs, small differences do exist and sertraline and escitalopram appear to have good profiles of efficacy and safety.

2 Selective serotonin and noradrenaline reuptake inhibitors (SNRIs) include venlafaxine and duloxetine. These drugs block both 5-HT and NA reuptake and there is evidence that venlafaxine is more effective than some SSRIs but also more likely to cause adverse effects.

3 Tricyclic antidepressants. Tricyclic antidepressant drugs (e.g. imipramine, amitriptyline) were the first group of effective antidepressants and were the standard therapy for many years (see p. 120). These drugs are slightly more effective in severe depressive disorders than SSRIs, but less well tolerated. The side effects and hazards of the tricyclic antidepressants are described on p. 120. The anticholinergic side effects are a frequent reason why patients stop taking these drugs. The main hazards are in patients who have heart disease, glaucoma, prostatic hypertrophy, or epilepsy.

4 Monoamine oxidase inhibitors (MAOIs). MAOIs (e.g. phenelzine, tranylcypromine, moclobemide) are generally less effective than tricyclics for severe depressive disorders, but some patients with less severe disorders with atypical features (p. 226) respond better to MAOIs than other drugs. MAOIs potentiate the effects of naturally occurring pressor amines including tyramine, found in some common foods (see p. 121), and of synthetic amines used as decongestants and vasoconstrictors (see p. 121), and these interactions can cause dangerous increases in blood pressure. Although these reactions can be avoided by careful choice of diet and by avoiding prescription of synthetic amines, it is better not to use MAOIs as the first treatment, but to reserve them for patients who have not improved with adequate dosage of an SSRI or a tricyclic drug. The reversible MAOI, moclobemide, is less likely to cause a tyramine reaction than the conventional MAOI drugs.

5 Other antidepressants. There are many other antidepressants (see also Chapter 13). Some are useful in treating patients resistant to standard drug therapy. They are not discussed here because specialist psychiatric advice should generally be sought before prescribing them.

Combined drug regimens

Combined treatment may be useful when patients have not responded to monotherapy, although there is limited evidence on their efficacy. Combinations of drugs are more likely to lead to interactions and adverse effects and should generally be initiated by a specialist, used cautiously, and monitored carefully.

The most commonly recommended combination treatment is lithium plus antidepressant, which is effective in some patients who have not responded to the antidepressant alone. Combinations of tricyclics and MAOIs and tricyclics and an SSRI may be effective in some patients unresponsive to either drug given separately.

Electroconvulsive therapy (ECT)

ECT is described more comprehensively on p. 127. The antidepressant action of ECT is quicker than that of antidepressant drugs, but it causes more adverse effects, especially impairment of short-term memory. For these reasons, ECT is mainly used to treat severe depressive illness when:

1 the depressive disorder has not responded to adequate antidepressant drug treatment; *or*

2 rapid response is necessary because of high suicidal risk or severe psychomotor retardation.

ECT is probably most effective in severe depressive disorders with delusions and/or psychomotor retardation.

Psychological treatment

Supportive and problem-solving treatments. All depressed patients and their families need supportive care to sustain them until improvement takes place. Persistent interpersonal problems maintain depression, and problem solving can resolve the difficulties. The least severe illnesses can usually be treated by problem solving and psychological and social support; more severe depressive disorders are usually treated with drug treatment with psychological and social support (though a few receive cognitive therapy—see below).

Dynamic psychotherapy. Although depressed patients often express guilt and regrets about experiences in their recent or remote past, these feelings generally resolve as mood improves and there is no evidence that dynamic psychotherapy speeds this process. Indeed, it is generally better not to dwell on past events in the early stages of treatment, as this may only increase the patient's guilty introspection.

Cognitive therapy (see p. 137) is as effective as antidepressant drugs in the treatment of moderate depressive disorders and may also prevent relapse. Cognitive therapy is increasingly available, particularly via telephone and Internet versions, and many patients prefer a psychological approach. Cognitive therapy may be useful for helping residual depressive symptoms that remain after antidepressant treatment, and there is evidence that the combination of drugs plus cognitive therapy is more effective than monotherapy.

Interpersonal psychotherapy is a standardized form of brief psychotherapy that focuses on improving the patient's interpersonal functioning and identifying the problems associated with the onset of the depressive episode.

Tailoring the treatment according to the severity of the disorder

The appropriate treatment for a person with depressive disorder depends on the severity of the disorder. All treatments have adverse effects and financial costs as well as benefits and so it is important to make sure that the likely benefits are worth the costs. There is little point in providing an intensive and expensive psychotherapy, or a drug with a high frequency of adverse effects, to a patient with a mild disorder which is likely to resolve spontaneously and quickly. On the other hand, a patient with a severe disorder may need early, intensive drug treatment, or inpatient care, and is likely to need urgent referral to the specialist mental health services.

Mild depressive disorders

Mild depressive disorders seldom require treatment with antidepressant drugs or an intensive psychological treatment, especially when they are clearly reactions to stressful life events that have resolved. Patients should receive a clear explanation of the problem and their part in overcoming it, and be encouraged to talk about their feelings and discuss their problems. The patient should be encouraged to eat well, take exercise, and try to get sufficient sleep. Such help is particularly important after bereavement or other kinds of loss (see p. 281). Self-help reading materials may also be helpful.

A hypnotic drug may be given for a few days to restore sleep, but such treatment should not be prolonged. If the depressive symptoms do not respond quickly to social and psychological measures, and if sleep problems persist, sedative antidepressants should be prescribed to be taken at night.

Should the patient remain at work? When the disorder is mild, work can be a valuable distraction from depressive thoughts, and can provide companionship.

Moderately severe and severe depressive disorder

All except mild depressive disorders should be treated with antidepressant drugs or with specific psychological treatments. The decision about which treatment to try first should be made jointly by the doctor and patient and will depend on the severity of the symptoms, the patient's preferences, and the availability of the treatments.

Is antidepressant drug treatment required? Antidepressant drugs are effective for most patients with a depressive disorder of at least moderate severity, and particularly those with 'biological' symptoms. A history of previous response to medication and severe symptoms both suggest a good response to treatment. No single antidepressant is clearly more effective than another, and the choice for a particular patient depends on:

• response to any previous antidepressant medication;

• adverse effects;

• concurrent medical illnesses;

• concurrent medication;

- toxicity in overdose;

- cost.

Doctors should become familiar with the use of one or two drugs from each group.

Is psychiatric referral appropriate? Moderately severe depression is usually treated by non-specialists, for example, general practitioners. However, it is essential to consider in every case whether psychiatric referral is required (Table 21.4) and, if so, whether the referral should be for outpatient treatment, or whether immediate inpatient or day-patient care is required (see below).

Should the patient remain at work? When the disorder is more severe, retardation, poor concentration, and lack of drive are likely to impair performance, and this failure may add to feelings of hopelessness. Sometimes, poor performance at work may endanger other people, and when the potential for such danger is great (as in the case of driving a heavy goods vehicle) the patient should not work even if the risk of failure is small.

What information do the patient and family need about medication? It is essential that the drugs are taken in the full prescribed dose. A depressed patient's adherence to antidepressant treatment can be improved by informing the patient and the family about the nature of the medication, its potential benefits and side effects, any possible toxic effects, and the importance of continuing a full dosage for an adequate period of time. It is important to explain that

although side effects will appear quickly, the therapeutic effect is likely to be delayed for 2 to 3 weeks. Patients should be warned about the sedative effects of taking alcohol. They should be advised about driving, particularly that they should not drive while experiencing sedative or any other side effects that might impair their performance.

Failure to respond to treatment

Around 30% of patients with a depressive disorder do not respond within 6 weeks to a combination of antidepressant drugs, graded activity, and psychological treatment. In these cases the treatment plan should be reviewed at 6 weeks, and earlier in severe cases (Table 21.5).

- **Is the diagnosis correct?** The diagnosis should be reviewed carefully.

- **Have stressors been overlooked?** A check should be made for stressful life events or continuing difficulties that may have been overlooked (Table 21.5).

- **Is the patient taking the full prescribed dose of medicine?** Check again that the patient has been taking the medication in the full amount. If not, the reasons should be sought. Some patients are convinced that no treatment can help, while others are unable to tolerate drug side effects.

- **Should the dose be increased?** If the preceding enquiries reveal nothing, the dose of antidepressant may be increased if it is not already maximal.

- **Should the medication be changed?** If the patient cannot tolerate the drug, or there has been no response to the maximum tolerated dosage, an antidepressant drug from another group may be tried.

- **Frequent supportive interviews** should be continued with monitoring of severity, and the patient reassured that depressive disorders almost invariably eventually recover. Meanwhile, provided that the patient is not too depressed,

Table 21.4 Referral for specialist advice

- In all severe and some moderately severe cases, especially when there is a substantial risk of suicide or harm to the welfare or life of another person (particularly dependent children)
- When the diagnosis is in doubt
- When a patient has failed to respond to antidepressant treatment
- When day or inpatient care is required
- When cognitive behaviour therapy (CBT) may be required

Is hospital care needed?

In deciding the need for inpatient or day-patient care, consideration is given to:

- Severity and risk to the self and to others, especially to any dependent children
- The patient's ability to look after him- or herself
- The availability of social support. (A patient living alone may need hospital care for a disorder that could be treated at home if there was a supportive family member who could be present day and night)

Table 21.5 Lack of response to antidepressant treatment

- Review diagnosis
- Check compliance with present treatment
- Review psychological and social causes
- Increase dose to maximum
- Consider change to antidepressant of a different group*
- Obtain specialist opinion concerning need for hospital admission and further treatment*
- Combined drug treatment*
- Consider ECT*

* These steps usually require a specialist opinion (see text).

any problems contributing to the depressed state should be discussed further.

- **Is a specialist opinion required?** If serious depression persists, specialist advice should be obtained concerning the need for combined antidepressant drug treatment, day care or admission to hospital, or, in the most severe cases, ECT.

Continuing failure to respond

Disorders that do not fully respond to at least two adequate courses of antidepressant medicine are called treatment resistant. In these cases, it is usually worth trying alternative treatments. For example, cognitive therapy may be effective in patients with residual symptoms of depression following antidepressant treatment. For most patients, however, the next step is combination therapy. The best established combinations are:

- Lithium augmentation of an antidepressant drug. Particular care is required if lithium is added to a 5-HT uptake blocker since this produces neurotoxic side effects in a few cases.

- Thyroid hormone augmentation of antidepressant drug, usually with tri-iodothyronine, although the evidence on this is limited.

- MAOI augmentation of a tricyclic drug. The reverse procedure of adding a tricyclic drug to MAOI should not be used because it is more likely to cause serious toxic effects.

Specialist advice should be sought before using any of these drug combinations.

ECT should also be considered in the treatment of patients with depressive disorders that do not respond to drugs.

Continuation therapy

The continuation phase of treatment focuses on maintaining the improvement during the first 6 months or so following the successful treatment of the acute phase. After recovery from a depressive disorder the patient should be followed up for several months, either by the family doctor or by a psychiatrist. At this stage it is often valuable to discuss possible precipitants of the illness with the patient and also in joint interviews with close relatives. This discussion is particularly important when there have been repeated depressive disorders provoked by life events.

Some residual symptoms may take several months to disappear and many patients are particularly vulnerable to relapse during this period. With antidepressant medicines, the same dose of the successful treatment should be continued during the continuation phase. Patients will need encouragement to continue with treatment and deal with any adverse effects, and advice about the appropriate level of activity and about returning to work.

Prevention of relapse

Maintenance medication. Patients who have responded to acute-phase treatment, remained well during the continuation phase, and are at moderate or high risk of relapse (for example, those with a history of relapse relatively soon after successful treatment of depression, or on the ending of continuation therapy) will benefit from long-term therapy for at least 2 years with antidepressants at the same dose that was effective in the acute phase. Long-term drug treatment will halve the risk of relapse.

Cognitive therapy (see p. 137) may also reduce the relapse rate after a moderately severe depressive disorder but there is less evidence than for drug maintenance. Cognitive therapy is sometimes tried for patients who have repeated episodes of depression despite maintenance medication, and apparently related to depressive forms of thinking.

Life changes. If the depressive disorder was clearly related to stressors such as overwork or complicated social relationships, the patient should be helped to change his lifestyle in the hope that this will reduce recurrence.

Recognizing early signs of relapse. It can also be helpful to have a written, agreed care plan should depressive symptoms recur. The patient should be fully involved in this process by being helped to understand the risk of relapse, taught to recognize warning signs, and by agreeing on an appropriate action plan. When appropriate, the patient's relatives should be involved.

Management of mood disorders following childbirth
Baby blues

The patient and her partner should be reassured that the condition is common and short-lived. No other treatment is needed.

Postnatal depressive disorder

Postnatal depression is assessed in the same way as other depressive disorders, with attention to any ideas that suggest a risk to the child (see p. 166). The Edinburgh Postnatal Depression Scale (Box 21.2) can aid assessment and suggest topics to be explored further in the interview. If there is doubt about the risk to the child, or when the risk is judged to exist, a specialist opinion should be obtained. Patients need a clear explanation of the nature of the condition and the plan of treatment, together with support from the medical team and if possible from the extended family. The general practitioner should liaise with the midwife, health

BOX 21.2 Edinburgh Postnatal Depression Scale (EPDS)

The EPDS was developed for screening postpartum women in outpatient or home-visiting settings, or at the 6–8 week postpartum examination. It has been utilized among numerous populations, including US women and Spanish-speaking women in other countries. The EPDS consists of 10 questions, and can usually be completed in less than 5 minutes. Responses are scored 0, 1, 2, or 3 according to increased severity of the symptom. Items marked with an asterisk (*) are reverse scored (i.e. 3, 2, 1, or 0). The total score is the sum of the scores for each of the 10 items. Validation studies have utilized various threshold scores to determine which women were positive and in need of referral. Cut-off scores ranged from 9 to 13 points. Therefore, to err on the safe side, a woman scoring 9 or more points or indicating any suicidal ideation—scoring 1 or higher on question 10—should be referred immediately for follow-up. Even if a woman scores less than 9, if the clinician feels she is suffering from depression, an appropriate referral should be made. The EPDS is only a screening tool. It does not diagnose depression—that is done by appropriately licensed healthcare personnel. Users may reproduce the scale without permission providing the copyright is respected by quoting the authors' names, the title, and the source of the paper in all reproduced copies.

Instructions for users

1 The mother is asked to underline 1 of 4 possible responses that comes the closest to how she has been feeling the previous 7 days.

2 All 10 questions must be completed.

3 Care should be taken to avoid the possibility of the mother discussing her answers with others.

4 The mother should complete the scale herself, unless she has limited English or difficulty reading.

Name: **Date:**
Address: **Baby's age:**

As you have recently had a baby, we would like to know how you are feeling. Please **underline** the answer which comes closest to how you have felt **in the past 7 days**, not just how you feel today.

Here is an example, already completed:
I have felt happy
   Yes, all the time
   <u>Yes, most of the time</u>

No, not very often
No, not at all

This would mean: 'I have felt happy most of the time during the past week'. Please answer the following 10 questions in the same way.

In the past 7 days:

1 I have been able to laugh and see the funny side of things
   As much as I always could
   Not quite so much now
   Definitely not so much now
   Not at all

2 I have looked forward with enjoyment to things
   As much as I ever did
   Rather less than I used to
   Definitely less than I used to
   Hardly at all

*3 I have blamed myself unnecessarily when things went wrong
   Yes, most of the time
   Yes, some of the time
   Not very often
   No, never

4 I have been anxious or worried for no good reason
   No, not at all
   Hardly ever
   Yes, sometimes
   Yes, very often

*5 I have felt scared or panicky for no good reason
   Yes, quite a lot
   Yes, sometimes
   No, not much
   No, not at all

*6 Things have been getting on top of me
   Yes, most of the time I haven't been able to cope at all
   Yes, sometimes I haven't been coping as well as usual
   No, most of the time I have coped quite well
   No, I have been coping as well as ever

*7 I have been so unhappy that I have had difficulty sleeping
   Yes, most of the time
   Yes, sometimes
   Not very often
   No, not at all

BOX 21.2 Edinburgh Postnatal Depression Scale (EPDS) (*Continued*)

*8   I have felt sad or miserable
    Yes, most of the time
    Yes, quite often
    Not very often
    No, not at all

*9   I have been so unhappy that I have been crying
    Yes, most of the time
    Yes, quite often
    Only occasionally
    No, never

*10   The thought of harming myself has occurred to me
    Yes, quite often
    Sometimes
    Hardly ever
    Never

Cox J. L., Holden, J. M., & Sagovsky, R. (1987). Edinburgh Postnatal Depression Scale (EPDS). *British Journal of Psychiatry* **150**: 782–6.

---

visitor, and any specialist mental health services involved in the case to ensure necessary support and frequent monitoring. Additional help with childcare may be needed. If the severity of the disorder is more than mild, or if a mild disorder persists for longer than a few weeks, treatment with antidepressant drugs may be indicated. The psychological components of the treatment plan resemble those for other depressive disorders (see above). Most cases can be treated in the community. However, when the disorder is severe or if there is a risk of self-harm or harm to the baby, hospital treatment may be required. If admission is necessary, especially if it is likely to be prolonged, then there are advantages to treatment in a specialist mother and baby unit if one is available.

Puerperal psychosis

The treatment of puerperal psychosis is the same as that for psychotic disorders occurring outside pregnancy (see pp. 238–239). When the disorder is not severe and the mother has no ideas of harming herself or the baby, treatment can be at home along the lines described above for non-psychotic postnatal depressive disorder. When the disorder is severe, or there are ideas of harm to the self or the baby, the mother should usually be admitted to hospital, if possible to a special mother and baby unit. If antidepressant or antipsychotic drugs or lithium have to be prescribed, then breast-feeding will have to be stopped. Electroconvulsive therapy is often used because it has a rapid effect, which if successful enables the mother to resume the feeding and other care of her baby.

Women who have had a puerperal psychosis should be referred to a psychiatrist if they become pregnant again and monitored closely during the subsequent delivery. Patients who have a history of bipolar disorder and who are taking long-term lithium therapy will need specialist assessment. In some cases, the lithium can be gradually stopped before the first trimester, to minimize the risk of fetal abnormality, or before the delivery and restarted soon after but with no breast-feeding. Patients with schizoaffective disorders may need continued antipsychotic therapy; conventional antipsychotics are usually favoured.

■ Bipolar disorder

Bipolar disorder (bipolar affective disorder, manic depressive disorder) is characterized by marked mood swings between mania (mood elevation) and bipolar depression that cause significant personal distress or social dysfunction, and are not caused by drugs or known physical disorders.

The features of mania are elevated mood, overactivity, and poor judgement. Mania occurs as part of bipolar disorder in which there may also be episodes of depression. Mania is considerably less common than depressive disorder; it is important that mania is recognized in its early stages because in the later stages the patient becomes increasingly unwilling to accept treatment. Long-term maintenance drug treatment to prevent relapse should be considered in the management of patients with recurrent bipolar illnesses.

Mania

Mania, a syndrome which is in some ways the reverse of depression, occurs as part of bipolar disorder. The term bipolar disorder implies episodes of both mania and depressive disorder, but the diagnostic category also includes those who, at the time of diagnosis, have suffered only manic illnesses (most patients with mania eventually develop a depressive disorder). When manic symptoms occur without significant psychosocial impairment, the syndrome is called hypomania.

Clinical features

The central features of the syndrome of mania are elation or irritability, increased activity, and self-important ideas (Table 21.6).

- **Elevated mood** may appear as elation, euphoria, cheerfulness, undue optimism, and infectious gaiety. In other cases, it appears as irritability or a tendency to become angry. Mood often varies during the day, although usually not with the regular diurnal rhythm characteristic of severe depressive disorders (see p. 224). Sometimes elation is interrupted by sudden, brief episodes of depression.

- **Appearance** often reflects the prevailing mood. Patients often select brightly coloured and ill-assorted clothes. When the condition is severe, they may appear untidy and dishevelled.

- **Behaviour.** Patients are overactive, often for long periods, leading to physical exhaustion. Manic patients are distractible, starting activities and leaving them unfinished as they turn repeatedly to new ones. Behaviour may be socially inappropriate due to a combination of increased activity, disinhibition, and grandiosity. The patient may go on unrestrained buying sprees, dramatically increase their sexual activity, or increase their consumption of alcohol and/or drugs.

- **Libido.** Sexual activity is often increased.

Table 21.6 Clinical features of mania

Mood
- Euphoria
- Irritability

Appearance

Behaviour
- Overactivity
- Distractibility
- Socially inappropriate behaviour
- Reduced sleep
- Increased appetite
- Increased libido

Thinking and speech
- Flight of ideas
- Expansive ideas
- Grandiose delusions
- Hallucinations

Impaired insight

- **Sleep** is often reduced but the patient wakes feeling lively and energetic and may often rise early and engage in noisy activity, to the surprise and distress of other people.

- **Appetite** is increased, and food may be eaten greedily with little attention to conventional manners.

- **Speech** is often rapid and copious, reflecting thoughts that occur in quick succession ('pressure of speech'). When severe, the rapid succession of thoughts is difficult to follow; the term 'flight of ideas' is used.

- **Thinking.** Expansive (grandiose) ideas are common. Patients believe that their ideas are original, their opinions important, and their work is of outstanding quality. Many patients become extravagant, spending more than they can afford, for example, on expensive cars or jewellery. Others make reckless decisions to give up good jobs or embark on plans for risky business ventures. In severe cases there may be grandiose delusions, for example the patient may believe that he is a religious prophet or an expert destined to advise statesmen about great issues. At times there are delusions of persecution, the patient believing that people are conspiring against him because of his special importance. Delusions of reference and passivity feelings may occur. The delusions often change in content over days.

- **Hallucinations** also occur in severe cases. They are usually consistent with the mood and fluctuating in content, taking the form of voices speaking to the patient about his special powers or, occasionally, of visions with a religious content.

- **Insight** is invariably impaired. Patients may see no reason why their grandiose plans should be restrained or their extravagant expenditure curtailed. They seldom think themselves ill or in need of treatment.

Most manic patients can exert some control over their symptoms for a short time. Many do so when the interviewer is assessing the need for treatment, with the result that the severity of the disorder may be underestimated. For this reason it is important, whenever possible, to interview an informant as well as the patient.

Clinical patterns

- **Hypomania.** This term refers to a state in which manic symptoms are present and noticeable, but they do not cause a serious degree of functional impairment.

- **Mild mania.** Physical activity and speech are increased, mood is labile, mainly euphoric but at times irritable, ideas are expansive, and the patient often spends more than he can afford. By definition, there is significant social impairment in this and the other patterns of mania.

- **Moderate mania.** There is marked overactivity with pressure and disorganization of speech, the euphoric mood is

BOX 21.3 DSM-IV diagnostic criteria for mania

A A distinct period of abnormally and persistently elevated, expansive, or irritable mood, lasting at least 1 week (or any duration if hospitalization is necessary).

B During the period of mood disturbance, three (or more) of the following symptoms have persisted (four if the mood is only irritable) and have been present to a significant degree:

1 Inflated self-esteem or grandiosity

2 Decreased need for sleep (e.g. feels rested after only 3 hours of sleep)

3 More talkative than usual or pressure to keep talking

4 Flight of ideas or subjective experience that thoughts are racing

5 Distractibility (i.e. attention too easily drawn to unimportant or irrelevant external stimuli)

6 Increase in goal-directed activity (either socially, at work or school, or sexually) or psychomotor agitation

7 Excessive involvement in pleasurable activities that have a high potential for painful consequences (e.g. engaging in unrestrained buying sprees, sexual indiscretions, or foolish business investments).

C The symptoms do not meet criteria for a Mixed Episode.

D The mood disturbance is sufficiently severe to cause marked impairment in occupational functioning or in usual social activities or relationships with others, or to necessitate hospitalization to prevent harm to self or others, or there are psychotic features.

E The symptoms are not due to the direct physiological effects of a substance (e.g. a drug of abuse, a medication, or other treatment) or a general medical condition (e.g. hyperthyroidism).

Note: manic-like episodes that are clearly caused by somatic antidepressant treatment (e.g. medication, electroconvulsive therapy, light therapy) should not count towards a diagnosis of bipolar I disorder.

BOX 21.4 DSM-IV diagnostic criteria for hypomania

A A distinct period of persistently elevated, expansive, or irritable mood, lasting throughout at least 4 days, that is clearly different from the usual undepressed mood.

B During the period of mood disturbance, three (or more) of the following symptoms have persisted (four if the mood is only irritable) and have been present to a significant degree:

1 Inflated self-esteem or grandiosity

2 Decreased need for sleep (e.g. feels rested after only 3 hours of sleep)

3 More talkative than usual or pressure to keep talking

4 Flight of ideas or subjective experience that thoughts are racing

5 Distractibility (i.e. attention too easily drawn to unimportant or irrelevant external stimuli)

6 Increase in goal-directed activity (either socially, at work or school, or sexually) or psychomotor agitation

7 Excessive involvement in pleasurable activities that have a high potential for painful consequences (e.g. engaging in unrestrained buying sprees, sexual indiscretions, or foolish business investments).

C The episode is associated with an unequivocal change in functioning that is uncharacteristic of the person when not symptomatic.

D The disturbance in mood and the change in functioning are observable by others.

E The episode is not severe enough to cause marked impairment in social or occupational functioning, or to necessitate hospitalization, and there are no psychotic features.

F The symptoms are not due to the direct physiological effects of a substance (e.g. a drug of abuse, a medication, or other treatment) or a general medical condition (e.g. hyperthyroidism).

Note: manic-like episodes that are clearly caused by somatic antidepressant treatment (e.g. medication, electroconvulsive therapy, light therapy) should not count towards a diagnosis of bipolar II disorder.

increasingly interrupted by periods of irritability, hostility, and depression, and grandiose and other preoccupations may become delusional.

- **Severe mania.** There is frenzied overactivity, thinking is incoherent and delusions become increasingly bizarre, and hallucinations are experienced. Very rarely, however, the patient becomes immobile and mute instead of over-active and talkative (manic stupor).

Mixed and alternating mood states

Occasionally, manic and depressive symptoms occur together, as a mixed mood state. For example, an over-active and overtalkative patient may have profound depressive thoughts including suicidal ideas.

In alternating mood states, mania and depression follow one another in a sequence of rapid changes. Thus, a manic patient may be intensely depressed for a few hours and then quickly become manic. Occasionally, states of mania and depression follow one another regularly with intervals of a few weeks or months between them. The disorder is called rapid cycling when four or more epi-sodes of mood disorder (depressive, manic, or mixed) occur within a 12-month period.

Differential diagnosis of manic disorders

Manic disorders have to be distinguished from:

- **Schizophrenia.** The differential diagnosis from schizo-phrenia can be most difficult. In manic disorders, auditory hallucinations and delusions can occur, including some delusions that are characteristic of schizophrenia such as delusions of reference. In mania these symptoms usually change quickly in content, and seldom outlast the over-activity. When there is a more or less equal mixture of features of the two syndromes, the term **schizoaffective** (or **schizomanic**) is used. These conditions are discussed further in Chapter 22.

- **Dementia** should always be considered, especially in mid-dle-aged or older patients with expansive behaviour and no past history of affective disorder. In the absence of gross mood disorder, extreme social disinhibition (e.g. urinating in public) strongly suggests frontal lobe pathology. In such cases, appropriate neurological investigation is essential.

- **Endocrine disorders.** Hyperthyroid states may cause symptoms suggestive of mania. Physical signs of elevated thyroid hormones should be sought and blood levels of thyroid hormones estimated.

- **Abuse of stimulant drugs.** The distinction between mania and excited behaviour due to abuse of amphetamines

depends on the history together with examination of the urine for drugs before treatment with psychotropic drugs is started. Drug-induced states usually subside quickly once the patient is in hospital and free from the drugs (see Chapter 29).

Epidemiology of bipolar disorders

The prevalence is between 1 and 6 per 1000 and the lifetime risk is rather less than 1 in 100. First-degree rela-tives are at much higher risk: a 12% lifetime risk of bipolar disorder, a 12% lifetime risk of recurrent depres-sive disorder, and a 12% risk of dysthymic or other mood disorders.

A primary care doctor responsible for 2000 patients of all ages may expect to see 20 to 30 patients a year present-ing with major depression and perhaps one or two patients presenting with an episode of mania.

Course and prognosis of bipolar disorders

Bipolar disorders usually begin in the first half of life, 90 per cent starting before the age of 50 years. They run a recurring course with recovery between episodes of illness. Each episode generally lasts several months—on average about three. Most patients experience depressive as well as manic episodes, but a few have only manic epi-sodes.

Suicide is substantially more frequent among patients with affective disorder than among the general popula-tion. Among patients with severe depressive disorder, about 1 in 10 eventually commit suicide.

Puerperal psychosis. Most patients recover fully from a puerperal psychosis but a few (mostly those with a schizo-phrenic psychosis) remain chronically ill. At a subsequent birth, the recurrence rate for puerperal depressive illness is between 1 in 2 and 1 in 3 (compared with 1 in 500 for those without a previous puerperal psychosis). At least half the women with a puerperal depressive illness go on to develop a depressive illness unrelated to childbirth.

Management of bipolar disorder

Assessment

The assessment of a depressive episode in a patient with bipolar disorder is essentially the same as the assessment of a unipolar depressive episode (see above), although the treatment is different as described below.

The assessment of a manic patient may need the help of a specialist. In the assessment of mania, the steps are those already outlined for depressive disorders, that is:

(i) decide the diagnosis; (ii) assess the severity of the disorder; (iii) form an opinion about the causes; (iv) assess the patient's social resources; and (v) judge the effect on other people.

Diagnosis depends on a careful history and examination. Whenever possible, the history should be taken from relatives as well as from the patient because the patient seldom recognizes the full extent of the abnormal behaviour. Differential diagnosis has been discussed earlier in this chapter; it is important to remember that mildly disinhibited behaviour can result from intoxication with drugs or alcohol, or, rarely, from frontal lobe lesion causes (e.g. by a cerebral neoplasm).

Severity and the degree of psychosocial dysfunction should be carefully considered because they have important implications for diagnosis (e.g. for discriminating between hypomania and mania, see p. 239) and management. For this purpose it is essential to interview another informant. Manic patients are able to exert a degree of self-control during an interview with a doctor, and then behave in a more disinhibited and grandiose way immediately afterwards. At an early stage of the disorder it is easy to be misled by patients in this way and to miss the opportunity to persuade them to enter hospital before causing difficulties for themselves, for example through ill-judged decisions at work or unaffordable extravagance.

Usually, the causes of a manic disorder are largely endogenous; some cases follow physical illness, treatment by drugs (especially steroids), or an operation. It is important to identify any life events that may have provoked the onset and also to identify maintaining factors.

The patient's resources and the effects of the illness on other people should be assessed along the lines already described for depressive disorders. Even for the most supportive family, it is extremely difficult to care for a manic patient at home for more than a few days unless the disorder is exceptionally mild. The patient's responsibilities for the care of dependent children or at work should always be considered carefully.

Treatment of mania

General aspects of the treatment of mania

It is important to commence treatment for a manic episode as quickly as possible because of the high likelihood of serious personal and social consequences that might follow from the errors of judgement that are characteristic of the disorder. The general practitioner will need to contact the specialist services urgently, and should commence effective drug treatment if the diagnosis is clear and the patient is agreeable. Milder manic episodes may be treated as an outpatient, but more severe disorders with associated loss of judgement will almost always need initial treatment as an inpatient. When the disorder is more severe, compulsory admission is likely to be needed.

Almost all patients with a manic episode will need drug treatment and, because it is important to commence this as soon as possible, many patients with a previous bipolar disorder keep a small supply of antipsychotic medication to take if they experience prodromal symptoms of mania (see below).

The clinical status should be monitored frequently. Progress is judged not only by the mental state and general behaviour, but also by the pattern of sleep and by the regaining of any weight lost during the illness. As progress continues, antipsychotic drug treatment is reduced gradually. It is important, however, not to discontinue the drug too soon, otherwise relapse may occur.

During treatment a careful watch should be kept for the appearance of depressive symptoms because transient but profound depressive mood change and depressive ideas are common among manic patients. Also, the clinical picture may change rapidly from mania to a sustained depressive disorder. In either case, suicidal ideas may appear. A sustained change to a depressive syndrome may require treatment, including with antidepressant drugs which should be used cautiously to avoid precipitation of a manic relapse. Following recovery, regular follow-up is necessary to detect relapse into mania or the onset of depression. Patients should be helped to deal with or to come to terms with any precipitating causes of the episode, and with the consequences of any ill-judged actions during the acute illness.

Specific treatments for mania

Antipsychotic drugs

Antipsychotic drugs have an established place in the treatment of mania. The older, conventional antipsychotics are frequently used, but there is now more evidence for the effectiveness of the newer atypical antipsychotics, which are also better tolerated in the short term. An atypical antipsychotic, such as olanzapine, quetiapine, or risperidone, is therefore usually the first-choice treatment. Antipsychotics should generally not be used to control behaviour because the doses required for this effect are high and adverse effects are therefore more likely. A benzodiazepine such as lorazepam or diazepam should be used instead.

Lithium

Lithium is effective in mania, but less so than antipsychotic drugs, and it can be difficult to use safely in severely disturbed patients. The effect in mania may take several days to begin. Lithium is therefore used mainly in patients with milder manic episodes, especially when it is intended to continue the treatment in the long term to prevent relapse. Lithium is also used in combination with antipsychotics—caution is required when used in combination with haloperidol because extrapyramidal effects occur commonly.

Anti-epileptic drugs

Valproate is effective in acute mania. It is slightly less effective than antipsychotics, but causes fewer adverse effects. Thus, it may be particularly useful in patients who are not currently taking a long-term mood stabilizer, and who have a mild manic illness without psychotic features. An advantage of valproate over lithium in the acute phase is that a high loading dose can be given, which leads to a more rapid response and shorter hospital stays.

Carbamazepine is another anti-epileptic drug that can be used in mania.

Electroconvulsive therapy

Although there is no evidence from randomized trials, clinical experience indicates that ECT has a powerful therapeutic effect in mania. Nevertheless, ECT is not a first-line treatment; its use is mainly in the uncommon cases when antipsychotic drugs are ineffective and the patient is so seriously disturbed that to spend time trying further medication or awaiting natural recovery is not justified.

Treatment of bipolar depression

General aspects of the treatment of acute bipolar depression

Depressive episodes cause more disability then manic episodes in most people with bipolar disorder. The general aspects of treatment are the same as those described above for unipolar depression, but there are important differences in both the effectiveness of treatments and the risks associated with treatment. As with the treatment of mania, the clinical status of the patient should be monitored frequently because rapid mood fluctuations are common.

Specific treatment for acute bipolar depression

Antidepressant drugs

Although there is less evidence than for unipolar depression, it appears that antidepressant drugs are reasonably effective in bipolar depression and that there are no differences in efficacy between the classes of drug. About 5–10% of patients with bipolar depression develop a manic episode following treatment with an antidepressant drug and the risk is worse with tricyclics than with SSRIs. For this reason antidepressant medication should usually be given only with the cover of an effective antimanic drug such as an antipsychotic, lithium, or valproate.

Antipsychotic drugs

There is good evidence that quetiapine is effective in acute bipolar depression and, because it carries little risk of inducing manic symptoms, it is not recommended as a first-line treatment.

There is some evidence that olanzapine is modestly effective in bipolar depression, but is more effective when added to an SSRI.

Lithium

Lithium is less effective in depression than in mania, but it is sometimes used in less severe but recurring cases when it is planned to use lithium for prophylaxis after the acute episode has recovered. Also when a depressive episode occurs in a patient who is already taking long-term lithium, one treatment option is to increase the dose of lithium.

Anti-epileptic drugs

There is no good evidence that valproate or carbamazepine are effective treatments for bipolar depression. Lamotrigine, another anti-epileptic, may be effective.

Electroconvulsive therapy

As in other severe or resistant depressive episodes, ECT is indicated when alternative therapies have not been effective.

Psychological treatments

There is some evidence that cognitive behavioural therapy and interpersonal psychotherapy are effective in bipolar depression.

Treatment of mixed mood episodes

Manic symptoms usually predominate over depressive symptoms in mixed states, and treatment of mixed states is therefore usually the treatment of a manic episode, with antipsychotics alone or in combination with a mood stabilizer. Mood stabilizers may also be used alone. Antidepressants should not be used when manic symptoms predominate, although they may be used when depressive symptoms are prominent.

Continuation therapy

This term refers to prevention of relapse in the first few weeks and months following recovery from mania or depression (i.e. return of symptoms after initial improvement during a single episode of illness). Following resolution of mania, the acute-phase treatment is usually continued for several weeks or months and then gradually discontinued (unless relapse prevention with the same agent is being considered; see below). Following the resolution of bipolar depressive disorders, it is uncertain whether antidepressants should be continued, because prolonged use of antidepressants could precipitate a manic episode.

Prevention of relapse

Bipolar disorder has a strong tendency to relapse. Following the first severe episode of mania, the risk of a serious manic relapse occurring in any year is about 10–20%. The risk is greater when patients have suffered multiple previous episodes, for example after three previous episodes the annual risk of relapse is about 20–30%.

Long-term drug treatment

Long-term drug treatment can substantially reduce the risk of relapse. There are several available treatments and the choice will depend on adverse effects and previous response to treatment. At present, the comparative efficacy of the drugs is largely unknown. Combinations of drugs are frequently used in practice, and there is now some evidence to support this.

Lithium

Lithium reduces the risk of relapse and is more effective at preventing manic than depressive episodes. The benefits outweigh the risks of adverse events for most patients who are at least at moderate risk of relapse (those with three or more previous episodes, very severe previous episodes, or a strong family history of recurrent bipolar disorder). Because lithium treatment is associated with several adverse effects, the plasma levels should be monitored regularly (see p. 123).

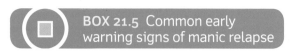

BOX 21.5 Common early warning signs of manic relapse

Reduced need for sleep
Increased physical activity
Racing thoughts
Elated mood
Irritability or rage if plans or wishes are not satisfied
Unrealistic plans
Overspending

Anti-epileptic drugs

Valproate reduces the risk of relapse, although it is uncertain how it compares with lithium. Carbamazepine may also be useful for some patients, although it is probably less effective than lithium. Lamotrigine is effective at preventing depressive relapses.

Antipsychotic drugs

Long-term treatment with antipsychotic drugs is usually reserved for patients with recurrent psychotic symptoms or for when alternative treatments have not proved effective.

Education to recognize early signs of relapse

Many patients develop characteristic prodromal symptoms before a relapse (see Box 21.5). These patients can be helped to recognize these symptoms and given an agreed plan of action to use when the prodromal signs occur. This approach can help patients avoid manic episodes, but it is less certain that it helps avoid depressive episodes.

Psychological treatments

Family therapy can help prevent relapse. The evidence that cognitive therapy prevents relapse in bipolar disorder is equivocal.

Further reading

Anderson, I. M., Ferrier, I. N., Baldwin, R. C., *et al.* (2008). Evidence-based guidelines for treating depressive disorders with antidepressants: A revision of the 2000 British Association for Psychopharmacology guidelines. *Journal of Psychopharmacology* 22: 343–96.

Goodwin, G. M., *et al.* (2009). Evidence-based guidelines for treating bipolar disorder: revised second edition recommendations from the British Association for Psychopharmacology. *Journal of Psychopharmacology* 23: 346–88.

NICE (2006). *National Clinical Practice Guideline 38. Bipolar Disorder: the Management of Bipolar Disorder in Adults, Children and Adolescents, in Primary and Secondary Care.* http://guidance.nice.org.uk/CG38.

NICE (2009). *National Clinical Practice Guideline 90. Depression: the Treatment and Management of Depression in Adults.* http://guidance.nice.org.uk/CG90.

CHAPTER 22

Schizophrenia and related disorders

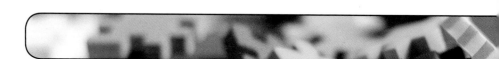

Chapter contents

Schizophrenia and related disorders are characterized by psychotic symptoms such as delusions and hallucinations. There is a spectrum of severity. In **schizophrenia**, the patient suffers from psychotic symptoms and functional impairment. In **delusional disorders**, the patient experiences delusions, but there is no evidence of hallucinations or any of the other symptoms characteristic of schizophrenia.

Schizophrenia can be a particularly disabling illness because its course, although variable, is frequently chronic and relapsing. The care of patients with schizophrenia places a considerable burden on all carers, from the patient's family through to the health and social services. General practitioners may have only a few patients with chronic schizophrenia on their lists but the severity of their problems and the needs of their families will make these patients important.

This chapter aims to provide sufficient information for the reader to be able to recognize the basic symptoms of schizophrenia and related disorders and to be aware of the main approaches to treatment.

■ Diagnosis and clinical features

As the clinical presentation and outcome of the disorder vary, schizophrenia can be a confusing illness to understand. It is best to start by considering simplified descriptions of two common presentations: (i) the acute syndrome; and (ii) the chronic syndrome. It is then easier to understand the core features as well as the diversity of schizophrenia.

The acute syndrome (positive symptoms)

The main clinical features of the acute syndrome can be illustrated by a short case study of a patient (Case study 22.1), which illustrates the following common features of acute schizophrenia:

- hallucinations
- persecutory ideas
- the false idea of being referred to (a delusion of reference, see p. 35).
- social withdrawal
- impaired performance at work.

The term **positive syndrome** is sometimes used to refer to these features (Table 22.1). It refers to the appearance of hallucinations and delusions, in contrast to the loss of function in the chronic syndrome—the **negative syndrome**.

Appearance and behaviour

Many patients with acute schizophrenia appear entirely normal. Some appear awkward in their social behaviour, preoccupied and withdrawn, or otherwise odd. Others smile or laugh without obvious reason, or appear perplexed by what is happening to them. Some are restless and noisy, and a few show sudden and unexpected changes in behaviour. Others retire from company, spending much time alone in their room, perhaps lying immobile on the bed apparently deep in thought.

Mood

Abnormalities of mood are common. There are three main kinds:

1 Mood change such as depression, anxiety, irritability, or euphoria. Depressive symptoms in the acute syndrome may develop in one or more of three ways:

   (i) as an integral part of the disorder—caused by the same processes that cause the other symptoms such as the delusions and hallucinations;

Table 22.1 The acute syndrome (positive symptoms)

Appearance and behaviour	Preoccupied, withdrawn, inactive
	Restless, noisy, inconsistent
Mood	Mood change
	Blunting
	Incongruity
Disorders of thinking	Vagueness
	Formal thought disorder
	Disorders of the stream of thought
Hallucinations	Auditory
	Visual
	Tactile, olfactory, gustatory
Delusions	Primary
	Secondary (especially persecutory)
Orientation	Normal
Attention	Impaired
Memory	Normal
Insight	Impaired

   (ii) as a response to insight into the nature of the illness and the problems to be faced;

   (iii) as side effects of antipsychotic medication.

2 A reduction in the normal variations of mood, which is called blunting (or flattening) of affect. A patient with this disorder may seem indifferent to others because of unchanging mood.

3 Emotion not in keeping with the situation, a condition known as incongruity of affect. A patient may, for example, laugh when told about the death of his mother.

Speech and form of thought

Speech may be difficult to follow. In the early stages, a patient's talk may be vague so that it is difficult to grasp the

Case study 22.1 Acute schizophrenia

A previously healthy 20-year-old male student had been behaving in an increasingly odd way. At times he appeared angry and told his friends that he was being followed by the police and secret services; at other times he was seen to be laughing to himself for no apparent reason. For several months he had spent more time on his own, apparently preoccupied with his own thoughts, and his academic work had deteriorated. When seen by the family doctor he was restless and appeared frightened. He said that he had heard voices commenting on his actions and abusing him. He also said that the police had conspired with his university teachers to harm his brain with poisonous gases and take away his thoughts, and that the police had arranged for items referring to him to be inserted into television programmes.

meaning. Later there may be more definite abnormalities (formal thought disorder). These abnormalities are of several kinds. Some patients have difficulty in dealing with abstract ideas (a phenomenon called concrete thinking) while others become preoccupied with vague pseudoscientific or mystical ideas. There is a lack of connection between the ideas expressed by the patient (loosening of associations). The links between ideas may be illogical, or they may wander from the original theme. In its most extreme form, loosening of association leads to totally incoherent thought and speech (word salad).

There may be disorders of the stream of thought, such as pressure of thought, poverty of thought, and thought blocking (all of which are described on p. 32).

Perception

Auditory hallucinations are among the most frequent symptoms of schizophrenia. They may be experienced as simple noises or complex sounds of voices or music. Voices may utter single words, brief phrases, or whole conversations. The voices may seem to give commands to the patient. A voice may speak the patient's thoughts aloud, either as he thinks them or immediately afterwards. Sometimes, two or more voices may seem to discuss the patient in the third person. Other voices may comment on his actions. As explained later, these last three symptoms have particular diagnostic value (see p. 39).

In schizophrenia, **visual hallucinations** are less frequent than auditory ones, and seldom occur without other kinds of hallucination. A few patients experience **tactile**, **olfactory**, **gustatory**, and **somatic** hallucinations, which are often interpreted in a delusional way; for example, hallucinatory sensations in the lower abdomen may be attributed to unwanted sexual interference by a persecutor.

Abnormalities of the content of thought

Delusions occur commonly in schizophrenia. Primary delusions (see p. 33) occur occasionally and when present are important because they occur seldom in other disorders and are therefore of value in diagnosis. Most delusions are secondary, that is they arise from a previous mental change. Delusions may be preceded by so-called delusional mood (see p. 34), which is seldom found in conditions other than schizophrenia, or by hallucinations. Several kinds of delusion occur. Persecutory delusions are common, but not specific to schizophrenia. Less common but of greater diagnostic value are delusions of reference (false beliefs that objects, events, or people have a special personal significance, see p. 35), delusions of control (the feeling of being controlled by an outside agency, see p. 35), and delusions about the pos-

session of thought (the idea that thoughts are being inserted into or withdrawn from the person's mind, or 'broadcast' to other people, see p. 35).

Insight

Insight is usually impaired. Most patients do not accept that their experiences result from illness, often ascribing them instead to the malevolent actions of other people. This lack of insight is often accompanied by unwillingness to accept treatment.

The combination of disturbed behaviour, hallucinations, and delusions is often referred to as **positive symptoms**. Schizophrenic patients do not necessarily experience all these symptoms. The clinical picture is variable, as explained later in this chapter (see p. 250).

The chronic syndrome (negative symptoms)

The **chronic syndrome** is characterized by the following 'negative' symptoms (Table 22.2):

- underactivity or disorganized behaviour;
- lack of drive;
- social withdrawal;
- emotional apathy;
- thought disorder;
- cognitive impairment.

Table 22.2 The chronic syndrome (negative symptoms)

Lack of drive and activity	
Social withdrawal	
Abnormalities of behaviour	
Abnormalities of movement	Stupor and excitement
	Abnormal movements
	Abnormal tonus
Speech	Reduced in amount
	Evidence of thought disorder
Mood disorder	Blunting
	Incongruity
	Depression
Hallucinations	Especially auditory
Delusions	Systematized
	Encapsulated
Orientation	Age disorientation
Attention	Normal
Memory	Normal
Insight	Variable

Case study 22.2 The chronic syndrome

A middle-aged man lives in a group home for psychiatric patients and attends a sheltered workshop. In both places he withdraws from company. He is usually dishevelled and unshaven, and cares for himself only when encouraged to do so by others. His social behaviour is odd and awkward. His speech is slow, and its content vague and incoherent. When questioned, he says that he is the victim of persecution by extraterrestrial beings who beam rays at him. He seldom mentions these ideas spontaneously and he shows few signs of emotion about them or about any other aspects of his life. For several years, this clinical picture has changed little except for brief periods of acute symptoms, which are usually related to upsets in the ordered life of the group home.

The syndrome can be illustrated by a brief case study of a typical patient (Case study 22.2). This description illustrates several of the features of what is sometimes called a 'schizophrenic defect state'.

Impairment of volition

The most striking feature is diminished **volition**, that is, a lack of drive and initiative. Left to himself, the patient may be inactive for long periods, or may engage in aimless and repeated activity.

Impairment of daily living skills

Social behaviour often deteriorates. Patients neglect personal hygiene and their appearance. They may withdraw from social encounters. Some behave in ways that break social conventions, for example talking intimately to strangers, shouting obscenities in public, or behaving in a sexually uninhibited manner. Some patients hoard objects, so that their surroundings become cluttered and dirty.

Movement disorders

A variety of disturbances of movement occur which are often called **catatonic**. They will be described only briefly here (they are detailed in the *Oxford Textbook of Psychiatry*). **Stupor** and **excitement** are the most striking catatonic symptoms. A patient in stupor is immobile, mute, and unresponsive, although fully conscious. Stupor may change (sometimes quickly) to a state of uncontrolled motor activity and excitement.

Patients with chronic schizophrenia sometimes make repeated, odd, and awkward movements. Repeated movements that do not appear to be goal directed are called **stereotypies**; repeated movements of this kind that do appear to be goal directed are called **mannerisms**. Occasionally, patients have a disorder of muscle tone, which can be detected by placing the patient in an awkward posture; when the sign is present, the patient maintains this posture without apparent distress for much longer than a healthy person could without severe discomfort (waxy flexibility). When catatonic symptoms are prominent the illness is referred to as catatonic schizophrenia.

Speech and form of thought

Speech is often abnormal, reflecting **thought disorder** of the same kinds as those found in the acute syndrome (see above).

Affect and perception

Affect is generally blunted, and when emotion is shown, it may be incongruous. **Hallucinations** are common, and any of the forms occurring in the acute syndrome may occur in the chronic syndrome.

Thought content

In chronic schizophrenia, **delusions** are common and often systematized. They may be held with little emotion. For example, patients may be convinced that they are being persecuted but show neither fear nor anger. Delusions may also be 'encapsulated' from the rest of the patient's beliefs. Thus, a patient may be convinced that his private sexual fantasies and practices are widely discussed by strangers, but his remaining beliefs are not influenced by this conviction, nor is his work or social life affected.

Cognitive function

It is now recognized that people with schizophrenia frequently suffer from a variety of cognitive impairments and that these impairments are associated with important aspects of functional outcome, such as the acquisition of social skill and the chances of successful employment. Many areas of cognitive functioning appear to be affected; the best established are deficits in working and semantic memory, attention, and executive functioning. Verbal fluency and motor functioning also appear to be affected, although to a lesser extent.

Insight

Insight is often impaired; the patient does not recognize that his symptoms are due to illness and is seldom fully convinced of the need for treatment.

Factors modifying the clinical features

In schizophrenia several factors can interact with the disease process to modify the clinical picture.

Age of onset

The symptoms of adolescents and young adults often include thought disorder, mood disturbance, and disrupted behaviour. With increasing age, paranoid symptoms are more common, and disrupted behaviour is less frequent.

Gender

The course of the illness is generally more severe in males.

Sociocultural background

Sociocultural factors may affect the content of delusions and hallucinations. For example, delusions with a religious content are more common among patients from a religious background. Recent technological innovations are often used to explain symptoms. For example, a patient thought that his auditory hallucinations were due to nanotechnology.

The amount of social stimulation has a considerable effect on the type of symptoms. *Understimulation* increases 'negative' symptoms such as poverty of speech, social withdrawal, apathy, and lack of drive, and also catatonic symptoms. *Overstimulation* induces 'positive' symptoms such as hallucinations, delusions, and restlessness. Modern treatment is designed to avoid understimulation; as a result, 'negative' features including catatonia are less frequent than in the past. This policy can, however, result in a degree of overstimulation, leading to more positive symptoms.

High emotional expression by people with whom the patient is living is one form of social stimulation that increases symptoms. Overt expressions of criticism seem to be particularly important. The more time the patient spends in the company of highly critical people, the more likely he is to relapse. This is a reason why some patients are less disturbed when living in a hostel than with their family.

Diagnosis

The diagnosis of schizophrenia is based entirely on the clinical presentation (history and examination). The only diagnostic tests used are those needed to exclude other disorders when there is clinical suspicion. Because the diagnosis is based on clinical findings, it is made more reliable when **diagnostic criteria** are used to specify patterns of symptoms which must be present to make the diagnosis.

The currently most widely used diagnostic criteria are those in the International Classification of Diseases (ICD-10) and the Diagnostic and Statistical Manual of the American Psychiatric Association (DSM-IV) (see Box 22.1). Both these systems include:

1 Individual symptoms that have been found to be highly specific for schizophrenia and therefore have a high **positive predictive value**. These are called **Schneider's 'first-rank' symptoms** after the clinician who first described them (Table 22.3 and described more fully in Chapter 5). They occur in about 70 per cent of patients who meet the full diagnostic criteria for schizophrenia.

2 Symptoms that are more frequent but less discriminating than first-rank symptoms (e.g. prominent hallucinations, loosening of association, and flat or inappropriate affect).

3 Impaired social and occupational functioning.

4 A minimum duration (6 months in DSM-IV but, unfortunately, a different period—1 month—in ICD-10).

5 The exclusion of (i) organic mental disorder, (ii) major depression, (iii) mania, or (iv) the prolongation of autistic disorder (which is a mental disorder of childhood, see p. 430).

Classification of psychotic disorders which do not meet the diagnostic criteria for schizophrenia

Both ICD-10 and DSM-IV provide categories for disorders that resemble schizophrenia but fail to meet the diagnostic criteria for schizophrenia in one of the following three ways.

1 Duration is too short. Cases lasting for less than 1 month are called acute psychotic disorders in both classifications. DSM-IV has an extra category for cases lasting less than the 6 months required in this classification for the diagnosis of schizophrenia. These cases are called schizophreniform. (Since ICD-10 requires a duration of only 1 month, it does not require this extra category.)

2 Prominent affective symptoms. These cases are called schizoaffective in both classifications.

3 Delusions without other symptoms of schizophrenia. These are called delusional disorders (in ICD-10 the term is persistent delusional disorder). Delusional disorder is described later in the chapter.

Differential diagnosis

Schizophrenia needs to be distinguished from four other types of disorder.

BOX 22.1 DSM-IV diagnostic criteria for schizophrenia

A Characteristic symptoms: two (or more) of the following, each present for a significant portion of time during a 1-month period (or less if successfully treated):

1 delusions;

2 hallucinations;

3 disorganized speech (e.g. frequent derailment or incoherence);

4 grossly disorganized or catatonic behaviour;

5 negative symptoms, i.e. affective flattening, alogia, or avolition.

Note: only one Criterion A symptom is required if delusions are bizarre or hallucinations consist of a voice keeping up a running commentary on the person's behaviour or thoughts, or two or more voices conversing with each other.

B Social/occupational dysfunction: for a significant portion of the time since the onset of the disturbance, one or more major areas of functioning, such as work, interpersonal relations, or self-care, are markedly below the level achieved prior to the onset (or when the onset is in childhood or adolescence, failure to achieve expected level of interpersonal, academic, or occupational achievement).

C Duration: continuous signs of the disturbance persist for at least 6 months. This 6-month period must include at least 1 month of symptoms (or less if successfully treated) that meet Criterion A (i.e. active-phase symptoms) and may include periods of prodromal or residual symptoms. During these prodromal or residual periods, the signs of the disturbance may be manifested by only negative symptoms or two or more symptoms listed in Criterion A present in an attenuated form (e.g. odd beliefs, unusual perceptual experiences).

D Schizoaffective and mood disorder exclusion: schizoaffective disorder and mood disorder with psychotic features have been ruled out because either (i) no major depressive episode, manic episode, or mixed episode has occurred concurrently with the active-phase symptoms, or (ii) if mood episodes have occurred during active-phase symptoms, their total duration has been brief relative to the duration of the active and residual periods.

E Substance/general medical condition exclusion: the disturbance is not due to the direct physiological effects of a substance (e.g. a drug of abuse, a medication) or a general medical condition.

F Relationship to a pervasive developmental disorder: if there is a history of autistic disorder or another pervasive developmental disorder, the additional diagnosis of schizophrenia is made only if prominent delusions or hallucinations are also present for at least a month (or less if successfully treated).

ICD-10 criteria for schizophrenia differ in requiring only one of the category A symptoms (if very clear-cut) and a minimum duration of 1 month.

Table 22.3 Schneider's 'first-rank' symptoms of schizophrenia*

- Hearing thoughts spoken aloud
- 'Third-person' hallucinations
- Hallucinations in the form of a commentary
- Somatic hallucinations
- Thought withdrawal or insertion
- Thought broadcasting
- Delusional perception
- Feelings or actions experienced as made or influenced by external agents

*The terms used in this list are explained in Chapter 5.

1 **Organic syndromes.** In younger patients the most relevant organic diagnoses are:

(i) **Drug-induced states.**

Drugs of abuse, especially that induced by amphetamines (see p. 405), but also phencyclidine, cocaine, ecstasy, and LSD. Cannabis intoxication may cause perceptual distortions but rarely frank psychosis. Cannabis may, however, precipitate relapse in patients with established schizophrenia.

Prescribed drugs: many prescribed drugs can rarely cause psychotic reactions, but steroids and the dopamine agonists used in the treatment of Parkinson's disease are probably the most commonly implicated drugs.

(ii) **Temporal lobe epilepsy** should be considered when the condition is brief and there is evidence of clouding of consciousness. (In a few patients, chronic temporal lobe epilepsy gives rise to a persistent state resembling schizophrenia more closely.)

In older patients, the organic brain diseases which should be excluded include the following.

(i) **Delirium** can be mistaken for an acute episode of schizophrenia, especially when there are prominent hallucinations and delusions; the cardinal feature

Science box 22.1 What is schizophrenia?

When Eugen Bleuler coined the term 'schizophrenia' in 1911, he was trying to describe the splitting of psychological functions—particularly the loosening of associations—that he observed in his patients at the Burghölzli Clinic in Zurich. Bleuler felt that schizophrenia was a better description of the serious mental disorder characterized by psychotic symptoms in the absence of coarse brain pathology that had been called **dementia praecox** by his German contemporary, Emil Kraepelin. Gradually, the term schizophrenia prevailed and achieved worldwide use in clinical psychiatry. It was always seen as being somewhat unsatisfactory, however, as it referred to an uncertain psychological process and led to popular misunderstanding that the illness was 'split-mind' or even multiple personalities. Gradually, the adjective 'schizophrenic' became a commonly used description of unpredictable or inconsistent thinking. Moreover, the clinical boundaries and fundamental symptoms of schizophrenia remain uncertain, which has led some to suggest that it does not exist and/or that it is simply a catch-all for labelling people who do not fit into society.

Until recently, attempts to replace the term have been resisted in the absence of reliable knowledge about aetiology, which would allow a classification rationally based on causes. Instead, the reliability of the diagnosis has been improved by the introduction of operational diagnostic criteria—exemplified by DSM-IV. This has fulfilled the need for a clinically valid and reliable diagnosis and has allowed the gradual development of a scientific basis for effective treatment.

Nonetheless, there has remained widespread dissatisfaction about the term schizophrenia because of the rather imprecise and arbitrary nature of the diagnostic boundaries (between both normality and other disorders), the failure of the term to provide a good description of either the neurobiology or the clinical features of the disorder, and the stigma which has gradually attached itself to the label.

The problem is what to replace it with. One proposal is **salience dysregulation syndrome**, admittedly a bit of a mouthful, but this describes the difficulty in deciding which stimuli are important that is characteristic of the disorder.[1,2] We shall see—but we predict that schizophrenia's days as a diagnosis are numbered!

References

1 Kapur, S. (2003). Psychosis as a state of aberrant salience: a framework linking biology, phenomenology, and pharmacology in schizophrenia. *American Journal of Psychiatry* **160**: 13–23.

2 van Os, J. A. (2009). Salience dysregulation syndrome. *British Journal of Psychiatry* **194**: 101–3.

---

of this disorder is clouding of consciousness (see p. 315).

(ii) **Dementia** can resemble schizophrenia, particularly when there are prominent persecutory delusions; the finding of memory disorder suggests dementia.

(iii) Some other **diffuse brain diseases** can present a schizophrenia-like picture without any neurological signs or gross memory impairment; for example, **general paralysis of the insane**, a form of neurosyphilis.

To exclude organic disorders, history taking and mental state examination should focus on cognitive impairment (including disorientation and memory deficit) which tends to be more severe in organic disorder but not in schizophrenia, and a thorough physical examination should be done, including a neurological examination.

2 **Psychotic mood disorder.** The distinction between mood disorder and schizophrenia depends on:

(i) the degree and persistence of mood disorder;

(ii) the congruence of any hallucinations or delusions with the prevailing mood;

(iii) the nature of the symptoms in any previous episodes (if previously predominantly mood, then current mood disorder is more likely).

Sometimes, mood and schizophrenic symptoms are so equally balanced that it is not possible to decide whether the primary disorder is affective or schizophrenic. As explained above these cases are diagnosed as schizoaffective disorder (see below).

1 **Personality disorders.** Differential diagnosis from personality disorder may be difficult, especially when there have been insidious changes of behaviour in a young person who does not describe hallucinations or delusions. As well as interviewing relatives it may be necessary to make prolonged observations for first-rank and other features of schizophrenia before a definite diagnosis can be reached.

2 **Schizoaffective disorder.** Some patients have, at the same time, definite schizophrenic symptoms and definitive affective (depressive or manic) symptoms of equal prominence. These disorders are classified separately because it is uncertain whether they are a subtype of schizophrenia, or of affective disorder. Schizoaffective disorders

usually require both antipsychotic and antidepressant drug treatment. When they recover, affective and schizophrenic symptoms improve together, and most patients lose all their symptoms, although many have further episodes. Some of these subsequent episodes are schizoaffective, but others have a more typical schizophrenic or more typical affective form.

■ Epidemiology

Incidence

The annual incidence of schizophrenia is between 10 and 20 per 100 000 of the population. In men, schizophrenia usually begins between the ages of 15 and 35. In women, the mean age of onset of the disorder is later (Figure 22.1). Although the incidence of schizophrenia is similar worldwide, it may be higher in certain ethnic groups (e.g. Afro-Caribbean immigrants in the UK).

Prevalence

The point prevalence of schizophrenia is about 4 per 1000 (much higher than the incidence because the disorder is chronic). The lifetime risk of developing schizophrenia is about 10 per 1000. The prevalence of schizophrenia is higher in socio-economically deprived areas: in people who are homeless, the prevalence is 100 per 1000.

The general practitioner with an average list of 2000 may expect to have about eight patients with schizophrenia. An inner-city doctor, with a large homeless population, may have considerably more cases (50–100).

Although the numbers are usually small, the needs of these patients for medical care are great.

■ Aetiology

The aetiology of schizophrenia is uncertain, although there is evidence for several risk factors (Table 22.4). There is strong evidence for genetic causes, and good reason to believe that stressful life events may provoke the disorder. Structural changes have been found in the brains of some schizophrenic patients, particularly in the temporal lobes, but it is not yet certain how they are caused.

Genetic factors

There is strong evidence for the heritability of schizophrenia from three sources.

1 **Family studies** have shown that schizophrenia is more common in the relatives of schizophrenic patients that in the general population (where the lifetime risk is approximately 1 per cent). The risk is 10–15 per cent in the siblings of schizophrenics, among the children of one schizophrenic parent 10–15 per cent, and among the children of two schizophrenic parents about 40 per cent.

2 **Twin studies** indicate that a major part of this familial loading is likely to be due to genetic rather than to environmental factors. Among monozygotic twins, the concordance rate (the frequency of schizophrenia in the sibling of the affected twin) is consistently higher

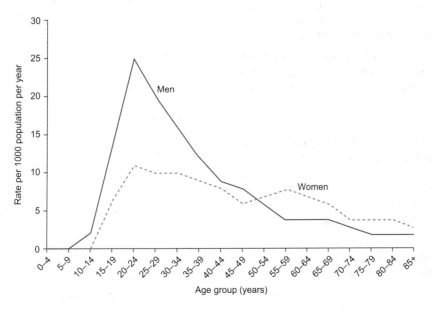

Fig. 22.1 Age- and gender-specific incidence rates for schizophrenia in men and women. Source: Information and Statistics Division, NHS Scotland, 1993.

Table 22.4 Risk factors for schizophrenia

	Risk factors	Relative risk of developing schizophrenia
Predisposing		
Genetic	Monozygotic twin of a schizophrenic patient	40
	Dizygotic twin of a schizophrenic patient	15
	Child of a schizophrenic patient	10–15
	Sibling of a schizophrenic patient	10–15
Environmental	Abnormalities of pregnancy and delivery	2
	Maternal influenza (second trimester)	2
	Fetal malnutrition	2
	Urban birth	2–3
	Migration	2
	Winter birth	1.1
Precipitating	Early cannabis consumption	2

(about 40 per cent) than among dizygotic twins (about 10–15 per cent). The heritability of schizophrenia is about 80 per cent.

3 **Adoption studies** confirm the importance of genetic factors. Among children who have been separated from a schizophrenic parent at birth and brought up by non-schizophrenic adoptive parents, the likelihood of developing schizophrenia is no less than that among children brought up by their own schizophrenic parent.

Specific genes and the mode of inheritance

Several susceptibility genes for schizophrenia have now been identified, which may have an effect on neurodevelopment and synaptic functioning (see Box 22.2).

These genes seem to be of small effect and the mode of inheritance of schizophrenia is still unclear but probably involves interaction between these, other genes, and

> **BOX 22.2 Susceptibility genes for schizophrenia**
>
> - DISC1
> - Dysbindin
> - Neuregulin-1
> - MHC locus
> - ZNF804A
> - G72

environmental factors. Rather than being specific for schizophrenia, these genes probably predispose to several mental disorders (including bipolar disorders)—the actual disorder will depend on the complex interaction between gene and environment in each individual's case (see below).

Environmental factors

Environmental factors can predispose to the development of schizophrenia, precipitate the onset, provoke relapse after initial recovery, and maintain the disorder in persisting cases.

- **Predisposing factors.** Some factors putatively implicated in the development of schizophrenia are summarized in Table 22.4. The role of most of the environmental factors remains uncertain. Abnormalities of pregnancy and fetal development are risk factors, although the size of the association is small. The mechanism of action remains obscure, although it may involve fetal hypoxia. There is also an association with low **social class** and this is probably both cause and effect: social deprivation increases exposure to several risk factors, and it is likely that people who develop schizophrenia tend to become increasingly socially deprived. There is some evidence that heavy cannabis consumption is associated with the development of schizophrenia.

- **Precipitating factors** of schizophrenia include stressful life events occurring shortly before the onset of the disorder.

- **Maintaining factors** include strongly expressed feelings, especially in the form of critical comments, among family members ('high emotional expression'). High expressed emotion may lead to increased relapse rates and can be modified by family therapy.

Finally, it has been suggested that inconsistent forms of **child rearing** predispose to schizophrenia, but such ideas are not supported by evidence. Such speculations have caused unjustified guilt in some parents.

Pathophysiology

The response of some schizophrenic symptoms to antipsychotic drugs suggests that they may have a biochemical basis. A disorder of dopaminergic function is implied by the efficacy of dopamine D_2-blocking antipsychotic drugs. Nonetheless, until recently, it has proved difficult to find direct evidence that there is abnormal dopaminergic transmission in schizophrenia. With the availability of more powerful brain imaging techniques, it is now clear that there is evidence of increased dopaminergic transmission in the basal ganglia in acute schizophrenia and diminished dopaminergic transmission in the prefrontal cortex. However, dopaminergic abnormalities are probably not the primary problem—these changes are probably the result of upstream alterations in glutamate transmission.

Schizophrenia as a disorder of brain development

It is currently thought that schizophrenia is a **neurodevelopmental disorder** caused by one or more genes—possibly interacting with environmental factors. This idea is based on several pieces of evidence.

1 Evidence of brain abnormalities has been consistently found in studies performing computed tomography (CT) and magnetic resonance imaging (MRI) scans of patients with schizophrenia. The most frequently observed abnormalities are reductions in the volumes of parahippocampus, temporal lobes, and amygdala/hippocampus, and increased lateral ventricular volumes. These abnormalities can be present before the illness and it remains uncertain to what extent they progress during the course of the disorder.

2 Patients with schizophrenia are more likely than controls to have dermatoglyphic abnormalities (sometimes associated with central nervous system developmental disorder) and separate 'soft' neurological signs.

3 Post-mortem studies have not found gliosis in the brains of schizophrenic patients. This means that it is likely that the brain abnormalities occurred early in life.

4 Subjects who subsequently develop schizophrenia are more likely than controls to have developmental problems during childhood.

Taken together, this evidence suggests a pathological process, which takes place early in life and results in abnormal neurodevelopment that is sometimes observable during childhood. The current neurodevelopmental model proposes a polygenetic susceptibility interacting with early environment and leading to abnormal brain maturation (in particular, synaptic pruning, myelination, and apoptosis). This process leads to the frequently observable childhood abnormalities and, in the presence of later environmental risk factors (psychoactive drugs, stress), leads to the onset of schizophrenia.

This model needs much more validation and testing but would integrate what is currently known and would also explain why there appears to be a spectrum of severity.

■ Course and prognosis

The *course* of schizophrenia is variable:

- Acute illness with complete recovery   20 per cent
- Recurrent course with some persistent deficits   50 per cent
- Chronic illness with persistent functional disability   20 per cent
- Suicide   10 per cent

In contrast to traditional views of a poor long-term prognosis in the majority of patients, it is now recognized that at least 30 per cent (and possibly as many as 50 per cent) of patients either recover completely or suffer minimal symptoms in the long term. This change to a more optimistic view of the prognosis is probably due to a combination of the increased recognition of milder illnesses and better treatment.

Patients with recurrent acute episodes often do not recover to the previous level after each relapse and so gradually deteriorate. The risk of *suicide* is high among young patients in the early stage of the disorder when insight is still present into the likely effect of the illness on the patient's hopes and plans.

The best *outcome* is in disorders of acute onset following stress. Other predictors of outcome, some related to the illness, others to the ill person, are listed in Table 22.5. Although of some value, these predictors cannot be used to make a definite prediction for an individual patient. For this reason, advice to patients and relatives should be given cautiously, especially in the first episode of illness. The factors listed in Table 22.5 are those operating before or at the onset of schizophrenia. Factors acting after the onset are discussed next.

Life events

As noted above, stressful life events can precipitate relapses, and patients exposed to many life events generally

Table 22.5 Factors predicting poor outcome in schizophrenia

Features of the illness
Insidious onset
Long first episode
Previous psychiatric history
Negative symptoms
Younger age at onset
Features of the patient
Male
Single, separated, widowed, or divorced
Poor psychosexual adjustment
Abnormal previous personality
Poor employment record
Social isolation
Poor compliance

have a less favourable course. In general, as explained above, an overstimulating environment increases positive symptoms, while an understimulating one increases negative symptoms. Prognosis depends, in part, on how far a balance can be achieved between these extremes.

Family environment

The risk of relapse is increased when relatives make many critical comments, express hostility, and show signs of emotional over-involvement. In such families the risk of relapse is greater if patients spend much time in contact with their close relatives (35 hours a week has been suggested as a cut-off point). Reducing this contact by arranging day care appears to improve prognosis, as may family therapy.

Cultural background

The outcome of schizophrenia may be better in less developed countries, perhaps because fewer demands are made on patients and there is greater family support, as part of a traditional rural way of life.

■ Assessment and management

The majority of people with schizophrenia will be treated by specialist mental health services, although the first evidence of schizophrenia is usually detected by general practitioners. Delay in starting treatment is associated with poorer outcome, and the importance of *early intervention* is increasingly recognized. General practitioners need to be familiar with the basic assessment and make a rapid referral for full assessment and management. The importance of early intervention has recently led to the development of specific services that aim to engage the patient with services and effective interventions as quickly as possible after the onset of symptoms.

Assessment of non-urgent cases

Sometimes the patient asks for help with the symptoms of schizophrenia, but more often relatives or other people draw attention to problem behaviours that could be caused by schizophrenia. For example, a general practitioner may be asked to help a young person who is becoming increasingly withdrawn and showing odd behaviour, or an elderly woman who is reclusive and suspicious. In these situations, family doctors are in a good position to make an initial assessment because they will often know the family and the patient's background. The doctor should try to:

- obtain a good description of the patient's symptoms and behaviour. When possible this should be supplemented by information from an informant;

- assess the patient's level of functional impairment. For example, is the patient still working? Is the patient having difficulties in his or her relationships?

- make an assessment of the degree of risk the patient poses to himself and others (see Chapter 9);

- clearly inform the patient of the results of the assessment and try to persuade the patient to accept referral to the specialist mental health services;

- when the patient will not accept referral, discuss the presentation with a psychiatrist. Treatment can then sometimes be commenced, although it is advisable to maintain contact with a psychiatrist in case the situation deteriorates.

Assessment and management of acutely disturbed patients

Disturbed behaviour may occur in the early stages of the disorder, or during a relapse of an established condition. If the patient has been, or seems likely to become, aggressive, special care should be taken. It is unwise to be alone with such a patient until an assessment of risk has been made. On the other hand, the doctor is sometimes called to see a patient who is being restrained by several people. An attempt should then be made to calm the patient and, if possible, remove the physical restraint while ensuring that helpers remain close at hand during the assessment.

Since not all overactive, aggressive, or otherwise disturbed behaviour is due to schizophrenia, the doctor's first task when assessing this problem is to make a provisional diagnosis. The main task is to exclude any acute organic disorder or non-psychotic disorder (such as personality disorder). At this stage the diagnosis between *schizophrenia* and *mania* may be difficult to make but the distinction does not affect the immediate management (Table 22.6).

If the cause of the behaviour disturbance appears to be a psychotic disorder, it is usually appropriate to refer for an urgent psychiatric opinion for assessment of the level of care required, including the need for hospital admission. Admission to hospital will depend on:

- the severity of the psychotic, mood, cognitive, or behavioural symptoms;

- the nature of the psychotic symptoms (e.g. command auditory hallucinations telling the patient to harm himself or others);

- the level of social support;

- the insight into illness and acceptance of need for treatment.

If the patient refuses admission to hospital when this is considered essential for his (or other people's) health or safety, compulsory powers for admission to hospital may be required (see Box 22.3 and p. 99). Increasingly,

Table 22.6 Assessment and management of acutely disturbed patients

1 Make a provisional diagnosis:
  - acute organic disorder
  - alcohol or drug intoxication or withdrawal
  - personality disorder
  - schizophrenia
  - mania
2 Appropriate examination and blood and urine specimens (if patient permits)
3 Antipsychotic drug treatment if needed
4 Decide the need for admission to hospital (may require Mental Health Act powers)

Table 22.7 Hospital management of an acute episode of schizophrenia

Antipsychotic medication

Appropriate activities

Counselling for patient and family

Good response and good prognosis:
  - continue medication for 6 months, gradual return to work and social activities
  - regular review and counselling

Incomplete response and/or poor prognosis:
  - long-term medication (consider depot)
  - counselling and support for family (reduce 'expressed emotion')
  - assess needs for sheltered work or housing

alternatives to hospital admission such as intensive community treatment are being developed because home treatment is often preferred by patients and their relatives (see Chapter 11).

Management of an acute episode of schizophrenia

If the diagnosis is uncertain, and if safe to do so, it may be desirable to withhold drug treatment for several days to allow the diagnosis to be clarified and to perform baseline investigations (e.g. prolactin) prior to treatment (Table 22.7).

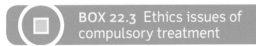

BOX 22.3 Ethics issues of compulsory treatment

Usually considered ethical when:

1 the patient is suffering from a severe mental disorder and does not consider himself ill and/or will not consent to treatment;

2 treatment is necessary for health or safety of the patient or to protect others.

Ethical issues include:

1 Nature of psychiatric diagnosis; for example, in the USSR and China, political dissidents were considered mentally ill and compulsorily detained and treated.

2 Balance between individual freedom and protection of others.

3 What is 'effective' treatment? Treatment may be defined vaguely as supportive care provided in hospital to prevent deterioration, or more specifically as a defined therapeutic intervention for which beneficial and adverse effects are known.

When the diagnosis is sufficiently clear, antipsychotic medication is started. The antipsychotic effect may not occur immediately, but antipsychotics also have a calming effect which may reduce the need for a sedative agent.

For treatment when a patient is very excited or abnormally aggressive see Chapter 16 on managing behavioural disturbance. Drug treatment may be needed for immediate behavioural control, in which case a sedative benzodiazepine such as diazepam or lorazepam (see p. 114) is usually used for behavioural control, often in combination with an antipsychotic. Escalating doses of antipsychotic drugs should not be used, because of increasing the risk of adverse effects.

Antipsychotic drug therapy

The most effective treatment for acute psychotic symptoms is antipsychotic drug therapy (see p. 116). Most antipsychotic drugs have an immediate sedative effect, followed by an effect on psychotic symptoms (especially hallucinations and delusions), which may take up to 3 weeks to develop fully.

There are many antipsychotic drugs, which differ more in side-effect profiles than in effectiveness. Equivalent doses of these drugs are shown in Table 22.8. These equivalents should only be used as a rough guide, and the manufacturer's instructions should be followed. Antipsychotic drugs should be started at a low dose and increased gradually. Second-generation 'atypical' agents are often used because of the lower risk of extrapyramidal side effects. However, the decision on which drug to be used should be tailored for the individual patient and take into account the patient's preference. For an acutely ill patient, effective treatment usually begins at a dose of olanzapine 10–20 mg, chlorpromazine 100 mg three times a day or an equivalent dose of another drug;

Table 22.8 Commonly used antipsychotic drugs with normal daily dose range

Conventional		Atypical	
Haloperidol	(2–30 mg)	Risperidone	(4–16 mg)
Chlorpromazine	(100–600 mg)	Olanzapine	(5–20 mg)
Trifluoperazine	(5–30 mg)	Quetiapine	(150–800 mg)
Sulpiride	(400–800 mg)	Clozapine	(100–900 mg)*

*Sometimes effective in schizophrenia resistant to conventional antipsychotics.

depending on side effects, the dose can be increased if there is no response, but not above 900 mg of chlorpromazine a day. Prescribers should follow the manufacturer's literature or a work of reference.

Choice of antipsychotic drug (see also p. 116)

There are many antipsychotic drugs (see Table 22.8), which are divided into two groups: the **conventional** (sometimes termed first-generation) and **atypical** (second-generation) antipsychotics. The conventional antipsychotics include chlorpromazine and haloperidol. They have been available for many years and are effective but cause troublesome extrapyramidal side effects (EPS). The second group, the atypical antipsychotics, cause fewer EPS but cause other adverse effects, including weight gain and hyperglycaemia. The atypicals include risperidone, olanzapine, and clozapine. Clozapine is currently the only drug that has been shown to be effective in illnesses which do not respond to adequate courses of conventional antipsychotics. The main problem with clozapine is that it causes agranulocytosis in less than 1 per cent of cases which, rarely, may be fatal. The main side effects of antipsychotics are shown in Table 22.9.

The different side-effect profiles will often determine which drug is used. For example, chlorpromazine is suitable when sedation is desirable, and trifluoperazine is appropriate when sedation is not required. Extrapyramidal side effects occur frequently when conventional antipsychotic drugs are used, and **anticholinergic medication** can be used to prevent the development of extrapyramidal symptoms, including acute dystonic reactions, akathisia, or parkinsonism. However, the goal of all drug treatment should be to avoid the side effects by adjusting the dose of the chosen antipsychotic. If the patient fails to respond to at least two trials of adequate doses of first-line antipsychotic given for an adequate duration, clozapine should be considered.

The effects of antipsychotics

Following commencement of an antipsychotic, symptoms of excitement, irritability, and insomnia usually improve within a few days. Hallucinations and delusions

may take longer to improve, often changing gradually over several weeks. If there is no improvement, a check should be made that the patient is taking the prescribed drugs. If not, the reason should be determined and an attempt made to ensure compliance. If the patient is taking the prescribed dose, this should be increased cautiously unless it is already at the top of the recommended range.

Table 22.9 Side effects of antipsychotic drugs

Conventional antipsychotics

Sedation, 70–80%

Anticholinergic and anti-adrenergic effects (including dry mouth, constipation, blurred vision, urinary retention, tachycardia), 10–50%

Extrapyramidal side effects (parkinsonism, dystonia, akathisia, neuroleptic malignant syndrome), 60%

Tardive dyskinesia: 4% per year of antipsychotic medication

Endocrine effects: galactorrhoea and oligomenorrhoea

Weight gain

Sexual dysfunction

Allergy

Atypical antipsychotics (e.g. risperidone, olanzapine)

Sedation

Weight gain

Orthostatic hypotension

Hyperglycaemia

Sexual dysfunction

Clozapine

Sedation

Weight gain

Hypersalivation

Tachycardia

Orthostatic hypotension

Seizures, 3%

Agranulocytosis, < 1%

Other aspects of hospital treatment

The patient should not be left unoccupied to become absorbed in his symptoms, nor overstimulated since this prolongs the acute symptoms. Nurses and occupational therapists should work together to arrange a suitable programme of activity.

As well as drug treatment, psychological support and education about the illness and treatment are needed to help the patient accept the limitations imposed by the effects of the illness on his day-to-day life, and on his hopes for the future. With the patient's permission, similar counselling should be offered to the family.

Electroconvulsive therapy (ECT)

ECT is not used regularly in the treatment of schizophrenia but there are two important indications:

1 when there are severe depressive symptoms accompanying schizophrenia;

2 in the rare cases of catatonic stupor.

ECT is often rapidly effective in both these conditions. ECT may be effective also in acute episodes of schizophrenia, even without severe depression or stupor, but it is seldom used because drug treatment is simpler and equally beneficial. The main exception is a postpartum psychosis, when a rapid response is particularly important (see p. 227).

Drug-resistant symptoms

In about 70 per cent of acute episodes, symptoms respond to antipsychotic drug treatment. Drug-resistant symptoms can be treated in two ways.

Alternative drug therapy. Clozapine is the only agent that has clearly been shown to be effective in patients where symptoms are resistant to treatment with conventional antipsychotics (see p. 116). In practice, if a patient does not respond to two or more courses of different first-line agents, than clozapine should be considered.

Psychological treatments. There is some evidence suggesting that cognitive therapy may reduce preoccupation with drug-resistant hallucinations and delusions.

Prevention of relapse

Preventing relapse in patients who recover fully from an acute episode

If the symptoms are well controlled on discharge from hospital, the dual aims of management are to continue to control symptoms with antipsychotic drugs, while making arrangements for daily living that protect the patient from too many stressors, and enable him to return as far as possible to his previous life. Even if the patient is free from symptoms, antipsychotic medication should be continued for 6 or more months, at a dose that does not produce intolerable adverse effects. For patients living with their families, family therapy aimed at reducing the number of critical comments, and improving the family's knowledge of the disorder, can reduce the relapse rate.

Long-term treatment of patients who do not fully recover from an acute episode

The general aims of treatment are similar to those for patients who recover in hospital, but more attention has to be given to the social aspects of care.

The main approach to management is based on a systematic assessment of the patient's medical and social needs. Patients with schizophrenia who do not fully recover may have multiple social needs (e.g. housing and occupation), which are best met by a multidisciplinary team (see p. 91). A **care plan** should be developed in which the problems are listed with the interventions proposed.

In caring for patients with chronic schizophrenia, an experienced community psychiatric nurse is often one of the key professionals. The roles of the community nurse include:

- acting as key worker responsible for coordinating the care plan;
- monitoring the mental state;
- administering depot neuroleptic medication;
- monitoring compliance with medication and the presence of side effects;
- arranging or carrying out specific behavioural and psychological interventions;
- education and support of the patient and relatives;
- liaison with other care workers.

Drug therapy

Continuation therapy reduces the risk of relapse. Since adherence to medication is often poor, intramuscular depot injections are often used instead of oral medication. There are two main problems. First, 20 per cent of patients remain well without drugs and secondly, long-term conventional antipsychotic medication leads to persistent tardive dyskinesia in 15 per cent of subjects after four years of treatment. Therefore, if all patients receive continuation treatment, some will be exposed unnecessarily to the risk of developing side effects. Unfortunately, it is not possible to predict which patients will benefit from continuing drug treatment. The clinician and patient therefore need to work together to judge the benefit of continuation treatment by reducing the drugs cautiously when the patient has been free from symptoms for several months. Patients taking long-term continuation therapy should be assessed every 6 months for signs of tardive dyskinesia, weight gain, and hyperglycaemia (see pp. 116–118).

Although anticholinergic drugs reduce parkinsonian side effects, they may increase the likelihood of dyskinesia. They should not be prescribed routinely but only if there are extrapyramidal side effects that cannot be avoided by adjusting the dose of antipsychotic drug.

Family therapy

Family psychoeducation aimed at reducing emotional involvement and criticism has been shown to reduce the rate of relapse in schizophrenic patients living with their families.

Treatment of associated depressive symptoms

Depressive symptoms in schizophrenia are common and may need specific treatment.

Antidepressants

When depressive symptoms are severe, antidepressant medication may be used although there is uncertainty about how efficacious antidepressants are in schizophrenia. Antidepressants are also indicated in schizoaffective disorder.

Lithium

Lithium may be beneficial for schizoaffective disorders, especially when there is a mixture of schizophrenic and manic symptoms (see pp. 123–126).

Psychosocial care and rehabilitation

The main aim of psychosocial care and rehabilitation is to reduce the long-term disability experienced by many patients with schizophrenia. In practice, psychosocial care is usually tailored to the individual patient needs. Skill is required to arrange a care plan which is optimally stimulating but not too stressful. The approach is a general one including supportive care from community nurses and others. There is only limited evidence for the effectiveness of specific methods that include:

Social skills training. Social skills training uses a behavioural approach to help patients to improve interpersonal, self-care, and coping skills needed in normal life.

Employment training. This includes a range of activities from help in developing the skills necessary to obtain and hold down a job, to the provision of sheltered employment or other occupational activities.

Cognitive remediation. Cognitive remediation therapy aims to help the neuropsychological impairments that are often associated with schizophrenia and, hence, improve psychosocial functioning.

Management of schizophrenia in primary care

In general, acute psychotic episodes should be dealt with by the specialist services because a successful outcome often needs multidisciplinary teamwork and/or admission to hospital.

After the acute episode, general practitioners provide the majority of care for up to 25 per cent of schizophrenic patients. As well as requiring care for their psychiatric disorder, schizophrenic patients are at increased risk of physical illness, particularly heart disease and metabolic problems. This is likely to be due to both increased exposure to risk factors such as smoking and also secondary to antipsychotic drugs, which are known to increase weight and blood glucose. The importance of this co-morbidity is increased because there is evidence that people with schizophrenia receive poorer treatment for physical illness.

To improve the care of schizophrenic patients in the community:

1 Hospital catchment areas should be based on primary care practices rather than administrative boundaries.

2 Psychiatrists and general practitioners should work closely together.

3 Responsibilities of the specialist and primary care teams should be defined clearly for both mental healthcare and management of physical illnesses.

4 Clear and consistent advice should be provided to patients and carers about diagnosis, treatment, and prognosis.

5 The training of general practitioners and psychiatrists in the care of these patients should be linked.

Management of aggressive behaviour in patients with schizophrenia

Overactivity and disturbances of behaviour are common in schizophrenia. There is an increased risk of violence to others, although this remains uncommon, and homicide is very rare. The risk of violence to others should be assessed in all cases; it is greater when there are delusions of control, persecutory delusions, or auditory hallucinations.

Threats of violence should be taken seriously, especially if there is a history of such behaviour in the past, whether or not the patient was ill at the time. The danger usually resolves as acute symptoms are brought under control, but a few patients pose a continuing threat and require regular, close supervision.

Treatment for a potentially violent patient is the same as for any other schizophrenic patient, although a compulsory order is more likely to be needed. While medication is often needed to bring disturbed behaviour under immediate control, much can be done by providing a calm, reassuring, and consistent environment in which provocation is avoided. A hospital with a special area with an adequate number of experienced staff is usually able to rely less on the use of large doses of medication.

■ Delusional syndromes

Delusional disorder

Delusional disorder is a chronic and unshakeable delusional system, developing insidiously in a person in middle or late life. The delusional system is encapsulated, and other mental functions are normal. The patient can often work and maintain a reasonable social life. Disorders conforming strictly to this definition are rare; most eventually turn out to be an early stage of schizophrenia.

Specific delusional syndromes

The remaining delusional syndromes can be divided into two groups: those with special kinds of symptoms, and those occurring in particular situations. Of the first group, only pathological jealousy is described, and of the second group, only induced psychoses are described.

Pathological jealousy

In pathological (or morbid) jealousy, the essential feature is an abnormal belief that the sexual partner is unfaithful. The condition is called 'pathological' because the belief, which may be an overvalued idea or a delusion, is held on inadequate grounds and is unaffected by rational argument. Jealousy is not classified as pathological because of strong feelings of jealousy or a violent response to a lover's infidelity; the condition is classified as pathological when the jealousy is based on unsound reasoning. Various other terms have been given to the syndrome, including sexual jealousy, erotic jealousy, morbid jealousy, psychotic jealousy, and the Othello syndrome.

Clinical features

Pathological jealousy is more common in men than women. The main feature is an abnormal belief in the partner's infidelity. This belief may be accompanied by other abnormal beliefs, for example that the partner is plotting against the patient. The mood is variable and includes misery, apprehension, irritability, and anger.

Commonly, there is intensive seeking for evidence of the partner's infidelity; for example, by searching in diaries and correspondence, and by examining bed linen and underwear for signs of sexual secretions. The patient may follow the partner about, or engage a private detective. Typically, the jealous person cross-questions the partner incessantly. This may lead to violent quarrelling and paroxysms of rage in the patient, and sometimes to a dangerous assault or murder. The partner may become worn out and even make a false confession in an attempt at pacification.

Aetiology

Pathological jealousy may be secondary to other psychiatric disorders, including schizophrenia, depressive disorder, alcoholism, and organic disorder. Pathological jealousy can also arise from a personality disorder, in which the person has a pervasive sense of his own inadequacy, and a vulnerability to anything that might increase this sense of inadequacy, such as loss of status. In the face of such threats, the person may project blame on to the partner, in the form of jealous accusations.

Prognosis

The prognosis is difficult to predict but generally poor, depending on the prognosis of any underlying psychiatric disorder, and on the patient's personality.

Assessment

Because of the risk of violence, the assessment of a patient with pathological jealousy should be particularly thorough, and specialist psychiatric advice is necessary. The partner should be seen alone to allow a much more detailed account of the patient's morbid beliefs and actions than may be elicited from the patient. In general practice, the partner may be the first person to seek help. The doctor should try to find out tactfully:

- the strength of the jealous person's belief in the partner's infidelity;
- the amount of resentment, and whether vengeful action has been contemplated;
- provoking factors for outbursts of resentment, accusation, or cross-questioning;
- the partner's response to such outbursts from the patient—an angry response may inflame the problem;
- the patient's response to the partner's behaviour;
- whether there has been any violence and if so, how it was inflicted, and whether there was any injury;
- further points about assessment of risk are described on p. 74.

In addition to these specific enquiries, the doctor should take a relationship and sexual history from both partners. It is also important to seek any evidence of an underlying psychiatric disorder (see Aetiology, above) as this will have important implications for treatment.

Treatment

The treatment of pathological jealousy is often difficult, because the jealous person is usually uncooperative. Specialist advice is usually needed. If there is a primary disorder (see above), it should be treated. If no primary disorder is identified, an antipsychotic drug, such as trifluoperazine or chlorpromazine, given in the dosage used for schizophrenia, may reduce the intensity of the jealous beliefs and the emotional disturbance.

Open discussion of the problem may help by reducing emotional tension. The partner should be encouraged to behave in ways that least provoke the patient's jealousy, avoiding argument and aggressive responses to the patient's questions.

If there is no response to such treatment, or if the risk of violence is high from the beginning, inpatient care may be necessary for the jealous patient. The doctor should warn the partner if there is a risk of serious violence.

If treatment fails, it may be necessary to advise temporary or lasting separation to protect the partner.

Induced psychosis (folie à deux)

An induced psychosis is a paranoid delusional system that develops in a healthy person who is in a close relationship with another person, usually a relative, who has an established, similar delusional system. The delusions are nearly always persecutory.

Induced psychosis is more frequent in women than in men. Before the induced psychosis appears, the person with the fixed delusional state has usually been dominant in the relationship, while the other person (who later develops the induced psychosis) has often been dependent and suggestible. Generally, the two have lived together for a long time in close intimacy, often cut off from the outside world. Once established, the condition persists until the two people are separated, when it usually improves gradually. This occurs sometimes without treatment but more often antipsychotic medication is required.

 Further reading

Harrison, P. J. & Weinberger, D. (2010). *Schizophrenia*, 3rd edn. Oxford University Press, Oxford. A comprehensive and definitive textbook covering aetiology, diagnosis, treatment, and prognosis.

National Collaborating Centre for Mental Health (2010). *Core Interventions in the Treatment and Management of*

Schizophrenia in Adults in Primary and Secondary Care, updated edition. British Psychological Society and Royal College of Psychiatrists, London.

Reactions to stressful experiences

In biological terms, stress literally means *a force from the outside world acting upon an individual,* and is a phenomenon we have all experienced. The term 'stress' was first used in the 1930s by the endocrinologist Hans Selye to describe the responses of laboratory animals to various stimuli. Originally Selye meant 'stress' to be the response of an organism to a perceived threat or 'stressor', but the term is now used to mean the stimulus rather than the response. When presented with a stressor of any type, everyone will produce a reaction to that stress, and this is a normal physiological event. However, if the reaction is prolonged, too intense, or atypical in some way, stress can become abnormal and cause problems.

Stressful events, even when reacted to normally, are important contributors to the causes of many kinds of psychiatric disorder. In this chapter we consider those psychiatric disorders that are specific reactions to stressful experiences. These include:

- disorders starting and ending very soon after stressful events (**acute stress disorder**);
- disorders following exceptionally severe stress (**post-traumatic stress disorder**);
- disorders occurring after a change in the circumstances of life (**adjustment disorders**);
- the normal and abnormal responses to bereavement (**grief reactions**).

There are also a variety of special types of acute stress to which people may react in a specific way (e.g. war, natural disasters). These are not individually named psychiatric conditions in their own right, and often patients will fit the criteria for one of the above disorders, but they are mentioned to highlight particular risks or management issues.

General practitioners encounter the vast majority of patients with stress disorders who present to the health services, but *all* clinicians will see these patients in their clinical specialties. The reasons for this are threefold:

1 acute physical illness and its treatment are stressful;

2 chronic illness or disability can result in substantial changes in life circumstances;

3 clinicians treat people involved in other kinds of stressful experiences.

Throughout the chapter, it is important to remember that the specific stress disorders described are not the only reactions to stressful events. Exceptionally severe stress or changes in life circumstances are also followed by anxiety and depressive disorders; indeed after road accidents, anxiety disorders are almost as frequent as post-traumatic stress disorder. These are discussed more fully in Chapters 21 and 24.

What is a stressful event?

Everyone reacts to stress differently, and what constitutes a stressful event is therefore a subjective matter. However, there are certain situations that are highly likely to be experienced as stressful by anyone. The Holmes and Rahe Stress Scale is a list of 43 life events which predispose to stress-related illnesses, weighted according to their respective probability of doing so. The list was compiled by asking a large sample of Americans which life circumstances or events they found stressful, and then giving them a ranking according to how difficult they were to adjust to. Table 23.1 shows a selection of these 43 life events.

■ The normal response to stressful events

The normal stress response has three components:

1 a somatic 'fight or flight' response;

2 an emotional response;

3 a psychological response that aims to reduce the potential impact of the experience and help to cope with the situation at hand.

The somatic response

Human physiology has evolved a variety of mechanisms to deal with perceived threats. The core components of

Table 23.1 Excerpt from life events table

Life event	Stress ranking*
Death of a spouse	100
Divorce	73
Marital separation	65
Imprisonment	63
Death of a close family member	63
Personal injury or illness	53
Marriage	50
Dismissal from work	47
Pregnancy	40
Child leaving home	29
Beginning or ending school	26
Change in residence	20
Minor mortgage or loan	17
Vacation	13
Christmas	12

* This is a rating where 100 is the most stressful event recorded, with relatively less stressful situations having progressively lower values. From Holmes, T. & Rahe, R. (1967). The Social Readjustment Rating Scale. *Journal of Psychosomatic Research* **11**: 213–18.

the stress response are the sympathetic nervous system and hypothalamic–pituitary–adrenal (HPA) axis. When a threatening situation occurs, the sympathetic nervous system is activated, releasing epinephrine (adrenaline) from the adrenal medulla. Epinephrine then causes the fight or flight response, which activates the body ready to flee from or deal with a threat. Both stress itself and firing of the locus coeruleus (pons) activate the HPA axis, which leads to release of glucocorticoids from the adrenal cortex. These two pathways alter the body to deal with a threat, and are outlined in Figure 23.1.

Emotional responses

Emotional responses to stressful events are of three kinds: the response to danger, the response to a threat, and the response to separation and loss.

- The response to danger is **fear.**
- The response to a threat is **anxiety.**
- The response to separation or loss is **depression**.

Typically the first two stresses are accompanied by sympathetic nervous system arousal as outlined above, whilst the latter leads to reduced physical activity.

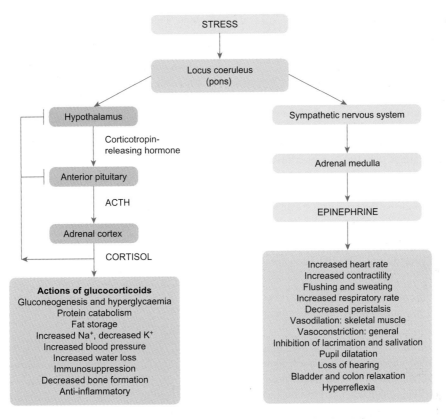

Fig. 23.1 The physiological response to stress. ACTH, adrenocorticotropic hormone.

Psychological changes that reduce the impact of stressful events

Difficulty in recall and numbing

People who have experienced stressful circumstances tend to have **difficulty in recalling** the details of the experiences. They may also experience an unexpected absence of feeling about the events (**numbing**). Freud suggested that both these responses are caused by an active but unconscious mental process, which he called **repression**.

Coping strategies

People cope with anxiety in a variety of ways. Their actions are of two kinds (Table 23.2): adaptive strategies, which reduce distress in both the short and long term, and maladaptive strategies, which are effective in the short term but lead to difficulties in the longer term.

Adaptive coping strategies include the avoidance of situations that cause distress, working through problems, and coming to terms with situations. Avoidance ceases to be adaptive when it is continued for so long that it prevents working through and coming to terms with the situation.

Table 23.2 Strategies for coping with stressful experiences

Potentially adaptive	Maladaptive
Avoidance	Excessive use of alcohol or drugs
Working through problems	Histrionic or aggressive behaviour
Coming to terms with situations	Deliberate self-harm

Maladaptive coping strategies include the excessive use of alcohol or drugs, discharging emotion through histrionic or aggressive behaviour, and deliberate self-harm. Avoidance that is at first adaptive becomes maladaptive if it is continued for too long, since this interferes with other adaptive responses.

Culturally determined coping strategies. In some cultures, open displays of extreme distress are a socially accepted and adaptive means of discharging emotion, for example, after the sudden death of a loved one. In cultures where such displays are not the norm, they may be maladaptive because they seem excessive and thereby lose the sympathy of potential helpers.

■ Acute stress disorder (acute stress reaction in ICD-10)

Acute stress disorder is *an abnormal reaction to sudden stressful events*. The basic response of the body is the same as in the normal stress reaction, but the symptoms are more severe and last for a longer period. It is generally accepted that having symptoms after a stressful event is normal for up to about 48 hours, but after this point the majority of people will have recovered. Table 23.3 shows the typical symptoms seen in acute stress disorder, but there are a few points that deserve further explanation.

1 **The emotional response** includes intense anxiety, restlessness, purposeless activity, insomnia, and panic attacks. Some patients experience depersonalization and derealization.

2 **Somatic symptoms** reflect the sympathetic activation (Figure 23.1); the most common are sweating, palpitations, and tremor.

3 **Dissociative symptoms.** This term is used to describe numbing and difficulty in recall, which are experienced as the feeling that the events have not really taken place, emotional numbing, being 'in a daze', and the inability to remember important aspects of the stressful events. The term **flashbacks** is applied to sudden and repeated re-experiencing of visual images of traumatic experiences, which usually cannot be recalled easily at other times. There may also be recurrent frightening **dreams** of these events.

4 **Coping strategies** include **avoidance** of reminders of the stressful events, and of talking or thinking about them. Social contacts may also be avoided, thus depriving the person of potential sources of support. **Maladaptive coping** responses include 'flight' (e.g. running away from the scene of a road accident), the release of emotion through histrionic or aggressive behaviour, excessive use of alcohol, or deliberate self-harm.

By definition, acute stress disorder lasts no more than 4 weeks. Cases that last longer are described as post-traumatic stress disorder. The diagnostic criteria are shown in Box 23.1.

Prevalence

Given the variety of experiences that can cause acute stress disorder, it is hard to be specific about the proportion of people who develop an abnormal reaction to a stressful event. However, there is good evidence that 13 to 14 per cent of road traffic accident survivors and 19 per cent of assault victims show reactions fitting diagnostic criteria. The highest values recorded are for witnesses of mass shootings, where one-third of people develop an acute stress reaction.

Co-morbidity

The most common co-morbidities in acute stress disorder patients are depression and substance misuse. People who have a psychiatric history, have had previous abnormal stress reactions, and suffer repeated traumatic events are at higher risk of an acute stress reaction.

Differential diagnosis

Post-traumatic stress disorder (PTSD). In DSM-IV, an acute stress disorder becomes PTSD when symptoms last for more than 4 weeks. Under ICD-10 criteria, PTSD is considered an alternative diagnosis to acute stress reaction. It requires an 'exceptionally threatening or catastrophic event', and symptoms to begin within 6 months of the event.

Adjustment disorder. This diagnosis refers to distress considered out of proportion to the severity of the stressor, and may be caused by any stressful event (i.e. it does not have to be an actual or perceived threat to life). The symptoms are more generalized, and usually less severe.

Table 23.3 Symptoms of acute stress disorder and post-traumatic stress disorder

Increased arousal
- Anxiety and panic attacks
- Restlessness, impaired concentration, and purposeless activity
- Irritability, depression, anger, or despair
- Insomnia

'Dissociative' symptoms
- Emotional numbness and 'being in a daze'
- Reduced awareness of surroundings
- Difficulty in recall of the stressful events
- Depersonalization and derealization

'Re-experiencing' symptoms
- Flashbacks
- Recurrent images or thoughts
- Disturbing dreams

Avoidance of reminders of the stressful events

Maladaptive coping strategies

Acute stress disorder is diagnosed when symptoms last from 2 days up to 4 weeks

Post-traumatic stress disorder is diagnosed when symptoms last for 4 weeks or longer

BOX 23.1 DSM-IV diagnostic criteria for acute stress disorder

A Exposure to a traumatic event in which the following were present:

1 actual or threatened death or serious injury, or a threat to the physical integrity of self or others;

2 the person's response involved intense fear, help-lessness, or horror.

B Due to the distressing event, the individual has at least three of the following dissociative symptoms:

1 a subjective sense of numbing, detachment, or absence of emotional responsiveness;

2 a reduction in awareness of his or her surroundings;

3 derealization;

4 depersonalization;

5 dissociative amnesia.

C The traumatic event is persistently re-experienced through recurrent images, thoughts, dreams, illusions, flashback episodes, or a sense of reliving the experience.

D Marked avoidance of stimuli that arouse recollections of the trauma.

E Marked symptoms of anxiety or increased arousal.

F The disturbance causes clinically significant distress.

G The disturbance lasts for a minimum of 2 days and a maximum of 4 weeks and occurs within 4 weeks of the traumatic event.

H The disturbance is not due to the direct physiological effects of a substance or a general medical condition, is not better accounted for by Brief Psychotic Disorder, and is not merely an exacerbation of a pre-existing Axis I or Axis II disorder.

ICD-10 F43.0 acute stress reaction

The main differences between the two classifications are:

- The symptoms must start within 1 hour of the stressor.

- Symptoms should begin to diminish within 48 hours.

- The clinical picture should change over time, with no one symptom lasting more than a few hours.

Brief psychotic disorder. The presence of hallucinations, delusions, disorganized speech, or grossly abnormal behaviour points to a psychotic disorder.

Dissociative disorders. These involve the presence of dissociative symptoms in the absence of a stressor.

Organic disorder. A head injury or space-occupying lesion in the brain can sometimes cause similar symptoms to acute stress disorder. History of a head injury, headaches, or the finding of neurological signs should raise suspicion, and appropriate imaging should be requested.

Aetiology

Many kinds of highly stressful event can provoke an acute stress disorder, for example involvement in an accident or fire, physical assault, or rape. Since the stress response does not become abnormal in everyone exposed to the same events, there must be some kind of personal predisposition, but it is not known what this is. Acute stress disorder can occur among bystanders as well as those directly involved, and among those involved in rescuing or caring for others.

Psychological theories. A variety of psychological mechanisms are probably at work in acute stress disorder, but dissociation is the most studied. It is thought that dissociation reduces the negative consequences of trauma by restricting awareness of the event and thereby preventing the person from being overwhelmed by the traumatic experience. Unfortunately, this prevents recovery as it does not allow the experience to be processed and integrated into existing coping mechanisms. A similar problem occurs when a person uses avoidance strategies excessively.

Biological theories. The main theory is based upon classical conditioning. When a traumatic event occurs (an unconditioned stimulus), people respond with fear (unconditioned response). As reminders of the trauma occur (conditioned stimulus), people then respond with fear reactions (conditioned response). It is thought that in some people, the stress response becomes sensitized to repeated stimuli, and a larger response is produced to each stimulus. Those people who suffer a panic attack during a traumatic event are very likely to experience increasing panic attacks in the few weeks afterwards.

Prognosis

In the DSM-IV, an acute stress disorder will either remit or become PTSD. It is currently unknown what proportion of patients with an acute stress disorder go on to develop PTSD, but one prospective study of road traffic accident survivors produced a figure of 50 to 60 per cent. However, this figures halves if only patients without dissociative symptoms are included.

Management

Most acute stress disorders can be managed by the family doctor, and only the most severe need treatment by a specialist. An outline of treatment strategies is shown in Table 23.4.

General measures

Provide emotional support. Usually the person can be comforted effectively by relatives or friends, and can talk to them about the stressful experience. If no close friend or relative is available, or if the response is severe, comfort may be offered by a healthcare professional. It is important to explain the course and prognosis of an acute stress disorder.

Provide practical support. The period after a traumatic event is usually very busy and confusing. The person involved will need advice regarding police procedures, support in obtaining medical care, help with insurance claims, assistance with dealing with the media, and help with domestic tasks.

Help with residual problems. Sometimes an acutely stressful situation results in lasting adversity to which the person has to adjust; for example, a serious car accident may lead to permanent disability. When this happens the treatment of an acute reaction should be followed by help in readjustment.

Psychological treatments

Encourage recall. As anxiety is reduced, the person is usually able to recall and come to terms with the experience. When memories of the events remain fragmented, help may be needed to remember the events and integrate them into memory.

Develop more effective coping strategies. As explained above, in a time of crisis some people will use maladaptive coping strategies such as using substances. It is important to try and help them develop more productive strategies—for example, provide a supportive atmosphere for working through problems, and encourage recall of events. Specific counselling is available in these situations and is called **crisis intervention**.

Debriefing. Until recently, a type of counselling known as debriefing was often made widely available after stressful events. The aim was to promote adaptation to the traumatic event, and it was usually given within 24 to 72 hours of the trauma. Subjects *talked* about the stressful events and were encouraged to express their thoughts and feelings at the time and since. However, despite the widespread routine use of debriefing, there was little good-quality evidence as to its efficacy. A Cochrane review of randomized controlled trials found that whilst the majority of people said they found the counselling useful, it did not reduce the proportion of patients developing PTSD. The authors concluded that compulsory debriefing of the victims of trauma should cease. UK guidance is now that debriefing should not be routinely offered to patients.

Cognitive behavioural therapy. CBT differs from debriefing crucially in its emphasis on integrating recovered memories with existing ones, and on self-help. Evidence suggests the most effective strategy is a brief intervention, typically five sessions of individual therapy. Studies vary in their results but on average CBT reduces the proportion of people developing PTSD by 20–50 per cent.

Pharmacological treatments

There has been very little research done on to which pharmacological interventions are effective in acute stress disorder.

Anxiolytics. A short course (3–5 days) of a benzodiazepine may be indicated in patients with a high level of anxiety immediately after the event. Occasionally, insomnia is severe, and a hypnotic drug (e.g. temazepam) should be given, but again only for a short period to avoid the development of tolerance and dependence.

Antidepressants. SSRIs are the most effective drug treatment for PTSD. Consider prescribing an SSRI if the symptoms continue to be severe, there is evidence of depression, or the patient is too unwell to engage in psychological therapy. It is also an option for those patients who fail to improve after CBT.

Prolonged reactions to stress

Prolonged reactions typically follow exposure to extremely stressful events including *natural disasters* such as earthquakes, *man-made calamities* such as major fires, serious accidents, and the circumstances of *war*, and serious physical *assault* or *rape*. Of these, the most frequent are road traffic accidents, and physical and sexual assault. Not all of those involved even in the most

Table 23.4 Treatment of acute reactions to stressful experiences

General measures
- Provide emotional support
- Provide practical support
- Help with residual problems

Psychological treatments
- Encourage recall of, and coming to terms with, the events
- Help with more effective coping
- Cognitive behavioural therapy

Pharmacological treatments
- Short-term anxiolytics
- Antidepressants

severe events develop a prolonged reaction; many recover within the month that is the arbitrary limit for acute stress disorder. The most frequent *long-term consequences* of stressful events are post-traumatic stress disorder, phobic disorder, and depressive disorders.

■ Post-traumatic stress disorder

Post-traumatic stress disorder (PTSD) is severe psychological disturbance following a traumatic event, characterized by the involuntary re-experiencing of the event combined with symptoms of hyperarousal, dissociation, and avoidance. It has been known for centuries that severe trauma can lead to psychological problems, but the first clinical descriptions of the syndrome were not published until the horrors of the World Wars and Holocaust forced the issue into mainstream practice. A variety of terms have been used to describe what we now call PTSD, including **railway spine, stress syndrome, shell shock, battle fatigue,** and **traumatic war neurosis.** Our modern understanding of PTSD began in the 1970s, when studies were undertaken in the forces that fought in the Vietnam War.

It is now recognized that PTSD is a relatively common disorder, with US citizens having a lifetime risk of developing the condition of 8 per cent. Effective treatments are available for PTSD, so it is an important condition to screen high-risk patients for, especially those who are being treated for physical injuries/diseases relating to the trauma.

What makes a stressful event traumatic?

As discussed in the introduction, stress is a subjective experience, which makes it hard to generalize as to the severity of a given situation. The DSM-III classification suggested that for a stressor to be called traumatic it must be outside the range of usual human experience *and* markedly distressing to almost anyone. However, this would discount relatively common events (e.g. road traffic accidents, divorce) as being traumatic, which is obviously not the case. The DSM-IV description was therefore much broader (Box 23.2). The ICD-10 classification gives a more general definition: '*a stressful event or situation ... of an exceptionally threatening or catastrophic nature ... which is likely to cause pervasive distress in almost anyone*'. This is probably the most useful working definition.

Clinical features

The symptoms of post-traumatic stress disorder are the same as those of acute stress disorder (Table 23.3), but they last for longer. The essential differences are that symptoms have *lasted for more than 4 weeks* and **dissociative symptoms** must be present. The reason for this change of diagnosis after 4 weeks is that cases lasting for more than this period generally run a chronic course and require rather different treatment from that used for acute stress disorder. As explained above, there are a number of characteristic features.

1 **Symptoms of increased arousal,** such as severe anxiety, irritability, insomnia, and poor concentration. There may be panic attacks and, occasionally, episodes of aggression. Anxiety increases further during flashbacks or reminders of the traumatic event.

2 **Avoidance and 'dissociative' symptoms,** such as difficulty in recalling the events at will, detachment, an inability to feel emotion ('numbness'), and a diminished interest in activities. There is avoidance of reminders of the events and sometimes there is depersonalization and derealization.

3 **Intrusions** in which memories of the traumatic events appear suddenly as repeated intense imagery ('flashbacks'), vivid memories, intrusive repetitive thoughts, or distressing dreams.

4 **Depressive symptoms** are common, and survivors of a major disaster often feel guilt.

5 **Maladaptive coping responses** include persistent anger (especially among those who believe they are innocent victims of others' misbehaviour), excessive use of alcohol or drugs, and episodes of deliberate self-harm, some of which end in suicide.

The full diagnostic criteria are shown in Box 23.2.

Prevalence

The US National Comorbidity Study found that 50 to 60 per cent of individuals experience at least one traumatic event (fitting DSM-IV criteria) in their lifetime. The most commonly experienced traumatic events are sudden death of a loved one, witnessing someone being killed or severely injured, accidents, and being involved in a fire. However, most of those affected by traumatic events do not develop PTSD. After a traumatic event of any type, the risk of developing PTSD is 8 per cent for men and 20 per cent for women.

The prevalence and incidence of PTSD vary markedly depending upon the geographical area studied. Socioeconomic conditions, natural disasters, wars, and violence are not equally distributed across the world, and most of the current epidemiological figures relate to economically more developed countries. In the USA, 7.8 per cent of the population will suffer PTSD at some point in their lives, but the risk is twice as great for women (10 per cent) as for men (5 per cent). The 1-year prevalence is 1 to 3 per cent.

BOX 23.2 DSM-IV diagnostic criteria for post-traumatic stress disorder

A The person has been exposed to a traumatic event in which the following were present:

  1 The person experienced, witnessed, or was confronted with an event or events that involved actual or threatened death or serious injury.

  2 The person's response involved intense fear, helplessness, or horror.

B The traumatic event is persistently re-experienced in at least one of the following ways:

  1 recurrent and intrusive distressing recollections of the event;

  2 recurrent distressing dreams of the event;

  3 acting or feeling as if the traumatic event were recurring;

  4 intense psychological distress at exposure to internal or external cues that symbolize or resemble an aspect of the traumatic event;

  5 physiological reactivity on exposure to internal or external cues that symbolize or resemble an aspect of the traumatic event.

C Persistent avoidance of stimuli associated with the trauma and numbing of general responsiveness, as indicated by three (or more) of the following:

  1 efforts to avoid thoughts, feelings, or conversations associated with the trauma;

  2 efforts to avoid activities, places, or people that arouse recollections of the trauma;

  3 inability to recall an important aspect of the trauma;

  4 markedly diminished interest or participation in significant activities;

  5 a feeling of detachment or estrangement from others;

  6 restricted range of affect;

  7 a sense of a foreshortened future.

D Persistent symptoms of increased arousal as indicated by two (or more) of the following: difficulty falling or staying asleep, irritability or outbursts of anger, difficulty concentrating, hypervigilance, or exaggerated startle response.

E Duration of the disturbance is more than 1 month.

F The disturbance causes clinically significant distress or impairment in social, occupational, or other important areas of functioning.
  Acute: if duration of symptoms is less than 3 months.
  Chronic: if duration of symptoms is 3 months or more.

ICD-10 F43.1 Post-traumatic stress disorder

The main differences are that the symptoms must occur within 6 months of the traumatic event (rather than being present for more than 4 weeks) and that the stressor criteria are as outlined in the text.

The types of trauma most likely to be associated with PTSD are:

- rape;
- exposure to combat during a war;
- sexual molestation (especially in childhood);
- being kidnapped or held hostage;
- having been a prisoner of war;
- Holocaust (and other genocide) survivors.

Co-morbidity

It is often difficult to determine if co-morbidities in patients with PTSD are primary disorders or secondary reactions to the traumatic event. The most common co-morbidities are depression, anxiety disorders, somatization, and alcohol or substance misuse. In the US National Comorbidity Study previously mentioned, 88 per cent of

patients with PTSD fitted the criteria for another psychiatric diagnosis.

Differential diagnosis

- **Acute stress disorder.** Symptoms have been present for less than 4 weeks.

- **Adjustment disorder.** This diagnosis refers to distress considered out of proportion to the severity of the stressor, and may be caused by any stressful event. The symptoms are more generalized, and usually less severe.

- **Depressive disorder.** Low mood, anhedonia, and lack of energy. Ask about biological symptoms and whether the symptoms pre-date the stressful event.

- **Anxiety disorder.** Usually the stressful event will not fit the criteria for being traumatic, and there will be no or few dissociative symptoms.

- **Obsessive-compulsive disorder.** Intrusive repetitive thoughts, dreams, and images are also found in OCD. The key is to identify rituals, and there should be resistance towards the obsessions and compulsions.

- **Brief psychotic disorder or schizophrenia.** The presence of hallucinations, delusions, disorganized speech, or grossly abnormal behaviour points to a psychotic disorder.
- **Dissociative disorders.** The presence of dissociative symptoms in the absence of an extreme stressor.
- **Substance-induced disorder.**

Aetiology

The necessary cause of post-traumatic stress disorder is an *exceptionally stressful event* in which the person was involved directly or as a witness. However, only a minority of those involved in the same event develop the disorder, and the reason for this is currently unknown. Post-traumatic stress disorder is more common among those involved most directly in the stressful events, but the variation in response is not accounted for solely by the *degree of personal involvement*. There are a variety of factors and theories surrounding the aetiology of PTSD, which are outlined in Table 23.5 and discussed further below.

Predisposing factors

1 **Genetics.** Twin studies have shown a higher concordance of PTSD amongst monozygotic than dizygotic twins. Studies of soldiers who fought in Vietnam also found that the risk of PTSD was significantly higher in those with affected first-degree relatives compared with other, non-related soldiers.

2 **Physiological reactions to stress.** Patients with PTSD appear to have greater physiological reactions to stressors than people without PTSD who experienced the same traumatic event. When stressed, patients show enhanced

Table 23.5 Aetiology of post-traumatic stress disorder

Predisposing factors	Precipitating factors	Maintaining factors
Genetics	Traumatic event	Conditioning theory
Enhanced physiological reactions to stress		Stimuli triggering memories of the event
Neuroanatomical abnormalities		Avoidance behaviours
		Maladaptive coping strategies
		Differing personal understanding of the event

secretion of epinephrine and corticotrophin-secreting hormone, although levels of cortisol are lower than usual. It seems that whilst the HPA axis is strongly stimulated, some abnormality occurs which enhances negative feedback. This may be an adaptation to reset the system in order to be able to respond quickly and strongly to new stressors. Neurotransmitters also seem to be deregulated; the adrenergic activity of the sympathetic nervous system is increased, whilst levels and activity of serotonin (5HT) are decreased. The fact that yohimbine (an alpha-receptor antagonist) provokes flashbacks whilst SSRIs decrease symptoms gives weight to this theory.

3 **Neuroanatomical abnormalities.** MRI studies have shown that adults with PTSD have a smaller hippocampus than the general population. Functional MRI has demonstrated that people with PTSD tend to show a heightened response to stress in the amygdala, hippocampus, and medial prefrontal cortex.

Maintaining factors

1 **Conditioning theory.** This theory suggests that the continued symptoms of PTSD are due to classical conditioning. When a traumatic event occurs (an unconditioned stimulus), people respond with fear (unconditioned response). As reminders of the trauma occur (conditioned stimulus), people then respond with fear reactions (conditioned response). It is thought that in some people, the stress response becomes sensitized to repeated stimuli, and a larger response is produced to each stimulus. Frequently, the variety of stimuli widens, thereby increasing the symptom load. Avoidance of stimuli reinforces the conditioning, as it leads to reduced discomfort in the absence of a stimulus.

2 **Differing personal understanding of the event.** People have widely different views as to why the same event occurred, or what the future holds because of it. Some individuals will shake off a traumatic experience as a one-off terrible event and move on. They tend to recover quickly. Patients with PTSD tend to have much more negative cognitions, often generalizing beyond the original event. Common examples are that the person starts to believe they were responsible for the accident that happened, or that nowhere is safe after being sexually assaulted. These negative cognitions reinforce themselves, similarly to those in patients with depression.

3 **Stimuli triggering memories of the event.** In a similar vein to the above, those patients who repeatedly come into contact with memories of the traumatic event tend to have symptoms for longer than those who do not. A good example of this is someone whose route to work passes the spot where a terrible car accident occurred.

4 **Behaviours that maintain symptoms.** Avoidance tends to stop people integrating the facts of the stressful

Science box 23.1 Is there a gene for stress?

When a group of people are exposed to the same stressor there is a wide range of individual response. In recent years, a variety of studies have been published looking for genetic predispositions to stress, especially for post-traumatic stress disorder (PTSD). One area of interest has been the glucocorticoid receptor (GR), which is a major regulator of HPA axis activity. In a cross-sectional study of 112 healthy people, Wust et al. demonstrated that three common polymorphisms of the GR were associated with differing responses to the standardized Trier Social Stress Test and a dexamethosone suppression test.[1] In particular, the patients with the Bcl1 polymorphism showed much lower cortisol and ACTH rises in response to stress than those with wild-type or N363S. A variety of other groups have replicated this work. Due to the negative feedback loop within the HPA axis, reduced functioning of the GR produces chronically increased cortisol levels. The GR is modulated by chaperone proteins, one of which is FKBP5. In 2008, Ising et al. demonstrated, using the Trier Social Stress Test, that in 64 healthy volunteers polymorphisms of the gene encoding FKBP5 lead to elevated cortisol levels.[2] Binder et al. have linked this work to PTSD.[3] They undertook a cross-sectional study of 900 non-psychiatric adult patients with a history of child abuse. The investigators interviewed each patient to determine the level of PTSD symptoms displayed and their genotype for FKBP5 polymorphisms. They found that the polymorphisms interacted with the level of child abuse experienced to predict the severity of PTSD symptoms. Those patients with polymorphisms showed enhanced GR sensitivity on a dexamethosone suppression test. It is therefore possible that people who have polymorphisms of GR or its chaperone proteins have both an elevated cortisol level when exposed to an acute stressor (e.g. child abuse), and abnormal sensitivity of the GR, which leads to long-term alterations to the HPA axis and affects the long-term consequences of the stressor.

It is likely that in the next decade, much more will be discovered about genetic predispositions to stress disorders, and hopefully this will be translated into ways to support those who are at risk of developing conditions such as PTSD.

1 Wust, S., Van Rossum, E. F., Federenko, I. S., et al. (2004). Common polymorphisms in the glucocorticoid receptor gene are associated with adrenocortical responses to psychosocial stress. *Journal of Clinical Endocrinology and Metabolism* **89**: 565–73.

2 Ising, M., Depping, A. M., Siebertz, A., et al. (2008). Polymorphisms in the FKBP5 gene region modulate recovery from psychosocial stress in healthy controls. *European Journal of Neuroscience* **28**: 389–98.

3 Binder, E. B., Bradley, R. G., Liu, W., et al. (2008). Association of FKBP5 polymorphisms and childhood abuse with risk of posttraumatic stress disorder symptoms in adults. *JAMA* **299**: 1291–305.

experience into their memory, so that they continue to be fearful of the symptoms and what happened. Safety behaviours (e.g. constantly checking the gas hob is off after a fire) prevent a return to normality, and cause an increase in PTSD symptoms. Maladaptive coping strategies tend to increase the feelings of numbness and separation from the event, and do not help the person to acknowledge what has happened and continue with their life.

Risk factors for post-traumatic stress disorder

These are shown in Table 23.6.

Course and prognosis

The majority of patients with PTSD will recover within 1 year of the traumatic event, but about 30 per cent will have symptoms for many years. Predictors of a poor long-term outcome include a history of multiple stressors, severe symptoms, and poor social support.

Table 23.6 Factors associated with developing post-traumatic stress disorder

Biological
Females
Age: children and older adults are particularly vulnerable
Ethnic minorities
Family or personal psychiatric disorder
Low intelligence
Psychological
Childhood abuse
Low self-esteem
Exposure to previous trauma
Social
Lack of social support
Difficult economic or legal circumstances

Assessment

A full psychiatric history should be taken, including information from the patient, a third-party informant, primary care physician, and previous hospital notes. Specific points to cover include:

- the nature and severity of the stressful event;
- current symptoms, including duration and severity;
- effect of symptoms upon life at home, work, school, etc.;
- the patient's beliefs about the nature of their condition;
- previous diagnoses of psychiatric conditions and treatments received for them;
- family history of psychiatric conditions;
- current medications (prescribed, illicit, over-the-counter, alcohol, caffeine, nicotine);
- premorbid personality traits;
- current social situation: accommodation, employment, finances.

It is important to exclude depressive disorder, and to start treatment for depression if it is present.

A risk assessment should be carried out (see p. 61), focusing specifically upon risk of self-harm.

Psychological evaluation should include use of standard scales for mood disorders (e.g. Beck Depression Index, Hospital Anxiety and Depression Scale) and assess the impact of symptoms on social and occupational functioning. Special scales for PTSD are available, but are not widely used. A physical examination should be undertaken, and baseline laboratory tests ordered as seems appropriate. If the traumatic event has included injury to the head (e.g. from an assault or a road accident), a neurological examination should be carried out to exclude an injury to the brain.

Because patients who have prolonged reactions to stress may engage in litigation, it is important to record the assessment fully.

Treatment

The National Institute of Health and Clinical Excellence (NICE) published guidance in 2005 regarding the management of PTSD. The treatment options below are based on this guidance, but the basic principles remain suitable for those working internationally. An outline of treatment is shown in Table 23.7.

Early interventions

Offer practical support and information. After any traumatic stressor, it is important to offer the patient emotional support, advice about adjusting to any new life circum-

Table 23.7 Treatment of post-traumatic stress disorder

General measures

- Provide support (practical, emotional, social, self-help materials)
- Information and education about PTSD
- Help with associated guilt, grief, or anger

Psychological

- Watchful waiting (symptoms for less than 4 weeks)
- Trauma-focused cognitive behavioural therapy
- Eye movement desensitization and reprocessing

Pharmacological

- Short-term hypnotics
- Antidepressants

stances, information about PTSD, and practical support. Leaflets and self-help materials are widely available.

Encourage talking about the event to friends and family, and finding ways to understand what has happened. This helps to integrate memories of the event with the rest of the person's experience and to find a way for them to continue with their life.

Psychological treatments

For patients presenting with symptoms that are severe or have persisted for 3 months after the trauma, psychological therapy should be offered. Occasionally, patients may have severe disabling symptoms soon after the event, and they should be offered psychological therapy too. There are two main types of therapy that are effective at reducing the symptoms of PTSD:

1 trauma-focused cognitive behavioural therapy (CBT);

2 eye movement desensitization and reprocessing (EMDR).

CBT is the first-line choice, and should be offered to all patients with PTSD. EMDR should be reserved for the more severe cases or those that fail to have an adequate response to CBT. It is extremely important to reassure all patients that the symptoms they are experiencing are part of PTSD, and are not a sign that they are going crazy.

Trauma-focused CBT. Specialized CBT for PTSD includes both *exposure* and *cognitive therapy*. The exposure element involves helping the patient to remember and put together memories of the events, and to relive the stressor with an emphasis on discussing their thoughts and feelings during the process. *In vivo* exposure is also used, in which the patient gradually works up to confronting situations they had avoided because they reminded them of the trauma. Common examples include visiting the site of an attack, or driving again after an accident. It is thought that exposure works in two ways: getting the patient used to being in the situation again (habituation), and organizing their memories such that they can identify that intrusive re-experiences are recollections, and are not happening right now. Cognitive therapy helps the patient to identify disbeliefs that they have formed about the events. For example, a rape victim may believe they are to blame for the rape, or a hostage survivor feels guilty that they survived capture when others did not. Frequently, patients develop fears that are out of proportion to the actual threat, for example, believing using any form of transport is dangerous after a car accident. The therapist helps the person to challenge these beliefs and to change their behaviours surrounding them. A completed course of CBT reduces symptoms to a clinically insignificant level in 60 per cent of patients.

Eye movement desensitization and reprocessing (EMDR). This is another specialized treatment that assists the patient to process memories of the traumatic event and feel more positive about it. The patient is told to track the therapist's finger as they move it rapidly back and forth in front of them, which induces saccadic eye movements. During this process the patient is supposed to focus on a trauma-related image, and then afterwards to discuss the thoughts and emotions that surround it. This is repeated many times while focusing on different images. The treatment is more effective than placebo treatment but its success has not been shown to depend on the specific eye movement component.

Pharmacological therapies

Drugs should not be used as the first-line treatment, but should be reserved for those patients who are unable to undertake therapy, fail to improve with therapy, or have co-morbid depression.

Hypnotics. A short-term course of a hypnotic can be given for insomnia, especially in the immediate aftermath of a traumatic event. A maximum of 3 weeks should be prescribed due to the risks of tolerance and dependence. A good choice is a short-acting benzodiazepine (e.g. temazepam).

Antidepressants. Approximately 60 per cent of patients will respond to an SSRI, although more than one may need to be tried to eliminate symptoms altogether. The first-line choice in the UK should be an SSRI, and paroxetine has the greatest evidence base. Mirtazapine and amitriptyline can be tried if an SSRI is not successful, but they should be initiated by a psychiatrist. The drug should be continued for at least 12 months after symptoms resolve, then tapered slowly. If a patient does not respond to medication, check their compliance, increase the dose of the drug, or try another class. Occasionally, patients will need to add an atypical antipsychotic (e.g. olanzapine) to their antidepressant.

■ Reactions to special kinds of acute stress

Road traffic accidents

Road traffic accidents (RTAs) are very common all over the world, with approximately 3 million people being involved in one each year. Only about 1 per cent of RTAs lead to a fatality, but a serious injury occurs in 20 per cent. Studies have consistently shown that about 20 per cent of those involved suffer an acute stress disorder; this

---

 Case study 23.1 Post-traumatic stress disorder

A 38-year-old man, originally from Rwanda, presented to his GP complaining of poor sleep. On questioning, he revealed that he had fled Rwanda after witnessing his entire family being massacred during the genocide that took place during the latter part of the civil war. He had entered the UK as a refugee, and was now working in a supermarket and living alone in a rented bedsit. He described having terrifying dreams where visions of the genocide returned to him, and was so scared of them that it became difficult to get to sleep. He also had frequent flashbacks of the killing of his family, and that combined with poor concentration and apathy meant he had trouble keeping in employment. The GP explained that PTSD was the likely diagnosis, and provided the details of how to get self-help materials in the patient's first language. She then made a referral for CBT, which the patient initially attended for, but his English was poor and he found it very difficult to discuss what had happened. At this stage the GP referred him to a psychiatrist, who decided to prescribe fluoxetine, and recommended a group CBT programme. The patient did not take up the therapy, but over the next year improved sufficiently on the fluoxetine to socialize more and to increase his English skills. He was then able to undertake a course of individual CBT, and whilst the symptoms did not totally resolve, they became much less intrusive.

Science box 23.2 Post-traumatic stress disorder after treatment in intensive care

The massive growth in medical technology in the past few decades has led to the development of specialized intensive treatment units (ITUs) in most hospitals. Approximately 1.4 million patients in the USA (140 000 in the UK) experience a stay on ITU in any given year. Management frequently includes assisted ventilation, multiple access lines, artificial feeding, and virtually complete loss of patient autonomy in the treatment process. It is starting to be realized that this (often unexpected) experience during a critical illness is traumatic for many, and that there are commonly psychological consequences of being 'saved' by ITU. Recently a number of studies have been published investigating this association further.

Wallen *et al.* conducted a prospective cohort study to determine the prevalence of PTSD after an ITU stay.[1] They enrolled 114 consenting adult patients being treated on ITU, and examined them via a questionnaire soon after discharge, and again 1 month later. They found 14 per cent of patients to fit the diagnostic criteria for PTSD at the 1-month follow-up. Similarly, Cutherbertson *et al.* published a prospective cohort study of 78 patients, reporting a 3 month after discharge prevalence of PTSD of 13 per cent.[2] A systematic review of 15 cohorts published (including 1200 patients) found a median value of 22 per cent of patients meeting criteria for PTSD at 1–9 months after ITU discharge.[3] It is therefore clear that PTSD is a common sequela of an ITU stay.

What are the risk factors for developing PTSD after being on ITU? Many of the studies alluded to above have addressed this question. The strongest association with PTSD is found for females, age less than 65 years, those with a pre-ITU history of depression or anxiety, and patients treated with high doses of benzodiazepines whilst on ITU. Lesser risk factors include delirium or agitation whilst in ITU, use of physical restraints, and longer duration of mechanical ventilation. Interestingly, the type of critical illness precipitating admission to ITU does not seem to affect the risk of developing PTSD.

At time of writing, there are still many unanswered questions as to who gets PTSD after ITU, why this occurs, and how they should be treated. Larger cohort studies are needed, including longer follow-up periods. Hopefully, time will tell.

1 Wallen, K., Chaboyer, W., Thalib, L., *et al.* (2008). Symptoms of acute posttraumatic stress disorder after intensive care. *American Journal of Critical Care* **17**: 533–45.

2 Cuthbertson, B., Hull, A., Strachan, M., *et al.* (2004). Posttraumatic stress disorder after critical illness requiring intensive care. *Intensive Care Medicine* **30**: 450–5.

3 Davydow, D. S., Gifford, J. M., Desai, S. V., *et al.* (2008). Post-traumatic stress disorder in general intensive care unit survivors: a systematic review. *General Hospital Psychiatry* **30**: 421–34.

includes drivers, passengers, witnesses, and close family or friends. Three months after an RTA, one-third of those injured in an RTA report symptoms fitting criteria for psychiatric disorders, with the majority of these persisting to 1 year. The most frequent conditions are PTSD (23 per cent), a phobia of travel in vehicles (22 per cent), general anxiety (17 per cent), and depression (5 per cent). Treatment should follow the usual guidelines for the specific disorder, but consider specialized trauma-focused CBT if symptoms are severe.

Reactions to natural disasters and acts of terrorism

Disasters such as earthquakes, floods, and terrorist attacks often cause significant psychological sequelae in those who are involved for a variety of reasons.

- Large groups of people are exposed to a severely traumatic event at the same time.

- There is often a high mortality rate and many severe injuries.

- If a whole community is involved, there may be few unaffected people who can comfort and support the victims.

- Those involved often not only lose family and friends, but also their homes, livelihoods, and culture.

- It often takes months to years for communities to recover, and returning to the pre-disaster lifestyle is frequently almost impossible.

In the setting of a major disaster, organized teams of trained therapists can play a useful role alongside doctors dealing with the physical consequences of the disaster. In the past, it has been routine to offer formal debriefing to as many people as possible, but as explained under acute stress disorder (p. 268), this is now no longer recommended.

In 2004, an earthquake off the coast of Indonesia caused a series of devastating tsunamis along the borders of the Indian Ocean, killing about 225 000 people and destroying coastal communities. Studies of survivors have showed that approximately 25 per cent of those involved had symptoms of anxiety, depression, and/or PTSD 3 years after the event.

Reactions to the stresses of war and torture, and among refugees

The current diagnostic syndrome of PTSD was developed from data gathered in the aftermath of World War Two and the Vietnam War, and is therefore an atypical reaction to those who have served in war zones. However, it is important that other stress reactions, depression, and anxiety disorders are also common. Similar reactions may develop among civilians in war zones, refugees, and victims of torture—any of whom may have additional problems of bereavement, remorse for the suffering of others, and the experience of rape. Some experience feelings of intense anger, shame, and humiliation. Treatment is similar to that for other post-traumatic disorders, but with attention to the special circumstances of the case.

Reactions to sexual assault (rape)

Sexual assault is more common than is widely appreciated, and often has serious psychological consequences for the victim, be they male or female. In the UK, only about one in seven sexual assaults are reported to the police, and up to 40 per cent of victims tell no one what has happened to them. Asking about sexual abuse of any type should be part of a standard psychiatric assessment process. Approximately one-third of people who have been sexually assaulted have long-term psychological problems relating to it.

In the 1970s the term 'rape trauma syndrome' became commonly used to describe the commonest psychological reaction to an assault. It is now recognized that this is a variant of PTSD, and it is more appropriate to use the terminology of acute stress disorder and PTSD. The symptoms are as outlined in Table 23.3. Rape is also associated with high levels of depression, suicidal ideation, anxiety, sexual dysfunction, and drug/alcohol misuse. There are a number of specific psychological reactions that are common in rape victims, and should be addressed in treatment:

- feeling humiliated, ashamed, and embarrassed about what happened;
- blaming themselves for having put themselves at risk;
- loss of confidence and poor self-esteem;
- difficulty in trusting others, especially in sexual relationships;
- feeling vulnerable to further attack.

After a sexual assault, it is important to give the person practical, emotional, and social support. It is helpful to talk over the problems, and to put them in touch with a victim support organization. These provide practical support and information, such as help in reporting the crime and understanding the criminal justice system. As with PTSD in other situations, watchful waiting is the best approach in the short term, but counselling or CBT from a therapist trained in managing sexual assault may be needed.

Long-term effects of sexual trauma in childhood

Sexually abused children frequently suffer psychological difficulties during the rest of their childhood, and in the longer term or as adults are at much higher risk of multiple psychiatric conditions (Table 23.8).

Most adults who were sexually abused as children retain some memory of the events, though these are often incomplete. Forgotten aspects are sometimes recalled again, for example after a chance encounter with some reminder of the events or when the person becomes sexually active as an adult. Memories may also return during the history taking and discussion involved in psychological treatment. Occasionally, an adult who is receiving counselling or psychotherapy suddenly recalls an episode of child abuse of which he was previously completely unaware. Sometimes such memories are confirmed by people who knew the patient at the time, but sometimes they are vigorously denied by others, including the alleged abuser. When this happens, it has to be decided whether the reports are true memories of actual events, or false memories induced by overzealous questioning, interpretation, or suggestion (the **false memory syndrome**). It is uncertain whether memories

Table 23.8 Conditions associated with childhood sexual abuse

- Anxiety
- Depression
- Post-traumatic stress disorder
- Eating disorders
- Functional disorders (somatization)
- Chronic pain
- Substance abuse (including alcohol)
- Poor educational and work performance
- Low self-esteem and poor confidence
- Problems with sexual relationships
- Violent and destructive behaviour
- Deliberate self-harm and suicide

of sexual abuse can be completely forgotten for many years and then recalled. It is, however, generally agreed that care should be taken during history taking, counselling, and psychotherapy to avoid questions or comments that could suggest childhood sexual abuse, and that any apparent recall of events of which the person had no previous recollection should be considered most carefully and supporting evidence sought, before concluding that it is a true memory.

Children who have suffered sexual abuse may present in a variety of ways, with secondary psychiatric problems, within the criminal justice system, or via social services. A full multidisciplinary assessment should be undertaken (see pp. 168–170), and then usually family and/or individual therapy is indicated. Some older children and adolescents can benefit from a support group as well.

Adults usually present for treatment with a secondary psychiatric problem (Table 23.8) and management should be aimed at the current symptoms, with consideration given to the sexual abuse being a causative factor. For example, a patient presenting with an eating disorder will require the same treatment as other patients (see Chapter 27), but in individual therapy the issues surrounding the sexual abuse should be discussed.

■ Normal and abnormal adjustment reactions

Normal adjustment

Adjustment refers to the psychological reactions involved in adapting to new circumstances. Like the physiological reaction to stress, it is a normal process that is expected after major life changes. Typical events where an adjustment period would be expected include divorce and separation, a change in job or home situation, transition between school and university, and the birth of a child. Symptoms of normal adjustment are mild short-lived anxiety, depression, irritability, and poor concentration.

Adjustment disorder

Adjustment is judged to be abnormal if the distress involved is:

- greater than that which would be expected in response to the particular stressful events (this judgement is subjective and the diagnostic manuals offer no objective criteria); *or*

- is accompanied by impairment of social functioning; *and*

- is close in time to the life change (ICD specifies within 1 month and DSM allows up to 3 months); *and*

- is not severe enough to meet the criteria for the diagnosis of another psychiatric disorder.

It is clear from the points above that adjustment disorders are really a bridge between normal behaviour and psychiatric conditions. It is usually a subjective matter as to where the line is drawn to consider a patient to have an adjustment disorder. Luckily, general practitioners and hospital doctors see many patients of this kind, often in relation to the life changes imposed by physical illness. These clinicians can usually judge better than a psychiatrist whether the patient's reaction is greater than that of most people with a similar illness. This shows the importance of gathering third-party information when assessing a patient.

Clinical features

There are no specific symptoms of an adjustment disorder, and patients usually present with mild symptoms of depression, anxiety, emotional or behavioural disturbance, or a combination of these. The diagnostic criteria are outlined in Box 23.3.

As making a diagnosis of adjustment disorder is often a judgement call, it can be useful to consider the following two questions:

1. Does the patient have a diagnosable mental disorder?
2. If there is a diagnosable mental disorder, does it fit criteria for another condition better than those for adjustment disorder?

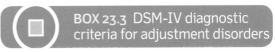

BOX 23.3 DSM-IV diagnostic criteria for adjustment disorders

A The development of emotional or behavioural symptoms in response to an identifiable stressor(s) occurring within 3 months of the onset of the stressor(s).

B These symptoms or behaviours are clinically significant as evidenced by either of the following:

1 marked distress that is in excess of what would be expected from exposure to the stressor;

2 significant impairment in social or occupational functioning.

C The stress-related disturbance does not meet the criteria for another specific Axis I disorder and is not merely an exacerbation of a pre-existing Axis I or Axis II disorder.

D The symptoms do not represent bereavement.

E Once the stressor (or its consequences) has terminated, the symptoms do not persist for more than an additional 6 months.

ICD-10 F43.2: Adjustment disorders

The only significant difference is that the symptoms must begin within 1 month of an identifiable stressor.

Prevalence

There have been few large epidemiological studies of adjustment disorder, partly due to the debates over time as to its exact diagnostic specifications. Figures range from 5 to 20 per cent of general hospital inpatients, and several large studies conclude about one-fifth of psychiatric inpatients have an adjustment disorder. The number of children and adolescents with adjustment disorders in psychiatric inpatient settings is much higher—approximately 60 to 70 per cent. Adjustment disorders are more common in women, and at the extremes of age.

Comorbidity

Alcohol and substance misuse frequently coexist with adjustment disorders.

Differential diagnosis

- **Acute stress disorder or PTSD.** The key to distinguishing between these and adjustment disorders is to decide if the stressor is extreme and traumatic, or a more routine change in life situation. If appropriate symptoms continue for more than 6 months, it is more likely to be PTSD.

- **Mood disorder.** Low mood, anhedonia, and lack of energy. Ask about biological symptoms and whether the symptoms pre-date the stressful event. Generally the symptoms of adjustment disorder are less severe than in depression.

- **Anxiety disorder.** Symptoms of anxiety which are severe enough to fit the diagnostic criteria for an anxiety disorder.

- **Alcohol or substance misuse.** Take a detailed history, including over-the-counter and Internet purchases, and recreational drugs. Sometimes it is necessary to see what happens when substances are stopped before making a diagnosis of a specific disorder.

- **Grief reaction.** Consider if the patient has recently lost a close friend or family member, and symptoms are severe and have lasted more than 6 months. Feelings of guilt and worthlessness, seeing or hearing the deceased in the house, and thoughts of death are all common in grief reactions.

- **Organic disorder causing psychological symptoms.** Again a full history is the key—it is common that psychological symptoms are attributed to an adjustment disorder after diagnosis of a severe physical illness, when actually the symptoms are being caused by the physical pathology itself.

Aetiology

Adjustment disorders may be caused by any identifiable stressful event. Typical examples include change of school or job, divorce or separation, death of a close family member, change in home situation, bankruptcy or high debt, relationship difficulties, or conflicts at work or in the home. It is thought that some people are more vulnerable to developing an adjustment disorder due to a lack of, or failure of existing, coping mechanisms. Individuals who have a broad range of flexible coping mechanisms usually adjust well to any change, whereas those who have more limited resources (especially poor problem-solving skills) fare less well.

Risk factors for an adjustment disorder are:

- age—young people have fewer established coping mechanisms;
- female gender;
- past experiences of stressful events;
- past psychiatric history;
- low self-esteem.

Course and prognosis

The majority of patients with an adjustment disorder will recover without any intervention within a few months. At 5-year follow-up of one large cohort, 70 per cent of adults and 40 per cent of adolescents had no remaining symptomatology. Approximately 20 per cent of adult patients go on to develop a more serious psychiatric disorder, usually depression or substance/alcohol misuse. Adolescents fare less well, in that 40 per cent develop a major psychiatric condition in the following years.

Management

Many patients with an adjustment disorder do not need any formal treatment; they recover spontaneously with the help of friends and family. The aim of any treatment is to help to relieve the acute symptoms caused by the stressor, and to teach the person a wider range of coping skills to protect against future episodes. An outline of treatment options is shown in Table 23.9.

Table 23.9 Management of adjustment disorders

General measures
- Practical support to manage the stressor
- Information about adjustment disorders
Psychological
- Self-help materials, including problem-solving techniques
- Supportive brief psychotherapy
Pharmacological
- Short-term anxiolytics
- Antidepressants

General measures

Practical support. It is important to try to relieve any stress that is still ongoing; for example, by providing financial support, childcare, helping to arrange a funeral, or getting an occupational therapy assessment.

Psychoeducation. Give the patient and their family information about adjustment disorders, and reassure them that it is not a serious psychiatric condition and that they are not going mad. Information leaflets, support groups, and websites can all be valuable.

Anxiety reduction can usually be achieved by encouraging patients to talk about the problems and to express their feelings to a sympathetic listener. A friend or family member can provide this, and many patients will not need any more formal therapeutic input.

Psychological treatments

Self-help materials. A good first step is to provide the patient with appropriate self-help materials, varied according to the predominant symptoms. CBT-based and problem-solving materials (e.g. books, computerized courses) are particularly useful.

Brief psychotherapy or counselling. Talking about the problems, understanding the meaning of the stressor to the patient, and addressing cognitive distortions are the mainstay of treatment. This can be delivered by many different health professionals, and longer formal CBT is not usually necessary. Options include individual or group psychotherapy, crisis intervention, family therapy, or specific counselling. The most effective approach is problem solving, in which the patient is helped to:

- list the problems and think of multiple ways of overcoming them;
- consider the advantages and disadvantages of various solutions to the problems;
- select an action and test it out;
- evaluate the action.

If the third step succeeds, the process is repeated with another problem; if it fails, the patient tries another approach to the first problem.

Crisis intervention. This approach is used when a patient has responded to an acute life change—such as the sudden breaking up of an intimate relationship—with a maladaptive coping mechanism such as deliberate self-harm. The approach resembles problem solving but with additional help in examining the maladaptive coping responses, recognizing their disadvantages, and considering other ways of dealing with similar problems in the future. Many mental health trusts have a crisis intervention team, who will provide daily telephone (or home visit) support to patients whilst they are at high risk in order to reduce the need for hospital admission.

Pharmacological treatments

Short-term anxiolytics. It may be necessary to provide a short-term supply (a few days) of an anxiolytic in the immediate aftermath of the stressful event. A low-dose relatively short-acting benzodiazepine is the best choice. They should not be continued longer term due to the risks of tolerance and dependence. Occasionally insomnia is a problem, and a few nights of a hypnotic (temazepam or a z-drug) are helpful.

Antidepressants. There is no good evidence that antidepressants are effective in relieving the symptoms of adjustment disorders. However, if there are prolonged/distressing mood or anxiety symptoms, a low-dose SSRI may provide some relief. Other antidepressants are not recommended as the risks outweigh the benefits.

■ Adjustment to special situations

Adjustment to physical illness

Being diagnosed with a serious physical illness is a stressor that many people experience and, as with any stressor, they may react in a variety of different ways. There are a number of characteristics that make having a diagnosis of illness stressful:

- problems and difficulties in accessing medical services;
- a diagnosis is usually unexpected;
- uncontrollability of what has happened, and what will occur in the future;
- poor understanding of what has caused the condition, and how it will progress;
- new treatments, which may be complex, unpleasant, and/or time consuming;
- there may be associated changes in other aspects of life (e.g. giving up work or sport).

Adjustment to having a physical illness involves a set of changes known as **illness behaviour.** This behaviour includes seeking medical advice, taking medication, accepting help, and giving up activities. Some people are able to make these changes easily, but others struggle. This may lead to an adjustment disorder, another psychiatric condition, or to **abnormal illness behaviour**. Illness behaviours are at first adaptive, but if they persist too long they may become maladaptive. Occasionally, people adopt illness behaviours when they have no physical disorder. They are said to display **abnormal illness behaviour**, though it is not the behaviour that is abnormal but the circumstances in which it occurs, namely without a medical reason.

The sick role is a related concept. Society allows sick people to adopt a special role, which comprises two privileges and two duties:

- **exemption** from some responsibilities;
- the **right** to help and care;
- the **obligation** to seek and cooperate in treatment;
- the **expectation** of a wish to recover and efforts to achieve this.

The sick role is usually adaptive. However, some people continue to adopt a sick role long after the illness is over, avoiding responsibilities and depending on others instead of becoming independent. Others adopt the sick role without ever having experienced any physical disorder.

Physical illness as a stressor. The stress associated with physical illness may lead to *anxiety* and *depression*, and sometimes to *anger*. Most of these reactions are short-lived, subsiding as the person adjusts to the new situation. The stressful effect of physical illness cannot be judged solely in terms of its objective severity; it depends also on the *patient's appraisal* of the illness and its likely consequences. This appraisal may be unrealistic and based on false assumptions. The latter may be shared by the relatives, thus reinforcing the patient's concerns, or contradicted by them, thus leading to family conflict.

Physical illness and its treatment as direct causes of psychiatric symptoms. As well as acting as a psychological stressor, physical illness may induce psychiatric symptoms directly. Anxiety, depression, fatigue, weakness, weight loss, and certain abnormal behaviours can all be caused in this way. Certain *medications* used in the treatment of physical illness may also affect mood, behaviour, and consciousness.

Denial. As in adjustment to other situations, adjustment to physical illness often involves an initial stage of denial, which protects against overwhelming distress. If denial persists beyond the early stage of adjustment it prevents the working through of problems and interferes with full engagement with treatment. Denial can be reduced by helping patients to discuss their concerns, and by providing information to correct misunderstandings, for example about the likely amount of pain.

Treatment

When adjustment to physical illness is slow and incomplete, support can usually be provided effectively by the primary care or hospital team dealing with the physical illness.

Psychoeducation. A doctor should explain the nature of the physical illness and its treatment, and provide as clear a picture of what the future holds as possible. Providing leaflets, books, and websites is useful as it is often hard for patients to remember everything that has been said in a consultation.

Supportive talking and listening. The patient needs someone to talk to about their anxieties, such as the effects of the illness on their family, or the threat of losing their job. It is important to provide a supportive person who has time to build up a trusting relationship with the patient. This may be a friend or family member, but sometimes more formal counselling is needed.

Counselling. This should address the issues above, but also consider any maladaptive behaviour (e.g. overdependence) that has developed. Teaching problem-solving techniques is important, in order for the patient to be able to adapt their life to the new situation.

Managing co-morbidities. Sometimes the stress of physical illness provokes an anxiety or depressive disorder. In this situation, the guidelines for these conditions should be followed as usual, including the use of medications if needed.

Adjustment to terminal illness

After terminal illness has been diagnosed, people tend to go through four stages in the journey to accepting their situation.

- **Denial** is usually the first reaction to the news of fatal illness. It may be experienced as a feeling of disbelief and a consequent initial period of calm. Denial usually reduces as the patient gradually comes to terms with the situation, but may return if there is progress of the disease which the patient is not ready to accept.

- **Displacement.** Anger about the situation may be displaced on to doctors, nurses, and relatives. All may find this anger difficult to tolerate unless they understand its origins. Without this understanding they may be less inclined to spend time with patients, thereby increasing their feelings of isolation and anger.

- **Dependency** is common among terminally ill people. It is adaptive at times when the patient is required to comply passively with treatment, but persisting or excessive dependency makes treatment more difficult, and increases the burden on the family.

- **Acceptance** is the final stage of adjustment. The aim is to help the patient to reach this state before the final stage of the physical illness.

At some point during their illness, many people become anxious, depressed, guilty, angry, or adopt maladaptive ways of coping. About half of patients who die in hospital have some emotional symptoms. Understandably, these emotional reactions are more common in the young than in the old, and less common in the religious. The following symptoms are particularly common among the dying:

- **Anxiety** may be provoked by personal concerns about pain, disfigurement, or incontinence, and by concerns about others, especially the family.
- **Depression** may be provoked by the loss of valued activities and the prospect of separation from loved ones. Depression and anxiety can also be the direct result of the physical disease or of the medication used to treat it.
- **Confusion** due to delirium is frequent among dying patients, and is caused, for example, by dehydration, drug side effects, and secondary infection.
- **Guilt** may be caused by the belief that excessive demands are being placed on relatives or friends.
- **Anger** may derive from ideas about the unjustness of impending death.

Treatment

Control of physical symptoms. The first steps in treatment are to control symptoms such as pain, vomiting, or confusion, as these distract patients from the psychological work needed to reach a satisfactory adjustment.

Explaining the illness and treatment. Carers sometimes worry that explaining the terminal nature of the illness will increase the patient's distress. While excessive detail, given unsympathetically and at the wrong time, can have this effect, it is seldom difficult to decide how much to say provided that *patients are allowed to lead the discussion*. When patients ask about the prognosis they should be told the truth; evasive answers undermine trust. Patients notice when answers to their questions are evasive. When people avoid talking to them, they infer the truth from this avoidance although they are not told directly. However, when patients do not at first indicate a desire to know the full extent of their problems, it is better to keep this information for a subsequent interview. The account should always be truthful, but the amount disclosed on a single occasion should be judged by the patient's reactions and by their questions. If necessary, the clinician should set aside time for further discussion when the patient seems ready for this. At an appropriate time, patients should be told what will be done to make their last days as comfortable as possible.

Help for relatives. Relatives may be anxious and depressed, and respond with denial, guilt, and anger. These reactions may make it difficult for them to communicate helpfully with the patient and with staff. Relatives need information about the disease and its treatment, and opportunities to talk about their feelings and to prepare for the impending bereavement.

Special nursing. In many places terminal care nurses work with the patient and the family, liaising with the family doctor, and with the hospital staff caring for the patient. These nurses are skilled in the psychological as well as the physical care of the dying.

Referral to a psychiatrist is indicated when:

- there is *doubt about the psychiatric diagnosis* (e.g. between adjustment disorder and depressive disorder);
- the patient has had a *previous psychiatric disorder*;
- the patient *refuses to discuss* the illness, or to make necessary decisions;
- the patient *refuses to cooperate* with treatment, in order to determine whether this refusal is for rational reasons or has a psychiatric cause.

Grief reactions

- **Bereavement** refers to any loss event, typically the death of a loved one but it may occur after loss of one's health, home, country, or wealth.
- **Grief** is the response to bereavement, encompassing the thoughts, feelings, and emotions surrounding the event.

Normal grief

Similarly to the stress response, grief is a normal physiological process that only becomes abnormal if it is prolonged, intense, or atypical. The classical theory of the grief response is the Küber–Ross model, published in 1969, which was originally modelled on people suffering from terminal illness, and later adapted to those suffering from a catastrophic personal loss. The model included five stages: denial, anger, bargaining, depression, and acceptance, not attached to any particular time-scales. More recent research suggests that this model is too restrictive, and that grief is typically more dynamic and multifactorial. However, it is relatively well accepted that there are three main stages to responding to bereavement, although these do not always occur in a restrictively linear order (Table 23.10).

The **first stage** lasts from a few hours to several days. There is a lack of emotional response ('numbness'), often with a feeling of unreality, and incomplete acceptance that the death has taken place.

The **second stage** lasts from a few weeks to 6 months. There may be extreme sadness, weeping, and often overwhelming waves of grief. Somatic symptoms of anxiety are common. The bereaved person is restless, sleeps poorly, and lacks appetite. Many bereaved people feel guilty that they failed to do enough for the deceased; some project these feelings on to clinical staff for failing to provide optimal care for the dead person. Some

Table 23.10 The normal grief reaction

Stage 1 (hours to days)

Denial, disbelief

'Numbness'

Stage 2 (weeks to 6 months)

Sadness, weeping, waves of grief

Somatic symptoms of anxiety

Restlessness

Poor sleep

Diminished appetite

Guilt, blame of others

Experience of the presence of the deceased

Illusions, vivid imagery

Hallucinations of the dead person's voice

Preoccupation with memories of the deceased

Social withdrawal

Stage 3 (weeks to months)

Symptoms resolve

Social activities resumed

Memories of good times

(Symptoms may recur at anniversaries)

bereaved people have an intense experience of being in the presence of the dead person, and may experience vivid imagery, illusions, or sometimes hallucinations of that person's voice. The bereaved person is preoccupied with memories of the dead person, and often withdraws from social relationships.

In the **third stage** these symptoms subside, and everyday activities are resumed. The bereaved person gradually comes to terms with the loss, and recalls the good times shared with the deceased in the past. Often, there is a temporary return of symptoms on the anniversary of the death.

Abnormal grief

Grief is said to be abnormal when the symptoms are:

- *more intense* than usual and meet the criteria for another psychiatric disorder;
- *prolonged* beyond 6 months;
- *delayed* in onset.

Typically, the patient will present with symptoms of a moderately severe depressive disorder (Box 23.4), and it is up to the clinician to link this to a recent loss event. There are a variety of circumstances that make it more likely that an individual will have an abnormal grief reaction; these are outlined in Table 23.11.

Assessment and management

The majority of patients who suffer a loss do not require any formal intervention, but for those who do, treatment resembles that for other kinds of adjustment reaction.

Assessment should address the death and its circumstances, the relationship, and the history and course of the bereaved one's symptoms. It is important to assess available social support, and take a full psychiatric history. If there are symptoms of anxiety, depression, or another psychiatric diagnosis that are affecting functionality, it is appropriate to treat them along condition-specific guidelines.

Emotional support. The first step is to provide empathic, compassionate support by *listening* while the bereaved person talks about the loss, and to enable him to express

BOX 23.4 Diagnostic criteria for grief reactions

There are no specific criteria in either the DSM-IV or ICD-10 diagnostic classifications, but both give guidelines that suggest a clinically significant reaction:

- Low mood, anhedonia, fatigue, and biological symptoms (weight loss, insomnia, poor appetite) severe enough to fit diagnostic criteria for a depressive episode.
- Symptoms persist for more than 2 months after the loss event.
- Guilt about actions done or not done around the time of the death.
- Suicidal ideation.

- A morbid preoccupation with worthlessness.
- Psychomotor retardation.
- Prolonged and marked functional impairment.
- Hallucinatory experiences other than thinking they hear the voice, or transiently see the image of the deceased person.

ICD-10 does not have a specific code for grief reactions, but say to code F43.22-26, which spans anxiety and depressive disorders, according to the most appropriate match of symptoms. Symptoms lasting more than 6 months should be coded as a prolonged depressive reaction.

Table 23.11 Risk factors for an abnormal grief reaction

Pre-existing vulnerabilities
- Avoidant or dependant personality traits
- Prior multiple losses
- Childhood separation anxiety
- Personal psychiatric history
- Family history of psychiatric disorders
- Co-morbid substance abuse

Nature of relationship
- Death of a child or partner
- Stillbirth, neonatal deaths, and cot deaths
- The survivor was dependent upon the deceased

Circumstances of the death
- Death was prolonged
- Sudden unexpected deaths
- People are missing, believed dead
- Homicide committed by a loved one

Lack of social support

Multiple other adversities

feelings of sadness or anger. When the person is seen soon after the loss, it is helpful to *explain* the normal course of grieving, and to forewarn about the possibility of feeling as if the dead person were present, or experiencing illusions or hallucinations. Without this warning, these experiences may be very alarming. As time passes, the bereaved person should be encouraged to resume social contacts, to talk to other people about the loss, to remember happy and fulfilling experiences that were shared with the deceased, and to consider positive activities that the latter would have wanted survivors to undertake.

Practical support. Help with death certification, funeral arrangements, and financial issues may be needed, and, following the loss of a partner, a parent may require help in caring for young children. The bereaved person may need help to move from the early stage of denial of the loss to *acceptance* of reality by viewing the body and by later putting away the dead person's belongings.

Supportive counselling. There is no evidence that one form of psychological intervention is better than another, so the choice is usually made on what is available locally. Options include:

- guided self-help programmes;
- bereavement counselling;
- specific brief CBT for traumatic grief;
- brief interpersonal psychotherapy.

Pharmacological treatments. If anxiety is severe or sleep disturbed in the first few days after a loss, then an anxiolytic or hypnotic drug may be appropriate. These should be prescribed in the short term only, due to the risks of tolerance and dependence, and the fact that in most cases distress can be reduced by the opportunity to talk and cry. Occasionally, grief is sufficiently intense to meet the criteria for depressive disorder—in this situation antidepressant drug treatment may be warranted.

Support groups are helpful, and the bereaved should be assisted and encouraged to make contact with one. The groups enable newly bereaved people to talk with others who have dealt successfully with the emotional and practical aspects of bereavement. Supportive counselling is also available through some charities, such as the organization CRUSE.

 Further reading

National Institute for Clinical Excellence (2005). *Posttraumatic Stress Disorder (PTSD): The Management of PTSD in Adults and Children in Primary and Secondary Care.* http://guidance.nice.org.uk/CG26 (accessed August 2010).

Ehlers, A., *et al.* (2009). Stress-related and adjustment disorders. In *New Oxford Textbook of Psychiatry*, 2nd edn. Ed.

Gelder, M., Andreasen, N., Lopez-Ibor, J, & Geddes, J, pp. 693–728. Oxford University Press, Oxford.

Bisson, J. (2007). Post-traumatic stress disorder. *British Medical Journal* 334: 789–93.

CRUSE Bereavement Care. www.crusebereavementcare.org.uk/ (accessed Aug. 2010).

CHAPTER 24

Anxiety and obsessional disorders

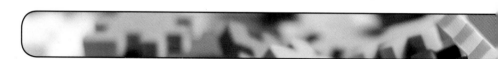

Chapter contents

Anxiety disorders are characterized by marked and persistent mental and physical symptoms of anxiety, that are not secondary to another disorder and that impact negatively upon an individual's life. They are the most common type of psychiatric disorder, with a 1-year prevalence of approximately 14 per cent. Anxiety disorders may be primary psychiatric conditions, or a secondary response to the stress associated with physical illness and its treatment. Given their frequency, and the fact that many patients present with physical rather than psychological symptoms, it is unsurprising that anxiety disorders are common in both primary care and general hospital medicine. Clinicians working in all branches of medicine should be able to diagnose anxiety disorders, arrange basic treatment, and know when to refer patients to a specialist.

Anxiety disorders are subdivided into generalized anxiety, phobic, and panic disorders, each with a characteristic pattern of symptoms and disabilities, and each requiring somewhat different treatment. Mixed states of anxiety and depression are common; these 'minor mood disorders' are described with depressive disorders, to which they are more closely related, and should be managed using the mood disorders treatment protocols (see p. 230).

Obsessive-compulsive disorders are also considered in this chapter. Currently, their relation to anxiety disorders is uncertain. They are classified with anxiety disorders in DSM-IV because there are many common features, but are classified separately in ICD-10 because there are some important differences.

What is normal anxiety?

Normal anxiety is the response to threatening situations. Feelings of apprehension are accompanied by physiological changes that prepare for defence or escape ('**fight or flight**'), notably increases in heart rate, blood pressure, respiration, and muscle tension. Sympathetic nervous system activity is increased, causing symptoms such as tremor, sweating, polyuria, and diarrhoea. Attention and concentration are focused on the threatening situation. Anxiety can therefore be a beneficial response in dangerous situations, and should occur in everyday situations of perceived threat (e.g. examinations).

Abnormal anxiety is a response that is similar but out of proportion to the threat and/or is more prolonged, or occurs when there is no threat. With one exception, the symptoms of anxiety disorders are the same as those of a normal anxiety response. The exception is that the focus of attention is not the external threat (as in the normal response) but the physiological response itself. Thus in abnormal anxiety, attention is focused on a symptom such as increased heart rate. This focus of attention is accompanied by concern about the cause of the symptom. For example, a common concern is that rapid heart action is a sign of heart disease. Another common concern is that other people will become aware of the symptom and think it strange, for example, that they will notice trembling of the hands. Because these concerns are threatening, they activate a further anxiety response thus adding to the autonomic arousal, generating further concern, and setting up a vicious cycle of mounting anxiety (Figure 24.1).

Anxiety disorders

Classification

Abnormal anxiety becomes clinically relevant when it causes distress or impairment of daily activities. Anxiety disorders are classified into those with continuous symptoms (**generalized anxiety disorder**) and those with episodic symptoms. The latter are divided into those in which episodes of anxiety occur in particular situations (**phobic anxiety disorders**) and those in which episodes can occur in any situation (**panic disorder**) (Figure 24.2). Phobic anxiety disorders are classified further into **simple phobia, social phobia,** and **agoraphobia** (these terms are explained later). Some patients have both episodes of anxiety in particular situations, characteristic of agoraphobia, and random episodes, characteristic of panic disorder. These mixed disorders are called **panic with agoraphobia** in DSM (unfortunately the term in ICD-10 is slightly different—agoraphobia with panic).

Prevalence

Anxiety disorders are common in the population, with a 1-year prevalence of about 14 per cent, or about 10 per cent

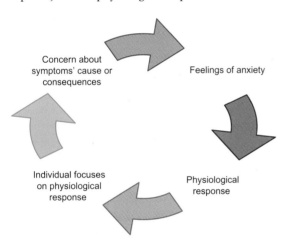

Fig. 24.1 Cycle of anxiety.

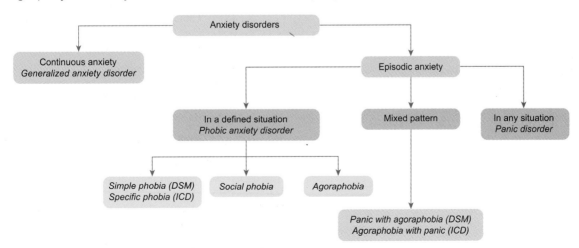

Fig. 24.2 Principles of classification of anxiety disorders.

Table 24.1 Approximate prevalence of anxiety disorders

Disorder	1-year prevalence (%)	Lifetime risk (%)
Any anxiety disorder	6.4	13.6
Generalized anxiety disorder	1.0	2.8
Agoraphobia	0.4	0.9
Social phobia	1.2	2.4
Simple phobia	3.5	7.7
Panic disorder	0.8	2.1
Obsessive-compulsive disorder	1.1	2.5

From Alonso, J. *et al.* (2004). Prevalence of mental disorders in Europe: results from the European Study of the Epidemiology of Mental disorders (ESEMeD) project. *Acta Psychiatrica Scandinavica* **109** (Suppl. 420): 21–7.

if simple phobias are excluded. The prevalence of the various kinds of anxiety disorder is shown in Table 24.1. The figures are approximate but nevertheless show the relative frequency of the disorders.

Generalized anxiety disorder

Generalized anxiety disorder (GAD) is characterized by excessive, uncontrolled, and irrational worry about everyday things that is out of proportion to the actual source of the worry. The worry impairs function, as the patient typically catastrophizes and becomes overly concerned with normal issues of health, money, work, and relationships.

The diagnostic criteria for generalized anxiety disorder are shown in Box 24.1 By convention, GAD is diagnosed only when symptoms of anxiety have been present for several months (6 months in DSM-IV). When symptoms have been present for a shorter time, the diagnosis is **stress** or **adjustment disorder** (see pp. 266 and 277).

Clinical features

Patients may complain directly of anxiety, or ask for help for one or more of the many physical symptoms of anxiety. It is also important to remember physical diseases can produce the same symptoms as anxiety disorders—see the differential diagnosis below for further information on how to tell these various conditions apart.

Appearance

The patient typically looks concerned about something, and is restless, sweaty, and shaky. Tearfulness, which may erroneously suggest depression, reflects a generally apprehensive state. However, it is important to remember that there may be no obvious outward physical signs of anxiety, and a full history must always be taken.

Psychological symptoms are listed in Table 24.2.

Physical symptoms reflect overactivity of the sympathetic nervous system and increased tension in skeletal muscles. The list of possible symptoms is long, but they can be grouped conveniently by the systems of the body, as shown in Table 24.2.

BOX 24.1 DSM-IV 300.02 generalized anxiety disorder

A Excessive anxiety and worry, occurring more days than not for at least 6 months, about a number of ordinary events or activities.

B The person finds it difficult to control the worry.

C The anxiety and worry are associated with three (or more) of the following six symptoms:

1 restlessness or feeling keyed up or on edge;

2 being easily fatigued;

3 irritability;

4 muscle tension;

5 difficulty falling or staying asleep, or restless unsatisfying sleep;

6 difficulty concentrating or the mind going blank.

Symptoms can also include nausea, vomiting, and chronic stomach aches.

D The anxiety, worry, or physical symptoms cause clinically significant distress or impairment in social, occupational, or other important areas of functioning.

E The disturbance is not due to the direct physiological effects of a substance or a general medical condition and does not occur exclusively during a Mood Disorder, a Psychotic Disorder, or a Pervasive Developmental Disorder.

ICD-10 F41.1 Generalized anxiety disorder

The only significant difference is that the symptoms must have been present for a minimum of several weeks (rather than 6 months).

Table 24.2 Symptoms of generalized anxiety disorder

Psychological	Fearful anticipation
	Irritability
	Sensitivity to noise
	Restlessness
	Poor concentration
	Depression
	Obsessions
	Depersonalization
Physical	Difficulty in swallowing
Gastrointestinal	Epigastric discomfort
	Excessive wind (due to air swallowing)
	Frequent or loose motions
Respiratory	Constriction in the chest
	Difficulty inhaling
	Overbreathing
Cardiovascular	Palpitations
	Discomfort in chest
	Awareness of missed beats
Genitourinary	Frequent or urgent micturition
	Failure of erection
	Menstrual discomfort
	Amenorrhoea
Neuromuscular	Tremor
	Prickling sensations
	Tinnitus
	Dizziness (unsteadiness rather than a rotational sensation)
	Bilateral headache
	Aching muscles (especially in the back and shoulders)
Sleep disturbance	Insomnia
	Night terrors

Sleep is disturbed in a characteristic way. On going to bed patients lie awake worrying; when at last they fall asleep, they wake intermittently. They often report unpleasant dreams, and occasionally 'night terrors' in which they wake suddenly feeling intensely fearful, sometimes remembering a nightmare, and sometimes uncertain why they are so frightened. Early waking with an inability to go back to sleep again is much less common among patients with a generalized anxiety disorder than among patients with a depressive disorder (see pp. 223–226). Therefore, early waking should always prompt a search for other symptoms of a depressive disorder.

Hyperventilation is a common symptom in generalized anxiety disorder—further information can be found in Table 24.3 and Box 24.2.

Panic attacks. Some patients with generalized anxiety disorder experience occasional panic attacks, that is, sudden episodes of very severe anxiety. However, panic attacks are more characteristic of panic disorder (see p. 297).

Prevalence

The lifetime risk of generalized anxiety disorder is 4 to 5 per cent, but in any given year approximately 3 per cent of the population will suffer from GAD. It is twice as common in women as in men, and seen more frequently in Caucasians and those in lower socio-economic groups. The average age of onset is 21 years, but there is a second peak of occurrence in the 40- to 59-year age group. The disorder is chronic and is therefore frequent among attendees in primary care.

Co-morbidity

It is usual for patients with GAD to suffer from other mood and anxiety disorders. Recent studies have shown that approximately 68 per cent of patients with a primary diagnosis of GAD meet criteria for another psychiatric disorder. The most common are depression, social phobia, and panic disorder, but alcohol and drug misuse also frequently occur.

Differential diagnosis

Generalized anxiety disorder needs to be distinguished from other psychiatric disorders in which anxiety may be prominent, and from physical illnesses that produce similar symptoms.

- **Depressive disorder** can present with symptoms of anxiety, and patients with chronic GAD may ask for help when they feel depressed. *Diagnostic errors can be reduced by routinely screening for depressive symptoms (p. 224) in patients presenting with anxiety.* Usually, the mood

Table 24.3 Symptoms and signs of hyperventilation

- Rapid shallow breathing
- Dizziness
- Tinnitus
- Headache
- Chest discomfort
- Weakness
- Faintness
- Numbness and tingling in the hands and feet
- Carpopedal spasm

BOX 24.2 Hyperventilation

Hyperventilation is overbreathing—usually in a rapid and shallow way—that results in a fall in the concentration of carbon dioxide in the blood and leads to a respiratory alkalosis. The resultant symptoms are listed in Table 24.3. Paradoxically, overbreathing produces a feeling of breathlessness, which causes the patient to breathe even more vigorously. It is common in all anxiety disorders and should be considered when a patient has appropriate unexplained symptoms. The diagnosis should be made on the definite occurrence of this group of symptoms, and on observations of the patient's respiration pattern. The finding that symptoms produced by deliberate overbreathing resemble those experienced spontaneously does not prove that involuntary hyperventilation is the cause of the latter.

• **To terminate an acute episode**, the patient should rebreathe expired air from a paper bag. This increases the alveolar concentration of carbon dioxide, correcting the acid–base abnormality and decreasing the feeling of breathlessness. Re-breathing during an episode is also an effective way of demonstrating that certain symptoms are caused by hyperventilation.

• **To prevent further episodes** of hyperventilation, patients should practise slow, controlled breathing, at first under supervision and then at home. A tape recording can be used to help the patient time their breathing appropriately. Such a tape can be made by the primary care team or obtained from a department of clinical psychology. It is important to identify and treat the underlying anxiety disorder/diagnosis.

---

symptoms are more severe than the anxiety symptoms and appeared first, and other symptoms of depressive disorder will be present. Rarely *agitation* occurring in a severe depressive disorder (see p. 224) is mistaken for anxiety.

• **Schizophrenia.** Occasionally patients with schizophrenia complain of anxiety before they reveal other symptoms of schizophrenia. Screen all patients for psychotic symptoms, including paranoia.

• **Dementia** may first come to notice when the patient complains of anxiety. When this happens, the clinician may overlook the accompanying memory disorder or ascribe it to poor concentration. For this reason, memory should be assessed appropriately, especially when older patients present with anxiety.

• **Drugs,** either prescribed or recreational, can cause anxiety-like symptoms. Alcohol, cannabis, antidepressants, antipsychotics, benzodiazepines, caffeine, and sedatives are frequent in psychiatry, but other common culprits include bronchodilators, antihypertensives, anti-arrhythmics, anticonvulsants, thyroxine, chemotherapy, and antibiotics.

• **Withdrawal from drugs or alcohol** can also cause anxiety, and the cause may be overlooked because patients wish to hide their drug or alcohol misuse. Reports that anxiety is particularly severe on awakening in the morning suggest alcohol dependence (see p. 382) or depressive disorder.

• **Physical illnesses** may present with symptoms similar to those of an anxiety disorder, especially if the symptoms are episodic.

  – Thyrotoxicosis leads to irritability, restlessness, tremor, and tachycardia. Patients should be examined for an enlarged thyroid, atrial fibrillation, and exophthalmos, and thyroid function tests should be arranged in appropriate cases.

  – Hypoparathyroidism.

  – Phaeochromocytoma.

  – Hypoglycaemia.

  – Arrhythmias.

  – Ménière's disease.

  – Temporal lobe epilepsy.

  – Respiratory disease.

  – Carcinoid tumours.

Any physical illness can also lead to the development of an anxiety disorder; clinicians should always be considering this when dealing with patients and families in whom a recent diagnosis of a severe illness has been made.

Aetiology

An overview of the causes of GAD is outlined in Table 24.4. **Predisposing factors** are of four kinds: genetic, neurobiological, childhood upbringing, and personality type.

1 **Genetic causes** are important in predisposing to all anxiety disorders. GAD is five times more prevalent in those with first-degree relatives with GAD than in the general population. The concordance for anxiety disorders of all kinds is greater among monozygotic than among dizygotic twins. However, most studies do not distinguish between the different kinds of anxiety disorder, so the size of the contribution of genetic factors to GAD is uncertain.

2 **Neurobiological mechanisms** have been implicated in the aetiology of anxiety disorders based on investigation

Table 24.4 Aetiology of generalized anxiety disorder

Predisposing factors	Precipitating factors	Maintaining factors
Genetics	Stressful events, e.g.	Continuing stressful life events
• Family history	• Relationships	
• Twin studies	• Unemployment	Depressive disorder
Neurobiological mechanisms	• Financial problems	
Personality	• Ill health	Cycle of anxiety (Figure 24.1)
Childhood upbringing	• Natural disasters	

of the stress response in animal models and patients. The response to stimulation of the autonomic nervous system is prolonged in patients with GAD, and negative feedback of the hypothalamic–pituitary–adrenal axis by cortisol is reduced.

3 **Childhood upbringing** is thought to predispose to GAD in adult life. Inconsistent parenting, poor attachments, and a chaotic lifestyle in childhood may cause apprehension and anxiety which persists into later life. However, despite much speculation, there is no good evidence for any specific causes currently.

4 **Personality traits.** Anxious and worry-prone personalities are linked to anxiety disorder but other personalities can predispose by making people less able to cope with stressful events.

Prognosis

By convention, the diagnosis of GAD cannot be made until the symptoms have been present for 6 months. Without treatment, about 80 per cent of patients still have the disorder 3 years after the onset, and for many it is a lifelong problem. Unemployment and separation/divorce are higher in those with GAD than the general population. Prognosis is worse when symptoms are severe, and when there is agitation, derealization, conversion symptoms, or suicidal ideas. Brief episodes of depression are frequent among patients with a chronic GAD and it is often during one of these episodes that further treatment is sought.

Assessment and management

Although there are differences in the features and treatment of the various types of anxiety disorder, there are also many common features. Treatments are tested on patients who meet formal diagnostic criteria, but many patients seek help before their symptoms meet these criteria, and it is usually appropriate to start treatment immediately based on clinical judgement. The following sections outline a general approach to all patients with anxiety disorders, plus individual guidance for GAD. Specific treatments for other disorders will be covered later in the chapter.

The National Institute for Clinical Excellence (NICE) published guidance on the management of anxiety disorders in 2004, which was amended in 2007. It is the standard reference for management within the UK, but the general principles will apply worldwide. A general plan of treatment is shown in Table 24.5 and a brief outline of psychological treatments for specific disorders in Table 24.6. It is rare for patients with anxiety disorders to need care that is more intensive than that provided in the outpatient setting. Generally, the primary care physician should make an assessment and try up to two different forms of treatment; failing this they should refer the patient to a mental health team for further management.

Assessment of anxiety disorders

A full psychiatric history should be taken, including information from the patient, a third-party informant, primary care physician, and old hospital notes (see Chapter 5). Specific points to cover include;

• current symptoms and their effect upon life at home, work, school, etc.;

• previous diagnoses of anxiety disorders, mood disorders, eating disorders, OCD, or other psychiatric conditions—are there current symptoms of these?

Table 24.5 General treatment plan for anxiety disorders

Assessment
• Make a diagnosis
• Detect any co-morbid depressive disorder

General measures
• Agree a clear plan
• Psychoeducation
• Problem-solving techniques and relaxation
• Manage hyperventilation (see Box 24.2)

Psychological treatment
• Self-help books, based on cognitive behavioural techniques
• Group/computerized cognitive behavioural therapy
• Individual cognitive behavioural therapy

Pharmacotherapy
• Antidepressants
• Short-term benzodiazepines

Social interventions

Table 24.6 Psychological treatments for anxiety disorders

Disorder	Therapy
General treatments	
Any anxiety disorder	Psychoeducation for patient and carers
	Relaxation training
	Problem-solving skills
	Self-help: books, website, telephone-guided treatment
	Computerized CBT
	Voluntary-sector group meetings and/or therapies
Specific therapies	
Generalized anxiety disorder	Cognitive behavioural therapy (CBT)
	• Group (in the UK, the mental health voluntary sector provides local CBT groups that patients can self-refer to)
	• Individual
Phobias	CBT: graded-exposure therapy
	• Group
	• Individual
Social phobias/ agoraphobia	CBT: graded-exposure therapy
	• Group
	• Individual
Panic disorder	Specialized CBT for panic disorder (usually individual sessions are required)
OCD	Mild to moderate: brief CBT, group/individual, based on 'exposure with response prevention techniques' Severe: full course of individual CBT

- previous psychiatric treatments and how successful they were;
- current medications (prescribed, illicit, over-the-counter, alcohol, caffeine, nicotine);
- premorbid personality traits;
- current social situation—accommodation, employment, finances.

A risk assessment should be carried out (see p. 61), focusing specifically upon risk of self-harm, exploitation, self-neglect, and driving.

Psychological evaluation should include use of standard scales for mood disorders (e.g. Beck Depression Index, Hospital Anxiety and Depression Scale) and assess the impact of symptoms on social and occupational functioning.

A physical examination should be undertaken, and baseline laboratory tests ordered as seems appropriate.

General measures

Agree a clear plan. Anxiety is prolonged by uncertainty, and a clear management plan, agreed with the patient, helps to reduce it. Try to limit contact to one named physician.

Provide and discuss information (psychoeducation). Anxiety disorders are maintained by fears about the nature and consequences of their symptoms. An explanation of the condition should be tailored to the particular concerns of the individual patient, but it is usually necessary to explain how fears that symptoms are caused by physical illness can cause vicious circles of anxiety. Providing written information is important, as anxious people often suffer from poor concentration, and involving a relative or carer can also facilitate understanding.

Identify and reduce or avoid any stressors. Learning problem-solving techniques is an important aspect of this (see p. 134).

Advice about self-help methods. Patients with anxiety disorders can help themselves in simple ways, for example time management, activity scheduling, taking time off to relax, and reducing caffeine intake. Relaxation training can be provided within a primary care team or at home using yoga or mindfulness exercises. To be effective it must be practised regularly; some patients are better motivated by training in a group rather than individually. Patients should be offered information about local support groups and national charities (e.g. Anxiety UK, www.anxietyuk. org.uk/).

Psychological treatments

Psychoeducation, support, and problem solving as outlined above are important for all patients, and may be all that is needed.

Self-help books or computer courses based on the principles of cognitive behavioural therapy may be useful prior to individual therapy. An example of this is dealing with worrying thoughts. A patient could:

- write down the worrying thoughts so that they can be considered more objectively;
- consider, for each problem, whether anything can be done to resolve the worrying problem;
- if possible take the appropriate action; if no action is possible, set aside a brief 'worry time' each day, and for the rest of the day endeavour to use distraction to prevent worrying (this procedure is described more fully by Butler and Hope (1995); see Further Reading).

Refer for cognitive behaviour therapy. The treatments described so far can all be carried out by generic members of a primary care team. Cognitive behaviour therapy is provided by a clinical psychologist or a specially trained psychiatric nurse, who may be based within primary or secondary care, and should be weekly sessions of 1 hour to a total of 16–20 hours delivered within 4 months. This may be quicker to access as a group treatment.

Pharmacotherapy

Antidepressants have been proven to be effective at reducing anxiety even in patients who do not have co-morbid depression. The main advantage of them over anxiolytic drugs is that they do not produce dependence, and therefore can be used long term. An SSRI should be the first-line medication; there is no evidence that any particular one is more efficacious than another. Tricyclic antidepressants are recommended for some anxiety disorders (these are discussed below). However, they are more toxic in overdose and have a less good side-effect profile than SSRIs. If there is no improvement after 12 weeks, another SSRI should be tried. Medication is usually continued for at least 6 months after the symptoms improve, and often longer. Patients who relapse can resume their medication or be referred for cognitive behaviour therapy. For GAD specifically, there is some evidence that paroxetine may be the best SSRI to use. Venlafaxine is also licensed for use in GAD, but should not be a first-line medication, and should be started by a specialist.

Limit the use of anxiolytics. Anxiolytic drugs (such as benzodiazepines) can bring rapid relief from anxiety at times of crisis, and are frequently used to cover the 2–3 weeks it takes for an antidepressant to work. While it is easy to prescribe them, this should not be done routinely but kept for more severe disorders or cases in which immediate relief is essential (for example, to fulfil an important commitment). Anxiolytics should not be prescribed for more than about 3 weeks because of the risk of dependency.

Buspirone is a non-benzodiazepine anxiolytic which can be used for short-term relief in GAD. It is less likely to cause dependence than a benzodiazepine, but does take up to 4 weeks to work.

Phobic anxiety disorders

The symptoms of phobic anxiety disorder are primarily the same as those of generalized anxiety disorder, but there are three distinguishing features.

1 **Anxiety occurs in particular circumstances only.** The amount of time the patient is anxious depends hugely on how frequently they come across the anxiety-provoking circumstances. Examples include *situations*, such as crowded place, *living things*, such as spiders, and *natural phenomena*, such as thunder.

2 **Avoidance** of circumstances that provoke anxiety.

3 **Anticipatory anxiety** when there is the prospect of encountering such circumstances.

Phobic disorders are classified in three groups: simple phobia, social phobia, and agoraphobia. As explained above, some patients have both agoraphobia and non-situational panic.

Simple phobia

A person with simple phobia is inappropriately anxious in the presence of a particular object or situation, or when anticipating this encounter, and has the urge to avoid the object or situation. A list of common phobias is shown in Table 24.7. The urge to avoid the stimulus is strong, and in most cases there is actual avoidance. Anticipatory anxiety is often severe; for example, a person who fears storms may become extremely anxious when there are only black clouds, which might precede a storm. The diagnostic criteria for simple phobias are shown in Box 24.3.

Prevalence

Simple phobias are common but very few patients seek medical help. Recent studies report a lifetime prevalence of 12.5 per cent, and a 12-month prevalence of 8.5 per cent. The age at which phobias develop is highly variable; the mean onset of an animal phobia is age 7, whereas most situational phobias develop in early adulthood. Women present with phobias more frequently than men, but the exact gender ratio is unknown.

Co-morbidity

Of individuals with a simple phobia, 83.4 per cent will meet criteria for another psychiatric diagnosis at some time in their life. These are most commonly other anxiety disorders or depression.

Table 24.7 Common simple phobias

Objects that induce anxiety	Situations that induce anxiety
Blood (haematophobia)	Dentists (5% of adults; may lead to poor dentition)
Excretion	
Vomit or vomiting (emetopobia)	Darkness (scotophobia)
Needles or injections (trypanophobia)	Elevators
	Illness
Animals (zoophobia), e.g.:	Heights (acrophobia)
• Spiders (arachnophobia)	Storms or thunder
• Snakes (ophidiophobia)	Flying or aeroplanes

BOX 24.3 DSM-IV diagnostic criteria for specific phobia

A Marked and persistent fear that is excessive or unreasonable, cued by the presence or anticipation of a specific object or situation.

B Exposure to the phobic stimulus almost invariably provokes an immediate anxiety response, which may take the form of a situationally bound or situationally predisposed panic attack.

C The person recognizes that the fear is excessive or unreasonable. Note: in children, this feature may be absent.

D The phobic situation(s) is avoided or else is endured with intense anxiety or distress.

E The avoidance, anxious anticipation, or distress in the feared situation(s) interferes significantly with the

person's normal routine, occupational (or academic) functioning, or social activities or relationships, or there is marked distress about having the phobia.

F In individuals under age 18 years, the duration is at least 6 months.

G The anxiety, panic attacks, or phobic avoidance associated with the specific object or situation are not better accounted for by another mental disorder.

ICD-10 F40.2 Specific (isolated) phobias

There are no important differences between the ICD-10 and DSM-IV criteria.

Differential diagnosis

Some patients with long-standing simple phobias seek help when an unrelated depressive disorder makes them less able to tolerate the phobic symptoms. Apart from this association, simple phobia is seldom mistaken for another disorder.

Aetiology

Most of the simple phobias of adult life begin in childhood when simple phobias are extremely common. Why most childhood phobias disappear and a few persist into adult life is not known, except that the most severe phobias are more likely to do so. Simple phobias that begin in adult life often develop after a very frightening experience; for example, a phobia of horses following a dangerous encounter with a bolting horse.

One suggestion is that phobias are due to classical conditioning, the individual reinforcing a learned behaviour after a negative experience with an object or situation. The most important behaviour that maintains the fear and makes it hard to eliminate is avoidance.

There is robust evidence for a genetic component to simple phobias; one in three first-degree relatives of a person with simple phobia also meet diagnostic criteria for simple phobias. The concordance rates for animal phobias in monozygotic and dizygotic twins are 25 per cent and 11 per cent, respectively, but there are no data available for most other phobias.

Prognosis

There is little reliable information about the prognosis of simple phobias. Clinical experience indicates that simple phobias that began in childhood continue for many years,

while those starting after a stressful experience in adult life may improve with time. Often patients with simple phobias will adjust their lifestyle to avoid the object or situation, thus perpetuating the disorder. They may present for treatment only if the phobia becomes severe or if a change in circumstances leads to increased contact with the feared situation. An example of this is a new job that requires frequent air travel in a person with a fear of flying.

Treatment

The basic treatment approach is as for GAD, outlined on p. 290. It is worth noting that the majority of patients need no treatment beyond sensible advice unless the phobia is having a significant impact on their well-being.

Cognitive behaviour therapy. The treatment of choice for simple phobia is **graded exposure therapy**, which is a structured programme aiming to gradually reintroduce the patient to the phobic situation in a supportive manner.

Medication. Patients sometimes ask for immediate relief of symptoms when a long-standing phobia makes it difficult to fulfil a forthcoming important engagement (e.g. a claustrophobic person who requires an urgent MRI scan). In such circumstances, a benzodiazepine can be used, but in the short term only—the use of sedative medication in such circumstances is another way of avoiding the feared stimulus. It is not usually appropriate to prescribe an antidepressant, as the symptoms of simple phobia are by definition very intermittent.

Social phobia

Social phobia is incapacitating inappropriate anxiety in social situations which leads to the desire for escape or

Case study 24.1 Simple phobia

Louise, who had just left school and started work as a secretary, presented to her general practitioner with a friend. She had been afraid of entering lifts since her early childhood, fearing that she would become stuck inside and suffocate. Louise had always avoided using a lift, preferring to take the stairs or not change floors in a building. On one previous occasion, she had been forced to use a lift at the railway station and had had a panic attack. Unfortunately, her new job was on the 23rd floor of a large building, and it was impractical for her to climb the stairs multiple times daily. She had therefore come to the doctor to ask for help to

overcome her fear. The GP reassured her that simple phobias are common, and that it was nothing to be ashamed of. He gave Louise an advice leaflet, and recommended a self-help book to use whilst awaiting a referral for CBT. Louise found the book helpful in understanding her phobia, but did not make practical progress. She attended individual CBT sessions with a therapist, who took her through a graded exposure programme. First, Louise was supported to talk about lifts, then to look at pictures and videos of them. Finally, her therapist took her to see a lift, and gradually worked up to going inside and being able to use them.

avoidance. In the ICD-10 classification the term social phobia is preferred, whereas the DSM-IV uses the terms social phobia and social anxiety disorder interchangeably to describe the same condition. There are a number of principal features.

- **Specific concerns** (which they know to be irrational) about being observed critically by other people.
- **Situations** that provoke anxiety include restaurants, canteens, and dinner parties, seminars, board meetings, and other places where it is necessary to speak in public, and occasions when some action is open to scrutiny, for example writing, eating, or drinking in front of another person. The theme common to all situations is the potential for being observed and negatively evaluated.
- **Anticipatory anxiety.** People with social phobia also feel anxious when they anticipate entering such situations.
- **Avoidance** of these situations. Sometimes the avoidance is partial; for example, entering a social group but failing to make conversation, or sitting in an inconspicuous place in the group.
- **Symptoms** are similar to those of other anxiety disorders, although blushing and trembling are particularly frequent. Often people are concerned that these symptoms will be noticed by others, and provide evidence of their inadequacies.
- **Use of alcohol.** Some people take alcohol to relieve anxiety, and alcohol abuse is more common among social phobics than among people with other phobias.
- **Low self-esteem and perfectionism** are common traits amongst those with social phobia.

The formal diagnostic criteria for social anxiety disorder are shown in Box 24.4.

Onset and course

The condition usually *begins* with an acute attack of anxiety in some public place. Subsequently, anxiety occurs in

similar places, with episodes that become gradually more severe and with increasing avoidance.

Prevalence

The lifetime prevalence of social phobia is 12.1 per cent, whilst the 12-month prevalence is about 6.8 per cent. Social phobia is about equally common in men and women. Mean age of onset for the condition is 13–20 years, but often the patient will recall having had symptoms as far back as early childhood.

Co-morbidity

About 80 per cent of patients with social phobia will fit diagnostic criteria for another psychiatric disorder. The most common are other anxiety disorders, depression, post-traumatic stress disorder (PTSD), and alcohol use disorders.

Differential diagnosis

- **Generalized anxiety disorder.** Social phobia is distinguished by the pattern of situations in which anxiety occurs.
- **Depressive disorder.** Social phobia is distinguished by the pattern of situations and the absence of the core symptoms of low mood, anhedonia, and loss of energy (see p. 224). Sometimes people who have previously coped with social phobia seek help when they become depressed.
- **Schizophrenia.** Occasionally, patients with schizophrenia are anxious in, and avoid, social situations because of paranoid delusions.
- **Anxious/avoidant personality disorder,** characterized by lifelong shyness and lack of self-confidence, may closely resemble social phobia. However, personality disorder starts at a younger age and develops more gradually than social phobia.
- **Social inadequacy** is a primary lack of social skills with secondary anxiety. People with social phobia possess these social skills but cannot use them when they are anxious.

BOX 24.4 DSM-IV 300.23 Social anxiety disorder

A A marked and persistent fear of one or more social performance situations in which the person is exposed to unfamiliar people or to possible scrutiny by others. The individual fears that he or she will act in a way (or show anxiety symptoms) that will be humiliating or embarrassing.

B Exposure to the social or performance situation almost invariably provokes an immediate anxiety response.

C The person recognizes that their fear is excessive or unreasonable.

D The social or performance situation is avoided, although it is sometimes endured with dread (intense anxiety or distress).

E The avoidance, anxious anticipation of, or distress in, the feared social or performance situation interferes significantly with the person's normal routine, occupational (academic) functioning, or social life, or the person is markedly distressed about having the phobia.

F In individuals under age 18 years, the duration is at least 6 months.

G The fear or avoidance is not due to the direct physiological effects of a substance or a general medical condition and is not better accounted for by another mental disorder.

H If a general medical condition or another mental disorder is present, the fear in Criterion A or the avoidance in Criteria D is unrelated to it (e.g. the fear is not of stuttering, trembling in Parkinson's disease, or exhibiting abnormal eating behaviour in anorexia nervosa).

ICD-10 Diagnostic criteria F40.1 social phobia

There are no important differences between the ICD-10 and DSM-IV criteria.

- **Panic disorder with agoraphobia** can usually be distinguished from social phobia by the fact that panic attacks are typically unexpected, whereas the anxiety or panic that comes with social phobia occurs in anticipation of negative evaluation by others.

Aetiology

The cause of social phobia is uncertain. Symptoms usually start in late adolescence, a time when many young people are concerned about the impression they are making on other people. It is possible that social phobias begin as exaggerated normal concerns, which are then increased and prolonged by thoughts that other people will be critical of any signs of anxiety. It may be that styles of parenting and early childhood experiences influence the development of social anxiety. Patients with social anxiety often remember their mother being fearful in social situations, and frequently describe their parents as overprotective.

Genetics certainly play a role in the aetiology of social anxiety disorder, but the extent of this is currently unknown. Concordance rates for monozygotic twins (25 per cent) are higher than for dizygotic twins (15 per cent), and it is known (but not quantified) that first-degree relatives of those with the disorder have a greater risk of developing it than the general population.

Prognosis

There are no systematic data on the long-term course of social phobia. Clinical experience suggests that the phobia persists for many years, although most improve by mid life.

Treatment

The general measures are described in Tables 24.5 and 24.6.

Antidepressant medication. The best evidence is for the use of one of the SSRIs. Paroxetine, fluvoxamine, escitalopram, and sertraline have been reported to be effective in social phobia in the short term although the long-term benefits are less certain. A second-line option is the SNRI venlafaxine, which is of similar efficacy to SSRIs but has a poorer side-effect profile (see p. 120). Traditionally, the monoamine oxidase inhibitors (e.g. moclobemide) were used for social anxiety, but the strict dietary restrictions needed to use them safely combined with adverse side effects mean their use is only justified when other medications prove ineffective. *While taking any antidepressant medication, patients should be advised to practise exposure* to situations that they have previously avoided.

Anxiolytic medication provides immediate short-term relief, for example to help the patient deal with an important professional or social situation before more lasting treatment has taken effect. However, anxiolytics should not be used regularly because of the risk of dependence (see p. 114).

Beta-adrenergic antagonists (e.g. propranolol) are used occasionally to control tremor and palpitations unresponsive to anxiolytic treatment, but have not been shown to be better than placebo at controlling social anxiety when used on a regular basis.

Agoraphobia

Agoraphobia is a condition in which the patient experiences anxiety in situations that are unfamiliar, from which they cannot escape, or in which they perceive they have little control. This anxiety leads to avoidance of those situations.

Clinical features

Agoraphobic patients are anxious when they are away from home, in crowds, in situations they cannot leave easily, in social situations, and in open spaces (this last fear explains the name—'agoraphobia' contains the Greek word for 'marketplace'). Patients experience *anticipatory anxiety* and *avoid* situations that cause anxiety. *Anxious thoughts* are common, with themes of fainting and loss of control. The anxiety symptoms are any of

Table 24.8 Situations feared and avoided by patients with agoraphobia

Common themes	Distance from home
	Crowding
	Confinement
	Open spaces
	Social situations
Examples	Public transport
	Crowded shops
	Empty streets
	School visits
	Cinemas, theatres

those shown in Table 24.2 together with *panic attacks*, *depression*, and *depersonalization*.

Situations that typically provoke anxiety and avoidance are listed in Table 24.8. As the condition progresses, patients avoid more and more of these situations until in severe cases they may be almost confined to their homes. The anxiety experienced in these situations is reduced by the reassuring presence of a trusted companion, or a reassuring object such as a few anxiolytic tablets, which are carried but never taken.

Anticipatory anxiety may be severe and appear several hours before the person has to enter a feared situation.

In both DSM-IV and ICD-10, agoraphobia is not a codable disorder on its own. In either criteria, the diagnosis must be related to the presence or absence of panic disorder, expressed as being either **panic disorder with agoraphobia** (DSM-IV)/**agoraphobia with panic disorder** (ICD-10) or **agoraphobia without a history of panic disorder.** The full diagnostic criteria are shown in Box 24.5.

Course and outcome

The median age of onset for agoraphobia is 20 years, but there are two peaks; 15–30 years and 70–80 years. (This is in contrast to the peak of onset of simple phobias in childhood and of social phobias in late teenage years.) The *first episode* of agoraphobia often occurs while the person is away from home, waiting for public transport, or shopping in a crowded store. Suddenly, the person develops an unexplained panic attack, and either hurries home or seeks immediate medical help. This first episode subsides before long, but there is another when the same or similar situation is encountered again, and another hurried escape is made. This sequence recurs over and over again and the person begins to avoid the situations. It is unusual to discover any immediate cause for the first panic attack, although some patients describe a background of problems at the time (e.g. worry about a sick child). The devel-

---

 BOX 24.5 DSM-IV Agoraphobia without panic disorder

A Anxiety about being in places or situations from which escape might be difficult (or embarrassing) or in which help may not be available in the event of having an unexpected or situationally predisposed panic attack or panic-like symptoms. Agoraphobic fears typically involve characteristic clusters of situations that include being outside the home alone, being in a crowd, or standing in a line, being on a bridge, and travelling in a bus, train, or automobile.

B The situations are avoided (e.g. travel is restricted) or else are endured with marked distress or with anxiety

about having a panic attack or panic-like symptoms, or require the presence of a companion.

C The anxiety or phobic avoidance is not better accounted for by another mental disorder.

ICD-10 F40.0 Agoraphobia

There are no important differences between the ICD-10 and DSM-IV criteria.

opment of agoraphobic symptoms late in life is often linked to physical frailty, and the fear that an accident or major medical illness will occur.

As the condition progresses, patients become increasingly *dependent on the partner or other relatives* for help with activities, such as shopping, that provoke anxiety. These demands on the partner sometimes lead to arguments, and serious marital problems are common.

Prevalence

The 1-year prevalence of agoraphobia without panic disorder is about 18 per 1000, whilst the lifetime risk is 1–2 per cent. Approximately twice as many women as men are affected. As described above, the age of onset follows a bimodal distribution.

Co-morbidity

The most common co-morbid condition is panic attacks, but agoraphobia is also associated with other anxiety disorders, depression, and alcohol misuse disorders. Approximately 50 per cent of patients with agoraphobia will fit the diagnostic criteria for social phobia as well.

Differential diagnosis

- **Generalized anxiety disorder**, although this does not have the pattern of avoidance characteristic of agoraphobia. The patient usually has excessive worries about all aspects of life, not just those that fit into the common themes of distance from home, crowding, and confinement.

- **Social phobia**. Although agoraphobic patients feel anxious in social situations and some social phobics avoid crowded buses and shops, the overall pattern of anxiety-provoking situations is different.

- **Simple phobias** may involve panic attacks, but they only occur in the presence of a specific situation or object, and do not fit into the common themes outlined above.

- **Depressive disorder**. Sometimes a person with long-standing agoraphobia seeks help when depressed. They will show the typical core symptoms of low mood, anhedonia, and lack of energy.

- **Schizophrenia**. Rarely, patients with paranoid delusions avoid meeting people in a way that suggests agoraphobia. If they hide the delusions, diagnosis may be difficult but a thorough history and mental state examination usually show the true diagnosis.

Aetiology

The development of anticipatory anxiety and avoidance after the first panic attack can be understood in terms of conditioning. The cause of the first panic attack is uncertain. It could be caused by panic disorder (see below) in which case agoraphobia is simply a variant of panic disorder. Alternatively, the first panic attack could have another cause such as an accumulation of stressful events, in which case agoraphobia and panic disorder are separate conditions. The matter is undecided and there may be different causes in separate cases. It is agreed, however, that agoraphobia is *maintained by avoidance*, which prevents deconditioning, and by *apprehensive thoughts*, such as fears of fainting or social embarrassment, which set up vicious circles of anxiety.

Prognosis

Agoraphobia that has been present continuously for a year is likely to persist for at least 5 years. Brief episodes of depressive symptoms often occur in the course of chronic agoraphobia.

Treatment

Treatment begins with the general measures described in Tables 24.5 and 24.6.

Antidepressants are of value not only for their general anxiolytic effect but also because some have anti-panic effects. SSRIs are the first-line choice, with the best evidence being for fluoxetine, fluvoxamine, citalopram, and sertraline. Their use should be combined with exposure, either as a self-help procedure or as part of cognitive behaviour therapy.

Anxiolytics (e.g. benzodiazepines) should be avoided, except for the short-term alleviation of incapacitating symptoms or when waiting for an SSRI to take effect.

There is some evidence that the most effective treatment for agoraphobia is a combination of cognitive behaviour therapy and medication.

Panic disorder

In Greek mythology the mischievous god Pan was said to be able to inspire fear in people and animals when they were in lonely places. He could do this without warning, very suddenly, and the emotions that people experienced when he did this became known as panic. The unprovoked, spontaneous nature of panic attacks is their defining quality, and is essential for their recognition and diagnosis. Panic attacks are very common—9 per cent of the population experience at least one in their lifetime—and are associated with significant social and occupational disability.

A panic attack is a period of intense fear characterized by a cluster of typical symptoms that develop rapidly, last a few minutes, and during which the person fears that some kind of catastrophe will occur. Panic attacks may occur in all anxiety disorders, as well as other psychiatric and physical disorders.

Panic disorder is a condition in which a person experiences recurrent panic attacks that occur unexpectedly (i.e. not in response to a phobic stimulus), and are not associated with substance abuse, medical conditions, or another psychiatric disorder.

Clinical features

The typical symptoms of a panic attack are listed in Table 24.9, and the formal diagnostic criteria are shown in Box 24.6. The characteristic feature of a panic attack is that it occurs spontaneously and without provocation. Anxiety increases over a few minutes to a severe level, during which the patient fears some kind of catastrophic outcome such as a heart attack. The frequency and severity of panic attacks vary between patients, but one or two attacks per week is usual. Panic attacks are a terrifying experience, and patients often become scared of having more attacks, and of being in situations where an attack previously occurred. This can lead to agoraphobia, as discussed above.

Panic disorder patients often seek advice from general practitioners, cardiologists, and other physicians to whom they complain not of anxiety, but of accompanying physical symptoms such as palpitations. It is therefore important to take a thorough history, including both physical and psychological symptoms.

Prevalence

If formal diagnostic criteria are used then the prevalence of panic disorder averages 7 to 9 per cent of the population. However, a looser definition produces much higher numbers—approximately 15 to 20 per cent. Panic disorder is at least twice as frequent among women as among men, and other risk factors include urban living, divorce, limited education, and physical or sexual abuse. There are two peaks of onset: 15 to 24 years and 45 to 55 years. It is rare for the disorder to begin after the age of 65.

Differential diagnosis

Panic attacks occur in many conditions other than panic disorder, both psychiatric and physical. Common examples include:

- other anxiety disorders (GAD, phobias, social anxiety, agoraphobia);
- depression;
- post-traumatic stress disorder;
- obsessive-compulsive disorder;
- drugs—intoxication or withdrawal—e.g. caffeine, cocaine, cannabis, theophylline, amphetamines, steroids;

Table 24.9 Symptoms of a panic attack (in order of frequency)

- Palpitations
- Tachycardia
- Sweating and flushing
- Trembling
- Dyspnoea
- Chest discomfort
- Nausea
- Dizziness or fainting
- Fears of an impending medical emergency
- Depersonalization

BOX 24.6 DSM-IV Panic disorder with (or without) agoraphobia

A Both (1) and (2):

1 recurrent unexpected panic attacks;

2 at least one of the attacks has been followed by 1 month (or more) of one (or more) of the following:

- persistent concern about having additional attacks;
- worry about the implications of the attack or its consequences;
- significant change in behaviour related to the attacks.

B The presence (or absence) of agoraphobia.

C The panic attacks are not due to the direct physiological effects of a substance or a general medical condition.

D The panic attacks are not better accounted for by another mental disorder, such as social phobia, specific phobia, obsessive-compulsive disorder, post-traumatic stress disorder, or separation anxiety disorder.

ICD-10 F41.0 Panic disorder (episodic paroxysmal anxiety)

A diagnosis of panic disorder can only be made if the patient does not fit the criteria F40—specific phobia, social phobia, or agoraphobia without panic.

- endocrine disorders (hyperthyroidism, hypoglycaemia, Cushing's syndrome, carcinoid tumours, and phaeochromocytoma);
- cardiovascular disorders (arrhythmias, chest pain, mitral regurgitation);
- respiratory disorders (chronic obstructive pulmonary disease, asthma).

Usually, the key to making the correct diagnosis is to take a full history, and consider which symptoms developed first. For example, did depression precede or follow the onset of panic? It is important to recognize and treat the underlying cause of the attacks.

Co-morbidity

About three-quarters of patients with panic disorder have concurrent agoraphobia, and half fit the diagnostic criteria for depression.

Aetiology

The causes of panic disorder are uncertain. There are three main areas of current research.

1 **Genetics.** There is good evidence that the rates of panic disorders amongst first-degree relatives of those with the disorder are seven to eight times higher than average. Unfortunately, there is currently insufficient evidence from twin studies to provide accurate concordance figures. Heritability of panic disorder is estimated to be around 40 per cent.

2 **The biochemical hypothesis** suggests that panic disorder is due to an imbalance in neurotransmitter activity in the brain. Certain chemical agents can induce panic attacks more readily in panic disorder patients than in healthy people—these agents include yohimbine (an alpha-adrenergic antagonist), isoproterenol (a beta-adrenergic agonist), and inhaled carbon dioxide. It is thought that the serotonin (5HT) and GABA systems are also involved, because SSRIs and benzodiazepines are effective at reducing panic attacks.

3 **The cognitive hypothesis** is based on the observation that compared with other anxious patients, patients with panic disorder more often have fears concerning physical symptoms of anxiety. They fear, for example, that palpitations will be followed by a heart attack. This produces a vicious cycle, as shown in Figure 24.1. There is experimental evidence in support of this hypothesis; for example, reducing fearful cognitions reduces panic.

Prognosis

Systematic follow-up data have not been reported but clinical observation indicates that some patients who experience panic attacks recover within weeks of the onset. However, in those with panic disorder that has persisted for 6 months or more the disorder usually runs a prolonged, although often fluctuating, course which may last for many years.

Treatment

The general guidance for anxiety disorders on p. 290 and in Tables 24.5 and 24.6 all applies to panic disorder and forms the basis of treatment, but there are specific additional points listed below, and in Table 24.10. The evidence for the efficacy of psychological, pharmacological, or self-help treatments is all robust—the patient should be involved in choosing the most appropriate approach for them.

Psychological treatment

Information. Clinicians who see patients soon after an initial panic attack should attempt to prevent progression to panic disorder by explaining that the physical symptoms are caused by anxiety and that, while frightening, they are harmless. When panic attacks are already established, it is often useful to compare them to a house alarm that is too sensitive so that it goes off when there is no real danger. Patients should be advised how safety behaviours prevent them from discovering that panic attacks are similarly a warning of non-existent danger (see above). They should be warned that if they avoid situations in which panic attacks have occurred they may develop agoraphobia.

Psychological therapies. See Table 24.6.

Table 24.10 Management plan for panic disorder

Assessment
- Make a diagnosis and detect any co-morbid depressive disorder

General measures
- Agree a clear plan
- Psychoeducation
- Problem-solving techniques and relaxation
- Manage hyperventilation (see Box 24.2)

Psychological treatment
- Self-help books, computerized cognitive behavioural therapy
- Cognitive behavioural therapy

Pharmacotherapy
- Antidepressants

Social interventions

Antidepressant drugs. As explained above, antidepressants are effective anxiolytics, and in high doses also have anti-panic effects. SSRIs are the first-line choice for panic disorder—there is no evidence that any one drug is more effective than another, but the most studied are fluvoxamine, paroxetine, and sertraline. If SSRIs are contraindicated or not effective after a 12-week trial, imipramine or clomipramine should be considered. Imipramine is historically used in panic disorder, and is probably the most effective, but its anticholinergic and cardiac side effects limit usage in many patients. The antidepressant should be continued for at least 6 months after symptoms resolve.

Anxiolytic drugs. As explained above, the general rules in treating anxiety disorders are that anxiolytics should be used only for short periods, usually while other treatment is being initiated.

■ Obsessive-compulsive disorder

Obsessive-compulsive disorder (OCD) is a condition characterized by obsessions and/or compulsions that the person feels driven to perform according to specific rules in order to prevent an imagined dreaded event. OCD is the fourth most common psychiatric disorder and is usually a chronic condition—it therefore represents a high burden of morbidity within the population. Effective treatment is available, so prompt diagnosis and referral are essential.

Clinical features

OCD is characterized by obsessional thinking, compulsive behaviour, and varying degrees of other psychiatric symptomology. An overview of the symptoms that may be experienced is shown in Figure 24.3, and explanations follow below. The formal diagnostic criteria for OCD are shown in Box 24.7.

Obsessions are recurrent persistent thoughts, impulses, or images that enter the mind despite efforts to exclude them. The feeling of being compelled to undergo the intrusion of a thought, impulse, or image and the resistances produced against them are key characteristics of an obsession. They may come in the form of any of the following.

- **Obsessional thoughts** which intrude forcibly into the patient's mind and the patient attempts to exclude them. Obsessional thoughts may be single words, phrases, or rhymes; they are usually unpleasant or shocking to the patient, obscene, or blasphemous.

- **Obsessional images** typically appear as vividly imagined scenes, often of violence or of a kind that disgusts the patient, such as abnormal sexual practices.

- **Obsessional ruminations** are internal debates in which continuous arguments are reviewed endlessly.

- **Obsessional doubts** are thoughts about actions that may have been completed inadequately, such as failing to turn off a gas tap completely, or about actions that may have harmed other people.

- **Obsessional impulses** are urges to perform acts, usually of a violent or embarrassing kind; for example, leaping in front of a car or shouting blasphemies in church. The urges are resisted strongly, and are not carried out, but the internal struggle may be very distressing.

- **Obsessional rituals** are repeated but senseless activities. They may be *mental activities*, such as counting repeatedly in a special way or repeating a certain form of words, or *behaviours*, such as excessive handwashing or lock checking. Rituals are usually followed by temporary release of distress. The ritual may be followed by doubts whether it has been completed in the right way, and the sequence may be repeated over and over again. Patients are aware that their rituals are illogical, and usually try to hide them.

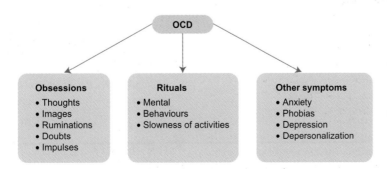

Fig. 24.3 Symptoms of obsessive-compulsive disorder.

BOX 24.7 Diagnostic criteria for obsessive-compulsive disorder

Obsessions

1 Recurrent and persistent thoughts, impulses, or images that are experienced as intrusive and that cause marked anxiety or distress.

2 The thoughts, impulses, or images are not simply excessive worries about real-life problems.

3 The person attempts to ignore or suppress such thoughts, impulses, or images, or to neutralize them with some other thought or action.

4 The person recognizes that the obsessional thoughts, impulses, or images are a product of his or her own mind, and are not based in reality.

Compulsions

1 Repetitive behaviours or mental acts that the person feels driven to perform in response to an obsession, or according to rules that must be applied rigidly.

2 The behaviours or mental acts are aimed at preventing or reducing distress or preventing some dreaded event or situation; however, these behaviours or mental acts are not actually connected to the issue, or they are excessive.

In addition to these criteria, at some point during the course of the disorder, the individual must realize that his or her obsessions or compulsions are unreasonable or excessive. Moreover, the obsessions or compulsions must be time-consuming (taking up more than 1 hour per day), cause distress, or cause impairment in social, occupational, or school functioning. OCD often causes feelings similar to those of depression.

ICD-10 F42.0 Obsessive-compulsive disorder

There are no important differences between the ICD-10 and DSM-IV criteria.

Anxiety and depressive symptoms are often present in patients with OCD. In some patients these are an understandable reaction to the obsessional symptoms, but in others there are recurring depressive moods that arise independently of the other symptoms. *Depersonalization* occurs sometimes, adding to the patient's disability.

Obsessional personality is described on p. 422. Although they share the same name, obsessional personality and OCDs do not have a simple one-to-one relationship. Obsessional personality is over-represented among patients who develop OCD, but about a third of obsessional patients have other types of personality. Moreover, although people with obsessional personality may develop OCDs, they are more likely to develop depressive disorders.

Prevalence

The lifetime prevalence of OCD in the general population is 2 to 3 per cent, whilst the 1-year prevalence is about 8 to 10 per 1000. Men and women are affected about equally. The mean age of onset of clinically relevant symptoms is 20 years, but many patients start developing symptoms earlier, in their teens.

Co-morbidity

Patients with OCD frequently fit the diagnostic criteria for other psychiatric disorders. The lifetime risk for a major depressive episode in these patients is 60 to 70 per cent. Other common co-morbidities include alcohol use disorders, eating disorders, phobias and PTSD.

Differential diagnosis

- **Anxiety disorders.** Obsessional symptoms are less severe than those of anxiety and develop later in the course of the disorder.

- **Phobias.** The fears in OCD tend to relate to concerns of harming others, rather than that harm will come to themselves. The stimuli in phobias are usually specific avoidable situations (e.g. lifts, spiders, crowds) whereas phobic symptoms in OCD are more generalised (e.g. bacteria, dirt).

- **Depressive disorder.** Obsessional symptoms follow the depression in depressive disorders and precede it in obsessional disorder. The correct diagnosis is important because obsessional symptoms in depressive disorders usually respond well to antidepressant treatment.

- **Schizophrenia.** When obsessional thoughts have a peculiar content, the clinical picture may suggest schizophrenia. Repeated mental state examinations will reveal other symptoms of schizophrenia and an informant may describe other behaviours that suggest this diagnosis.

- **Organic cerebral disorders.** Although obsessional symptoms may occur in dementia, they are seldom prominent and other features of dementia are present.

■ Aetiology

An overview of the aetiology of OCD is shown in Table 24.11.

Table 24.11 Causes of Obsessive-compulsive disorder

Predisposing factors	Precipitating factors	Maintaining factors
Genetics	Stressful events, e.g.:	Checking and rituals
• Family history	• Relationships	Cycle of anxiety (see Figure 24.1)
Neurobiological mechanisms	• Unemployment	Continuing stressful life events
• Structural	• Financial problems	Depressive disorder
• Neurotransmitters	• Ill health	
• Autoimmune		
Early experiences		
Psychological		
Obsessive-compulsive personality		

Predisposing causes

1 **Genetics.** The lifetime risk for OCD is increased tenfold in first-degree relatives of patients diagnosed with OCD. It is not certain whether this familial pattern indicates genetic causes rather than family environment, because the necessary large-scale twin and adoption studies have not been carried out.

2 **Structural organic abnormalities.** Parents with OCD have an increased rate of minor, non-localizing neurological signs but no specific neurological lesion has been identified. Positron emission tomography (PET) and functional MRI have shown increased activity in the frontal lobes, caudate nucleus, and cingulum in OCD patients.

3 **Neurotransmitters.** The clinical benefits of SSRIs in OCD suggest that a dysregulation of the 5HT pathways may play a role in its aetiology. A variety of randomized controlled challenge studies have been undertaken and have shown that giving a 5HT antagonist increased anxiety levels in OCD. Evidence for the involvement of dopaminergic pathways in OCD comes from the fact that disorders of the basal ganglia (e.g. Tourette's, post-encephalitic parkinsonism) show a high level of obsessive symptoms.

4 **Autoimmune factors.** For many years it has been known that Sydenham's chorea—an autoimmune disease of the basal ganglia—is associated with OCD in two-thirds of cases. These patients have autoantibodies to the caudate nucleus. More recently, an association has been made between Group A streptococcal infections and OCD/tic disorders (see Science box 24.1).

5 **Early experience.** Obsessional mothers might be expected to transmit a tendency to obsessional symptoms to their children through social learning.

6 **Psychological causes.** Obsessions can be thought of as a conditioned response to an anxiety-provoking event. The patient develops avoidant behaviours (of which compulsions are part) to try and avoid experiencing the anxiety-provoking event. Sigmund Freud's psychoanalytic approach suggests that the symptoms of OCD reflect unsolved conflicts or impulses of a violent or sexual nature. These impulses create anxiety, which is avoided by the use of defence mechanisms.

Prognosis

About two-thirds of obsessional disorders improve within a year; the remaining third run a prolonged and usually fluctuating course with periods of partial or complete remission lasting a few months to several years.

Treatment

NICE published guidance for the management of OCD in 2005, the content of which is outlined in Table 24.12.

Table 24.12 Management of Obsessive-compulsive disorder

Assessment
- Make a diagnosis and detect any co-morbidities

General measures for all patients
- Psychoeducation
- Problem-solving techniques and relaxation
- Self-help books

Mild functional impairment
- Offer brief cognitive behavioural therapy

Moderate functional impairment
- SSRI *or*
- Full course of cognitive behavioural therapy

Severe functional impairment
- Combined treatment with SSRI and cognitive behavioural therapy
- Consider clomipramine

BOX 24.8 Screening questions for Obsessive-compulsive disorder

Do you wash and clean a lot?

Do you check things a lot?

Are there any thoughts that keep bothering you that you would like to get rid of but can't?

Do your daily activities take a long time to finish?

Are you concerned about putting things in a special order or are you very upset by mess?

Do these problems trouble you?

Patients who are at higher risk of OCD and should be screened (Box 24.8) include those presenting with:

- depressive disorder;
- anxiety disorders;
- alcohol or substance misuse;
- eating disorders;
- body dysmorphic disorder.

A risk assessment should specifically focus on the risk of self-harm or suicide.

The guidelines suggest different management strategies according to the level of functional impairment the OCD is causing to the patient. This is obviously a subjective matter, but as a general rule the simpler treatments should be tried initially before moving on to the more intensive ones, unless the patient is unable to function (e.g. housebound, unable to work, causing themselves physical harm) at a basic level due to the OCD. Most of the measures can be initiated in primary care, but more severe cases or non-responders should be referred to a mental health specialist.

General measures

All of the general measures to reduce anxiety, described on pp. 289–291, are relevant to OCD. It is especially important to detect and treat any co-morbid depressive disorder.

Science box 24.1 Obsessive-compulsive disorder in adults: an autoimmune disease?

Sydenham's chorea is the archetypical condition demonstrating molecular mimicry; in response to streptococcal infection, the body produces antineuronal antibodies, which attack the streptococci but also cross-react with the basal ganglia producing choreoathetoid movements. It has been suggested that a childhood OCD and tic disorders may be a similar autoimmune disease, now termed **paediatric autoimmune neuropsychiatric disorders associated with streptococcal infections (PANDAS)**.[1] This is further discussed on p. 455. However, in the last decade, a series of prospective cohorts has not found an association between the clinical symptoms of PANDAS and streptococcal infections, and studies searching for the presence of specific antibasal ganglia antibodies or cytokines have reported inconsistent results.[2,3] The controversy surrounding whether or not PANDAS exists continues.

Meanwhile, it remains that the majority of patients who present with OCD are adults. Could there be an autoimmune basis to (at least a subset of) these cases? Maina *et al.* conducted a study on 74 adult patients with OCD and 44 controls with a major depressive disorder. They measured the antistreptolysin O titres (ASOT) and an array of antitissue and antibrain antibodies. They found the proportion of patients with a positive ASOT was significantly greater in the OCD group. However, there was no difference for any of the other antibodies measured.[4] The results of this study mirror similar results published by other groups. There is currently no evidence that OCD in adults is an autoimmune condition, a disappointment for those searching for novel therapeutic approaches.[5]

1 Swedo, S. E., Leonard, H. L., Garvey, M., *et al.* (1998). Pediatric autoimmune neuropsychiatric disorders associated with streptococcal infections: clinical description of the first 50 cases. *American Journal of Psychiatry* **155**: 264–71.

2 Luo, F. *et al.* (2004). Prospective longitudinal study of children with tic disorders and/or Obsessive-compulsive disorder: relationship of symptom exacerbations to newly acquired streptococcal infections. *Pediatrics* **113**: 578–85.

3 Morer, A. *et al.* (2008). Antineuronal antibodies in a group of children with Obsessive-compulsive disorder and Tourette syndrome. *Journal of Psychiatry Research* **42**: 64–8.

4 Maina, G. et al. (2009). Anti-brain antibodies in adult patients with obsessive-compulsive disorder. *Journal of Affective Disorders* **116**: 192–200.

5 Shulman, S.T. (2009). Pediatric autoimmune neuropsychiatric disorders associated with streptococcal infections: update. *Current Opinion in Pediatrics* **21**: 127–30.

Case study 24.2 Obsessive-compulsive disorder

A 32-year-old woman who was 28 weeks pregnant was referred to psychiatry by her general practitioner. Since becoming pregnant, she had become excessively concerned that she might be harming her baby by letting germs enter her body. This had led to her washing her hands over 50 times per day, and to showering at least 10 times per day. When finishing washing she was never quite sure she had done it adequately, and would repeat the process multiple times. She described having visions of her baby covered in bacteria popping uncontrollably into her mind, and the urge to cut herself to release any germs in her blood. Each day she called her doctor to ask for an ultrasound to be done to check she had not harmed the baby. The GP had given her self-help materials and offered an SSRI, which had been refused on the grounds that drugs might cause the baby damage. The psychiatrist organized an intensive course of individual CBT, which helped her to reduce the behaviours slightly. She gave birth to a healthy girl at 39 weeks, after which her symptoms improved greatly. She continued to receive CBT for another 6 months, after which she was able to return to work.

Psychoeducation. The provision of information is the important first step in treatment. Patients with an OCD find their thoughts and actions so strange and irrational that they often fear that they are 'going mad' and could act on the impulses they are resisting. It is important to explain that OCD does not progress in this way.

Self-help methods. It is important that patients resist rituals for although these produce short-term relief from distress, they maintain the disorder. Patients need a lot of support and encouragement to resist the very strong urge to carry out rituals. If the patient agrees, a relative or close friend can help, but most patients are ashamed of the rituals and are therefore reluctant to accept such help. Books, computerized resources, and self-help groups can be powerful tools in either starting the process of change or maintaining it.

Treatment for patients with mild functional impairment

Brief cognitive behavioural therapy (CBT) based on exposure with response prevention is the treatment of choice, and can be delivered in a variety of ways:

- brief individual CBT (up to 10 hours) with structured self-help materials;
- CBT by telephone;
- group CBT.

Treatment for patients with moderate functional impairment

The patient should initially be offered a choice between individual CBT and medication.

Antidepressants. There is robust evidence that 5HT reuptake inhibitors suppress Obsessive-compulsive symptoms, and the action is independent of their antidepressant effect. Effective drugs include the SSRIs (fluoxetine, citalopram, sertraline, paroxetine) and the tricyclic drug clomipramine, which is a non-specific inhibitor of 5HT uptake. The efficacy of SSRIs and clomipramine is similar, with about half the patients improving substantially, although clomipramine may be slightly superior. All these drugs are slow to act, taking up to 6 weeks to reach their full effect. Medication is continued for at least 12 months after symptoms recede. SSRIs are the usual first choice because clomipramine has to be given in high dosage, which is liable to produce anticholinergic and cardiac side effects.

Anxiolytic drugs are not recommended to be used routinely in OCD, although they may be used in the short term whilst waiting for an SSRI to take effect.

Treatment for patients with severe functional impairment

These patients should be offered combined treatment with an SSRI and a full course of individual CBT. The details of treatment are the same as outlined above.

Clomipramine should be considered in physically healthy patients who have shown no improvement on adequate trials of two SSRIs. A referral to a mental health specialist should be made if this approach fails.

Rarely, a patient with OCD may need more intensive treatment, such as an inpatient admission. This should only occur if there is a serious risk of self-harm/suicide, dangerous self-neglect, or co-morbid severe depression, anorexia nervosa, or schizophrenia.

Psychosurgery is not recommended for the treatment of OCD.

Further reading

National Institute for Clinical Excellence (2005). *Obsessive-Compulsive Disorder: Core Interventions in the Treatment of Obsessive-Compulsive Disorder and Body Dysmorphic Disorder.* http://guidance.nice.org.uk/CG31/.

National Institute for Clinical Excellence (2004, amended 2007). *Anxiety: Management of Anxiety in Adults in Primary, Secondary and Community Care.* http://guidance.nice.org.uk/CG22/ .

Butler, G. & Hope, T. (1995). *Manage your Mind: the Mental Fitness Guide.* Oxford University Press, Oxford. A useful account of self-help methods for anxiety disorders and other conditions.

Gale, C. & Davidson, O. (2007). Generalised anxiety disorder. *British Medical Journal* **334**: 579–81.

Kroenke, K., Spitzer, R. L., Williams, J. B. *et al.* (2007). Anxiety disorders in primary care: prevalence, impairment, comorbidity and detection. *Annals of Internal Medicine* **146**: 317–25.

Soomro, G. M., Altman, D. G., Rajagopal, S., & Oakley, B. M. (2008). Selective serotonin reuptake inhibitors versus placebo for Obsessive-compulsive disorder. *Cochrane Database of Systematic Reviews*, Issue 1. http://mrw.interscience.wiley.com/cochrane/clsysrev/articles/CD001765/frame.html

Medically unexplained physical symptoms

Concern about physical symptoms is a common reason for people to seek medical help. Many of these symptoms, such as headache, chest pain, weakness, dizziness, and fatigue, remain unexplained by identifiable disease even after extensive medical assessment. Several general terms have been used to describe these types of symptom—somatoform, medically unexplained, and functional. We prefer the terms 'medically unexplained physical symptom' or 'functional symptom', because they imply a disturbance of some kind in bodily functioning without implying that the symptom is psychogenic. Patients and doctors often assume that a physical symptom implies that a physical pathology exists. However, commonly experienced and often severe, distressing, and disabling symptoms, such as menstrual pain or 'tension headache', indicate that this is not always the case. By assuming that a physical symptom is explained by physical disease/pathology, we may be subjecting the patient to unnecessary tests and hospital visits, adding to patient distress, and failing to deliver the kind of integrated management that is needed.

There are many kinds of these symptoms (Table 25.1), and they are seen in primary care and across the full range of secondary care. They are considered in this psychiatry textbook because psychological factors (including, at times, psychiatric disorder) are important in the aetiology and because psychological and behavioural interventions have an important role in treatment.

A major obstacle to effective management of patients with functional symptoms is that they feel their doctors do not believe them. They are concerned that they may be thought to be 'putting it on'. It is crucial to note that the

Table 25.1 Some common physical symptoms that are often 'functional'

Pain syndromes:

  abdominal pain

  non-cardiac chest pain

  headache

  atypical facial pain

  muscular pain

  low back pain

  pelvic pain

Chronic fatigue

Non-ulcer dyspepsia

Irritable bowel

Palpitations

Dizziness

Tinnitus

Dysphonia

Premenstrual tension

Food intolerance

deliberate manufacture or exaggeration of symptoms or signs is quite different (see p. 313).

■ Classification of medically unexplained physical symptoms

Classification in this area is, unfortunately, not straight-forward. Diagnoses of three kinds may be given.

Descriptive physical syndromes. These include fibromyalgia, chronic fatigue syndrome, non-cardiac chest pain, chronic pain syndrome, and irritable bowel syndrome. Although the specific terms are useful in everyday medical practice, there is substantial overlap, and many patients with, for example, fibromyalgia will also have irritable bowel syndrome.

Psychiatric syndromes that are a primary cause of the functional symptoms. Well-recognized psychiatric syndromes, such as depression, anxiety, and adjustment disorders, are common **primary causes** of functional symptoms, and commonly present via them, sometimes via the general hospital's A&E department or cardiology outpatient clinic. For example, a patient with generalized anxiety disorder has multiple autonomic symptoms of anxiety (which are an integral part of the diagnostic criteria), including palpitations; the palpitations are themselves alarming, and trigger negative automatic thoughts about possible cardiac illness and its outcomes, thereby maintaining anxiety, autonomic arousal,

and physical symptoms. The physical symptoms may resolve with effective treatment of these psychiatric disorders. Psychiatric disorders such as anxiety disorder may also be **secondary** to functional symptoms, which are then exacerbated and maintained by the psychiatric disorder.

Psychiatric syndromes comprising health concern and functional symptoms. The appropriate psychiatric diagnosis is a somatoform disorder. These are conditions characterized by (i) *persistent abnormal concern* about physical health, and (ii) one or more *physical symptoms unexplained by physical pathology*. Within the somatoform disorders, there are several specific disorders (see Box 25.1) of which you should be aware. However, this area of classification is a vexed one, and is likely to be substantially revised in DSM-V and ICD-11, which are due for publication in the near future.

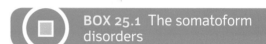

BOX 25.1 The somatoform disorders

Somatoform autonomic dysfunction. Common. A large, ill-defined, category of patients who present repeatedly with one or more unexplained physical symptoms, attributable to a system under autonomic control (cardiovascular, gastrointestinal, respiratory, urogenital), which persist in spite of negative investigation and reassurance.

Somatization disorder. Uncommon. *Multiple*, recurrent and changing unexplained physical symptoms, with multiple presentations to medical care, often over a period of many years. Usually begins in early life. Chronic and often fluctuating course.

Hypochondriasis. Severe persistent anxiety about ill health and conviction of disease, with repeated presentation of concern about the possibility of one or more specific diseases (such as cancer, heart disease), despite negative medical investigations and appropriate reassurance.

Body dysmorphic disorder. Persistent, inappropriate concern about the appearance of the body (e.g. about the shape and size of the nose or breasts), despite reassurance. Some patients demand cosmetic plastic surgery, which is helpful only in those with clear and reasonable expectations.

Persistent somatoform pain disorder. The intensity and duration of pain cannot be accounted for by any primary physical or mental disorder.

Dissociative (conversion) disorder. Partial or complete loss of the normal integration between (i) memories of the past, (ii) awareness of identity and immediate sensations, and (iii) control of movements, in the absence of a medical explanation. Examples of symptoms include amnesia, aphonia, paralysis, and anaesthesia. (See further description on p. 311.)

Epidemiology

Functional symptoms are common, occurring in about one-fifth of the population in all countries and communities. In primary care only a small proportion of people with functional symptoms ever receive a specific physical diagnosis (Figure 25.1). Most functional symptoms are transient, and are therefore not usually brought to medical attention. However, a sizeable minority persist and are often disabling. Up to half will remain disabled by the symptoms at the 12-month follow-up. Outcome is poorest for patients with more intractable problems who are referred to specialist care.

Functional symptoms may occur alone, but also commonly accompany serious physical illness. For example, following a heart attack or cardiac surgery, minor muscular chest aches and pains in the chest may be misinterpreted as evidence of angina, and lead to unnecessary worry and disability. It is, therefore, important not to assume that all chest pain in someone with chest pathology is due to that pathology. Explanation, and advice about how to respond to the pain, and perhaps in the context of a psychologically informed cardiac rehabilitation programme, may result in significant improvement in quality of life.

Aetiology

Functional symptoms are often put down to *either* physical *or* psychological causes. This 'mind–body dualism' is unhelpful to us, as it prevents us from using more effective, integrated models to explain aetiology or to plan

treatment. It is also often unacceptable to patients. By implication, in the absence of physical pathology, a symptom is 'all in the mind', and in the presence of physical pathology, a symptom is not influenced at all by psychological or social factors.

An alternative approach uses an integrated model in which *physical*, *psychological*, and *social* factors all contribute to the formation of symptoms (Figure 25.2). This approach suggests that functional symptoms arise initially from minor physiological or pathological bodily sensations, triggered by a multitude of usually benign causes, such as a hangover, autonomic effects of anxiety, lack of sleep, prolonged inactivity, overeating, fatigue, sinus tachycardia, or minor arrhythmias.

The key next step is attribution—the process of assigning a putative cause to the symptom. Attributions may be **normalizing** (assigning benign causes such as the effects of a hangover or tiredness), **psychologizing** (assigning causes such as stress or depression), or **somatizing** (assigning more serious physical causes such as tumour, endocrine disease, or cardiac disease). Whether an individual normalizes, psychologizes, or somatizes is influenced by several factors, including the person's usual 'attributional style', which may be seen as a feature of their personality, that is it is relatively static through time, and their personal situation at that time—if they are undergoing a period of interpersonal stress, or excessive demands at work, they may be emotionally aroused and more likely to somatize. Other factors may influence an individual's response to a physical sensation, including:

- their family medical history—a middle-aged man with a family history of heart disease may be understandably concerned about the implications of a chest pain which is, in fact, of musculoskeletal origin;

- their personal medical history, including experience of illnesses and their management, whether successful or unsuccessful;

- their knowledge of illnesses of possible relevance, derived from multiple sources including healthcare professionals, family, friends, and media coverage, whether accurate or inaccurate;

- their family and friends' response to the physical sensation;

- their doctor's (or other healthcare professionals') response.

Finally, patients' understandable attempts to alleviate their symptoms may paradoxically exacerbate them. For example, excessive rest to reduce pain or fatigue may actually prolong it, by leading to physical deconditioning, and by increasing the patient's focus on their symptoms and disability, rather than on their abilities and their

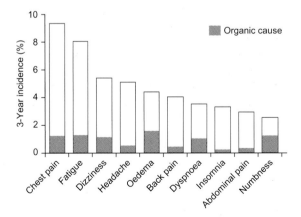

Fig. 25.1 Three-year incidence of 10 common presenting symptoms and proportion of symptoms with a suspected organic cause in US primary care attenders. Reproduced with permission from Kroenke, K. & Mangelsdorff, A. D. (1989). Common symptoms in ambulatory care, *American Journal of Medicine* **86**: 262–8.

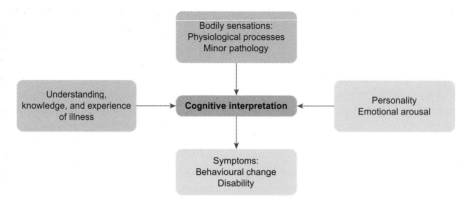

Fig. 25.2 Aetiology of medically unexplained symptoms.

opportunities. Furthermore, they may devote great energy to seeking 'the answer' on the Internet, to the extent that their life becomes defined by their illness. Disability benefits may act as an understandable disincentive for some patients to return to productive employment, and ongoing litigation can maintain the patient's focus on their disabilities rather than their abilities. Doctors may also unintentionally maintain symptoms by failing to address patients' concerns, or by excessive investigation or multiple referrals within secondary care, as they seek a physical explanation.

■ Management

Although it is always essential to consider physical disease as the cause of the patient's symptoms, an approach exclusively devoted to this can lead to difficulties if no disease is found. It is better to adopt a more integrated, biopsychosocial approach from the start. Explain that physical symptoms are often only fully explained by considering physical, psychological, and social factors relating to the individual's health, and use examples to illustrate this—a stressed businessman facing a deadline who presents with chronic, debilitating headache, for example, or a head teacher with chronic bowel symptoms which worsen as the school's annual inspection looms. This keeps open the option of a wider discussion of causes, either initially or in due course, and allows psychological treatment to be presented as a part of *usual* medical care rather than as an *alternative* that the patient may feel does not take his physical symptoms seriously.

Assessment

A thorough physical assessment is essential, both to exclude the possibility of physical disorder, and to emphasize to the patient that you are taking their concerns seriously. This should include:

- listening carefully to the patient's history;
- conducting a focused physical examination;
- organizing any medically indicated physical investigation. Be aware that tests should be justified in terms of the likelihood and value of new information. Investigations that cannot be medically justified may increase the patient's anxiety, increase disease conviction, and reinforce illness behaviours.

In addition, a more psychological approach should be taken, from the start, to include:

- identifying the patient's concerns about the symptoms and belief about their cause;
- reviewing any previous history of 'unexplained' symptoms;
- investigating how the patient reacts to, and attempts to cope with, the symptoms, e.g. activity avoidance, work sickness absence; are these behaviours likely to help or hinder?
- using screening questions for depression, anxiety, and alcohol and substance misuse.

In psychiatry, we interview routinely a corroborant such as a close relative, and this can be helpful here, by ascertaining their views on the cause of the symptoms, and possible ways forward.

Treatment

The assessment as treatment

A thorough, patient-focused, integrated assessment, as described above, is the first step in effective management, and should be followed by careful explanation and reassurance.

Provide explanation and reassurance

Most patients are reassured by being told that:

- the symptoms they have are common;
- the symptoms they have are rarely associated with serious disease;
- the symptoms they have are real, and their doctor is familiar with them;
- the symptoms they have often settle with time;
- the symptoms they have need not be an impediment to an active life;
- they can be reviewed again should the symptoms persist.

A positive explanation for symptoms is more helpful than a statement that no disease is present. A positive explanation outlines how behavioural, psychological, and emotional factors may exacerbate physiologically based physical symptoms. Most patients accept integrated explanations, which include psychological and social factors as well as physiological ones, provided they feel the symptoms are accepted as real. The explanation can usefully show the link between these factors, for example how anxiety leads to physiological changes, which are experienced as somatic symptoms, which, if attributed to disease, lead to increased anxiety.

Simple advice on self-help techniques can then be given, including how to control negative thoughts (see p. 137), using physical relaxation techniques (see p. 135), and increasing activity levels (see p. 135). A self-help book which uses evidence-based, cognitive behavioural approaches should be recommended.

Reassurance needs to be given carefully. It is essential to elicit the patient's specific concerns before offering reassurance, and to target this appropriately. Reassurance that fails to address a patient's concerns is ineffective. When anxiety about disease is severe (hypochondriasis), repeated reassurance is not only ineffective but may even perpetuate the problem.

Communicate effectively

Effective communication is crucial to success. Tips include the following.

- Discuss and agree the treatment plan with the patient.
- Agree follow-up arrangements, and be specific—when, who, and why.
- Involve key carer(s) in your decision making.
- Involve primary care—they will have useful perspectives, and have an important 'gate-keeper' role in accessing health services.
- Communicate the treatment summary clearly in writing to the patient, carer, and key clinician(s).

Encourage a graded return to normal activity

Reduced activity levels are not only a consequence of functional symptoms, but also a cause. It follows, therefore, that a graded increase in activity is not only a goal of treatment but also a part of treatment. The patient can make a list of activities which they used to undertake, but which they no longer engage in, or which they engage in less frequently. They should then choose one or two and plan a phased return to those activities. It is important that the patient is realistic about what can be achieved in the short term. Diaries can be helpful for planning and recording activities.

Identify and treat any psychiatric disorder

In particular, consider the possibility of anxiety, depression, and alcohol and substance misuse. Explain to the patient how the psychiatric disorder is contributing to the maintenance of their physical symptoms. Offer simple treatments as part of a stepped care approach to their management.

Review medicines

Medicines should be reviewed, and consideration should be given to reducing or stopping those that do not have a clear medical indication.

Consider prescribing antidepressants

Antidepressants may be appropriate for two different reasons. The first is because of their *antidepressant* function—depressive illness is common in patients with functional symptoms. The second is because of their *neuromodulating* function—antidepressants may help people with functional symptoms by modifying nerve action and, thereby, the extent to which physiological disturbance in the 'soma' is manifested in the 'psyche'. There is good evidence, for example, for the role of antidepressants in some pain syndromes.

Refer if appropriate

It is often tempting to refer difficult patients to another doctor but this can result in greater long-term difficulties without achieving a more effective treatment plan. When there is a clear reason for further medical or psychiatric referral, this should be discussed with the patient. The referral letter should clearly explain what is required of the specialist; for example, confirmation or negation of the diagnosis or advice on management.

Address social factors

These may include, for example, relationship conflict financial problems, and unemployment, and may be potent maintaining factors.

Consider further psychiatric treatment

Help from psychiatric services might include:

- advice on more complex antidepressant drug regimens;
- specialist psychological interventions, including:
  - **anxiety management;**
  - **cognitive therapy** to modify thoughts and beliefs, by reducing catastrophization, and facilitating normalizing attributions;
  - **behavioural therapy** to increase activity and reduce illness-related behaviours, such as symptom monitoring, and searching for medical evidence;
  - **cognitive behavioural therapy (CBT),** which combines elements of cognitive and behavioural therapies; CBT has been shown to be effective in randomized controlled trials for hypchondriasis, and for a variety of functional syndromes, including non-cardiac chest pain and irritable bowel syndrome;
- illness-specific interventions, such as graded activity to treat physical deconditioning in chronic fatigue syndrome;
- management of complex associated social and psychological problems.

■ Some common clinical problems

Irritable bowel syndrome

In primary care, about half of the patients seen with gut complaints have functional disorders, the most common type being irritable bowel syndrome. Most patients have relatively mild symptoms and can be managed effectively in primary care through the provision of information on self-help that includes diet, physical activity, and first-line, symptom-targeted medication (e.g. laxatives, antimotility agents). One-third of patients seen in primary care with irritable bowel syndrome are referred to gastrointestinal specialists for further assessment and treatment. Other treatment options include the following.

- **Antidepressants.** Tricyclic antidepressants are indicated at low dose as second-line agents, and SSRI antidepressants as third-line agents. Here, these medications are not being used as antidepressants, but (as has been described above), as modifiers of nerve function and, thereby, of intestinal motility.
- **Psychological interventions.** There is evidence to support the use of cognitive behavioural therapy and hypnotherapy.
- **Management of associated psychiatric disorder,** such as anxiety and depression.

Musculoskeletal pain and chronic pain

Musculoskeletal symptoms (for example, neck pain, limb pain, low back pain, joint pain, and chronic widespread pain) are frequent reasons for consultation in primary care. Most patients can be effectively managed using the following general measures:

- explaining the difference between 'hurt' and 'harm', using for example menstrual pain or tension headache as examples;
- reassuring patients about the benign nature of their symptoms;
- helping patients regain control over the pain, rather than the pain controlling them;
- encouraging early progressive mobilization, and an early return to work, with increases in activity in small graded stages;
- advice that analgesic drugs should be taken on a regular rather than a pain-contingent basis;
- setting of realistic goals;
- agreeing rewards for success; for example, engaging in a favourite activity when a specific target is reached.

The treatment of severe chronic pain is difficult, and patients are often referred to specialist pain clinics. Many have physical disease, but experience more pain, distress, and disability than can be accounted for by the pathology. Analgesia should be made as effective as possible and patients should be encouraged to try other ways of coping with the pain. These approaches include:

- distraction, by engaging in non-pain-related activities;
- reducing any behaviour that focuses attention on the pain (e.g. repeatedly rubbing or checking the area);
- cognitive approaches, such as identifying and challenging negative thoughts and beliefs relating to the pain;
- antidepressant medication, when used either as an antidepressant or as an analgesic/neuromodulator;
- intensive multidisciplinary pain management programmes, which integrate physical therapies, graded rehabilitation, medication, psychological techniques, and active involvement of patients and their families in planning treatment and monitoring progress.

Chronic fatigue syndrome/myalgic encephalomyelitis

Depression, fatigue, and malaise are common following influenza, hepatitis, infectious mononucleosis, and other viral infections, but these usually improve over days and weeks. Chronic fatigue syndrome, which is also known as myalgic encephalomyelitis, and shortened to CFS-ME, is characterized by (i) more persistent fatigue, and aching limbs with muscle and joint pains, and (ii) the absence of physical or mental disorder sufficient to explain the symptoms. Mild physical exertion is often followed by increased fatigue and pain so that patients alternate brief periods of activity with prolonged rest, in a 'stop–start' pattern. Many patients are convinced that their symptoms are caused by a chronic virus infection or another, as yet undetected, medical condition. However, after thorough physical assessment, few cases are found to have a specific medical cause such as anaemia, persistent infection, or endocrinopathy.

In most cases, the causes of the syndrome are neither wholly psychological nor wholly physical, but a mixture of the two, with psychological factors becoming increasingly common over time. A common triad at the outset is a viral illness (physical), presenting at a time of personal stress (social), in an individual with a driven personality (psychological). Recovery from the viral illness is slow, and inactivity and resultant physical deconditioning start to play an important role. As the person senses that they are recovering, they may suddenly return to their former lifestyle, only to relapse quickly because their physical condition is still impaired. Morale may well suffer and, in some, a depressive syndrome may emerge, which may merit antidepressant treatment.

The treatment of this disorder is challenging, not least because it arouses passionate feelings among sufferers and their carers. The clinician should explain that the syndrome is real, common, and familiar, and that although there is no specific medical treatment, there are ways of improving outcome. A graded programme of slowly increasing activity should be started with regular monitoring. Considerable effort is needed to ensure that patients practise progressively rather than alternating erratically between excessive activity and resting in bed. It is often appropriate to seek specialist advice for these patients. Cognitive behavioural therapy and graded exercise therapy have both been shown to be helpful in randomized controlled trials. The role of pacing, in which patients adapt their lifestyle to the energy that they have available, is currently uncertain, but a large trial funded by the UK's Medical Research Council will provide helpful evidence in the near future.

Multiple chronic functional symptoms

Patients who have multiple functional symptoms over long periods are said to have somatization disorder. They are difficult to treat and management is often focused on 'coping' (limiting distress and unnecessary investigation) rather than 'curing'. The general approach already described for the treatment of functional symptoms is used, with an emphasis on avoiding inappropriate investigation and ensuring a consistent approach. If possible, this should be by a single doctor, usually based in primary care, who can act as a 'gatekeeper' to ensure that specialist care is accessed only when indicated. A psychiatric assessment may be useful in establishing a treatment plan, although specialist psychiatric interventions are seldom of much value.

Management may include:

- reviewing the (often large) medical notes, and discussion with the (often many) doctors currently involved;
- negotiating with other doctors to simplify the medical care:
  - limit the number of healthcare staff involved;
  - agree who has primary responsibility;
  - minimize the use of psychotropic and other drugs;
  - ensure that referrals and investigations are arranged only in response to a clear medical indication;
- arranging brief, regular appointments with the lead clinician (proactive versus reactive appointments);
- avoiding repeated reassurance about the symptoms;
- focusing on coping with disability and psychosocial problems;
- encouraging/planning a graded return to normal activities;
- involving relatives in the treatment plan;
- being realistic about outcomes.

Dissociative and conversion disorders

These are fascinating disorders. The Greeks coined the term **hysteria** ('disease of the womb') for these disorders, and the term persists in use to this day. However, its use is clearly inappropriate now that we understand that both men and women may suffer from these disorders, and that the aetiology is entirely unconnected with the reproductive system. Conversion disorder refers to unexplained sensory and motor symptoms; dissociative disorder refers to unexplained amnesia, fugue (amnesic wandering), stupor, or identity disorder. The conditions are classified differently in DSM-IV and ICD-10, reflecting uncertainty in this field. In DSM-IV, conversion disorder is listed among somatoform disorders and there is a separate category for dissociative disorder, whereas in ICD-10 both conditions are grouped together in a single category—dissociative disorder.

Conversion and dissociative *symptoms* also occur in many psychiatric disorders other than conversion and dissociative disorders, notably in anxiety, depressive, and organic mental disorders. A conversion (or dissociative) symptom is one that suggests physical illness but occurs in the absence of relevant physical pathology and is produced through unconscious psychological mechanisms. There are two obvious practical difficulties in applying this concept. First, it is seldom possible to exclude physical pathology completely at the time when a patient is first seen. Second, it is difficult to be certain that the symptoms are produced by unconscious mechanisms rather than consciously and deliberately. (The deliberate feigning of symptoms is known as malingering.)

The *prevalence* of conversion and dissociative disorder varies between countries, being reported more often in less industrialized societies. In Western societies, the prevalence is believed to be between 3 and 6 per 1000 for women, and substantially less for men. Most dissociative and conversion disorders of recent onset seen in general practice or hospital emergency departments recover quickly. Those that persist for longer than a year are likely to continue for many years more. Occasionally, organic disease may be present but undetectable when these patients are first seen, becoming obvious later. For this reason, patients should receive a thorough physical assessment, and should be followed up most carefully.

Clinical features

Although conversion and dissociative symptoms are not produced deliberately, they are nevertheless shaped by the patient's concepts of illness. Sometimes, the symptoms resemble those of a relative or friend who has been ill. Sometimes they originate in the patient's previous experience of ill health; for example, dissociative memory loss may appear some years after head injury. Usually, there are obvious discrepancies between signs and symptoms of conversion and dissociative disorder and those of organic disease; for example, a pattern of sensory loss that does not correspond to the anatomical innervation of the part. These discrepancies are important in diagnosis.

Motor symptoms include paralysis of voluntary muscles, tremor, tics, and abnormalities of gait. **Sensory symptoms** of conversion disorder include anaesthesiae, paraesthesiae, hyperaesthesiae, pain, deafness, and blindness. In general, the sensory changes are distinguished from those in organic disease by (i) a distribution that does not conform to the known innervation of the part, (ii) their varying intensity, and (iii) their responsiveness to suggestion.

Dissociative symptoms are less common. Dissociative amnesia starts suddenly. Patients are unable to recall long periods of their life and sometimes deny any knowledge of their previous life or personal identity. In a dissociative fugue the patient loses his memory and wanders away from his usual surroundings. In dissociative stupor, the patient is motionless and mute and does not respond to stimulation, but he is aware of his surroundings. Multiple personality is a rare condition, of uncertain diagnostic validity, in which there are sudden alterations between the patient's normal state and another complex pattern of behaviour, which constitutes a 'second personality'.

Management

Diagnosis depends partly on the exclusion of physical causes, but also on psychological assessment to identify psychological reasons for the onset and course of the symptoms. A vital differential diagnosis is from physical disease. This depends on careful physical assessment highlighting any discrepancies in physical signs that are unlikely to have a physical basis. It is important to keep an open mind and to remember that conversion symptoms are common accompaniments to physical disorder, and that is it is not necessarily an 'either/or' diagnosis.

Acute disorders seen in general practice or hospital emergency departments often respond to simple measures (Table 25.2). For *persistent cases* the general approach is similar, although the results are less satisfactory. Attention is directed away from the symptoms and towards problems that have provoked the disorder. Staff should show sympathetic concern for the patient, but at the same time encourage self-help and avoid reinforcing the disability. For example, a patient who complains of paralysis of the legs should be encouraged to return to walking, not offered a wheelchair. The main emphasis should be to try and concentrate the patient's attention on understanding problems and methods of solving them. More intense psychological exploration seldom produces results better than those of the simple measures described above.

Table 25.2 Treatment of acute conversion disorder

- Medical and psychiatric history from patient and informants
- Full examination and appropriate investigation to exclude physical causes
- Sympathetic but positive reassurance that the patient is suffering from an acute temporary condition, with which the doctor is familiar, and which is not a serious medical disorder
- Discussion of the expected rapid recovery
- Avoidance of reinforcement of disability or symptoms
- Offer continuing assessment and treatment of related psychiatric or social problems

BOX 25.2 Some ethical issues in the management of factitious disorders

Confidentiality

- Disclosure of diagnosis to other parties, e.g. employers such as the NHS
- Circulation between hospitals of details of patients with suspected factitious disorder

Invasion of privacy

- Searching patients' belongings for evidence to support the diagnosis
- Covert videotaping to provide evidence to support the diagnosis

■ Self-inflicted and simulated illness

Factitious disorder

The term factitious disorder refers to the intentional production of physical pathology or the feigning of physical or psychological symptoms, with the apparent aim of being diagnosed as ill. Factitious disorder differs from malingering in that it does not bring any external reward such as avoidance of military or other occupational duties, or financial compensation.

Common symptoms include skin lesions ('dermatitis artefacta') and pyrexia of unknown origin. Sometimes the patient deliberately worsens an existing physical disorder; for example, preventing the healing of varicose ulcers or neglecting the care of diabetes. At other times the whole condition is induced; for example, by self-inflicted damage to the skin.

There is no specific treatment. Supportive counselling is often offered, and helps some patients but many do not take up the treatment. If deliberate feigning of symptoms and signs is established, patients should be told sympathetically what has been discovered and offered help with whatever problems might have led to the behaviour. This should be part of a sympathetic plan that also offers psychological help. Box 25.2 summarizes the ethical issues.

Munchausen syndrome is an extreme and uncommon form of factitious disorder, in which a patient gives a plausible and often dramatic history of an acute illness, with feigned symptoms and signs. Symptoms may be of any kind, including psychiatric symptoms. These patients often attend a series of hospitals, giving different names to each. Frequently, strong analgesics are demanded for pain. Patients often obstruct efforts to obtain additional information about them and may interfere with diagnostic investigations. It has a poor prognosis.

Munchausen syndrome by proxy refers to a form of child abuse in which a parent (or occasionally another adult, such as a nurse) gives a false account of symptoms in a child, and may fake physical signs (see p. 170).

Malingering

Malingering is the fraudulent simulation or exaggeration of symptoms with the intention of gaining financial or other rewards. It is the obvious external gain that distinguishes malingering from factitious disorder (see above). When clinically significant malingering occurs it is most often among prisoners, the military, and people seeking compensation for accidents. However, more minor malingering, such as feigning illness to secure extra holiday from work, is common.

Malingering should be diagnosed only after a full investigation of the case. When the diagnosis is certain, the patient should be informed tactfully of this conclusion and encouraged to deal more appropriately with any problems that contributed to the behaviour.

Further reading

Mayou, R., Sharpe, M., & Carson, A. (2003). *ABC of Psychological Medicine.* BMJ Publishing Group, London. Includes general and more specific chapters on practical management.

CHAPTER 26

Delirium, dementia, and other cognitive disorders

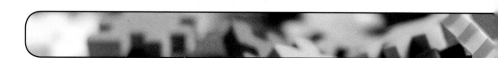

■ Introduction

Organic psychiatric disorders result from brain dysfunction caused by organic pathology inside or outside the brain. Dementia is the most common condition, with Alzheimer's disease alone affecting 1 per cent of the population at 60 years, rising to 40 per cent over 80 years. Many of the rarer organic psychiatric disorders tend to affect a wider age range, but present in similar ways. Given the changing demographics of most developed countries, disorders producing cognitive impairment in older adults are becoming increasingly important for provision of healthcare services and in daily clinical practice. This chapter will cover the more common causes of cognitive impairment, and there is additional information in Chapters 18 and 20 on psychiatry of older adults and psychiatry and medicine.

There are three common clinical presentations of organic psychiatric disorders:

1 **Delirium**—an acute generalized impairment of brain function, in which the most important feature is impairment of consciousness. The disturbance of brain function is generalized, and the primary cause is often outside the brain; for example, sepsis due to a urinary tract infection.

2 **Dementia**—chronic generalized impairment, in which the main clinical feature is global intellectual impairment. There are also changes in mood and behaviour. The brain dysfunction is generalized, and the primary cause is within the brain; for example, a degenerative condition such as Alzheimer's disease.

Table 26.1 Classification of organic psychiatric disorders causing brain disease

Global syndromes

- Delirium
- Dementia

Specific syndromes

- Amnesic syndrome
- Organic mood disorder
- Organic delusional state
- Organic personality disorder

3 **Specific syndromes**, which include disorders with a predominant impairment of memory only (amnesic syndrome), of thinking, or of mood, or personality change. These include neurological disorders that frequently result in organic psychological complications; for example, epilepsy.

Table 26.1 lists the main categories of psychiatric disorder associated with organic brain disease. The following sections describe these syndromes and the psychiatric consequences of a number of neurological conditions. Organic causes of other core psychiatric conditions (e.g. anxiety, psychosis) are covered in the relevant specific chapters.

■ Delirium

Delirium is characterized by an acute impairment of consciousness producing a generalized cognitive impairment. The word delirium is derived from the Latin, 'lira', which means to wander from the furrow. Delirium is a common condition, affecting up to 15 per cent of patients in general medical or surgical wards, with the primary cause often being a systemic illness. The term '**acute confusional state**' is a synonym for delirium.

Clinical features

The features of delirium differ widely between patients, but there are eight main themes within the presentation (Table 26.2).

1 **Impairment of consciousness** is the most important symptom, and is seen as a deficit of attention, concentration, and awareness. Often the patient will not be able to follow or engage in a logical conversation. The features *fluctuate in intensity* and are often *worse in the evening*.

2 **Disorientation**—uncertainty about the time, place, and identity of other people.

Table 26.2 Clinical features of delirium

Impaired consciousness

- Disorientation
- Poor attention and concentration
- Loss of memory

Behaviour

- Overactive
- Underactive

Thinking

- Muddled (confused)
- Ideas of reference
- Delusions

Mood

- Anxious, irritable
- Depressed
- Perplexed

Perception

- Misinterpretations
- Hallucinations, mainly visual
- Acute onset, fluctuating course, worse in the evening

3 **Behaviour** may be either overactive, with noisiness and irritability, or underactive. Sleep is often disturbed.

4 **Thinking** is slow and confused but the content is often complex. Ideas of reference and delusions are common.

5 **Mood** may be anxious, perplexed, irritable, or depressed and is often labile.

6 **Perception** may be distorted with misinterpretations, illusions, and visual hallucinations. Tactile and auditory hallucinations occur but are less frequent.

7 **Memory.** Disturbance of memory affects registration, retention, and recall, as well as new learning.

8 **Insight** is impaired.

The diagnostic criteria for delirium are shown in Box 26.1.

Prevalence

Delirium is an extremely common condition and may occur in all age groups. Those at the extremes of age, with pre-existing dementia, or who have a serious physical illness make up the majority. On a general medical or surgical ward, 10 to 15 per cent of patients will be admitted with delirium, and another 10 to 15 per cent will have an episode during their hospital stay. The highest incidence is in intensive care units, where 40 to 60 per cent of

BOX 26.1 DSM-IV diagnostic criteria for delirium

A Disturbance of consciousness with reduced ability to focus, sustain, or shift attention.

B A change in cognition or the development of a perceptual disturbance that is not better accounted for by a pre-existing, established, or evolving dementia.

C The disturbance develops over a short period of time and tends to fluctuate during the course of the day.

D There is evidence from the history, physical examination, or laboratory findings that the disturbance is caused by the direct physiological consequences of a general medical condition.

The above refers to delirium caused by a general medical condition, and is the same in the ICD-10. There are separate diagnostic codes for delirium due to substance intoxication/withdrawal, or multiple aetiologies. The ICD-10 has a specific code for delirium superimposed upon pre-existing dementia.

patients meet the criteria, including many young people. The prevalence of delirium in the community is unknown.

Co-morbidity

Half of all cases of delirium occur in patients with an underlying (diagnosed or undiagnosed) dementia

syndrome. Delirium is also more common in those with primary mood or anxiety disorders.

Differential diagnosis

The key differentials of delirium are dementia, depression, and non-organic psychoses. Table 26.3 outlines the key differences between these conditions.

Aetiology

There are many causes of delirium, the most important of which are listed in Table 26.4. However, few episodes of delirium are caused by one single aetiological factor; usually three or four factors can be identified, each of which may be relevant at different points in the illness. The neuropathology of delirium is poorly understood, although the relatively consistent clinical presentation suggests a common pathological pathway for all the aetiological processes. A diffuse slowing is seen upon the EEG, and there are global changes in the cerebral circulation. Neuroimaging suggests involvement of the prefrontal cortex, thalamus, posterior parietal lobe, and subcortical regions. It is unclear currently why some functions (e.g. speech, motor, sensory) remain intact in delirium, whilst others are badly deranged. Laboratory studies have shown an imbalance of neurotransmitters in delirium, with a relative deficit of cholinergic action compared with an excess of dopaminergic action.

Delirium is more frequent in children and older adults, among people with previous brain damage of any kind, in conditions of low sensory input (such as deafness and poor vision), or in malnutrition. Isolation, immobility,

Table 26.3 Differential diagnosis of delirium

Characteristic	Delirium	Dementia	Depression	Psychosis
Onset	Acute	Gradual (often insidious)	Usually gradual	Variable
Level of consciousness	Impaired	Normal	Usually normal	Normal
Attention	Poor	Intact	Mildly impaired	Poor
Memory	Impaired	Impaired (primary problem)	Inconsistent (pseudodementia)	Intact
Mood	Variable	Normal	Low and flat	Incongruous
Hallucinations*	Usually visual	Visual or auditory	Auditory	Auditory
Delusions	Persecutory, but fleeting	Paranoid, fixed	Mood congruent	Complex, systematized, often paranoid
Reversibility	Usually	Not usually	Usually	Sometimes
Course	Fluctuating	Progressive	Diurnal variation	Chronic relapsing and remitting

* Hallucinations may be experienced in any of the five senses for all diagnoses; the table above merely gives the mostly commonly encountered for comparison.

Table 26.4 Some causes of delirium

| Systemic infection, e.g. urinary tract, chest, cellulitis, IV lines |
| Neurological infection: meningitis or encephalitis |
| Stroke or myocardial infarction |
| Trauma or head injury |
| Metabolic failure: cardiac, respiratory, renal, or hepatic |
| Hypoglycaemia |
| Electrolyte abnormalities |
| Nutritional deficiencies: vitamin B_{12}, thiamine, nicotinic acid |
| Drug intoxication or withdrawal |
| Alcohol withdrawal |
| Raised intracranial pressure or space-occupying lesions |
| Post-ictal states or status epilepticus |

stress, use of restraints, and the intensive care environment have also been shown to be risk factors.

Assessment

Assessment should aim to identify the underlying physical cause of delirium, and to place this in the context of the patient's premorbid level of cognition and functioning. The diagnosis is clinical and is usually obvious upon talking to the patient. Typically, a standard medical and surgical history is taken, rather than a formal psychiatric interview. Often little history can be obtained from the patient, so it is essential to contact relatives, carers, friends, and other clinicians in order to gather the story. Include a comprehensive list of medications, including over-the-counter remedies, alcohol, and smoking. A full examination of all physical systems should be undertaken, including a detailed neurological examination. Physical investigations should include the following:

- blood for full blood count, urea and electrolytes, liver function tests, thyroid function tests, calcium, phosphate, magnesium, glucose, lactate, troponin, albumin, paracetamol and salicylate, haematinics;
- blood and urine cultures;
- arterial blood gas;
- ECG;
- urinalysis;
- chest X-ray;
- consider further tests, e.g. CT head, lumbar puncture, EEG.

Complex cognitive investigations are usually not needed, but the following are useful simple tests to quantify the level of impairment.

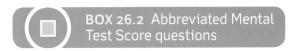

BOX 26.2 Abbreviated Mental Test Score questions

What is your age? (1 point)

What is the time to the nearest hour? (1 point)

Give the patient an address, and ask him or her to repeat it at the end of the test. (1 point) e.g. 42 West Street

What is the year? (1 point)

What is the name of the hospital or number of the residence where the patient is situated? (1 point)

Can the patient recognize two persons (the doctor, nurse, carer, etc.)? (1 point)

What is your date of birth? (day and month sufficient) (1 point)

In what year did World War 2 begin? (1 point) (other dates can be used, with a preference for dates some time in the past)

Name the present monarch/dictator/prime minister/ president. (1 point)

Count backwards from 20 down to 1. (1 point)

- Abbreviated Mental Test Score (AMTS)—out of 10 points, a score of 6 or less is taken as delirium (Box 26.2).
- Mini Mental State Examination (MMSE)—30 points, with more than or equal to 25 taken as normal, mild dementia 21–24, moderate 10–20, and severe less than 10 points.

The AMTS is often used sequentially to monitor for improvement or decline in functioning. The MMSE is primarily used for dementia, but may be helpful in delirium.

Management

Treatment of delirium is directed both to dealing with the underlying physical cause and with measures to treat the patient's anxiety, distress, and behavioural problems.

1 **Treat the underlying cause.** This obviously depends on the exact aetiology, but frequently involves giving oxygen, fluids, antibiotics, and pain relief, as well as any specific treatments. Intravenous access (and other invasive procedures) should only be undertaken if there is a valid indication.

2 **Reassurance and reorientation.** Patients need reassurance to reduce anxiety and disorientation; this should be repeated frequently. A clock should be visible at all times, and the patient reminded of the time, place, day, and date regularly.

Case study 26.1 Delirium

As a general hospital duty doctor you are called in the middle of the night to see a 79-year-old man who has become disturbed and distressed 3 days after major abdominal surgery. The nursing staff, who have not known the patient before, say the patient has been attempting to pull out his drip, has been shouting incoherently, and seems frightened. He has accused them of being guards in a prison. You look at the case notes, which contain routine medical information, but find that in the nursing notes the patient has been intermittently rather drowsy and that during the day his relatives reported that he seemed confused.

You find it difficult to interview the patient, who seems unable to concentrate on your questions and makes disconnected comments about being in prison and having been attacked by people who want to kill him. He is unable to say where he is or to tell you the date. He is bewildered and fearful. You diagnose delirium. You notice that he has pyrexia and the nurses tell you that he appears to be developing a wound infection. You examine the

wound, and find it red, hot, and painful. You continue IV fluids, start antibiotics, and take a swab for culture from the wound.

You arrange for the patient be moved to a quiet, well-lit side room. You explain to the patient that he is safe in hospital and that you will be able to help him feel better. One of the nurses takes responsibility for looking after the patient and for repeatedly reassuring him that all is well. Despite reassurance, the patient remains very agitated. Your prescribe 3 mg of haloperidol, which the patient is willing to take as syrup.

In the morning you review the patient, who is calmer. You discuss a consistent, reassuring regime with the day nursing staff, explain to the relatives what has happened, and encourage them to spend time with the patient explaining and reassuring him about what is going on.

You also discuss the response of the patient and your treatment with the responsible medical team so that they are able to continue with a consistent long-term plan.

3 **Predictable, consistent routine.** On the ward the patient should be nursed either in a quiet side room or next to the nursing station. It should be reasonably dark at night and light during the day. Meals and activities should occur at standard times each day. Relatives and friends should be encouraged to stay or to visit frequently.

4 **Avoid unnecessary medications.**

5 **Explain to relatives and friends** what delirium is and what has caused it. This helps them to reassure and reorientate the patient.

6 **Sleep** is often disturbed, and it is reasonable to give small doses of hypnotics (e.g. zopiclone 3.75 mg) or benzodiazepines (e.g. temazepam 10 mg) at night to promote sleep. Benzodiazepines should be avoided during daytime as their sedative effects may increase disorientation. The exception to this is in alcohol withdrawal or in order to treat seizures.

7 **Disturbed, violent, or distressed behaviour** may be treated with carefully monitored antipsychotic medications. There is good randomized controlled evidence supporting the use of antipsychotics in delirium, with a consistent two-thirds of patients experiencing clinical improvement. Haloperidol is the traditional choice, 0.25–2 mg every 4 hours, although atypical antipsychotics are becoming more commonly used. Haloperidol is available in oral, intramuscular, and intravenous preparations. Olanzapine has been shown to be just as effective at relieving agitation as haloperidol, but the intramuscular formulation is not

widely available. Lorazepam is also effective, but has a moderate risk of worsening the mental state. If a patient is acutely distressed or agitated, an IM dose is usually needed, with follow-on treatment orally for as long as necessary. This should be regularly reviewed, and never used unless other methods of management have been exhausted.

■ Dementia

Overview of dementia

Dementia is *a generalized decline of intellect, memory, and personality, without impairment of consciousness, leading to functional impairment.* It is a clinical syndrome, rather than a diagnosis in itself, which may be caused by a variety of pathologies. This section will outline common features of the dementias, and further information on specific diagnoses follows in the latter part of the chapter.

Dementia is an acquired disorder, as distinct from learning disability in which impairments are present from birth (see Chapter 19), although the onset may be at any age. Onset before the age of 65 is called presenile dementia. Although most cases of dementia are irreversible, small but important groups are remediable, meaning that the assessment process must aim to exclude reversible causes before making a diagnosis of a progressive condition. Dementia is on the increase, largely due to an ageing population, and managing patients effectively is a large part of a junior doctor's job in general medical and surgical rotations.

Clinical features (Table 26.5)

Dementia usually presents with impairment of memory. Although the onset is typically insidious, it may come to notice after an acute deterioration. This may be triggered by a change in social circumstances or an intercurrent illness. There may also be uncharacteristic aggressive behaviour or sexual disinhibition. In a middle-aged or older person any social lapse that is out of character should always suggest dementia. The clinical picture depends in part on the patient's premorbid personality; for example, neurotic and paranoid traits may become exaggerated. People who are socially isolated or deaf may be less able to compensate for failing intellectual abilities. On the other hand, a person with good social skills may maintain a social facade despite severe intellectual deterioration.

Cognitive function. A decline in cognitive function is the key feature of dementia. Forgetfulness usually appears early and is prominent; difficulty in new learning is a conspicuous sign. Memory loss is more obvious for recent than for remote events. Patients often make excuses to hide these memory defects, and some confabulate. In some cases there is aphasia, agnosia, or apraxia. Attention and concentration are also impaired. Disorientation for time, and at a later stage for place and person, are almost invariable once dementia is well established (but in contrast to delirium are not usually prominent in the early stage).

Behaviour may be disorganized, restless, or inappropriate. Typically, there is loss of initiative and reduction of interests. Some patients become restless and wander about by day and sometimes at night. When patients are taxed beyond their restricted abilities, there may be a sudden change to tears or anger (a '**catastrophic reaction**'). As dementia worsens patients care for themselves less well and may become disinhibited, neglecting social conventions. Behaviour becomes aimless. Eventually, the patient may become incontinent of urine and faeces.

Changes of mood. In the early stages, changes of mood include anxiety, irritability, and depression. Low mood is a common feature at presentation, and it is important to distinguish dementia from the 'pseudodementia' of depression, seen in those with psychomotor retardation. As dementia progresses, emotions and responses to events become generally blunted, though there may be sudden changes of mood without apparent cause or the catastrophic reactions noted above.

Thinking slows and becomes impoverished in content. There may be difficulty in abstract thinking, reduced flexibility, and perseveration. Judgement is impaired. Persecutory and paranoid delusions are common. In the later stages, thinking becomes grossly fragmented and incoherent. Disturbed thinking is reflected in the patient's *speech*, in which syntactical errors and nominal dysphasia are common. Eventually, the patient may utter only meaningless noises or even become mute.

Perceptual disturbances may develop as the condition progresses. Hallucinations are often visual.

Insight is usually lacking into the degree and nature of the disorder.

There are no generic criteria in the DSM-IV or ICD-10 for dementia as a clinical syndrome; specific criteria for the common and important pathologies are included below.

Prevalence

Dementia currently affects about 25 million people worldwide, with the numbers set to increase dramatically as life expectancy increases further. In the UK, 850 000 people have dementia, with 19 000 of these being younger than 60 years at time of diagnosis. Table 26.6 gives an idea

Table 26.5 Clinical features of dementia

Cognition
- Poor memory
- Impaired attention
- Aphasia, agnosia, and apraxia
- Disorientation
- 'Personality change'

Behaviour
- Odd and disorganized
- Restless, wandering
- Self-neglect
- Disinhibition
- Social withdrawal

Mood
- Anxiety
- Depression

Thinking
- Slow, impoverished
- Delusions

Perception
- Illusions
- Hallucinations

Insight
- Impaired

Table 26.6 Global prevalence of dementia. Extract from Ferri, C. P., Prince, M., Brayne, C., *et al.* (2005). Global prevalence of dementia: a Delphi consensus study. *Lancet* 366: 2112–7.

Age (years)	Prevalence (%)
40–60	0.01
60–65	0.5
65–70	1.0
70–75	2.0
75–80	4.0
80–85	10.0
85≥	40.0

of the prevalence of dementia at different ages. It is four times more common in men than in women.

Differential diagnosis

The main differentials are those shown in Table 26.3, including the key differences between delirium and dementia. However, always consider that symptoms (especially isolated forgetfulness) may be a feature of normal ageing or, in a young person, that the diagnosis could be a learning disability.

A common diagnostic problem is presented by so-called depressive pseudodementia. In this syndrome, a depressed patient complains of poor memory and appears intellectually impaired because poor concentration leads to inadequate registration. Depressed mood may lead to slowness and self-neglect. Characteristic features are:

- a history from another informant that the depressed mood preceded the memory problems;
- memory testing shows that the poor performance improves when interest is aroused;
- the patient is retarded and unwilling to cooperate in the interview; by contrast, patients with dementia are usually willing to reply to questions but make mistakes.

Conversely, an organic disorder can present with mood disorder or behaviour change that suggests a functional disorder. The points in favour of an organic cause are:

- the cognitive disorder preceded the mood or other disorder;
- cognitive defects occur in specific areas of intellectual function;
- neurological signs;
- the presence of symptoms seldom found in non-organic disorder, such as visual hallucinations.

It is important to consider a possible organic cause in every case of acute psychological or behavioural disturbance, especially when there are atypical features. The diagnosis of functional disorder is partly by exclusion of organic causes but also by the finding of positive evidence of psychological aetiology, since organic causes may be undetectable in the early stages of disease.

Aetiology

Dementia has many causes, of which the most important are listed in Table 26.7. Among older patients, the majority of cases are caused by Alzheimer's disease (55 per cent), vascular dementia (20 per cent), and Lewy body dementia (15 per cent). Although these and many other causes are irreversible, when assessing a patient the clinician needs to keep in mind the whole range of causes so as not to miss any that might be partly or wholly treatable, such as an operable cerebral neoplasm.

Assessment

In the UK, the assessment and management of dementia (of any cause) is guided by the guideline from the National Institute for Clinical Excellence (NICE), last updated in

Table 26.7 Causes of dementia

Irreversible causes	Potentially reversible causes
Primary degenerative conditions	Neurological
• Alzheimer's disease	• Normal-pressure hydrocephalus
• Lewy body dementia	• Intracranial tumour
• Frontotemporal dementia (Pick's disease)	• Chronic subdural haematoma
• Huntingdon's disease	Vitamin deficiencies:
• Wilson's disease	• Vitamin B_{12}
• Multiple sclerosis	• Folic acid
• Motor neuron disease	• Thiamine
Traumatic head injury	Endocrine:
Infections: HIV, encephalitis, CJD	• Hypothyroidism
	• Cushing's
Vascular: multi-infarct dementia	
Toxins: alcohol	
Anoxia: cardiac arrest, carbon monoxide poisoning	
Metabolic: hepatic encephalopathy, diabetes mellitus	

2006. Memory assessment clinics are the single point of access to services in the UK. The aim should be to perform the minimum of investigations to reveal the cause of the disorder, whether acute or chronic. Assessment should include the following:

1 **Detailed history taking.** Any suspicion of dementia should lead to detailed questioning about intellectual function and neurological symptoms. It is important to interview other informants, since patients are often unaware of the extent of the change in themselves. An assessment of mood should be made.

2 **Full physical examination,** focusing on the neurological system.

3 **Cognitive testing.** Standardized procedures for assessing cognitive state may be of value, but in interpreting the results it is essential to take account of previous education and achievement. The Mini Mental State Examination (MMSE) is used widely in assessment; it combines standard questions with tests of spatial ability, and has high sensitivity and specificity.

4 **Laboratory investigations.** Basic haematology, biochemistry, liver function, thyroid function, vitamin B_{12}, folate, thiamine, calcium, and glucose should be carried out. Special investigations (e.g. HIV, syphilis testing) should not be done unless there is high clinical suspicion from history and examination.

5 **Imaging.** A CT or MRI brain scan may be needed, as they are valuable in the diagnosis of both focal and diffuse cerebral pathology. It should be requested if there is any suspicion of organic brain disease in patients up to late middle age, or if there is any suggestion of a focal brain lesion in the over-65s.

Management of dementia

The initial step in the management of dementia is to treat any physical disorder, be it causal or co-morbid. After this, treatment aims to reduce disability and provide support. Whenever possible, care is outside the hospital, either with relatives or in residential accommodation. Admission to hospital should be reserved for those few patients at risk of harming themselves or others, or those with complex physical or psychiatric co-morbidities.

The aims of treatment are to:

• maintain any remaining ability as far as possible;

• relieve distressing symptoms;

• arrange for the practical requirements of the patient;

• support the family.

A summary of treatment approaches is shown in Table 26.8.

Table 26.8 Management of dementia

General measures
• Treat any physical disorders
• Psychoeducation of patient, family, and carers
• Promote and maintain independence with a written care plan
• Provide training courses and support groups for carers
• Respite care
• Palliative care input

Psychological
• Structured group cognitive stimulation programme
• For agitation: aromatherapy, dance/music therapy, animal therapy
• Psychological support for carers

Pharmacological (see text for UK limitations on prescribing)
• Acetylcholinesterase inhibitors
• Memantine
• For agitation: antipsychotics and benzodiazepines
• For depression: antidepressants

Psychoeducation should begin at the time a diagnosis of dementia is made and continue throughout the illness. The patient, their relatives, and carers should all be actively informed of the following: symptoms of dementia, course and prognosis, treatments, support groups, financial and legal considerations (e.g. capacity and driving), and where to look for further information.

A written care plan is the recommended way of ensuring consistent high-quality treatment tailored to the individual's needs. This can be drawn up soon after the diagnosis is made, and includes important decisions such as views on residential accommodation, end-of-life care, and resuscitation. Input from an occupational therapist, physiotherapist, and dietitian should be offered.

Support for carers is as important as treatment of the patients themselves. There are many training courses and support groups for carers available, many of which are run by the voluntary sector and are free of charge. Having respite care available for short-term use is invaluable to carers, especially in the later stages of dementia. Frequently, carers may suffer distress themselves during the illness; psychological interventions such as CBT or counselling should be given where appropriate.

Structured group cognitive stimulation programmes have been shown to improve MMSE scores and quality of life in patients with mild to moderate dementia in the medium term.

Agitation and challenging behaviour are common in patients with dementia. Carers and healthcare professionals working with patients should be taught how to manage these situations. NICE recommends aromatherapy, music/dance therapy, animal-assisted therapy, and massage as effective ways of reducing agitation. These should always be first-line management, rather than drugs.

Medications do not yet play a prominent role in the treatment of dementia. There are four main groups of drug used in dementia:

1 **Acetylcholinesterase inhibitors** (donepezil, galantamine, rivastigmine) increase the concentration of and duration of action of acetylcholine in the central nervous system. There is evidence that in moderately severe Alzheimer's disease, these drugs improve cognitive function and behaviour for up to a year. There is no current evidence that these drugs halt or delay the progression of disease. In the UK, acetylcholinesterase inhibitors are licensed for use in patients with Alzheimer's disease and an MMSE score of 10–20 points, or those with agitation not controlled by non-drug measures or antipsychotics. These drugs should only be prescribed by specialists, and should be stopped after 6 months if there is no clinical benefit. Acetylcholinesterase inhibitors are not recommended for non-Alzheimer's dementia.

2 **Memantine** is a glutamine NMDA receptor antagonist which improves cognition, mood, and behaviour in moderate to severe Alzheimer's. Memantine is currently not recommended for use in the UK because the benefit is small and has not been shown to be cost-effective. However, it is widely available in other countries.

3 **Antipsychotics should generally be avoided whenever possible** and only have a role in patients with severely distressing symptoms or agitation causing risk to self or others. They should be avoided in those with mild–moderate dementia, as there is a slight increase in the risk of cerebrovascular events. Before using an antipsychotic, the above non-pharmacological methods should be used, and the patient nursed in a safe, low-stimulation environment (e.g. a quiet bedroom or side-room on the ward). Oral medications should be offered before parenteral drugs are given. The recommended drugs are haloperidol and olanzapine. A few patients need long-term oral antipsychotics to manage their behaviour at home.

4 **Benzodiazepines should be avoided wherever possible**, especially during the day. Intramuscular lorazepam is a suitable alternative to an antipsychotic for extreme agitation, and should be tried if antipsychotics do not relieve the symptoms.

Depression is common in patients with dementia, and should be treated along usual guidelines (see Chapter 21).

Specific dementia syndromes

The most common causes of dementia are Alzheimer's disease, vascular dementia, and Lewy body dementia. These are described below. The main clinical features of less common causes are outlined in Table 26.9, more detail on which can be found in the Further reading on p. 331. The section on management above is relevant to all causes of dementia.

Alzheimer's disease

Alois Alzheimer, a German psychiatrist and neuropathologist, described the salient features of what is now known as Alzheimer's disease in 1906. Alzheimer's disease is the most common cause of dementia, accounting for 50–60 per cent of cases worldwide. It is a condition which not only affects the patient, but also their family and carers, and therefore represents a huge financial, social, and emotional burden on society.

Pathology

Post-mortem (and more recently neuroimaging) investigations have shown that a brain affected by Alzheimer's is significantly smaller than age-matched controls, with widened sulci and enlarged ventricles. There is cell loss, shrinkage of the dendritic tree, proliferation of astrocytes, and increased gliosis. There are two key histological findings.

- **Amyloid plaques** are areas of dense, insoluble beta-amyloid peptide surrounded by abnormal neuritis filled with highly phosphorylated tau protein.

- **Neurofibrillary tangles** are made up of helical filaments of the microtubule-associated protein, tau, in a highly phosphorylated state. These are found throughout the cortical and subcortical grey matter (Figure 26.1).

Beta-amyloid is derived from a larger protein, APP, which is encoded by the *APP* gene on chromosome 21. Mutations in this gene have been found which produce an early-onset autosomal dominant form of Alzheimer's, although this is exceptionally rare. Mutations in the *presenilin* genes, which encode proteins involved in the cleavage of APP to beta-amyloid, also cause an autosomal dominant form of the disease. The exact method by which plaques and tangles are formed is poorly understood, and a large amount of research at the molecular and cellular levels is currently under way.

The plaques and tangles occur initially in the hippocampi, and then spread more widely. The occipital lobe and cerebellum tend to remain relatively unscathed.

It has been shown that the neurons lost tend to be primarily cholinergic, leading to the 'cholinergic hypothesis',

Science box 26.1 Are antipsychotics safe and effective to use in dementia?

Over 90 per cent of patients with Alzheimer's disease have behavioural and/or psychiatric problems at some point in their illness. The most common are psychosis, agitation, and aggression. These can make managing the patient (especially in a domestic environment) challenging, and are upsetting and difficult for both patient and carer to experience. There are a variety of behavioural and psychological interventions available, but pharmacological options for agitation and aggression are popular. Typical antipsychotics have been the traditional choice, but is there evidence that the newer 'atypical' antipsychotics are effective in reducing aggression, agitation, or psychosis in Alzheimer's disease?

The Cochrane Collaboration published a systematic review and meta-analysis on this question in 2008, attempting to summarize the multiple studies published.[1] They identified 16 randomized controlled trials, primarily using olanzapine and risperidone. They report that there was a significant improvement in aggression and psychosis with olanzapine and risperidone compared with placebo. No conclusions about other antipsychotics could be drawn. This study added to a previous Cochrane review which reported the efficacy of haloperidol in reducing agitation in dementia.[2] The Clinical Antipsychotic Trials of Intervention Effectiveness–Alzheimer's Disease (CATIE-AD) was a randomized controlled trial of olanzapine, risperidone, quetiapine, or placebo for up to 36 weeks in 421 patients with aggression or agitation. They report that olanzapine and risperidone showed greater clinical improvement than the comparison groups. Several other large, well-conducted RCTs have been published giving similar results; it therefore appears there is evidence that atypical antipsychotics can be effective in this patient group.

One problem has consistently arisen throughout research in this area. Atypical antipsychotics seem to be associated with a greater risk of both cardiovascular events and all-cause mortality when used in Alzheimer's patients. Ballard and Howard reported a threefold increase (odds ratio 3.64) in cardiovascular events (primarily ischaemic stroke) in a meta-analysis of RCTs of risperidone.[3] In 2005, the US FDA issued a warning regarding the significant increase in mortality (odds ratio 1.7) for patients with Alzheimer's taking atypical antipsychotics. Systematic reviews of the evidence have found this to be true; no difference was found between individual drugs.[4] There are clearly safety issues surrounding the use of atypical antipsychotics. The consensus view is that it is appropriate to prescribe them for aggression or agitation causing distress, but only in the short term at the lowest possible dose.[5]

1 Ballard, C. G., Waite, J., & Birks, J. (2008). Atypical antipsychotics for aggression and psychosis in Alzheimer's disease. *Cochrane Database of Systematic Reviews,* Issue 1: CD003476. DOI: 10.1002/14651858.CD003476.pub2.

2 Lonergan, E., Luxenberg, J., Colford, J., & Birks, J. (2005). Haloperidol for agitation in dementia. *Cochrane Database Systematic Review,* 4.

3 Ballard, C. & Howard, R. (2006). Neuroleptic drugs in dementia: benefits and harm. *Nature Review Neurosciences* 7: 492–500.

4 Schneider, L. S., Dagerman, K. S. & Insel, P. (2005). Risk of death with atypical antipsychotic drug treatment for dementia: meta-analysis of randomised placebo-controlled trials. *JAMA* 294: 1934–43.

5 Ballard, C., Corbett, A., Chitramohan, R., & Aarsland, D. (2009). Management of agitation and aggression associated with Alzheimer's disease: controversies and possible solutions. *Current Opinion in Psychiatry* 22: 532–40.

which suggests that the cognitive impairment in Alzheimer's is due to a deficit of cholinergic neurotransmission. This is what has led to the development of the acetylcholinesterase inhibitors.

Clinical features

Alzheimer's disease represents the 'classical' presentation of dementia, so the descriptions of clinical features on p. 319 are all relevant. It is usual that medical advice is sought either due to an intercurrent physical illness, or because of a sudden worsening, leading to inability of the patient/family to cope at home.

- **Forgetfulness** is the first symptom to emerge. This is initially for short-term memories, but later remote events will also be lost.

- **Disorientation** is usually an early sign and may be evident for the first time when the person is in unfamiliar surroundings; for example, on holiday.

- **Mood variations.** Mood may be predominantly depressed, euphoric, flattened, or labile.

- **Poor sleep**, with multiple awakenings and wandering.

- **Social behaviour declines** and self-care may be neglected, although some patients maintain a good social facade despite severe cognitive impairment.

Table 26.9 Rare degenerative neurological diseases causing dementia

Condition	Pathology	Epidemiology	Clinical features
Frontotemporal dementia (group of conditions including Pick's disease)	Preferential atrophy of the frontal and temporal lobes Ubiquitinated inclusion bodies, loss of cortical neurons, gliosis, and spongiform change	20–60/100 000 Onset 45–60 years Male = female 50% have a family history	Abnormal social behaviour/conduct Change in personality Reduction of speech Mood symptoms Dietary changes Stereotyped behaviour Hallucinations, delusions
Huntington's chorea	Autosomal dominant degenerative disorder of frontal lobes and caudate nucleus	70 per million in Europe Onset 35–44 years Male = female	Choreiform movements Dysarthria Ataxia Dementia Persecutory delusions
Prion disease (includes CJD, vCJD, Kuru)	Deposits of prion protein throughout the brain causing a spongiform encephalopathy Majority sporadic, may be acquired or iatrogenic	Sporadic CJD: 1 per million per year Onset 15–60 years Male = female	Rapidly progressive dementia Myoclonus Focal neurological signs Death within 6 months
HIV-associated dementia (AIDS–dementia complex)	Metabolic encephalopathy caused by the HIV lentivirus, and activation of macrophages in the brain which secrete neurotoxins	10–20% of patients with untreated AIDS Recent decline in numbers following widespread use of HAART	Insidious onset, memory loss, poor attention and concentration Apathy and social withdrawal Depression or psychosis Focal neurology (motor), ataxia and tremor Myoclonus and seizures

- **Personality change** may occur, often with an exaggeration of less favourable traits.

- In the later stages of the disorder, the above features progress, and signs of **parietal lobe dysfunction**—such as dysphasia, dyspraxia, and agnosia—may occur.

The diagnostic criteria for Alzheimer's disease are shown in Box 26.3.

Prevalence

The prevalence in developed countries of moderate and severe Alzheimer's disease is about 5 per cent of individuals aged 65 years and over, and 40 per cent of those aged over 85 years. Therefore, as life expectancy increases in developing countries so the number of patients with Alzheimer's disease increases. About 80 per cent of these demented people live in the community rather than institutions. The disease is more common in men.

Aetiology

The cause of Alzheimer's disease is unknown. Some of the known risk factors are shown in Table 26.10. **Genetic factors** play a role, especially in those with early onset of the disease. A family history of Alzheimer's is the single most important risk factor; first-degree relatives of those with late-onset Alzheimer's disease have a risk of developing the disorder that is three times that of the general population. A small number of families with mutations in the APP, presenilin, and Apo E4 genes have inherited autosomal dominant forms of the disease, but most cases are thought to be sporadic.

Course

There is a progressive decline, the rate of which is not necessarily steady. Incidental physical illness may cause a superimposed delirium resulting in a sudden deterioration in cognitive function from which the patient may not recover fully. Death occurs usually within 5–8 years of the first signs of the disease, and is most frequently from bronchopneumonia.

Treatment

Assessment and management are considered on pp. 320–322.

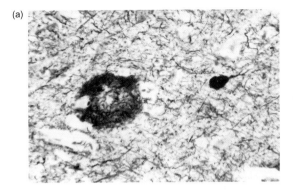

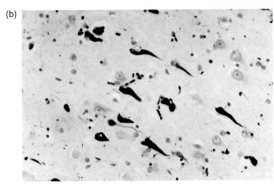

Fig. 26.1 (a) Amyloid plaque and neurofibrillary tangle from the brain of a patient who died of Alzheimer's disease. The plaque shows denser outer staining with an inner core. (b) Characteristic flame-shaped neurofibrillary tangles from the brain of a patient who died from Alzheimer's disease. The tangles are stained with an antibody to hyperphosphorylated tau protein. (Reproduced by permission of Professor Margaret Esiri.)

Vascular dementia

Vascular dementia (also known as **multi-infarct dementia**) is the second most common cause of dementia, accounting for 15–20 per cent of cases. It is a clinical syndrome caused by a variety of different cerebrovascular pathologies, including but not confined to infarctions.

Table 26.10 Risk factors for Alzheimer's disease

- Age
- Family history
- APP, presenilin, or apoE4 gene mutation carrier
- Previous head injury
- Down's syndrome
- Hypothyroidism
- Parkinson's disease
- Cardiovascular disease (including hypertension)
- Low level of education, lower IQ

Pathology

Vascular dementia is associated with ischaemic and non-ischaemic changes in the brain. Both large and small blood vessels may be involved. Neuroimaging has identified that in patients with vascular dementia the following typically occur:

- multiple infarctions and ischaemic lesions in the white matter;
- atrophy of old infarcted areas;
- infarcts tend to be bilateral;
- lesions involve the full thickness of the white matter;
- changes in blood flow in unaffected regions;
- the entire brain is smaller and the ventricles expanded.

Clinical features

Vascular dementia usually presents in the late sixties or early seventies, with a more sudden onset than

---

 BOX 26.3 DSM-IV diagnostic criteria for dementia of the Alzheimer's type

A The development of multiple cognitive deficits manifested by both memory impairment and at least one of aphasia, apraxia, agnosia, or a disturbance in executive functioning.

B The cognitive deficits cause significant impairment in social or occupational functioning and represent a significant decline from a previous level of functioning.

C The course is characterized by gradual onset and continuing cognitive decline.

D The cognitive deficits are not due to any of the following: other central nervous system conditions that cause progressive deficits in memory and cognition; systemic conditions that are known to cause dementia; substance-induced conditions.

E The deficits do not occur exclusively during the course of a delirium.

F The disturbance is not better accounted for by another Axis I disorder.

There are no major differences in the ICD-10 classification system.

Table 26.11 Clinical features of Alzheimer's disease and vascular dementia

Alzheimer's disease	Vascular dementia
Insidious decline	Stepwise progression
Poor memory	Patchy impairment of cognitive function
Progressive disorientation	
Mood change	Poor memory
Restless activity	Episodes of confusion
Insomnia	Mood change
Decline in social behaviour	Personality change
	Seizures
Personality change	Neurological signs
Dysphasia, dyspraxia	

Alzheimer's disease. Patients may present after a stroke, or due to a sudden unexplained decline in function. Unlike Alzheimer's, emotional and personality changes tend to occur early, before memory loss becomes apparent. The symptoms are characteristically fluctuating, and episodes of confusion are common, especially at night. Depression is a prominent feature. Fits, transient ischaemic attacks, or other signs of cerebral ischaemia may occur. On examination there may be focal neurology, often upper motor neuron deficits, and signs of cardiovascular disease elsewhere.

Diagnosis

The diagnosis from Alzheimer's disease is difficult to make with certainty unless there is a clear history of stroke or neurological localizing signs (Table 26.11). Suggestive features are patchy defects of cognitive function, stepwise progression of the condition, and the presence of hypertension and of arteriosclerosis in peripheral or retinal vessels. The diagnostic criteria for vascular dementia are shown in Box 26.4.

Prevalence

The prevalence of vascular dementia is 1–4 per cent of individuals aged 65 and over, depending mainly upon geographical location. Incidence is 6–12 per 1000 per year over 70 years. It is more common in men than women.

Aetiology

Risk factors include:

- personal history of cardiovascular disease, including hypertension and high cholesterol;
- smoking;
- family history of cardiovascular or cerebrovascular disease;
- atrial fibrillation;
- diabetes mellitus;
- coagulopathies;
- polycythaemia;
- sickle-cell anaemia;
- carotid disease.

Prognosis

From the time of diagnosis the lifespan averages 4–5 years, although the variations are wide. About half the patients die from ischaemic heart disease, while others die from cerebral infarction or renal complications.

Lewy body disease

Frederick Lewy was a German neuropathologist who worked with Alzheimer, and in 1912 described the spherical neuronal inclusion bodies found in some patients with dementia. These 'Lewy bodies' are characteristic of Lewy body disease, which has three main clinical manifestations:

1 Parkinson's disease;

2 dementia with Lewy bodies;

BOX 26.4 DSM-IV criteria for the diagnosis of vascular dementia

A The development of multiple cognitive deficits manifested by both:

1 memory impairment;

2 one or more of the following cognitive disturbances: aphasia, apraxia, agnosia, disturbance in executive functioning.

B The cognitive deficits cause significant impairment in social or occupational functioning and represent a significant decline from a previous level of functioning.

C Focal neurological signs and symptoms or laboratory evidence indicative of cerebrovascular disease that are judged to be aetiologically related to the disturbance.

D The deficits do not occur exclusively during the course of a delirium.

E The course is characterized by sustained periods of clinical stability punctuated by sudden significant cognitive and functional losses.

3 autonomic failure associated with degeneration of sympathetic neurons in the spinal cord.

There is a cross-over between the three syndromes, as many patients with Parkinson's develop both dementia and autonomic dysfunction in their latter years.

Pathology

There is usually a mixture of Lewy bodies and Alzheimer-type amyloid plaques and tangles. Lewy bodies are dense, intracytoplasmic inclusions made of phosphorylated neurofilament proteins, associated with ubiquitin and alpha-synuclein. These are primarily found in the basal ganglia, and later spread into the cortex. Neuronal loss is prominent, and there is a slight reduction in total brain volume. The significance of the Alzheimer's-like pathology is unknown.

Clinical features

- **Dementia**—relative sparing of memory, with *fluctuating* cognitive ability and level of consciousness is typical.

- **Parkinsonism**—postural instability and shuffling gait; only 20 per cent have a tremor.

- **Visual hallucinations.**

- **Falls.**

- **Depression.**

- **Sleep disorders**—daytime somnolence.

Prevalence

Lewy body dementia accounts for 10–15 per cent of dementia cases. The prevalence is 0.7 per cent in over 65s, rising to 5.0 per cent in over 85s. It is more common in men than women.

Aetiology

The cause of Lewy body dementia is unknown, but once again family history is a key risk factor, and rare familial types have been found. No environmental risk factors have been identified.

Course and prognosis

Life expectancy for Lewy body dementia is 4–10 years, with the rate of cognitive decline similar to that in Alzheimer's. Frequently, the early stages are only recognized in retrospect, but function can be much more impaired than in other dementias due to pronounced parkinsonism affecting movement. Perceptual and behavioural disturbance can be severe in the later stages of the illness, with antipsychotic medications often needed. A high proportion of these patients will enter residential care by this stage.

Treatment

The principles of treatment remain as previously outlined, but there are a couple of specific points relating to Lewy body dementia. Parkinsonism should be treated with L-DOPA and other antiparkinsonian medications. Anticholinergics should be avoided as there is evidence that they can increase confusion and visual hallucinations in these patients. If needed, atypical antipsychotics should be used before typical antipsychotics, because Lewy body dementia carries a higher risk of neuroleptic malignant syndrome than other conditions.

■ Other organic psychiatric syndromes

Brain pathology may give rise to several specific psychiatric syndromes as well as the generalized disorders described above. These include:

- transient global amnesia;

- amnesic syndrome;

- organic mood disorders;

- organic personality disorders.

Transient global amnesia

This syndrome is an occasional but important cause of episodes of unusual behaviour, which may present as emergencies to general practitioners and the emergency department. Doctors who are not familiar with the syndrome may misdiagnose it as an dissociative disorder (see p. 311). The condition occurs in middle or late life, and more commonly in men. There are abrupt episodes, lasting several hours, of global loss of recent memory. The patient apparently remains alert and orientated, and usually asks repeated questions about what is going on. There is complete recovery, except for amnesia for the episode. The cause is unknown, but there is some evidence that episodes may be associated with migraines or acute physical or emotional stress.

There is no specific treatment.

Amnesic syndrome

The amnesic syndrome is characterized by a prominent disorder of recent memory, in the absence of the generalized intellectual impairment observed in dementia or the impaired consciousness seen in delirium. The condition usually results from lesions in the posterior hypothalamus and nearby midline structures, but occasionally results from bilateral hippocampal lesions. It is often described as **Korsakov's syndrome,** after the Russian neurologist who first described the clinical features, or as the **Wernicke–Korsakov syndrome,** because the amnesic syndrome may accompany an acute neurological syndrome described by Wernicke (**Wernicke's encephalopathy**) characterized by impairment of consciousness, memory defect, disorientation, ataxia, and ophthalmoplegia. The prominent causal factor in most cases appears to be thiamine deficiency.

Clinical features

The central feature of the amnesic syndrome is a profound **impairment of recent memory** (Table 26.12). The patient can recall events immediately after they have occurred, but cannot do so even a few minutes thereafter. Thus, on the standard clinical test of remembering an address, immediate recall is good but grossly impaired 10 minutes later. One consequence of the profound disorder of memory is an associated **disorientation in time**. Gaps in memory are often filled by **confabulation.** The patient may give a vivid and detailed account of recent activities that, on checking, turn out to be inaccurate. It is as though he cannot distinguish between true memories and the products of his imagination or recollection of events from times other than those he is trying to recall. Such a patient is often suggestible; in response to a few cues from the interviewer, he may give an elaborate account of taking part in events that never happened.

Other cognitive functions, including remote memory, are relatively well preserved. Unlike the patient with dementia, the patient with an amnesic syndrome seems alert and able to reason or hold an ordinary conversation, so that the interviewer may at first be unaware of the extent of the memory disorder.

Aetiology

Alcohol abuse is the most frequent cause, and seems to act by causing a deficiency of thiamine. Other causes include carbon monoxide poisoning, vascular lesions, encephalitis, and tumours of the third ventricle.

Treatment

For cases that may be due to **thiamine deficiency,** this vitamin should be prescribed in the hope of limiting

Table 26.12 Clinical features of amnesic syndrome

- Recent memory severely impaired
- Remote memory spared
- Disorientation in time
- Confabulation
- Other cognitive functions preserved

further damage. Oral thiamine is sufficient in non-urgent situations, but patients admitted to hospital should be given parenteral B vitamins (Pabrinex®). Otherwise, there is no specific treatment and the general measures are those described above for dementia.

Course and prognosis

The course is chronic. Prognosis is better when the condition is due to thiamine deficiency, provided that thiamine treatment was started promptly.

Organic personality disorder

Brain damage may result in **personality change** and this may be severe enough to be classified as **personality disorder.** An example is the distinctive syndrome associated with **frontal lobe damage** in which behaviour is disinhibited, over-familiar, and tactless. Patients may be over-talkative, make inappropriate jokes, and engage in pranks. They may make errors of judgement and commit sexual indiscretions, and disregard the feelings of others. The patient is often euphoric, with poor concentration and attention. Measures of formal intelligence are generally unimpaired, but special testing may show deficits in abstract reasoning. Insight is impaired.

■ Neurological syndromes

A variety of primary neurological conditions may also cause cognitive decline and/or other neuropsychiatric symptoms. The common and important ones are briefly described below, with more detailed information to be found in the references on p. 331.

Normal-pressure hydrocephalus

In normal-pressure hydrocephalus (NPH) there is dilatation of the ventricles in the absence of a mechanical block within the ventricular system. Instead, there is an obstruction in the subarachnoid space. At lumbar puncture, the CSF pressure measurement is usually high normal, representing the fact there is little rise in intracranial pressure. NPH can be idiopathic (50 per cent), or be caused by meningitis, subarachnoid haemorrhage, a head injury, or a CNS tumour. It can usually be diagnosed with a combination of neuroimaging and a lumbar puncture.

The characteristic features are a triad of gait ataxia, dementia, and urinary incontinence. Gait disturbance is due to the ventricular dilatation stretching the corona radiata holding the motor fibres which innervate the lower limbs. It presents similarly to parkinsonism, but without the other typical features. The dementia is progressive, with worsening memory, inattention, apathy, and fatigue.

Acetazolamide and repeated lumbar punctures can be used as holding measures to halt progression of symptoms. Definitive treatment requires surgical insertion of a ventriculoperitoneal shunt to improve the circulation of cerebrospinal fluid. This procedure arrests the condition and sometimes the dementia improves. It is important to differentiate this treatable condition from the primary dementias, as well as from depressive disorder with mental slowness.

Cerebrovascular disease

Among people who survive a stroke, about half return to a fully independent life. The rest may have psychological as well as physical problems. The psychological changes are often the more significant, preventing a return to a normal life when the physical disability has ceased to be a serious obstacle. A wide range of psychiatric symptoms may occur after a stroke.

- **Cognitive defects.** Stroke can cause dementia as well as specific deficits of higher cortical function, such as dysphasia and dyspraxia. If the stroke is repeated the dementia may progress to the syndrome of vascular dementia. Amnesic disorders have also been described.

- **Personality change.** Irritability, apathy, or lability of mood may occur after a cerebrovascular accident. Difficulties in coping with everyday problems are common and failure may result in a 'catastrophic reaction'. Such changes are probably due more to associated widespread arteriosclerotic vascular disease than to a single stroke, and they may continue to worsen even though the focal signs of the stroke are improving.

- **Depression** occurs in 50–60 per cent of patients in the first 2 years after a stroke. It is partly a psychological reaction to the handicap caused by the stroke but may in part be a direct consequence of any localized brain damage. It can contribute to the apparent intellectual impairment and is often an important obstacle to rehabilitation.

- **Lability of mood** is frequent and may be a significant clinical problem.

- **Psychosis** is a very rare complication of stroke, usually after a right hemispheric infarct.

Even though biological factors may contribute to aetiology, depressed mood should be treated with antidepressant medication. Lability of mood is also frequently helped by antidepressant treatment. Practical help is frequently required by both the patient and carers.

Cerebral tumours

Many cerebral tumours cause psychological symptoms at some stage, and in a significant minority these symptoms are the first to appear. Fast-growing tumours are more likely to cause a delirium, especially if there is raised intracranial pressure; slow-growing tumours are more likely to present with dementia or, occasionally, depressive symptoms.

Multiple sclerosis

Mood symptoms are the predominant psychiatric disturbance seen in multiple sclerosis. Two-thirds of patients experience symptoms of low mood, with half of these reaching criteria for a major depressive episode. Pathological euphoria with prominent crying and laughing attacks is relatively common later in the disease. Some degree of cognitive impairment is seen in 40 per cent of patients with multiple sclerosis, and a few of these suffer from a rapidly progressive dementia.

Head injury

Major head injuries are common all over the world, the majority being associated with road traffic accidents and/or the use of alcohol. The peak age for head injuries is 15 to 24 years, and they are more common in males. It is difficult to predict the likelihood of brain injury from the size of the injury. The neuropsychiatric consequences are highly variable, both in severity and the type of symptoms.

In the acute phase (hours to days) after a head injury, the following are common:

1 **Post-traumatic amnesia:** loss of memory for the period of the injury and until normal memory is resumed afterwards. Amnesia for longer than 24 hours is associated with a high risk of longer-term cognitive impairment.

2 **Retrograde amnesia:** loss of memory for a distinct period of time leading up to the injury.

3 **Acute post-traumatic delirium:** confusion, anxiety, mood lability, paranoia, and hallucinations occurring soon after the patient regains consciousness.

In the longer term, more typical psychiatric syndromes are seen.

- **Cognitive impairment.** This may be a global dementia picture, or more focal deficits in memory, attention, and concentration or speech. Some more minor head injuries cause less obvious cognitive impairments that may significantly impair functioning and behaviour for many months. Patients returning to demanding occupations who complain of difficulties following head injury require full neurological review. Repeated minor blows to the head, such as occur in **boxing**, can lead to progressive deterioration in intellectual function.

- **Personality change** is often the most serious long-term complication after severe head injury, particularly after damage to the frontal lobe. There may be irritability, loss of spontaneity and drive, some coarsening of behaviour, and occasionally reduced control of aggressive impulses. These changes often cause serious difficulties for the patient and his family.

- **Emotional symptoms** may follow any kind of injury. Depression is frequent in those with severe physical disability following the accident. Whatever the severity of the injury, there may also be a combination of anxiety, depression, and irritability, with headache, dizziness, fatigue, poor concentration, and insomnia. This **post-concussional syndrome** is probably due to an interaction of minor brain damage with anxiety and depression.

Assessment and management

A plan for long-term treatment should be made as early as possible after head injury. Three aspects of the problem should be assessed:

1 neurological signs and the degree of physical disability;
2 any neuropsychiatric problems and their likely future course;
3 social circumstances, social support, the possibility of return to work, and the effect of the injury on the patient's responsibilities in the family.

Specialist rehabilitation should include not only physiotherapy and graded increase in physical activity, but work with the patient and family to try and minimize disabilities in everyday life and to find ways of dealing with specific cognitive deficits such as impaired memory. Late deteriorations in cognitive function after brain injury should be taken seriously, and reversible causes such as normal-pressure hydrocephalus, subdural haematoma, or epilepsy considered. Depression, psychosis, or agitation should be treated along usual guidelines.

■ Psychiatric manifestations of epilepsy

Epilepsy is a very common condition, with a lifetime risk of 3.4 per cent for males and 2.8 per cent for females, and is therefore seen frequently in all medical specialties.

People with epilepsy suffer from the misconceptions and prejudices of other people about epilepsy as well as

Table 26.13 Associations between epilepsy and psychological problems of epileptic individuals

Effects of stigma and social restrictions
Psychiatric disorder due to the cause of epilepsy
Behavioural disturbance associated with the seizure
• Before: tension, irritability, depression
• During: complex partial seizures
• After: automatism (rarely)
Disorders between seizures
• Cognitive impairment
• Personality disorder
• Paranoid disorder
• Sexual dysfunction
• Increased self-harm and suicide

from the condition itself. Epilepsy can be restricting; for example, the inability to drive or to go swimming unsupervised. The prevalence of psychiatric disorders in people with epilepsy is four times greater than in the general population, but there is a wide variation depending upon the type of epilepsy. There are several ways in which epilepsy predisposes to psychiatric disturbance (see Table 26.13).

Psychiatric disorder associated with the cause of epilepsy

When epilepsy is a consequence of brain damage, this damage may also cause intellectual impairment or personality problems.

Behavioural disturbance associated with the seizure

Before a seizure (prodromal) there may be a period of increasing tension, irritability, and depression lasting for hours or sometimes a few days.

During seizures (ictal) of the complex partial type there may be automatic behaviours. Occasionally, such seizures are prolonged for days as 'complex partial status', in which there may be an abnormal mental state, abnormal behaviour, or social withdrawal.

After the seizure (post-ictal) there may occasionally be a prolonged period of confusion (post-ictal delirium), during which the patient is disorientated, inattentive, and agitated. It usually only lasts a few hours, and tends to recur with further seizures. Post-ictal psychosis tends to be confined to patients with severe epilepsy who experience a sudden increase in seizure frequency or severity. There is a sudden onset of hallucinations and delusions, which may last from days to months.

Psychiatric disorder occurring between seizures

Cognitive dysfunction. In some patients, there is persistent abnormal electrical activity in the brain between seizures, and this activity can be associated with poor attention and memory. The drugs used to treat epilepsy may also cause impaired attention.

Personality. Most people with epilepsy are of normal personality. When personality disorder does occur, it is not of any single kind. The causes are multiple: social limitations imposed on the epileptic person during childhood and adolescence, self-consciousness, and the reactions of other people. In cases where brain damage has caused the epilepsy, the former may contribute to the personality disorder.

Chronic inter-ictal psychosis occurs in patients who have had poorly controlled epilepsy for at least a decade. The symptoms are hard to distinguish from those of schizophrenia, and should be treated with antipsychotics.

Depression and anxiety. Affective disorder is more common in people with epilepsy than in the general population.

Sexual dysfunction. This problem is more common in epileptics than in non-epileptics. Reduced libido, a decrease in activity, and sexual dysfunction are all seen. The causes include difficult relationships and the effects of anti-epileptic medication. There may also be neurophysiological causes in some cases since sexual problems are more common with temporal lobe epilepsy than with other kinds.

Suicide and deliberate self-harm. Among people with epilepsy, suicide is five times more frequent, and deliberate self-harm is seven times more frequent, than in the general population.

Crime is associated with epilepsy—males with epilepsy are three times more likely to receive a criminal conviction than matched controls. There are many confounding factors (lower IQ, low socio-economic status) so it is currently unclear how much of this increase is due to the epilepsy itself.

Management

Collaboration with a neurologist to maximize seizure control with anticonvulsants is the most important part of treatment. Specific symptoms such as depression or psychosis should be treated with antidepressants or antipsychotics, respectively. Many of the mood stabilizers (e.g. lamotrigine, carbamazepine) also have anticonvulsive properties.

Further reading

Gelder, M., Andreasen, N., Lopez-Ibor, J, & Geddes, J. (eds) (2009). *New Oxford Textbook of Psychiatry*, 2nd edn. Section 4.1: Delirium, dementia, amnesia, and other cognitive disorders, pp. 325–419. Oxford University Press, Oxford.

David, A., Fleminger, S., Kopelman, M., *et al.* (2009). *Lishman's Organic Psychiatry: A Textbook of Neuropsychiatry*, 4th edn. Blackwells, Oxford.

National Institute of Clinical Excellence (2006). *Dementia: Supporting People with Dementia and their Carers in Health and Social Care.* http://guidance.nice.org.uk/CG42.

Burnes and Iliffe (2009). *Alzheimer's Disease. British Medical Journal* **338**:b158.

CHAPTER 27

Eating disorders

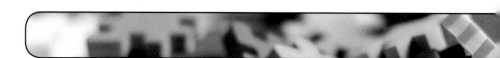

Chapter contents

■ Introduction to eating disorders

The formal definition of an eating disorder is a disturbance of eating habits or weight-control behaviour that results in clinically significant impairment of physical health and/or psychosocial functioning. The take-home message from this chapter is that eating disorders are serious conditions, which affect every aspect of an individual's life; they are not simply a problem of eating too much or too little, or an attempt to look like models in glossy magazines. Anorexia nervosa has the highest mortality of any psychiatric disorder, and it is notoriously difficult both to engage eating-disordered patients, and to treat them successfully.

Eating disorders have been increasingly conspicuous in the last 30 years, both in clinical practice and in the public domain. It is uncertain whether the changes in presentation reflect a true increase, with epidemiological research consistently reporting the lifetime risk of an eating disorder to be 5 to 7 per cent for women and 2.5 per cent for men in the developed world. However, many eating disorders remain undiagnosed—it is estimated that general practitioners recognize only 12 per cent of cases of bulimia nervosa and 45 per cent of cases of anorexia nervosa, although this is steadily improving.

There are a variety of reasons why all clinicians should have a good working knowledge of the characteristics and management of eating disorders.

- Eating disorders are common, and associated with high morbidity and mortality.

- The earlier the diagnosis of the disorder, the better the prognosis.

- Patients frequently present to specialties other than psychiatry, e.g. gastroenterology, gynaecology, cardiology, Accident and Emergency, and neurology.

- The physical consequences of eating disorders can be short term (hypokalaemia, dehydration, bradycardia) or long term (osteoporosis, infertility), and may only become evident many years after the acute illness.

- The majority of less severe eating disorders can be successfully treated in the community by a supportive primary care team, without the need for intensive specialist input.

- Eating disorders are relatively common amongst colleagues working within the medical profession.

Classification of eating disorders

There are three main types of eating disorder recognized by the DSM-IV classification system:

1 anorexia nervosa (AN);

2 bulimia nervosa (BN);

3 eating disorder not otherwise specified (EDNOS).

The criteria and characteristics of each disorder are discussed in the sections below, with specific information about childhood eating disorders on p. 445. The ICD-10 classification includes 'atypical anorexia nervosa' and 'atypical bulimia nervosa' rather than EDNOS, and a separate category for 'overeating associated with other psychological disturbances' (e.g. bereavement, mood disorders, and stress). Figure 27.1 illustrates the relationship between the three main disorders.

The classification above assumes that eating disorders are categorical in nature, and that the separate behavioural

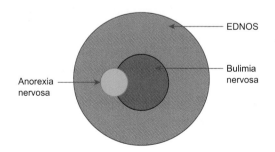

Fig. 27.1 Venn diagram illustrating the relationship between the diagnoses of anorexia nervosa, bulimia nervosa, and eating order not otherwise specified (EDNOS). Reproduced from Fairburn *et al.* (1993). The classification of recurrent overeating: the 'binge eating disorder' proposal. *International Journal of Eating Disorders* **13**: 155–9.

conditions represent different underlying psychopathology. This way of thinking has been used to develop separate treatment methods and guidelines for anorexia nervosa compared with bulimia nervosa. However, a recent **transdiagnostic theory** suggests that all eating disorders share the same characteristic psychopathology, and the differing syndromes merely represent patients moving along a spectrum of potential symptoms over time. For example, the major difference between anorexia nervosa and bulimia nervosa would be the balance of total energy intake being negative in the former and neutral or positive in the latter, whilst the underlying psychological process remain the same. One of the major pieces of evidence for this theory is the propensity for anorexia nervosa patients to cross over into bulimia nervosa, and that when looked at over a lifetime, the majority of eating-disordered patients exhibit behaviours from both disorders at different points.

Anorexia nervosa

Anorexia nervosa is a clinical syndrome characterized by low body weight, amenorrhoea, a distorted body image, and an intense fear of gaining weight. The term 'anorexia nervosa' was first used by William Gull in 1874, and his original description of the essence of the condition contains all of the core elements of the diagnostic criteria that we use today. At the same time, the French physician Charles Lasegue published a similar work, and whilst Gull and Lasegue were very explicit in their descriptions of the physical findings in anorexia nervosa, both were cautious about extrapolating to describe the psychopathology underlying it, and how to fit this into the classification of other psychiatric conditions. Our understanding has improved in the last century, but there are still many unanswered questions.

Anorexia nervosa is a relatively common condition which may present to almost any clinical specialty with a multitude of presenting complaints. The role of the general practitioner (GP) in the management of anorexia nervosa is especially important for a number of reasons:

- to make an initial diagnosis and risk assessment;

- to develop a trustworthy relationship with the patient, and assist them to decide whether they are ready to make changes to their behaviour, and then to support them in doing so;

- to provide easy access to healthcare for the very many people with less severe anorexia nervosa;

- to make referrals and then effectively coordinate between mental health services and specialties dealing with physical complications;

Science box 27.1   Should amenorrhoea be included in the diagnostic criteria for anorexia nervosa?

The upcoming publication of the latest version (V) of the *Diagnostic and Statistical Manual of Mental Disorders* has led to some debate as to the validity of the current criteria for anorexia nervosa (AN). Specifically, should the requirement for 'the absence of at least three consecutive menstrual cycles' remain necessary for the diagnosis of AN? In recent years, a large number of studies have been published attempting to decide if amenorrhoea is a useful criterion, principally asking: is it a specific enough sign to diagnose anorexia nervosa? And is amenorrhoea a reliable indicator of disease severity?

A strong argument for keeping amenorrhoea in DSM-V is the objective nature of it as a measure, compared with psychopathological criteria. However, it is only useful for some patients, as amenorrhoea is irrelevant to males, females on hormonal contraceptives, and prepubertal and postmenopausal patients. Currently, those patients who fit all criteria for AN except for being amenorrhoeic are classed as EDNOS; this often has implications for what treatment they are eligible for.

Clinicians across medicine frequently use menstrual disturbance as a proxy measure of poor physical health. Amenorrhoea could therefore be useful in anorexia nervosa to distinguish those individuals who are at higher physical risk because of their illness. It may also separate those females who are constitutionally thin from those with an eating disorder. However, whilst there is a definite link between body weight or body fat percentage and amenorrhoea, the widely believed 'critical percentage' to be reached for menarche to occur has not been substantiated. Athletes, healthy controls, and those with AN show a wide variation in BMI/body fat percentage at which their menses cease. Many other factors may also cause amenorrhoea, e.g. exercise, stress, and thyroid disease. Amenorrhoea therefore does not have high specificity for diagnosing AN.

A series of large, retrospective chart reviews have shown that there is little clinical difference in presentation between those patients with and without amenorrhoea. Age of onset, length of illness, lowest weight, presenting BMI, and psychological parameters all consistently do not predict amenorrhoea reliably. In one-fifth of patients, amenorrhoea precedes weight loss and in many menses do not return for some time after weight restoration. It is already known that leptin (and other energy-regulatory peptide) levels are low in AN, but are comparable to those with similarly low BMIs for other reasons. No correlation has been found between leptin levels and menstrual status. Similarly, whilst low oestrogen levels and low weight independently predict a reduction in bone mineral density (and therefore increased risk of fractures), cross-sectional data have not shown a correlation between amenorrhoea and bone mineral density. There is, therefore, no strong evidence that amenorrhoea is a reliable measure of physical health in AN.

The options for those writing DSM-V are threefold; leave the amenorrhoea criterion as it currently stands, remove it completely, or alter it in some way. It is clear that amenorrhoea is a characteristic feature of AN. Therefore it might be proposed that it should be moved from being a necessary criterion to a supplementary sign supporting a diagnosis on the other criteria. The debate continues.

American Psychiatric Association (1994). *Diagnostic and Statistical Manual of Mental Disorders*, 4th edn.

Attia, E. & Roberto, C. O. (2009). Should amenorrhoea be a diagnostic criterion for anorexia nervosa? *International Journal of Eating Disorders* **42**: 581–9.

Watson, T. L. & Anderson, A. E. (2003). A critical examination of the amenorrhoea and weight criteria for diagnosing anorexia nervosa. *Acta Psychiatrica Scandinavica* **108**: 175–82.

- to monitor physical risk and medications prescribed by secondary care regularly;

- to provide support for those caring for the individual with anorexia nervosa.

Diagnostic criteria

The diagnostic criteria are shown in Box 27.1. These describe the core clinical features required for a diagnosis of anorexia nervosa, and are a good summary of the major presenting features.

Clinical features

The classical presentation of anorexia nervosa is a young female who has reduced her food intake and lost weight over the preceding few months, and who is brought to medical attention by a concerned member of the family. However, this is a stereotypical view and should not be relied upon, as there is significant heterogeneity in presentation. The most striking features of anorexia nervosa are excessive concern with shape and weight together with a relentless pursuit of thinness, but these are often only picked up on detailed questioning, with the actual

BOX 27.1 DSM-IV diagnostic criteria for anorexia nervosa

A Refusal to maintain body weight at or above a minimally normal weight for age and height: body mass index (BMI) < 17.5 or ideal body weight (IBW) < 85 per cent of expected value*.

B Intense fear of gaining weight or becoming obese.

C Disturbance in the way in which one's body weight or shape is experienced, undue influence of body weight or shape on self-evaluation, or denial of the seriousness of the current low body weight.

D The absence of at least three consecutive menstrual cycles (amenorrhoea) in women who have had their first menstrual period but have not yet gone through menopause.

*In children there may just be failure to make expected weight gain during a period of growth, leading to body weight less than 85 per cent of that expected.

Furthermore, the DSM-IV-TR specifies two subtypes:

- Restricting type: during the current episode of anorexia nervosa, the person has not regularly engaged in binge-eating or purging behaviour (that is, self-induced vomiting, over-exercise, or the misuse of laxatives, diuretics, or enemas).
- Binge-eating type or purging type: during the current episode of anorexia nervosa, the person has regularly engaged in binge-eating or purging behaviour (that is, self-induced vomiting, over-exercise, or the misuse of laxatives, diuretics, or enemas).

ICD-10 F50.0 anorexia nervosa

There are no clinically significant differences between the two classification systems.

reason for consultation being physical symptoms relating to starvation.

The main features of anorexia nervosa can be divided into four categories (Figure 27.2):

1 core psychopathology;

2 behaviours in pursuit of thinness and low weight;

3 psychiatric co-morbidities;

4 physical consequences of starvation, including physical signs and biochemical disturbances.

Food and eating habits

Patients with anorexia nervosa usually eat very little, and may show a particular avoidance of carbohydrates and foods containing fats. However, make no assumptions as to eating habits, as again there is great variation— a food diary is the best method of collecting data on intake. Patients frequently describe eating almost entirely fruits and vegetables, with copious quantities of calorie-free liquids (black unsweetened tea and coffee, water, diet sodas). Most set daily calorie limits, and eat alone at particular times of the day. Patients may eat extremely slowly, with elaborate rituals of how each food must be eaten, including cutting up the food into minute pieces and making unusual combinations. Most patients with anorexia nervosa are preoccupied with thoughts of food, and some will enjoy cooking complex meals or cakes for others, but refuse to eat any themselves. Excessive use of chewing gum and cigarettes as appetite suppressants is very common. Patients often weigh

themselves frequently, sometimes multiple times per day.

Up to half of patients describe episodes of uncontrollable overeating (known as **binge eating** or **bulimia**). During binges, the patients may eat very large amounts of the foods they usually avoid; for example, a whole loaf of bread or a large pizza. After overeating the patient feels bloated and may induce vomiting. Binges may be followed by remorse and intensified efforts to lose weight.

Patients with anorexia nervosa sometimes develop fears that calories may be able to enter the body in a variety of everyday situations. Licking stamps, using moisturizers or sun-creams, and taking medications in tablet form are common examples.

Additional harmful behaviours

Patients with anorexia nervosa use a variety of methods to lose weight, which are often secretive and need to be asked about directly. Self-induced vomiting is common, and often occurs without the episode of overeating seen in bulimia nervosa. Laxative abuse—most frequently with senna or bisacodyl—is (mistakenly) used to accelerate weight loss, often with increasing quantities of laxatives being taken as the gut becomes tolerant of them. In the long term this can lead to chronic constipation. Excessive exercise is usually overt—hours in the gym, long walks, or aerobic classes—but may be more secretive. Many patients will exercise in the privacy of their bedroom at night, or walk a long distance to school instead of taking the bus.

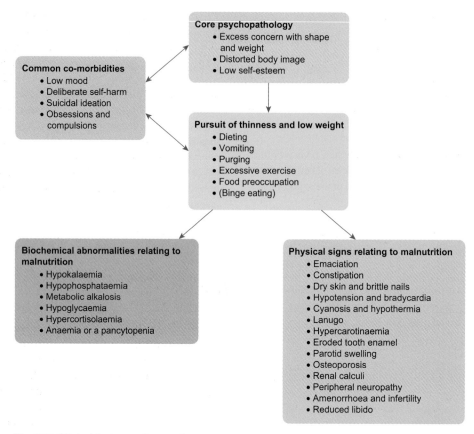

Fig. 27.2 Clinical features of anorexia nervosa.

Psychopathology

The core psychopathology in anorexia nervosa has the following features:

- a disturbance of body image, such that the emaciated patient believes that she is overweight despite all evidence to the contrary;

- a fear (and sometimes hatred) of fatness;

- valuation of self-worth as a function of weight and body shape, rather than by the usual values of the society they live in.

The patient will usually see themselves as fat when put in front of a mirror, and will be able to point out specific areas of their body which are perceived as fat/unattractive/disgusting or inadequate. The abnormal thoughts surrounding weight and shape are conventionally described as an **overvalued idea** rather than a delusion.

Other extremely common features include:

- a preoccupation and obsession with food, weight, and shape in themselves, and often in friends and family;

- body checking; repeatedly checking specific areas of the body in mirrors, shop windows, or by touch to reassure themselves they are not fat;

- denial of the severity of the condition and its possible implications for physical and mental health. The patient may also deny symptoms of hunger, fatigue, and amenorrhoea—it is often hard to tell if this is deliberate or unintentional denial;

- low self-esteem;

- perfectionism in activities, e.g. academic work, cleaning, playing a musical instrument.

Other psychiatric symptoms

Low mood, which frequently fits criteria for a moderate or severe depressive episode, is common in anorexia nervosa. Low mood is a symptom of starvation in itself, but is also independently found in eating disorders. Patients frequently express extreme guilt after eating, and may believe they do not deserve food. Social withdrawal often occurs as mood drops, and patients may spend much of their time alone. Deliberate self-harm is very common, especially scratches or cuts on the wrists, forearms, and lower calves. Suicide is the most frequent mode of death in anorexia nervosa, and all patients with severe and/or enduring disorders should be considered at high risk.

Obsessive-compulsive symptoms are characteristic of many of the eating habits seen in anorexia, but OCD as a clinical diagnosis in itself is also frequently present. Obsessive exercise routines, cleaning, and studying are typical themes.

Physical consequences of starvation

Low weight is essential for the diagnosis, with a cut-off of BMI 17.5 (or weight less than 85 per cent of expected) being the usual limit. See Box 27.3 on p. 342 for how to calculate BMI.

Amenorrhoea is an important feature, and the only physical sign apart from weight to be included in the diagnostic criteria. It occurs early in the development of the condition and in about one-fifth of cases it precedes obvious weight loss. Amenorrhoea is a common presenting complaint, and represents a global impairment of the hypothalamic–pituitary–gonadal axis. In the undernourished state, concentrations of follicle-stimulating hormone (FSH), luteinizing hormone (LH), and oestrogen in the blood are very low or even undetectable. The secretion pattern of the pituitary hormones is also abnormal, with the 24-hour cycle of LH secretion being more similar to the prepubertal than adult pattern. This almost always reverses with weight gain. Pelvic ultrasound in an underweight woman will show small ovaries, with no sign of the heterogeneity of follicles seen during a typical menstrual cycle. In males, testicular function is reduced, with a decreased level of testosterone production. The patient is infertile until endocrine function recovers with weight gain. Hypercortisolaemia and low thyroxine may also be seen, and are adaptive measures to reduce metabolic rate and deal with the stress of malnutrition.

Severe malnutrition produces emaciation and cold, blue extremities. Some patients have signs that are secondary to the low food intake, namely constipation, low blood pressure, bradycardia, sensitivity to cold, and hypothermia. Myopathy is common, and characteristic of that seen in any cause of protein–energy malnutrition. Proximal muscle groups are affected first, with the patient having trouble climbing stairs or rising unaided from a squatting position. Osteoporosis is the inevitable consequence of a combination of low calcium and vitamin D intake, low weight, and low circulating oestrogen levels.

Biochemical abnormalities

Patients who vomit, use laxatives, or take diuretics are at high risk from dehydration and electrolyte disturbances. Vomiting produces a loss of gastric acid, leading to a metabolic alkalosis and hypokalaemia. Cardiac arrhythmias are not uncommon in this situation, and can lead to sudden death. Laxative abuse can cause dehydration, hypokalaemia, hyponatraemia, and a metabolic acidosis. Diuretics produce dehydration and hyponatraemia. Hypoglycaemia is rare, but is another recognized cause of sudden death. Reduced haemoglobin and leucocyte levels can occur, but they are not nearly as common as the electrolyte disturbances, and are a marker of severe starvation.

Peripheral oedema is a relatively frequent occurrence in severely emaciated patients. It is unclear currently what leads to the retention of fluid in starvation, but it can lead to pulmonary oedema and congestive cardiac failure, and therefore should be taken seriously. The exception to this is re-feeding oedema, seen in inpatients on very high-calorie diets—this is usually benign and does not need investigating.

Epidemiology

The prevalence of anorexia nervosa is 0.5 to 1 per cent in adolescent and young adult women, and approximately 0.1 per cent in adolescent males. Lifetime risk is 5 to 7 per cent for women and 2.5 per cent for men. The ratio of affected females to males is reportedly 10:1, although it is thought many cases of anorexia nervosa in men go unrecognized. The average age of onset is 15–17 years for females and 12–13 years for males. However, anorexia nervosa may present at any age; one survey of a US inpatient unit had patients aged 7 to 78 years undergoing treatment at that time.

It has been suggested that the incidence of anorexia nervosa has risen dramatically since the 1950s—or is it just that better diagnosis is picking up previously unrecognized cases? Epidemiological studies from Scandinavia and the USA show that the incidence did increase between the 1950s and 1980s, but this was confined to female patients aged 15 to 24 years. Since the 1980s, the figures appear to have reached a plateau.

Co-morbidity

Depressive disorder (and/or deliberate self-harm) is seen in 40–60 per cent of patients with anorexia nervosa. Other frequently occurring conditions include obsessive-compulsive disorder, body dysmorphic disorder, sleep disorders, anxiety disorders, and chronic fatigue syndrome.

Differential diagnosis

- **Bulimia nervosa** is characterized by episodes of uncontrolled overeating, compensatory methods of weight control, and a fear of becoming fat. Technically, it is distinguished from anorexia nervosa on weight criteria; if the patient has a BMI greater than 17.5, experiences binges, and does not fit criteria for anorexia nervosa then the diagnosis is bulimia nervosa. If their BMI is 17.5 or lower, the diagnosis is anorexia nervosa binge–purge subtype.

- **EDNOS** describes those patients with disordered eating that is clinically significant, but which does not fit criteria for a specific eating disorder; for example, a patient with all the features of anorexia nervosa, but who is not amenorrhoeic.

- **Klein–Levin syndrome** is a sleep disorder seen in adolescent males, characterized by recurrent episodes of binge eating and hypersomnia.

- **Mood disorder.** Core features include low mood, fatigue, and anhedonia. Loss of appetite and weight loss are common, but the patient will not show the specific psychopathology and other weight control behaviours seen in anorexia nervosa.

- **Substance abuse.** Patients with chemical dependencies (especially intravenous opioid users) may present extremely underweight, but do not show the other characteristics of an eating disorder.

- **Iatrogenic drugs.** Many drugs may cause weight loss, through either loss of appetite or a direct effect on metabolism; for example, SSRIs, stimulants (methylphenidate, metamphetamine), slimming pills (e.g. orlistat, sibutramine).

- **Organic disorders.** These can usually be identified by a clear history and lack of associated core psychopathology, but specific investigations may need to be done:

  - **gastrointestinal disorders:** inflammatory bowel disease, coeliac disease, chronic pancreatitis;
  - **endocrine disorders:** hyperthyroidism, diabetes mellitus, insulinoma;
  - **neurological disorders:** brain tumours affecting the hypothalamus, dementia, chronic degenerative conditions (e.g. motor neuron disease);
  - **cancer.**

Aetiology

Like most psychiatric disorders, there is no one cause of anorexia nervosa. A multidimensional model including biological, psychological, and social factors is the best explanation at the current time. It is likely that factors interact with one another, such that, at a specific point, a vulnerable individual becomes ill. Table 27.1 outlines the major aetiological factors known for anorexia nervosa. These causal factors may also be considered under the categories of predisposing, precipitating, and maintaining factors.

Predisposing factors

Biological

1 **Genetics.** Genes undoubtedly play a large role in the aetiology of anorexia nervosa, but it is not a simple hereditary

Table 27.1 Aetiology of anorexia nervosa: predisposing factors

Biological factors	Psychological factors	Social factors
• Genetics:	Personality traits	Childhood upbringing and home environment
• Gender, ethnicity	Parental eating disorders	
• Family history	Adverse events in early life	Occupation
• Twin studies		Socio-economic status
Cerebral abnormalities	Childhood sexual abuse	
Serotonin dysregulation		Societal pressures and norms*
Zinc deficiency*		

*These are proposed causative factors which remain controversial.

pattern such as is found in single gene disorders. The heritability of anorexia nervosa is thought to be 50 to 70 per cent, with female first-degree relatives of a patient with the illness having an eightfold increased risk compared with the general population. Many patients have a positive family history, or detailed questioning will reveal a propensity towards or subclinical illness in a relative. Twin studies show the concordance of anorexia nervosa is 65 per cent and 35 per cent in monozygotic and dizygotic twins, respectively.

2 **Cerebral abnormalities.** Rare cases of presumed anorexia nervosa have later been discovered to have actually been organic in nature, typically caused by a tumour involving the hypothalamus. Neuroimaging has shown atrophy of the brain, with widening of the sulci and enlargement of the ventricles. However, this reverses in 50 per cent of patients with weight gain. Hypoperfusion of the temporal lobes has been demonstrated in anorexic children using fMRI, but further research remains to be done to substantiate this in adults.

3 **Serotonin dysregulation** is postulated to be a causative factor in many psychiatric illnesses, and anorexia nervosa is no exception. Serotonin (5HT) is known to play a role in appetite, mood, anxiety, and impulse control. It is known that activation of serotonin in the brain leads to the inhibition of food consumption. While still underweight, patients have reduced levels of serotonin metabolites in the CSF, which normalize with weight gain. However, recent meta-analyses of trials of SSRIs in anorexia nervosa have not shown them to be of benefit in reducing core psychopathology.

4 **Zinc deficiency.** Since the 1970s, there have been advocates of the theory that zinc deficiency plays a major role in the aetiology of anorexia nervosa. Lack of zinc is clearly documented to cause loss of appetite, and one randomized

controlled trial showed zinc supplementation doubled the rate of weight restoration in anorexic patients. However, the issue remains controversial.

Psychological

1 **Personality traits.** Certain personality traits are extremely common in patients with anorexia nervosa—these include obsessive–compulsive thoughts and behaviours, clinical perfectionism, and high levels of personal restraint (the ability to fight temptation). Approximately 30 per cent of patients in large studies were said to have a 'normal' personality in childhood before their illness, with the others having anxious, obsessive, or perfectionistic traits. One cohort study found 72 per cent of inpatients on an eating disorders unit to fit criteria for a personality disorder under the DSM-III criteria.

2 **The influence of parental eating disorders.** Aside from the genetic vulnerability passed to the offspring of those with eating disorders, there is also the problem that many anorexic mothers extend their abnormal concern with weight and shape to their children. Children pick up cues from others easily, and the mother's verbal concerns and behaviours will soon be taken on board by the child. There have also been numerous cases of children suffering from food deprivation, due to their mother consciously or unconsciously restricting their intake. This is not child abuse, merely a representation of the mother's ongoing psychopathology. The abnormal beliefs surrounding food, weight, and shape may then be carried into later life by the child.

3 **Previous adverse experiences** such as the loss of a parent, divorce, illness in the family, or difficulties at school. Males with anorexia nervosa often report having sexual problems, and many are relieved by the loss of libido that occurs with weight loss.

4 **Childhood sexual abuse.** Studies consistently report that approximately one-third of patients hospitalized for anorexia nervosa give a history of sexual abuse in childhood.

Social

1 **Childhood upbringing and environment.** Growing up in a household where parents are overprotective, rigid in thoughts and actions, and place high expectations (be these personal, musical, sporting, or academic) is a strong risk factor for anorexia nervosa. Families with an anorexic child are often poor at resolving conflict, such that conflict is avoided or when it does occur the child is involved and placed between the parents. They also tend to be close families, with strong relationships between family members.

2 **Societal pressures and the 'cult of thinness'.** In the last few decades, it has become increasingly fashionable for women to be thin; there are copious magazines, slimming books, weight-loss clubs, television adverts, and diet foods surrounding everyone in the Western world. The fashion industry has been highly criticized for supporting a 'size zero culture' in which models (and therefore what young people aspire to) are displayed at unhealthily low weights. None of these things cause an eating disorder; however, they may help to reinforce underlying abnormal beliefs in a vulnerable individual.

Precipitating factors

There are a multitude of different events that may precipitate the onset of anorexia nervosa in a vulnerable individual. These include bereavement, parental divorce, change of school or the move to university, academic stress surrounding exams, serious physical illness in the patient or family, bullying, physical or sexual abuse, and loss of weight for other reasons. In some cases no obvious stress or triggering event will be found.

Maintaining factors

There are five main aspects to the forces that may cause anorexia nervosa to continue in a patient.

1 Starvation itself causes many of the symptoms of anorexia nervosa. Odd eating behaviours, an obsession with food, and excessive exercise are all seen in starved individuals in other contexts.

2 The precipitating factors in the illness may be ongoing; for instance, dealing with the sequelae of sexual abuse.

3 Denial is common in anorexia nervosa, and it is impossible for the illness to recede unless the patient accepts that there is a problem.

4 The transdiagnostic model of eating disorders (see Further reading) proposes that all eating disorders share the same psychopathology, and that patients move between different diagnoses (and therefore exhibit different symptomatology) over time. The authors of this theory, Fairburn *et al.*, have put forward a cognitive theory of the maintenance of anorexia nervosa, which is shown in diagrammatic form in Figure 27.3.

5 Anorexia nervosa becomes part of the patient, and they may not be able to envisage themselves without it. This combined with the general benefits that the sick role provides may provide great inertia towards recovery.

Course and prognosis

In its early stages, anorexia nervosa often runs a fluctuating course with periods of partial remission. The most

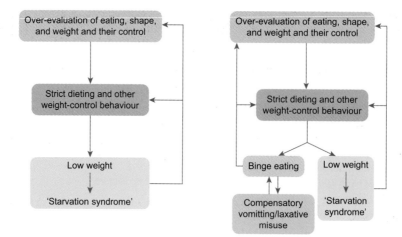

Fig. 27.3 A schematic representation of the maintenance of eating disorders. Reproduced with permission from Fairburn *et al.* (2003). Cognitive behaviour therapy for eating disorders: A transdiagnostic theory and treatment. *Behaviour Research and Therapy* **41**: 509–28.

sensitive *predictor of poor outcome* is a long history at the time the patient is first seen by a doctor. The long-term prognosis is variable:

- one-third of patients make a full recovery;
- one-third remain severely ill;
- one-third attain a partial recovery; among those with improved weight and menstrual function, some continue to have abnormal eating habits, some become overweight, and some others develop bulimia nervosa;

The aggregate mortality rate from anorexia nervosa has been shown in meta-analyses to be 0.5 per cent per annum. Complications of starvation account for 50 per cent of deaths, with suicide making up the majority of the remaining half. Table 27.2 shows the main factors associated with a poor prognosis.

Table 27.2 Poor prognostic factors in anorexia nervosa

- Long length of illness at first presentation
- BMI less than 14 at diagnosis
- Older age of onset
- Bulimic features (bingeing and purging)
- Presence of anxious, obsessive, or dependent traits in childhood
- Personality disorder
- Relationship difficulties within the family
- Anxiety when eating with others
- Male sex

Screening

Screening in primary care and in the general hospital environment is very important, especially in those patients who present with physical rather than psychological problems. The high-risk groups that should be targeted include:

- adolescent females, especially those from higher socio-economic classes;
- ballet dancers;
- gymnasts;
- models and modelling students;
- type 1 diabetic patients;
- medical students and doctors.

The questions that should be asked are known as the SCOFF questionnaire, and are shown in Box 27.2. The questionnaire is valid for both anorexia nervosa and bulimia nervosa, but has a low sensitivity, such that a score of more than or equal to 2 should lead to further history and investigations.

■ Assessment of an eating disorders patient

The following assessment of eating disorders can be used for anorexia nervosa, bulimia nervosa, or EDNOS. Assessment may initially be carried out within the primary care team, but usually specialist input is required. More than one interview may be needed to obtain all relevant

BOX 27.2 The SCOFF* questionnaire

- Do you make yourself **Sick** because you feel uncomfortably full?
- Do you worry you have lost **Control** over how much you eat?
- Have you recently lost more than **One** stone in a 3-month period?

- Do you believe yourself to be **Fat** when others say you are thin?
- Would you say that **Food** dominates your life?

Morgan, J.F., Reid, F., & Lacey, J.H. (1999). The SCOFF questionnaire: assessment of a new screening tool for eating disorders. *British Medical Journal* **319**: 1467–8.

---

information and to gain the patient's trust. The specific questions to ask eating-disordered patients are presented before the generic psychiatric history, but this order may need to be reversed depending upon the clinical situation.

Specific eating disorder questions

- What is a typical day's eating? To what degree is the patient attempting restraint?
- Do they stick to particular calorie limits?
- Is there a pattern? Does it vary? Is eating ritualized?
- Do they avoid particular foods? And if so, why?
- Do they restrict fluids?
- What is the patient's experience of hunger or of any urge to eat?
- Do they binge? Are these objectively large binges? Do they feel out of control?
- Are the binges planned? How do they begin? How do they end? How often?
- Do they make themselves vomit? If so, how? Do they vomit blood? Do they wash out with copious fluids afterwards?
- Do they take laxatives, diuretics, emetics, or appetite suppressants? With what effects?
- Do they chew and spit? Do they fast for a day or more?
- Can they eat in front of others? Who is there at mealtimes?
- Do they exercise? Is this to 'burn off calories'? Ask for a typical weekly schedule.
- What does the patient feel about their body and weight? Do they think they are fat? Which parts of the body do they particularly dislike, and why?
- What do they think would happen if they did not control their eating/weight?
- Ask for an idea of how weight has fluctuated over time.
- Are they amenorrhoeic?

Psychiatric history

A full psychiatric history should be taken, including information from the patient, a third-party informant, primary care physician, and previous hospital notes. Specific points to cover include:

- current eating-disordered symptoms and their effect upon life at home, work, school, etc.; ask about the context in which the problems have arisen;
- depressive and obsessive-compulsive symptoms;
- previous diagnoses of eating disorders, anxiety disorders, mood disorders, OCD, or other psychiatric conditions;
- previous treatments, hospitalizations, therapy—how successful were these?
- known physical complications of the eating disorder, e.g. infertility, osteoporosis, damaged tooth enamel;
- current medications (prescribed, illicit, over-the-counter, alcohol, caffeine, nicotine, diet pills, and supplements);
- personality history: childhood eating problems, school bullying, educational achievement, etc.; age of pubertal onset and menarche;
- premorbid personality traits—perfectionism?
- family history of eating disorders and other psychiatric problems;
- current social situation—accommodation, employment, finances.

Physical examination

As the physical consequences of starvation can be very dangerous, it is important to undertake a full physical examination. **Weigh** the patient in their underclothes after having used the toilet. Be alert for the propensity of patients to hide weights in their clothes, or water-load before being weighed. Calculate a **body mass index** (BMI; see Box 27.3) and record it clearly in the notes. If it is a follow-up, record the change in weight from the previous appointment.

Look at the patient walking, climbing stairs, and rising from a chair. Next ask them to squat down on the floor and then get up. Patients with proximal myopathy will not be able to do so without using their hands— this is called the **'stand and squat test'**.

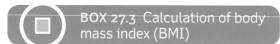

BOX 27.3 Calculation of body mass index (BMI)

$$BMI = \frac{weight\ (kg)}{height\ (cm)}$$

BMI 19.5–25   ideal body weight range
BMI < 19.5   underweight
BMI < 17.5   anorexia nervosa
BMI < 14   life-threatening emaciation

Take pulse, postural blood pressures, and temperature. In severely emaciated patients, take a blood glucose measurement. Consider testing for urine specific gravity, which can be done on a conventional urinalysis stick and may suggest water-loading.

Do a **full physical examination**, looking specifically for bradycardia, arrhythmias, dehydration, peripheral oedema, lanugo, and anaemia. Be aware of the **signs of regular vomiting**, which include swollen parotid glands, poor dentition, and calluses on the dorsal aspect of the knuckles (**Russell's sign**).

Psychological tests

The most widely used questionnaire for detecting an eating disorder is the **Eating Attitudes Test** (EAT). There are many others, but as the diagnosis is clinical, they are mainly used in research. It is also worth giving all patients a **Beck Depression Index** and **Hospital Anxiety and Depression Scale**, to pick up any significant co-morbidities.

Investigations

An eating disorder is a clinical diagnosis, and investigations are done merely to pick up and treat complications, and to help risk stratify (Table 27.3).

Risk assessment

The main risks in anorexia nervosa are the effects of starvation (self-neglect) and deliberate self-harm or suicide. All patients should be considered at high risk of these. Driving is a particular issue in those with a very low BMI, poor concentration, or episodes of hypoglycaemia. The main medical risks are arrhythmias, electrolyte disturbances, anaemia, and GI bleeds. Patients with any of the characteristics shown in Box 27.4 are at extremely high risk, and admission to hospital should be considered.

Table 27.3 Investigations in eating disorders

Investigation	Typical abnormalities in severe starvation
Blood tests	
FBC	Anaemia, thrombocytopenia, leukopenia
U&Es	Increased urea and creatinine if dehydrated
	Low potassium, phosphate, magnesium, and chloride
TFTs	Increased T3 and T4
LFTs	Increased bilirubin and hepatocellular markers
Lipids	Increased cholesterol
Cortisol	Increased levels
Sex hormones	Decreased LH, FSH, oestrogens, and progestogens
Arterial blood gas	Metabolic alkalosis (vomiting), metabolic acidosis (laxatives)
ECG	Prolonged QTc interval
	Relating to hypokalaemia—flattened T-waves
Urinalysis	Reduced specific gravity in water loading
	Increased specific gravity in dehydration
Blood glucose	Low
DEXA scan	Osteopenia or osteoporosis

FSH, follicle-stimulating hormone; LH, luteinizing hormone.

Management of eating disorders

Successful treatment of anorexia nervosa is possible, but requires hard work on the part of the patient, their carers, and the professionals treating them. There is a lack of good evidence about treatment and management, reflecting the variable severity of the disorder and also the difficulties in evaluating complex interventions in an uncommon condition. This means that current views about treatment are based mainly on clinical experience. Success largely depends on making a good relationship with the patient, and gaining their collaboration.

The management of eating disorders within the UK is based upon the National Institute for Clinical Excellence (NICE) guidelines, published in 2004. These endorse a stepped care approach to management, with the lowest-intensity treatment appropriate to the situation being chosen first. An outline of management options is shown

BOX 27.4 Criteria for admission to hospital in anorexia nervosa

BMI < 14 (NB: BMI is unreliable in children and those with oedema)

Rapid weight loss (> 1 kg/week)

Electrolyte imbalances or hypoglycaemia

Bradycardia, arrhythmias

Hypotension or a postural drop

Hypothermia

Suicidal ideation or deliberate self-harm

Psychosis or another change in mental state

Refusal to engage with treatment

Failure of outpatient treatment

---

in Table 27.4. The general practitioner should coordinate care across specialties, and make appropriate referrals.

Choosing an appropriate treatment setting

The majority of patients with anorexia nervosa can be effectively treated as outpatients, and more intensive treatment should only be considered in the following situations:

- if the patient is at high physical risk (Box 27.3); *or*
- if the patient is at high risk of suicide or deliberate self-harm; *or*
- if there is significant deterioration during outpatient treatment, or there is no improvement on completing a course of psychological. therapy.

In the first two situations, it is probable that inpatient care will be required; in the third, a day-patient programme may be more appropriate. A day-patient programme typically runs on 4 or 5 days of the week from about 8 am to 5 pm. It includes supported meals, individual and group psychotherapy, physical monitoring, dietary advice, management of medications, and family interventions. Inpatient programmes provide 24-hour care, and may have more of an emphasis on medical stabilization, but otherwise are similar to day programmes. In the UK, the average inpatient stay is 10 weeks, with most patients 'stepping down' to day patient upon discharge. Psychological therapy and follow-up should be continued for at least a year after discharge from inpatient care. There is currently insufficient evidence to show that outpatient, day-patient, or inpatient treatment is more efficacious; however, it is clear that treatment of any type by a specialist eating disorders treatment is highly superior to treatment by non-specialists.

Psychoeducation

The patient and family should be told the nature of the disorder, the hazards of extreme dieting, and the nature and purpose of the proposed treatment. It should be

Table 27.4 Management of anorexia nervosa

Assessment

- Diagnosis of anorexia nervosa, co-morbidities, and complications
- Risk assessment
- Assess patient level of acceptance of and commitment to treatment
- Decide upon appropriate level of care:
- Primary care team
- Outpatient treatment in secondary care
- Specialist day-patient programme
- Inpatient treatment in an eating disorders unit
- Admission to general hospital for medical stabilization

General measures for all patients

- Agree a clear treatment plan and assign a care coordinator
- Psychoeducation
- Self-help resources
- Problem-solving and relaxation techniques
- Dietary advice
- Regular monitoring of physical health and mental state
- Consider preparation for treatment group

Elements of outpatient treatment

- Advice on and motivation towards weight gain
- Psychological therapy lasting at least 6 months
- Dietary advice
- Consider pharmacotherapy

Elements of day-patient and inpatient treatment

- Nutritional rehabilitation (re-feeding)
- Psychological therapy: individual and/or group based
- Family therapy
- Dietary advice
- Pharmacotherapy
- Management of co-morbidities and complications
- Assistance with return to school or work
- Follow-up outpatient therapy for at least 12 months

made clear that the maintenance of adequate weight is an essential first priority, but that help will be offered for any psychological problems as well. Highlighting the dangers of anorexia nervosa, and relating physical symptoms and complications that the patient is suffering from to their extreme malnutrition, is often helpful in motivating them towards change. It is now relatively common for patients to be offered a 'preparation for treatment' group, which helps to prepare them for challenging their eating-disordered behaviours, before committing to intensive treatment. Self-help materials such as books, leaflets, or supportive websites can be helpful, especially as undernourished patients have poor concentration and may not remember everything that is said to them.

Nutritional rehabilitation (re-feeding)

It is important to negotiate a reasonable dietary plan with the patient and to set this out clearly, together with a medically acceptable, but not overambitious, target weight. The aim should be to increase weight gradually via a balanced meal plan of three meals and three snacks per day. It is reasonable to aim for 0.7–1 kg gain per week in inpatients, and 0.5 kg gain per week in outpatients. Re-feeding is usually started at 1200–1500 kcal/day (to avoid re-feeding syndrome; Box 27.5), and titrated up to approximately 3000 kcal/day. Supplements may be used to increase caloric intake once a normal food intake has been achieved. Eating should be supervised, either by a nurse whilst in hospital or by a parent/carer at home. They have three important roles:

1 to reassure the patient that she can eat without the risk of losing control over her weight;

2 to be firm about the agreed targets;

3 to ensure that the patient does not hide food, induce vomiting, or take purgatives.

Oral re-feeding is possible in almost all patients; feeding by nasogastric tube should be seen as a last resort, and only initiated by specialist consultants. Exercise should be limited to short walks only whilst the patient is still underweight, gradually increasing to two to three sessions of moderate aerobic activity per week once the target weight is achieved.

Psychological therapies

The psychological therapies that are recommended by NICE for use in anorexia nervosa are cognitive behavioural therapy (CBT), cognitive analytical therapy (CAT), interpersonal therapy (IPT), focused psychodynamic therapy, and family interventions. It is recommended that therapy lasts at least 6 months, and continues for at least 12 months after an inpatient admission.

Cognitive behavioural therapy

CBT is the most common therapy used in adults with anorexia nervosa, although it is not backed up by a good evidence base. The most important aspect is a positive therapeutic alliance between patient and therapist. The theory behind CBT and its general use are discussed on p. 137. There are usually two themes to the treatment: firstly, examining and tackling the behaviours the patient has used to reduce their weight, and secondly, considering psychological problems such as low self-esteem, perfectionism, interpersonal relationships, and family issues. The therapist asks the patient the motivation behind their behaviours in order to discover the incorrect or abnormal beliefs they hold about weight, shape, food, and other problems. They help the patient to link these beliefs to

 BOX 27.5 Re-feeding syndrome

Re-feeding syndrome is a metabolic disturbance that occurs in the first few days of starting to re-feed a severely malnourished patient. It occurs when carbohydrate is suddenly provided, and metabolism shifts from fat to carbohydrate. Insulin increases, which leads to increased uptake of phosphate, and an increased metabolic rate can cause excessive cellular uptake of electrolytes. The main biochemical features include:

- hypophosphataemia;
- hypokalaemia;
- hypomagnesaemia;

- hypoglycaemia;
- thiamine deficiency.

Hypophosphataemia is common and may cause confusion, coma, fits, and sudden death. Shift of fluids may increase cardiac work and precipitate acute heart failure. Patients should be monitored for peripheral and pulmonary oedema daily.

Electrolytes should be checked regularly, and supplements given as appropriate. Prescribing daily thiamine, a vitamin B complex, multivitamins, and minerals is sensible.

thoughts, feelings, and behaviours, and to replace negative, unrealistic thoughts with positive realistic ones. The therapist will try to persuade the patient that starvation will prevent them from tackling their problems, and that by eating normally they will not 'lose control' and become overweight. It is often helpful to examine the pros and cons of anorexia for the patient's life, as considering the negative aspects can be motivational, and the positive aspects may reveal reasons why the illness has been maintained. The aim is to help the patient to become brave enough to gain weight, eat more normally, and stop their other eating-disordered behaviours.

Family-based therapy: the Maudsley method

Family-based therapy is the only treatment to have definitively been shown to be effective in anorexia nervosa, and so far only in children and adolescents. All children and adolescents should be offered family therapy, and it is often a helpful adjunct in adults as well. The family may be seen together, or the parents may have separate sessions with the therapist who sees the patient for individual sessions. There are usually 15–20 sessions over about a year. There are three stages to treatment.

Phase 1. The parents are urged to take control of the patient's eating, and help them to gain weight. The patient has no input in meal planning, shopping, food preparation, cooking, or serving meals. The expectation is that all food is consumed, and no eating-disordered behaviours are undertaken. The topics in the psychoeducation section are discussed, and some individual therapy work may be done. There will be much confrontation at this stage, and many tears may be shed.

Phase 2. The parents help their child to take more control over their eating again, whilst general family issues and relationship problems are dealt with.

Phase 3. This starts when the patient is able to maintain their weight in the healthy range, and has normal eating habits. Treatment then focuses on helping them to develop a normal relationship with their body, working on issues such as perfectionism and low self-esteem, and adjusting family life back to normality.

Pharmacotherapy

The majority of patients with anorexia nervosa do not need any medications, and there is no evidence for this use of any specific drugs in treatment. Depression, OCD, and anxiety disorders should be treated along usual guidelines with appropriate antidepressants, starting with an SSRI. Binge–purge behaviours can also be reduced with high-dose SSRIs. Some advocate the use of low-dose atypical antipsychotics (olanzapine, quetiapine) in severely depressed patients who continue to resist food,

but there is no convincing evidence for this currently (Science box 27.2). Prokinetics and laxatives may be useful in the early stages of re-feeding, and patients should be encouraged to take daily multivitamin supplements. Insomnia is a common problem, but avoid prescribing either benzodiazepines or z-drugs for longer than a few days, instead opting for sedating antidepressants at night (e.g. mirtazapine).

Compulsory treatment

In the UK, 5–15 per cent of inpatient admissions to specialist eating disorders units are for involuntary treatment. Section 3 of the Mental Health Act 1983 is typically used, allowing up to 6 months of treatment. Many of the patients admitted convert to voluntary status during the admission as their mental state improves. They are usually patients with severe emaciation, a long-standing illness, and outright rejection of treatment. However, given that 95 per cent of sufferers of anorexia are treated as outpatients, those needing compulsory treatment are few and far between. The majority of deaths from anorexia are in patients who have been treated involuntarily at some point.

■ Bulimia nervosa

Bulimia nervosa is an eating disorder characterized by recurrent episodes of uncontrolled excessive eating ('binges'), compensatory methods of weight control, and a fear of becoming fat. The term 'bulimia' refers only to the episodes of uncontrollable excessive eating, and may also be present in other forms of eating disorder. Unlike anorexia nervosa, for which there are historical accounts dating back to medieval times, bulimia nervosa was first described as a distinct clinical entity in 1979. Gerald Russell, a British psychiatrist, published a case series of 30 patients with bulimia nervosa and used them to describe the defining features of the condition. Since Russell's initial work, it has been realized that bulimia nervosa is a common condition, and effective treatments have since been developed to treat it.

Diagnostic criteria

The formal diagnostic criteria for bulimia nervosa are shown in Box 27.6, but the essential features can be summarized as follows:

1 recurrent episodes of binge eating, characterized by eating a large amount of food and by a sense of lack of control over eating;

2 recurrent inappropriate behaviour to prevent weight gain;

Science box 27.2 Atypical antipsychotics and anorexia nervosa

Since the 1960s, it has been suggested that antipsychotics could be of value in anorexia nervosa (AN). The rationale behind their use is that severe AN has features in common with psychotic disorders, as the abnormal belief system surrounding weight and shape is held strongly despite evidence to the contrary, is ego-syntonic and encompasses lack of insight. There is strong evidence from randomized controlled trials (RCTs) that atypical antipsychotics reduce anxiety and agitation and promote weight gain; could they therefore be a useful adjunct in AN?

There is a surprising lack of evidence on this topic. Only a handful of small RCTs have been conducted, and they relate almost entirely to olanzapine.[1] Bissada *et al.* undertook a double-blind placebo-controlled flexible-dose trial of olanzapine in anorexia nervosa patients attending a day hospital programme.[2] Both trial arms achieved a significant increase in BMI at the end of the trial, and the patients receiving olanzapine showed a greater increase compared with those receiving placebo. There was no difference in psychological improvement between the groups. However, it was a small study with a lack of follow-up data. In 2005, Mondraty *et al.* published a non-blinded RCT of olanzapine versus chlorpromazine in hospitalized patients with anorexia nervosa.[3] No significant difference in weight gain was seen between groups, but a significant decrease in psychological rumination was seen in the olanzapine arm. Open-label trials have given similarly conflicting results.

Multiple case reports in both adults and children have been published, almost all reporting significantly reduced psychopathology and ease of weight restoration when an atypical antipsychotic is prescribed. The majority of the patients included in these reports represent severe cases of AN who have failed multiple courses of intensive treatments. No serious side effects of using olanzapine or quetiapine have been described.

There is currently insufficient evidence to advise sensibly on the use of atypical antipsychotics in AN because the minimal evidence is conflicting and there are many unanswered questions. It seems as if some patients have a good physical and/or psychological response, but that atypicals do not promote weight gain in the majority. It is unknown which patients may benefit, at what stage in their illness the drug should be given, or for how long. The main hindrance to answering these questions is the difficulty of recruiting patients into clinical trials; a strategy needs to be worked out, in order to better guide clinical practice in the future.

1 McKnight, R. F.& Park, R. J. (2010). Atypical antipsychotics and anorexia nervosa: a review. *European Eating Disorders Review* **18**: 10–21.

2 Bissada, H., Tasca, G. A., Barber, A. M., & Bradwejn, J. (2008). Olanzapine in the treatment of low body weight and obsessive thinking in women with anorexia nervosa: A randomized, double-blind, placebo-controlled trial. *American Journal of Psychiatry* **165**: 1281–8.

3 Mondraty, N., Birmingham, C. L., Touyz, S., Sundakov, V., Chapman, L., & Beumont, P. (2005). Randomized controlled trial of olanzapine in the treatment of cognitions in anorexia nervosa. *Australasian Journal of Psychiatry* **13**: 72–5.

Case study 27.1 Anorexia nervosa

A 16-year-old girl called Susan is brought to the GP by her parents, who report that she has been eating poorly and losing weight for 6–9 months. They have tried to encourage her to eat more, but big arguments have ensued and now she is so thin they are scared she will die. Susan refuses to talk in the consultation, but allows herself to be examined and weighed. The GP finds her to weigh 38 kg (BMI 14), with dry cracked skin, downy hairs covering most of her body, and pallor of the conjunctiva. The GP told Susan and her parents that he thinks Susan may have anorexia nervosa, and that her weight is dangerously low. He refers Susan to the adolescent services as an emergency, and sends blood for haematology and biochemistry, which come back normal. Two days later, the adolescent team assesses Susan. Her parents tell the team that Susan is bright, achieving mostly A and Bs at school, and plays netball for the county team. She is very exact in her work, is obedient, and very neat and tidy. No one in the family has had an eating disorder, but Susan's grandmother had depression. Without her parents present, Susan tells the psychologist that she feels fat and that she wanted to be thinner to be better at netball. She started throwing away her lunch at school, and upon losing some weight felt so much better that she carried on. Recently, she has only been eating dinner, and has been hiding much of that in her sleeves. Susan last had a period 5 months ago. The adolescent psychiatrist confirms the diagnosis, and explains that family-based interventions are the most effective treatment. Susan and her parents meet with the dietician and a psychologist weekly, where they are helped to take control of Susan's eating and help her gain weight. It is successful, and Susan gradually gains weight to 50 kg (BMI 20), and her periods restart. Susan sees the psychologist alone for sessions, but refuses to engage much. Throughout the next 2 years, Susan remains at a stable weight, although her parents are still in charge of most of her meals. At age 18 she starts university—studying chemistry—and immediately starts to lose weight again. She cuts down to 200 kcal per day, starts going to the gym daily, and takes 30 senna tablets each night. In the middle of the second term, she faints during a practical class, and is taken to the emergency room. Susan's BMI is 12.8, heart rate 38 and potassium 2.9 mmol/l. She is admitted to the general hospital for medical stabilization, and the nearest eating disorder unit (EDU) contacted. Susan receives IV fluids with added

potassium, and is stabilized, but refuses to eat anything in the hospital. She is transferred to the EDU, and admitted as a voluntary inpatient. The specialist team start her on 900 kcal per day, monitoring carefully for re-feeding syndrome, then gradually increase the meal plan to promote weight gain. Susan is reluctant to start eating, and takes several weeks to comply with the programme. However, she does eventually and after 5 months is discharged back to her parents at BMI 17.8. Follow-up is arranged locally, and Susan takes time out of university to recover at home. She gets a part-time job in a chemist, and with the help of her mother manages to keep her weight stable. A year later she returns to university and finds a boyfriend, who is supportive and increases her self-esteem. Susan starts eating more, and increases her weight into the normal range.

BOX 27.6 DSM-IV diagnostic criteria for bulimia nervosa

A Recurrent episodes of binge eating. An episode of binge eating is characterized by both of the following:

1 eating, in a fixed period of time, an amount of food that is definitely larger than most people would eat under similar circumstances;

2 a lack of control over eating during the episode: a feeling that one cannot stop eating or control what or how much one is eating.

B Recurrent inappropriate compensatory behaviour to prevent weight gain, such as self-induced vomiting, misuse of laxatives, diuretics, or other medications, fasting, and excessive exercise.

C Self-evaluation is unduly influenced by body shape and weight.

D These symptoms occur at least twice a week on average and persist for at least 3 months.

E The disturbance does not occur exclusively during episodes of anorexia nervosa.

There are two subtypes of bulimia nervosa: purging and non-purging.

- Purging type: the patient uses self-induced vomiting and other ways to rapidly remove food from the body before it can be digested, such as laxatives, diuretics, and enemas.
- Non-purging type: occurring in approximately 6–8 per cent of cases, in which the patient uses excessive exercise or fasting after a binge to offset the caloric intake after eating. Purging-type bulimics may also exercise or fast, but as a secondary form of weight control.

ICD-10 F52.2 bulimia nervosa

There are no clinically significant differences between the classification systems.

---

3 evaluation of self-worth primarily based on weight and shape;

4 symptoms do not occur exclusively during episodes of anorexia nervosa.

The last point means that a diagnosis of anorexia nervosa effectively 'trumps' bulimia nervosa; if the patient has a BMI of less than 17.5, the diagnosis is always anorexia nervosa.

Clinical features

The main clinical features of bulimia nervosa are shown in Table 27.5. There is often a history of anorexia nervosa or EDNOS.

Food and eating habits

The eating habits of a patient with bulimia nervosa occur in a cycle of dieting, bingeing, and purging. The dieting

Table 27.5 Clinical features of bulimia nervosa

Weight control

- Strict dieting interspersed with episodes of binge eating
- Compensatory behaviours to prevent weight gain
    Self-induced vomiting
    Laxatives or diuretics
    Excessive exercise
    Diet pills

Psychopathology

- Excessive concern about shape and weight
- Distorted body image
- Low self-esteem and perfectionism

Physical consequences of weight control behaviours

- Normal body weight
- Hypokalaemia, hyponatraemia, hypochloraemia
- Menstrual abnormalities
- Swollen parotid glands
- Erosion of dental enamel
- Calluses of the dorsal aspect of the fingers (Russell's sign)
- Peripheral oedema
- Increased plasma amylase

Other co-morbid psychiatric conditions

- Depression
- Anxiety
- Deliberate self-harm
- Misuse of alcohol or drugs
- Borderline personality disorder

is similar to that seen in anorexia nervosa; it tends to be strict, with multiple rules surrounding what can be eaten, when, and with whom. The patients show the same preoccupation with food, and get severe cravings for particular food items. After a period of dieting, a binge occurs. This entails eating of an unusually large amount of food, and is accompanied by a feeling of loss of control over their eating. Patients vary widely in the amount to which they binge; it may range from several times a day to only once a month. Similarly, some individuals will find certain things trigger a binge (e.g. if the calorie limit for the day is exceeded, when at home alone, or after an emotionally charged situation), whilst in others binges will occur unprovoked. The foods eaten during a binge are usually high in carbohydrate and fats and are usually foods the patient avoids at other times. The majority of binges occur when the patient is at home and alone, as they tend to be embarrassed and disgusted by their behaviour.

Compensatory mechanisms of weight control

Self-induced vomiting is the most common method by which patients try to avoid weight gain, and usually occurs soon after a binge. The patient uses their fingers to stimulate a gag reflex, and repeats the act until they think all the food has been removed. Often patients will be very distressed if they are unable to vomit after a binge, and will avoid bingeing if they think they may not be able to purge. In severe bulimia nervosa (and anorexia nervosa), the patient may induce vomiting after normal meals, which usually leads to weight loss. **Laxatives** and **diuretics** may be taken in large quantities to try and counteract the effects of a binge. It is important to explain to all patients that these do not cause weight loss, but merely disrupt fluid and electrolyte balance. **Excessive exercise** is similar to that seen in anorexia nervosa.

Psychopathology

There is an extreme over-concern with weight and shape, such that the patient values themselves primarily in terms of their weight and shape. Like anorexics, they fear fatness and will go to any length to avoid it. The majority of patients have low self-esteem, and show similar perfectionistic traits to those with anorexia.

Depressive symptoms are present in almost all patients with bulimia nervosa, and may be severe. Patients tend to have negative cognitions (hopelessness, guilt, and helplessness), shame and embarrassment over their bulimia, and pronounced suicidal ideation. Unlike in anorexia nervosa, the patient is usually aware of the limitations the condition is having on their life (e.g. poor concentration, unable to eat out with friends, apathy, and anhedonia), and feels guilty about this. Deliberate self-harm can occur secondary to depression, but may also be independently caused by impulse-control problems, which may also lead to excessive use of alcohol or drugs. Occasionally, patients may meet diagnostic criteria for borderline personality disorder.

Physical consequences

Body weight is normal in the majority of patients, as dieting and purging compensates for the binges. However, repeated vomiting leads to several complications. Hypokalaemia is particularly serious, resulting in weakness, cardiac arrhythmia, and renal damage. Metabolic alkalosis and hypochloraemia may also occur. Regular vomiting may cause swelling of the parotid glands, erosion of dental enamel by stomach acid, and calluses on the back of the fingers which are used to induce emesis. Occasionally, patients present to the emergency room vomiting blood, often due to a Mallory–Weiss tear. Menstrual abnormalities are common, although these reverse if normal eating is resumed. Use of laxatives and diuretics may cause fluid shifts, hyponatraemia, and metabolic acidosis.

Epidemiology

Both the prevalence and lifetime risk of bulimia nervosa are between 1 and 2 per cent in women aged 15–40 years. The prevalence among men is unknown. In the 1980s and 1990s the number of presenting cases of bulimia nervosa increased dramatically—however, it is unclear if this is due to an actual increase in incidence or because of increased awareness and availability of treatment.

Co-morbidities

The following commonly coexist with bulimia nervosa:

- depressive disorder;
- deliberate self-harm;
- anxiety disorders;
- borderline personality disorder;
- alcohol misuse.

Differential diagnosis

- **Anorexia nervosa** can be differentiated from bulimia nervosa principally by a low body weight (BMI <17.5). Binges may occur in anorexia nervosa, but must be present for a diagnosis of bulimia nervosa.

- **EDNOS** describes those patients with disordered eating which is clinically significant, but which does not fit criteria for a specific eating disorder; for example, a patient with all the features of bulimia nervosa, except for the use of compensatory behaviours to prevent weight gain.

- **Klein–Levin syndrome** is a sleep disorder seen in adolescent males, characterized by recurrent episodes of binge eating and hypersomnia.

- **Mood disorder.** Core features include low mood, fatigue, and anhedonia. Weight gain and binge eating may occur, but the patient will not show the specific psychopathology and other weight control behaviours seen in bulimia nervosa.

- **Iatrogenic drugs.** Many drugs may cause weight gain, either through increased appetite or a direct effect on metabolism; for example, antipsychotics, lithium, steroids.

- **Organic disorders.** These can usually be identified by a clear history and lack of associated core psychopathology, but specific investigations may need to be done; for example, upper GI disorders with associated vomiting, brain tumours.

Aetiology

The main risk factors for bulimia nervosa are shown in Table 27.6.

Table 27.6 Risk factors for bulimia nervosa

Biological	Psychological	Social
Female sex	Critical comments in early life about eating, shape, or weight	Living in a developed country
Age (15–40 years)		
Family history of:		Cultures that encourage dieting and value thinness
• Mood disorders	Family environment with a focus on shape and dieting	
• Substance abuse		
• Eating disorder		
• Obesity	Sexual or physical abuse in childhood	Occupation (e.g. ballet dancer)
Type 1 diabetes	Low self-esteem	
Early menarche	Perfectionism	

Course and prognosis

The natural course of bulimia nervosa is not yet well understood. Part of the problem with obtaining accurate data is that many people with the disorder never present for treatment. As many patients present having had bulimia for many years, it is thought that the illness tends to be chronic and long term. One study in a cohort of patients who underwent treatment reported 30 per cent of patients had either bulimia nervosa or EDNOS at 10-year follow-up. Anorexia nervosa is a very rare outcome.

Assessment

Patients with bulimia nervosa should be assessed in the same way as those with anorexia nervosa, as outlined on p. 340.

Management

The management of bulimia nervosa is more evidence based than that of anorexia nervosa, and in the UK is again based on the guidance from NICE. The key elements are shown in Table 27.7.

Choosing an appropriate treatment setting

The majority (98 per cent) of patients with bulimia nervosa can be managed in the outpatient setting, and some may not even need input from secondary care providers. The GP is primarily in charge of monitoring physical health, and coordinating treatment. Patients should be offered guided self-help and/or antidepressant medications in primary care, and then if needed are referred for CBT delivered by a specialist therapist. If a patient fails to respond to a full course of CBT, consider either a break from treatment for a few months to avoid

Table 27.7 Management of bulimia nervosa

Assessment

- Diagnosis of bulimia nervosa, co-morbidities, and complications
- Risk assessment
- Assess patient level of acceptance of and commitment to treatment
- Decide upon appropriate level of care:
- Primary care team
- Outpatient treatment in secondary care
- Specialist intensive treatment: day-patient or inpatient care

General measures for all patients

- Agree a clear treatment plan
- Psychoeducation
- Problem-solving and relaxation techniques
- Dietary advice
- Regular monitoring of physical health and mental state

Psychological treatments

- Guided self-help
- Cognitive behavioural therapy for bulimia nervosa
- Interpersonal therapy

Pharmacotherapy

- Antidepressants: high-dose SSRI

Elements of day-patient and inpatient treatment

- Establishing regular eating and a healthy weight
- Psychological therapy: individual and/or group based
- Family therapy
- Dietary advice
- Pharmacotherapy review
- Management of co-morbidities and complications
- Assistance with return to school or work

therapist–patient 'burnout', a different psychological treatment, or medication. Day or inpatient treatment should be considered in the following situations:

- high suicide risk;
- high risk of serious deliberate self-harm;
- physical problems (e.g. symptomatic electrolyte disturbances);
- pregnancy (high risk of miscarriage in those who are actively vomiting);
- extreme refractory cases.

Psychoeducation

Psychoeducation is built into the standard format of CBT for bulimia nervosa and is essentially the same as for anorexia nervosa.

Self-help

A minority of patients will recover with a course of guided self-help based on the principles of CBT. Various books are available, containing information and a self-help programme, which the patient works through at home. The patient is allocated a self-help facilitator, who is a non-specialist therapist, whose role is to support and encourage the patient to follow the programme. If the patient does not respond in 6–8 weeks, they should be referred for formal CBT.

Cognitive behavioural therapy for bulimia nervosa (CBT-BN)

CBT-BN is based on the standard principles of CBT, but has been adapted to tackle the behaviours and psychopathology that are specific to bulimia nervosa. The treatment has four distinct stages:

1 **Stage 1.** This preliminary stage aims to educate the patient about the treatment and bulimia nervosa, engage the patient and develop a therapeutic relationship, and establish regular eating and weekly weighing. The therapist explains how the eating disorder is maintained (Figure 27.3), and encourages daily self-monitoring of food intake, compensatory behaviours, feelings, and emotions. The patient is encouraged to stick to three planned meals and two planned snacks per day, and not to eat between them. At each session there is a review of the previous week's progress, and discussion of how to overcome problems.

2 **Stage 2.** This is a review of stage 1, and identification of all the main problems still to be addressed.

3 **Stage 3.** This stage aims to identify and address the mechanisms maintaining the patient's eating disorder. The topics addressed include over-evaluation of weight and shape, body checking, feeling fat, considering the origins of the eating disorder, dealing with triggers to binge, and any other psychological problems.

4 **Stage 4.** The last stage is designed to reduce the risk of relapse, and allow the patient to manage long term. A plan for further work at home is devised, and mechanisms to cope with setbacks and problems.

CBT-BN has a large evidence base behind it, and meta-analyses show a mean reduction in the frequency of binges of 80 per cent. There is a relatively high dropout rate (20 per cent) but this is lower than for medication, or treatment of anorexia nervosa. Relapse rates are low in

Case study 27.2 Bulimia nervosa

Charlie, a 25-year-old type 1 diabetic, was referred to psychiatry from the endocrine services. Her consultant was concerned that Charlie had recently lost 10 kg in weight, and her HbA1$_c$ had increased to 11 per cent. He suspected she was omitting her insulin with the aim of losing weight. At the assessment, Charlie admitted she had only been taking one-third of her daily insulin, and had been bingeing regularly and making herself sick after meals. She felt self-conscious that she was not thin like her non-diabetic friends, and that she wasn't as good as the rest of her family, who had all been to university. Her mood appeared low, with a flat affect, and she admitted poor sleep, fatigue, and anhedonia. Charlie's BMI was 22.3, and there were no physical abnormalities on examination. Charlie was deemed to be stable, and therefore recommended for outpatient therapy. Fluoxetine was started, and she saw a dietician and had CBT weekly. Charlie managed to reduce her bingeing and purging, but was unable to give herself adequate insulin due to fears of excessive weight gain, and lost more weight. A joint meeting between the eating disorder and endocrine team was arranged, where it came to light that Charlie now had proliferative diabetic retinopathy and would need pan-retinal photocoagulation therapy. It was decided that Charlie needed extra support to manage her insulin, and she was admitted to the eating disorders unit as a day patient. She attended for 3 months, by which time her mood improved, weight had stabilized at BMI 21.5, she had stopped purging completely, and was able to take her daily insulin. At 1-year follow-up, Charlie had maintained these changes, and although she occasionally binged and purged, was managing her diabetes appropriately, and had applied to go to university.

the first year, but there are few long-term data beyond this. CBT-BN is more effective than antidepressants, other psychological treatments, or watching and waiting. Approximately one-half to two-thirds of patients achieve a full and lasting recovery.

Interpersonal psychotherapy (IPT)

IPT is the second-line therapy for bulimia nervosa, and helps patients overcome current interpersonal problems. It does not focus specifically on eating disordered symptoms, and is much less directive and interpretive. However, randomized controls have found that CBT-BN and IPT are equally effective in bulimia nervosa, but IPT takes several months longer to produce an effect.

Antidepressants

Antidepressants are the only medication recommended for use in bulimia nervosa by NICE, and the only ones with a positive evidence base. SSRIs, tricyclics, monoamine oxidase inhibitors, and atypical antidepressants have all been used, and are equally effective. **SSRIs** (specifically 60 mg fluoxetine in the morning) are the first-line drugs, as they have the best cost, side-effect, tolerability, and safety record. High doses are required for the effect, which is not dose dependent. Antidepressants produce a 50 per cent reduction in bingeing and purging frequency, and 20 per cent stop altogether. Patients who fail to respond to one antidepressant should be changed to another; there is currently no evidence to support augmentation with a second agent.

■ Eating disorder not otherwise specified (EDNOS)

EDNOS is the third major diagnostic category of eating disorders described in the DSM-IV. EDNOS is defined as *disorders of eating that do not meet the criteria for a specific eating disorder*, and is equivalent to the categories of 'atypical anorexia nervosa' and 'atypical bulimia nervosa' found in the ICD-10 system. Examples of patients with EDNOS in the DSM-IV include:

- a female fitting all the criteria for anorexia nervosa but who still has regular menses;
- all criteria for anorexia nervosa are met, but despite substantial weight loss, the BMI remains greater than 17.5;
- all criteria for bulimia nervosa are met, but bingeing and purging occur less frequently than twice a week, or have been present for less than 3 months;
- regular use of inappropriate compensatory mechanisms by an individual of normal body weight (e.g. vomiting after eating small amounts of food);
- repeatedly chewing and spitting, but not swallowing, food;
- binge-eating disorder (BED)—recurrent episodes of uncontrolled binge eating in the absence of inappropriate compensatory mechanisms characteristic of bulimia nervosa.

Patients with EDNOS should be assessed as for those with anorexia or bulimia nervosa. The NICE guidelines recommend that as there is no evidence base for the treatment of EDNOS, patients are managed using the elements of treatment for other eating disorders, which are aimed at the symptoms closest to their own.

Binge eating disorder (BED)

BED is not currently an independent diagnosis, but is considered to be part of EDNOS within the classification systems. However, opinion is divided and it may soon become a distinct category of eating disorder. Treatment includes self-help, an SSRI, CBT for binge-eating disorder, and nutritional advice.

■ Obesity

Obesity is defined by the World Health Organization (WHO) as the accumulation or presence of excess body fat to the extent that it may impair health. WHO has also defined obesity in terms of BMI: 'overweight' is a BMI of 25–30, and 'obesity' a BMI of greater than 30. Obesity is not an eating disorder in the conventional use of the term, and it does not figure in the DSM-IV or in the Mental Health section of the ICD-10. However, it is becoming increasingly recognized that the most effective treatment is a behavioural approach similar to that used in other eating disorders, and that adding a cognitive dimension to the therapy can significantly reduce the rate of relapse. It may therefore fit into the wider transdiagnostic approach to eating disorders, and this, combined with the epidemiological significance, is the reason why obesity is included in this chapter.

Consequences of obesity

Obesity is associated with significant mortality and morbidity, and some of the conditions it predisposes to are shown in Table 27.8. Smoking rates are higher in obese patients than in the general population, and the combined risk of most associated conditions is greater than the two separate risks added together.

Epidemiology

Almost 20 per cent of adults in the UK and 400 million adults worldwide are obese, and the figures are rising. Women are more likely to be obese than men. Rates of obesity gradually increase from age 5 to 60, and decrease rapidly from then on. Unfortunately, in the last decade the number of children in developed countries who are obese has doubled, and there are clear data to show that obese children tend to become obese adults.

Table 27.8 Mortality and morbidity of obesity

Mortality

- Life expectancy is reduced on average by 2–4 years if BMI is 30–40
- Life expectancy is reduced on average by 20 years for men and 5 years for women if BMI is greater than 40

Morbidity—an increased risk of:

- Ischaemic heart disease, hypertension, hyperlipidaemia, heart failure
- Deep vein thrombosis and pulmonary embolism
- Diabetes mellitus
- Menstrual disorders, infertility, obstetric complications, polycystic ovary syndrome
- Stroke, carpal tunnel syndrome, idiopathic intracranial hypertension
- Depression
- Gout, osteoarthritis, back pain
- Stretch marks, cellulitis, hirsuitism
- Gastro-oesophageal reflux, gallstones, fatty liver
- Cancers: breast, ovarian, oesophageal, colon, liver, pancreas, stomach, prostate, kidney, lymphoma, myeloma
- Obstructive sleep apnoea, asthma
- Complications during anaesthesia
- Erectile dysfunction, infertility

Aetiology

Most obesity can be attributed to genetic factors exacerbated by social factors that encourage overeating. However, the following may all contribute.

Diet. The availability of food has increased gradually over the last 100 years, so that the average person in a developed country has access to approximately 3770 kcal/day (recommended UK daily requirements are 1940 kcal/day for women and 2550 kcal/day for men). Although the majority of people do not eat this value, average daily kcal consumption has increased by 300–400 kcal/day since the 1970s. Sweetened soft drinks are thought to be a major contributing factor, making up 25 per cent of most American teenagers' daily energy intake.

Sedentary lifestyle. The change in our lifestyles towards office/sedentary work, routine use of motorized transport, televised entertainment, and a reduction in easy access to open spaces have meant that the population as a whole does less exercise. The recommended 30-minute sessions of cardiovascular exercise three times per week are only done by 20–30 per cent of the population, mostly under 35 years. Studies have shown a strong correlation between numbers of hours spent watching TV per day and rates of obesity in both adults and children.

5 **Genetics.** The heritability of obesity is estimated to be approximately 75 per cent, meaning the vast majority of the cause of obesity is genetic. Polymorphisms in several genes controlling appetite and metabolism have been linked to obesity when the person is put in an environment favouring it. There are rare genetic conditions—for example, lack of the *ob/ob* gene for leptin—which lead to severe obesity in all cases, and many syndromes (e.g. Prader–Willi, Down's) in which obesity is a frequent characteristic.

6 **Medical and psychiatric causes.** Certain physical, psychiatric, or pharmacological causes of obesity are common:

(i)   **physical:** hypothyroidism, Cushing's syndrome;

(ii) **psychiatric:** depression, BED, Klein–Felter syndrome;

(iii) **drugs:** antipsychotics, insulin, lithium, antidepressants, steroids, oral contraceptives, steroids.

7 **Psychological aspects.** Obesity is more common in those with significant levels of anxiety, depression, and low self-esteem. The core psychopathology seen in other eating disorders is not usually found, except for a distinct minority of patients who have a distorted body image.

8 **Social aspects.** There is a clear correlation between social class and obesity in almost every culture. In developed countries, lower social classes are more likely to be obese, whereas in developing countries the reverse is true. It is unclear why this occurs, as explanations such as cost of food or fashions do not hold true in research. Smoking tends to keep people's weight low; on average 5 kg is gained when someone stops smoking, and this may entrain them into poorer eating habits. Obesity is higher in urban areas, in mothers with more than three children, and if there was malnutrition in early life.

Assessment

The aim of assessing an obese patient is threefold;

- to detect any underlying physical or psychological cause;
- to detect any adverse consequences of being obese;
- to assess the patient's motivation for weight loss, current lifestyle, personal history, and preferred methods of treatment.

It is very important to exclude a physical cause of weight gain (e.g. hypothyroidism) and to manage another eating disorder (e.g. BED), or depression if it is present. Always take a physical and psychiatric history and do a full physical examination. Weigh the patient, calculate the BMI, and take their pulse and blood pressure. It may be useful to have a dietician's assessment of the situation, and run basic haematology, biochemistry, and liver function tests, and order an ECG. Always check the patient has not developed diabetes.

Management

The most important aspect of management is for the patient to be well informed about their situation, and to be motivated towards weight loss and a healthier lifestyle. The options for treatment are shown in Table 27.9, and further points elaborated on below.

Dieting and exercise

Dieting and exercise are the major aspects of losing weight in most people. There are endless different types of diet used, but evidence shows that no one method is better than the next. The only important factor is that the energy going into the body is less than that expended. In meta-analyses, low-fat, low-calorie, low-carbohydrate, and high-protein diets all produce a mean 2–4 kg loss over 3–6 months. NICE recommends that patients work out their maintenance energy needs, and aim for 600 kcal less than that per day, in order to achieve sustained weight loss of 0.5 kg per week. Patients should be advised against going on very low calorie diets (less than 1000 kcal/day) for longer than 12 weeks.

Most people can lose 5 per cent of body weight quite easily by dieting, and another 5 per cent if they are determined. Five per cent is enough to have significant health benefits, so should be the usual goal. Exercise is a good adjunct to dieting, but alone is not usually enough to enhance weight loss by much. They should aim to get at least 30 minutes cardiovascular exercise five times per week, and try to work more activity into their daily schedule (e.g. walk or cycle instead of taking the bus). The problem is that over the next 3 years, 80 per cent of people

Table 27.9 Treatment options for obesity

Psychoeducation on diet, exercise, and healthy living
Dietary modifications
Increased exercise
Behavioural modification programmes:
• Self-help
• Groups
• CBT
Medications
Surgery

will regain all the weight lost, and half of these will go beyond their previous weight.

Behavioural programmes

Behavioural programmes were first advocated as a means of treating obesity in the 1960s. They basically involve a low-calorie diet (typically 1200–1500 kcal/day), increased exercise, and education about healthy living. There are currently three main methods of providing a behavioural programme for obesity:

1 individual or guided self-help;
2 group programmes; for example, Weight Watchers, Slimming World;
3 cognitive behavioural therapy.

Self-help

The main aim of self-help is to educate the person about the causes of weight gain, and to guide them in making modifications to diet and lifestyle. This may be delivered by a book, computer program, or in person by a non-specialist therapist. Self-help is usually only effective for the overweight (as opposed to obese) patients who are highly motivated to make a change.

Group programmes

Organized group programmes have been popular since the 1960s, and are now found all over the world. Patients typically have to join a local group (which involves a membership fee), and attend regular meetings. At them they are helped to set a goal weight, devise suitable low-calorie meals, and educated about food, exercise, and healthy living. The members are weighed at each meeting, and give feedback to one another on their progress. There is an opportunity to discuss feelings around weight, shape, and food, and so the programme effectively works by using members to motivate one another, and using the fact that some therapy is usually better than none at all.

Cognitive behavioural therapy for obesity

In the last decade, it has become increasingly recognized that an approach similar to that used for other eating disorders is effective in treating obesity. The research group that proposed the transdiagnostic model for eating disorders has produced a CBT approach for obesity, which aims to avoid the weight regain that often occurs in the 3 years after a successful diet. The idea is to help the patient set more realistic targets for weight loss in the first place, to recognize success, and value any weight that is lost and see weight maintenance as the ultimate goal, rather than the weight loss itself. CBT for obesity takes

about a year, is delivered as individual sessions, and is divided into two phases.

Phase 1:

- weight loss (based on a daily meal plan of 1500 kcal);
- overcoming problems that might threaten weight maintenance;
- nutrition;
- increasing activity;
- body image (tackling misconceptions about body shape, body checking, etc.);
- weight goals (setting realistic goals for particular reasons).

Phase 2: helping the patient to acquire the skills and motivation for long-term weight maintenance. This includes appropriate cognitive responses to changes in weight, and how to adapt behaviours to cope with this.

Short-term studies have shown this treatment to be effective in producing weight gain and maintenance, but the long-term effects are currently unknown.

Medications

NICE recommends that drug treatment be considered only once dietary, exercise, and behavioural approaches have been tried, and the patient has failed to reach their target weight or reached a plateau. The two drugs licensed in the UK (and also by the US FDA) are orlistat (Xenical, Alli) and sibutramine (Meridia). Orlistat should only be used in adults with a BMI greater than 28, and only continued for longer than 3 months if the patient has lost at least 5 per cent of body weight. It acts by inhibiting lipase in the gut, and reduces absorption of fat by about a third. Sibutramine should only be prescribed in adults with a BMI of over 30, or a BMI of over 27 plus type 2 diabetes or hyperlipidaemia. Again it should only be used for longer than 3 months if effective, and not for more than 12 months in total. Sibutramine acts within the CNS to reduce appetite. These drugs should not be prescribed to patients with a BMI lower than those described above, and should not be used without behavioural modifications.

Bariatric surgery

Bariatric surgery refers to any surgical technique in which the aim is to treat obesity. It is only recommended for severely obese (BMI > 40) patients who have not lost weight using behavioural and pharmacological treatments. In the UK, surgery is only available to those who are generally fit and healthy enough for an anaesthetic and who commit to long-term specialist follow-up. The surgery generally involves reducing the size of the stomach (to increase early satiety) or decreasing the length of bowel through which food may be absorbed. Gastric banding is a reversible procedure, whereas gastric bypass is not. Weight loss is usually rapid, with vast amounts being lost in the 2 years following surgery. Complications from the operations are common, and patients are usually unable to eat 'normally' again. They often experience severe nausea and vomiting in the long term, and need to take multivitamin supplements to avoid deficiencies.

Further reading

National Institute for Clinical Excellence (2004). *Core Interventions in the Treatment and Management of Anorexia Nervosa, Bulimia Nervosa and Related Eating Disorder.* http://guidance.nice.org.uk/CG9.

National Institute for Clinical Excellence (2006, amended 2008). *Obesity: The Prevention, Identification, Assessment and Management in Adults and Children.* http://guidance.nice.org.uk/CG43.

Fairburn, C. G., Cooper, Z., & Shafran, R. (2003). Cognitive behaviour therapy for eating disorders: A 'transdiagnostic' theory and treatment. *Behaviour Research and Therapy* **41**: 509–28.

Morris, J. & Twaddle, S. (2007). Anorexia nervosa. *British Medical Journal* **334**: 894.

Fairburn, C. G. & Harrison, P. J. (2003). Eating disorders. *Lancet* **361**: 407–16.

McKnight, R. F. & Boughton, N. (2009) A patient's journey with anorexia nervosa. *British Medical Journal* **399**: 46–51.

Schmidt, U. & Treasure, J. (1993). *Getting Better Bit(e) by Bit(e): A Survival Guide for Sufferers of Bulimia Nervosa and Binge-Eating Disorder.* Psychology Press, 1st edn.

Sleep disorders

Chapter contents

The term sleep disorder (**somnipathy**) simply means a disturbance of an individual's normal sleep pattern. Doctors typically see patients in whom the disturbance is severe enough to be having a negative effect upon physical, mental, or emotional functioning, but subclinical disturbances of sleep are common and something almost everyone will suffer at some point in their life. Sleep disorders are a heterogeneous group, ranging from the frequently experienced insomnia to the extremely rare hypersomnias such as Kleine–Levin syndrome. However, there are many shared characteristics between all sleep disorders, and this chapter will concentrate mainly on providing a framework for assessment, diagnosis, and management in the generic sense, with some guidance on specific disorders in the latter sections.

A good working knowledge of basic sleep disorders is essential in all specialties of clinical medicine. As a general rule, sleep disorders within the general hospital environment tend to be poorly managed, with great detriment to the patient. There are a variety of reasons why it is important to understand sleep disorders.

- Sleep disorders affect all ages.
- Poor sleep leads to a reduced ability to cope with other difficulties (e.g. pain, physical symptoms, poor mobility).
- Poor sleep reduces the ability of the body to fight infection, heal wounds, and recover from surgery or anaesthesia.
- Sleep disturbance is often a prodromal symptom of psychiatric disorder.
- Medications (not just psychotropics) often affect sleep.

- Poor familiarity with sleep disorders can lead to them being misdiagnosed as primary psychiatric disorders.
- Physical disorders frequently cause sleep disorders.

Sleep disturbance is an important part of many primary psychiatric conditions (e.g. depressive disorders, bipolar disorder, anxiety disorders); further information on these can be found in the chapter relating to each disorder.

■ What is normal sleep?

Sleep is a natural state of bodily rest seen in humans and many animals and is essential for survival. It is different from wakefulness in that the organism has a decreased ability to react to stimuli, but this is more easily reversible than in hibernation or coma. Sleep is poorly understood, but it is likely that it has several functions relating to restoration of body equilibrium and energy stores. There are a variety of theories regarding the function of sleep, which are outlined in Table 28.1.

The state of sleep can be identified by electroencephalography (EEG), which records the net electrical activity of the brain. Two distinct sleep states have been defined according to their EEG patterns, muscle tone and various physiological parameters: **non-rapid eye movement (NREM)** and **rapid eye movement (REM)** sleep. NREM sleep is divided into four stages, and REM sleep typically precedes them: stage 1 → stage 2 → stage 3 → stage 4 → stage 3 → stage 2 → REM, which repeats in cycles throughout the night (Figure 28.1).

NREM sleep

Stage 1 occurs at sleep onset, or when aroused from another stage of sleep. Sudden twitches or hypnagogic jerks may occur at the onset of sleep. The EEG shows theta waves at 4–7 Hz, some muscle tone is lost and consciousness reduced. Stage 1 accounts for 4–16 per cent of total overnight sleep.

Table 28.1 Proposed functions of sleep

- **Recovery** of physical and psychological strength
- **Restoration**: repair, wound healing, immune system function, correction of metabolic disturbances, and temperature regulation
- **Energy conservation**
- **Preservation**: allows animals to remain silent and hidden when at risk from predation
- **Discharge of emotions**
- **Memory consolidation**

Stage 2 is characterized by high-frequency bursts on the EEG (**sleep spindles**) and accounts for 45–55 per cent of overnight sleep. Muscle tone is lost, and there is complete loss of conscious awareness of the environment.

Stage 3 only accounts for 4–6 per cent of total sleep, and shows delta waves (**slow wave**).

Stage 4 shows the slowest activity on the EEG (0.5–4 Hz), and is the deepest stage of sleep. This is when parasomnias, such as night terrors, sleep walking, and bed wetting, occur. It accounts for 12–15 per cent of sleep.

The combination of stages 3 and 4 is also known as **slow-wave** or **delta sleep**.

REM sleep

Rapid eye movement sleep accounts for approximately a quarter of normal sleep time in healthy adults, and shows an EEG pattern very similar to the awake state. Muscle tone is completely lost except for spontaneous movements of the extraocular and middle ear muscles. Respiration rate, heart rate, blood pressure, and core temperature regulation all become irregular. People who are awoken from REM sleep usually say they were dreaming, but unless the content of dreams is recalled they are quickly forgotten.

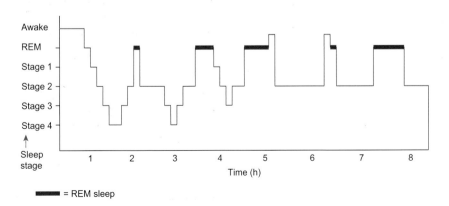

Fig. 28.1 An example of a normal hypnogram from an adult.

During a typical night, cycles of sleep lasting approximately 90 minutes occur. They start with NREM sleep for 80 minutes, followed by 10 minutes of REM sleep. As the night progresses, the REM stage tends to lengthen, with subsequent shortening of NREM. The quantity of stage 3 and 4 sleep is reduced gradually throughout the night. Total sleep time varies between individuals, but is usually somewhere between 5 and 9 hours. This pattern can be seen on a hypnogram (see Figure 28.1).

Circadian sleep–wake rhythms

The timing of when sleep occurs is regulated by the suprachiasmatic nucleus (SCN) in the anterior hypothalamus, whose neurons fire in a sinusoidal pattern across approximately 24 hours. Environment cues (**zeitgebers**) entrain the intrinsic rhythm of the SCN and include light, exercise, work schedules, and social interactions. The SCN controls temperature, cortisol, and growth hormone secretion, which it links into the sleep–wake cycle. The pineal gland secretes the hormone melatonin, which is related to the light–dark cycle rather than the sleep–wake cycle. Melatonin is secreted into the blood during darkness, so duration of melatonin secretion is a proxy measure of daylength. Melatonin is transported across the blood–brain barrier to act upon the SCN, thereby linking the light–dark and sleep–wake cycles.

Consequences of inadequate sleep

Prolonged sleep deprivation inevitably leads to death (usually due to loss of temperature regulation and overwhelming sepsis), which is clear evidence that sleep is essential to survival. Poor or disturbed sleep has a myriad of negative consequences, which are outlined in Table 28.2. It is worth keeping these in mind when considering the general hospital patient complaining of poor sleep.

■ Classification of sleep disorders

There are approximately 90 sleep disorders, many of which are poorly understood and subject to regular change in definition as research progresses. The result is that attempting to classify sleep disorders is challenging, and ultimately very confusing.

A simple way to approach it is to consider what can go wrong with sleep patterns; this reduces the field to four basic categories:

1 not enough sleep (**insomnia**);

2 sleeping too much (**hypersomnia**);

3 disturbed episodes during or related to sleep (**parasomnias**);

4 inappropriate timing of sleep, or the sleep–wake cycle loses synchrony with the rest of society (**circadian rhythm disorders**).

Making this distinction is adequate to allow most simple management strategies to be tried, but a thorough history and examination will usually allow you to be more specific as to the diagnosis if specialist help is likely to be needed.

Sleep disorders are covered by both the DSM-IV and the ICD-10 classifications, but the array of confusing terminology has led to the development of a third classification system. The **International Classification of Sleep Disorders** is now in its second edition (**ICSD-2**), and is published by the American Academy of Sleep Disorders based on international discussion and collaboration. It is the least confusing of the systems, as conditions are grouped into only seven major diagnostic categories. Table 28.3 outlines these categories, and compares them with the equivalent conditions in the DSM-IV and ICD-10.

Screening

It is very quick and simple to screen for sleep disorders; suggested questions are shown in Box 28.1. If any of the questions produce positive answers, a full assessment should be carried out. It is important to target the following high-risk groups:

- any patient presenting with psychiatric symptoms;
- patients with a psychiatric history;
- general hospital inpatients;
- patients with neurological, endocrine, or respiratory disease;
- patients with any other chronic disease.

Table 28.2 Consequences of sleep disturbance

Short-term consequences	Long-term consequences
Fatigue (mental, emotional, physical)	Decreased cognitive function
Irritability or depression	Memory loss
Poor concentration and attention	Reduced immune system function
Impaired judgement	Growth suppression
Increased reaction time, inaccuracy	Increased risk of type 2 diabetes, heart disease, and obesity
Yawning, aches, tremors, shivers	
Hallucinations, disorientation, persecutory ideas	

Table 28.3 Classification of sleep disorders: comparison of the three main classification systems. Bullet points show commoner conditions subclassified within a category of disorders.

ICSD-2	DSM-IV-TR	ICD-10
1 Insomnias	Insomnias	Non-organic insomnia
• Primary	• Primary	
• Secondary	• Secondary	
	• Related to another mental health disorder	
2 Sleep-related breathing disorders	Sleep-related breathing disorders	
• Obstructive sleep apnoea	• Obstructive sleep apnoea	
• Central apnoea		
3 Hypersomnias	Hypersomnias	Non-organic hypersomnia
• Primary	• Primary	
• Narcolepsy	• Narcolepsy	
• Kleine–Levin syndrome	• Hypersomnia related to another mental health problem	
4 Circadian rhythm disorder	Circadian rhythm disorder	Non-organic sleep–wake schedule disturbance
• Delayed sleep phase syndrome		
• Advanced sleep phase syndrome		
• Jet lag		
• Night-shift work disorder		
5 Parasomnias	Parasomnias	Parasomnias
• Sleep terrors	• Sleep terrors	• Sleep terrors
• Nightmares	• Nightmares	• Nightmares
• Sleepwalking	• Sleepwalking	• Sleepwalking
6 Sleep-related movement disorders	Dysomnia not otherwise specified	
• Restless leg syndrome	• Restless leg syndrome	
• Periodic limb movement disorder	• Periodic limb movement disorder	
7 Other sleep disorder related to physical health problem	Sleep disorder due to a general medical condition	
	Substance-induced sleep disorder	

■ Assessment of sleep disorders

Assessment

A full history should be taken, including information from the patient and their bed or room partner, as some forms of sleep disturbance are not known to the patient.

It may also be helpful to contact the primary care physician and look at old hospital notes.

Sleep history

• Precise nature of the sleep complaint (including onset, duration, course, frequency, severity). Were there any significant events or stressors around the time of the onset of the problem?

BOX 28.1 Screening for sleep disorders

• Do you sleep long enough and well enough?

• Are you very sleepy during the day?

• Do you do unusual things or have strange experiences at night?

• Pattern of symptoms, timing, and exacerbating or relieving factors (e.g. does it vary at weekends or during holidays?).

• Behaviour whilst asleep, dreams/nightmares, episodes of awakening, and perceived quality of sleep.

- Effect of symptoms upon mood, behaviour, work, social life, school, and bed partner or other family members.
- Previous sleep problems and treatments.

Daily routine

- Time and mode (natural, alarm) of waking; ease of getting up;
- Activities and level of alertness during the day;
- Daily naps;
- Preparations for bed;
- Time of going to bed;
- Activities in bed (reading, TV, sex, eating);
- Time of falling asleep;
- Night-time awakenings;
- Consumption of caffeinated drinks—how much and at what time?

Psychiatric history

- Previous diagnoses of psychiatric conditions;
- Previous psychiatric treatments and how successful they were;
- Current medications (prescribed, illicit, over-the-counter, alcohol, nicotine);
- Premorbid personality traits;
- Current social situation: accommodation, employment, finances.

A mental state examination should be carried out as for any other patient, as problems with sleep are common presenting complaints in other psychiatric conditions.

It is also important to include a full general review of systems to exclude any other symptoms that could be interfering with sleep (e.g. shortness of breath, pain, nocturia).

Physical examination. A full physical examination should be undertaken, focusing specifically on the respiratory, neurological, and endocrine systems.

Psychological evaluation. If an underlying psychiatric disorder is suspected, the usual methods of assessment should be used (e.g. Beck Depression Index).

Further investigations

The majority of patients presenting with sleep problems will need no investigations other than those above. However, if the diagnosis is unclear or it is difficult to get an accurate history, there are a variety of other methods of assessing sleep.

Sleep diaries are a more accurate way of understanding sleep patterns. The patient is provided with a booklet in which they record daily activities, sleeping, mealtimes, caffeine intake, and sleep-related symptoms over a 2-week period. These are often extremely revealing as to the cause of the problem.

Video recordings can be very useful in demonstrating the parasomnias. This may be done at home or in hospital.

Actigraphy. This is the monitoring of body movements (usually via a unit worn like a wrist watch) which can be used to quantify sleep–wake cycles. They can also be useful in detecting movement disorders occurring during sleep.

Polysomnography is more usually known as a sleep study, and involves the monitoring of various physiological parameters during sleep. Basic polysomnography includes the recording of EEG, electro-oculography (EOG), and electro-myography (EMG), but often ECG, pulse oximetry, oesophageal pH, and respiratory monitoring are added. This is combined with audio and video recording of the patient overnight, and is the most definitive method of diagnosing a specific sleep disorder. The downside is that it has to be done in a special sleep laboratory, which is expensive and may not be suitable for the very young, acutely disturbed patients, or the disabled.

The Multiple Sleep Latency Test (MSLT) is a method of assessing daytime sleepiness. The patient is put to bed at intervals throughout the day, and the length of time it takes them to fall asleep is recorded.

■ General principles of management

The majority of sleep disorders are secondary consequences of another problem, and the emphasis should always be on treating the primary condition. The quick and simple response to sleep problems (usually insomnia) is to prescribe hypnotics, but due to the high risk of tolerance and dependence these should be avoided wherever possible. Most sleep disturbances can be treated using behavioural regimes combined with treatment of the underlying condition.

Sleep education

Providing accurate information about normal sleep and the effects of external factors on sleep reduces the patient's feeling of being out of control. Irrespective of the underlying diagnosis, the following should be discussed with the patient:

- functions of sleep;
- how sleep changes with age;
- sleep as an active process with different stages;
- factors adversely affecting sleep (behaviour, drugs, work patterns, etc.);

- the effects of sleep loss (Table 28.2);
- how to keep a sleep diary;
- different types of sleep problems.

Sleep hygiene

Sleep hygiene refers to the behavioural and environmental factors preceding sleep that may interfere with it. Establishing appropriate sleep habits is a vital part of the treatment of sleep disorders. Components of good sleep hygiene are shown in Box 28.2, and again should be discussed with all patients, and a leaflet provided containing the same advice.

Table 28.4 shows the various treatment options available for sleep disorders, and more specific guidance for each condition is given in the sections below.

■ Specific sleep disorders

Insomnia

Insomnia is usually a symptom rather than a disorder, and refers to persistent problems falling asleep, maintaining sleep, or having a good quality of sleep. It is extremely common, with one-third of adults experiencing significant insomnia at some point. Sleep disruption may be a primary disorder, but is more often secondary to another medical or psychiatric condition.

Clinical features

The patient may complain of:

- not being able to get to sleep;
- repeated awakenings throughout the night;

Table 28.4 Treatment strategies for sleep disorders

General measures

- Treat the underlying cause of the problem (medical or psychiatric)
- Psychoeducation
- Ensure good sleep hygiene
- Advise on safety or protective measures (e.g. for sleepwalking)
- Relaxation therapy, yoga, mindfulness training

Psychological treatments (mainly used for insomnia)

- Supportive counselling
- Cognitive behavioural therapy
- Sleep restriction therapy

Pharmacological treatments

- Hypnotics (short term)
- Stimulants (narcolepsy, hypersomnias)
- Melatonin (sleep–wake disturbances)
- Antidepressants (underlying depression, narcolepsy)

Physical measures

- Continuous positive airway pressure (obstructive sleep apnoea)
- Light therapy (circadian rhythm disturbances)
- Chronotherapy (circadian rhythm disturbances)

- early morning awakening;
- perceived poor quality of or unrefreshing sleep;
- inadequate total quantity of sleep;

Inadequate sleep may lead to daytime sleepiness, irritability, fatigue, poor attention and concentration, and substandard performance at daily activities. The patient is usually distressed and preoccupied by sleep problems, and in severe cases social or occupational functioning is negatively affected. Rarely, the consequences will have been severe; for example, loss of a job due to poor performance secondary to fatigue. There are often co-morbid symptoms of anxiety related to the attempts to obtain adequate sleep.

Diagnosis

According to DSM-IV criteria, the following criteria must be met irrespective of the type of insomnia.

- The predominant complaint is difficulty initiating or maintaining sleep.
- It has been present for at least 1 month.
- It is accompanied by daytime fatigue or impaired daytime functioning.

BOX 28.2 Sleep hygiene

- Ensure the bedroom is comfortable; control light, temperature, and noise.
- Relax away from the day's stresses for at least 1 hour before bed.
- Avoid caffeinated drinks (and other stimulants) after 4 pm.
- Avoid smoking for an hour before bed.
- Ensure regular exercise (although not late at night).
- Eat a stable, regular, suitable diet.
- Moderate alcohol consumption.
- Have a milky (or other tryptophan-containing) snack before bed.
- Avoid daytime naps.

- Sleep disturbance causes clinically significant distress in social or occupational functioning.
- The disturbance is not better accounted for by another sleep disorder.

The insomnia can then be further classified as primary, related to another medical or psychiatric problem, or due to substance misuse. Severe and chronic insomnia requires a minimum duration of 6 months with problems on at least three nights of the week.

The ICD-10 classification defines non-organic insomnia as a *condition of unsatisfactory quantity and/or quality of sleep, which persists for a considerable period of time, including difficulty falling asleep, difficulty staying asleep, or early final wakening.*

Prevalence

Insomnia affects one-third of adults occasionally, and approximately 10 per cent on a clinically significant basis. A US national survey in 2003 reported 58 per cent of adults complained of poor sleep at least one night per week, but only 12 per cent felt it interfered with their daily commitments. Insomnia is more common in females, shift workers, professionals, and people with medical or psychiatric disorders. Age is an important risk factor; up to 25 per cent of elderly people sleep poorly, although it is unclear how much of this is due to other factors (e.g. drugs, nocturia, etc.).

Aetiology of insomnia

Table 28.5 contains an overview of the main causes of insomnia. This is not an exhaustive list, and more detailed information can be found in the further reading section. Secondary causes of insomnia constitute 98 per cent of cases, so take a careful history. A list of drugs that interfere with sleep can be found on p. 374.

Course and prognosis

There has been little research into the natural course of insomnia, as the myriad of aetiologies make it difficult to generalize. However, it is known that untreated primary insomnia is usually lifelong, and that insomnia of any cause tends to gradually worsen with time. For insomnia that is secondary to another diagnosis, improvement of the underlying cause is usually mirrored by an improvement in sleep patterns, but this is not universally the case. Although some cases of insomnia will run a prolonged course, the prognosis of an adequately treated episode of secondary insomnia is very good.

Assessment

Assessment should be carried out as outlined on p. 359. Special attention should be paid to taking an in-depth

Table 28.5 Classification of insomnia

Primary causes (rare)	
Primary (idiopathic) insomnia	No cause found (very rare)
Paradoxical insomnia	Complaint of poor sleep despite normal patterns
Psychophysiological insomnia	Learned sleep prevention behaviours
Sleep apnoea syndromes, e.g. obstructive sleep apnoea	Central alveolar hypoventilation syndrome (Ondine's curse)
Restless leg syndrome	Painful sensations in legs which prevent sleep (Ekbom's syndrome)
Periodic limb movement syndrome	Episodes of repeated, stereotyped leg movements which prevent sleep, common over 60 years
Secondary causes (common)	
Environmental	Poor sleep hygiene, stress
Hormonal	Menstruation or menopause related
Medical disorders	Pain, neurological, endocrine, respiratory disease
Psychiatric disorders	Depressive disorder, anxiety disorder, dementia, PTSD, OCD, schizophrenia, mania, eating disorders
Circadian rhythm disturbance	Jet lag, shift work
Substance use or misuse	Alcohol, caffeine, nicotine, stimulants
	Prescription drugs
	Rebound insomnia from overuse of hypnotics

description of daily routine, and include a full systems enquiry and physical examination.

Management

At the time of writing, there are no UK national guidelines on the general management of insomnia, so a practical and common-sense approach must be taken. The National Institute for Clinical Excellence (NICE) published a technology appraisal on the use of non-benzodiazepines in insomnia in 2004—this is discussed below.

The most important aspects of the management of insomnia are:

1 treating the secondary cause of the insomnia;

2 a clear explanation of what is causing the problem and how it will be treated;

3 ensuring good sleep hygiene (Box 28.2).

Table 28.6 Management of insomnia

General measures

- Identification and treatment of the cause of insomnia
- Psychoeducation
- Improve sleep hygiene

Psychological treatments (first line)

- Relaxation therapy
- Stimulus control therapy
- Sleep restriction
- Cognitive behavioural therapy

Pharmacological treatments (second line)

- Hypnotics
  - Benzodiazepines
  - Non-benzodiazepines
- Antihistamines
- Antidepressants

A general outline of management options is shown in Table 28.6. Psychological interventions should be used as a first line, as they are more effective and provide longer-term benefit than medications.

General measures

These are discussed in detail in the 'general principles of treatment' section on p. 360.

Psychological treatments

Stimulus control therapy. This form of treatment plays on the natural instinct to become sleepy when presented with a familiar pre-bedtime routine and environment. For someone with a normal sleep pattern, positive associations are made between time, feeling sleepy, getting into bed, and falling asleep. For the insomniac, these same stimuli are perceived negatively, and wakefulness and restfulness become a conditioned response. Stimulus control involves removing everything from the bedroom that might hinder sleep, and then reconditioning the person to associate the room with sleep. The individual is only allowed to go to bed when sleepy, and all other activities (with the exception of sex) are banned from the bedroom. Sleeping is forbidden in other rooms of the house. If sleep does not occur within 20 minutes, they should get up and go to another room until they are sleepy. There should be a regular time to get up, with no more than 60 minutes variation, even at weekends. This is continued until the patient is able to go to bed at a specified time and get to sleep quickly.

Sleep restriction therapy. This is especially helpful for patients who spend long periods in bed, but are awake for much of the time. Reducing the time spent in bed helps to consolidate the sleep, providing higher-quality rest. Sleep restriction involves the patient first keeping a sleep diary and calculating average sleep duration. For the first week, they are only allowed to spend this much time in bed per night, with no daytime naps. The sleep time can be slightly altered until an appropriate satisfactory amount of sleep is achieved. This treatment is hard work, and requires a highly motivated patient.

Cognitive behavioural therapy (CBT) is the most effective treatment for chronic insomnia. Around 70 per cent of patients with insomnia will benefit from CBT, and the effects are maintained in the long term. It acts by identifying thoughts that prevent sleep from occurring, and finds ways to challenge these and alter behaviour. Components of CBT for insomnia include:

- identifying intrusive thought patterns;
- addressing misconceptions about sleep;
- establishing a daily review and planning session in the early evening;
- relaxation training;
- distraction and thought blocking;
- challenging negative thoughts;
- motivation to maintain cognitive and behavioural change.

Pharmacotherapy

There are a large number of prescription and over-the-counter medications available that are designed to help people sleep. All products with an active psychotropic component have the potential to cause tolerance and dependence (psychological and/or physical) and so need to be used with caution. No drug should be prescribed for more than a **3-week** period, and they should be reserved for acutely distressed patients. Avoid using any hypnotic in patients with hepatic encephalopathy or severely impaired respiratory function. A quick guide to prescribing is shown in Box 28.3.

Benzodiazepines are the most commonly used class of hypnotic, and are highly effective at inducing sleep. They

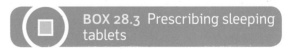

BOX 28.3 Prescribing sleeping tablets

Safest starting choices include:

- Temazepam 10 mg at night
- Zopiclone 3.75–7.5 mg at night
- Zolpidem 10 mg at night
  Note: Halve doses in the elderly or those with liver disease.

act on a benzodiazepine receptor, which increases GABA inhibition within the CNS. Unfortunately, tolerance and dependence occur within 14 days, and they may cause rebound insomnia if used regularly. Benzodiazepines are best used short term to supplement other therapies in severe, disabling insomnia. It is important to choose the benzodiazepine carefully, as the longer-acting drugs can lead to dangerous 'hangover' effects the following day.

- Ultra-short acting: midazolam, triazolam—not suitable for insomnia.
- Intermediate (*c.* 8 hours): temazepam—best for insomnia.
- Long-acting: diazepam—risk of 'hangover' the next day.

Non-benzodiazepine hypnotics ('Z-drugs') are a newer class of drugs which also potentiate GABA inhibition in the CNS. Examples include zopiclone, zolpidem, and zaleplon. Clinical trials have shown them to be as effective as benzodiazepines, but with a slightly lower risk of tolerance and dependence. However, they do cause morning sedation and are not currently licensed for long-term use.

Sedating antihistamines are widely available as off-prescription sleeping aids. Diphenhydramine (Benadryl, Nytol) and promethazine are the most common. Antihistamines are effective hypnotics, but the effects do tend to wear off with time, and often cause drowsiness the next day. The most frequent side effect is headache.

Antidepressants have traditionally had a role in the treatment of insomnia. A low dose of trazodone or mirtazapine is a good choice, but runs the risk of a number of side effects.

Atypical antipsychotics are being used more frequently for night sedation. Quetiapine has the best risk–benefit ratio when given at doses of 50–200 mg (the antipsychotic dose being 300–900 mg) at night. Current UK recommendations do not include the use of atypicals for sedation, but on a worldwide basis they are commonly used, especially in psychiatric inpatients.

Hypersomnias

Hypersomnia means **excessive daytime sleepiness**, and is a term used to cover a heterogeneous group of sleep disorders. Hypersomnias have a prevalence of 5 to 15 per cent (depending upon severity), and are a leading cause of road traffic accidents. Many of the syndromes can be effectively treated, so they are important conditions to diagnose and manage. In a general psychiatric text it is impossible to cover in detail all of the hypersomnias—the commoner and/or more important conditions are briefly outlined below, and in-depth resources and full diagnostic criteria can be found in references within the further reading section (p. 374).

General clinical features

Excessive daytime sleepiness manifests itself in a variety of different ways. Patients may present complaining of:

- bouts of sleepiness during the day;
- irresistible, unrefreshing episodes of sleep during the day;
- abnormally long length of night-time sleep;

(Q) Case study 28.1 Insomnia

A 46-year-old man, Peter, presented to his general practitioner complaining of poor sleep. He described difficulty in getting to sleep, frequent awakenings during the night, and waking up at 5–6 am daily. He had tried over-the-counter sleeping tablets and milky drinks at bedtime, but found them no use. On further questioning, he said that the problems had gradually worsened over the last year, and now he was feeling down, apathetic, and very tired during the day. Peter's wife said she had noticed him snoring extremely loudly at night and stopping breathing sometimes, which worried her. She had starting wearing earplugs at night. She also felt that Peter had become withdrawn, and mentioned he had been made redundant 6 months previously. The GP examined Peter, and apart from finding him to be rather overweight (BMI 38), there were no abnormalities. She also took a full psychiatric and sleep history, and decided that the causes of the insomnia were threefold: a depressive disorder, obstructive sleep apnoea, and poor sleep hygiene (high caffeine and nicotine intake in the evenings). The GP explained this to Peter, gave him some leaflets about insomnia and sleep hygiene, and discussed various treatments for depression. Peter felt he would like to try some medication, so the GP prescribed an SSRI. She also referred him to the sleep apnoea clinic, and warned him that it was not safe to take hypnotics as they cause respiratory depression. Over the next few months, Peter had a good response to the SSRI and his sleep improved slightly. Later that year he received a continuous positive airway pressure (CPAP) machine, which increased his sleep quality immensely, and allowed him to feel ready to look for another job.

- prolonged difficulty in waking up, often with disorientation ('sleep drunkenness');
- recurrent periods of almost continuous sleep for days on end, which occur every few months.

Other related symptoms may include irritation, decreased energy, restlessness, slow speech, psychomotor retardation, anorexia, and memory problems. Frequently, the patient will present to a doctor when the sleepiness is interfering with their work, studying, or family life. Fifty per cent of hypersomniacs will have an automobile accident due to their sleepiness, and many are unable to hold down full-time employment. In children, sleepiness can prevent academic progression and may mask a child's natural abilities. Often the patient may not be fully aware of their condition, and it is brought to medical attention by a family member, employer, or after an accident.

Prevalence

Severe sleepiness (which is daily, embarrassing, and impairs function) has a prevalence of 5 per cent of the general population. Another 10 to 15 per cent suffer occasional moderate sleepiness. Males and females are equally affected (with the exception of Klein–Levin syndrome, which is exclusively found in males). Hypersomnia is usually present from birth, but typically present between 10 and 30 years.

Aetiology

The major causes of hypersomnia are shown in Table 28.7 Further detail as to the drugs that cause hypersomnia can be found on p. 374. In an adult with new-onset sleepiness, the most common causes are an underlying psychiatric or medical condition, or the effects of substances.

Assessment

General assessment should be carried out as outlined on p. 360.

The Epworth Sleepiness Scale is a self-completed questionnaire which asks the patient to rate their chance of dozing off in eight daily situations. It has a high sensitivity and is therefore a good screening tool for hypersomnia.

The Multiple Sleep Latency Test is the gold standard for diagnosis of hypersomnia, and is based on the fact that the sleepier a patient is, the faster they fall asleep. The patient is put to bed every 2 hours throughout the day and a polysomnograph times how long it takes them to get to sleep. A mean time of less than 5 minutes across five readings is taken as pathological sleepiness.

Table 28.7 Aetiology of hypersomnia

Hypersomnia secondary to a psychiatric condition
- Unipolar or bipolar mood disorders
- Somatoform disorders
- Personality disorders

Hypersomnia due to a drug or substance
- Prescribed drugs (e.g. hypnotics, antidepressants, antipsychotics, antihistamines, antiparkinson drugs)
- Toxins (arsenic, bismuth, carbon monoxide, vitamin A, copper)
- Alcohol
- Recreational drugs (opiates)

Hypersomnia related to a breathing disorder
- Obstructive sleep apnoea

Hypersomnias of central origin
- Narcolepsy with or without cataplexy
- Idiopathic hypersomnia (no cause found)
- Recurrent hypersomnia (Klein–Levin syndrome)

Hypersomnias related to a general medical condition
- Neurological diseases (brain tumours, raised intracranial pressure, Parkinson's disease)
- Endocrine diseases (hypothyroidism, acromegaly)
- Infectious diseases (Epstein–Barr, hepatitis B, trypanosomiasis)
- Post-traumatic hypersomnia

Behaviourally induced insufficient sleep syndrome

Narcolepsy

Narcolepsy is characterized by excessive daytime sleepiness, extreme fatigue, and irresistible episodes of sleep. There are three subtypes.

1 **Narcolepsy with cataplexy.** The irresistible episodes of sleep are accompanied by a sudden bilateral loss of skeletal muscle tone, usually triggered by emotion or surprise.

2 **Narcolepsy without cataplexy.**

3 **Narcolepsy secondary to a medical condition.** The condition must be a significant underlying medical or psychiatric disorder which could account for the sleepiness. It is linked to low hypocretin levels in the CSF.

Narcolepsy is not particularly rare; the majority of cases are with cataplexy, and have a prevalence of 0.4 per 1000. Males and females are equally affected. Narcolepsy tends to be present from birth, and may present from 5 to 50 years of age. It is a chronic disorder which tends to be lifelong.

Clinical features

The classical tetrad of excessive sleepiness, cataplexy, sleep paralysis, and hypnagogic hallucinations is actually very rare. The sleepiness is present every day, and tends to worsen gradually until there is an irresistible and refreshing short episode of sleep. These are uncontrollable, and may occur at inappropriate times. The frequency of these naps is highly variable, from a few per day to one every couple of minutes. Cataplexy is triggered by specific emotional, stressful, or surprising stimuli in the environment, and all voluntary muscles except the respiratory and extraocular musculature are involved. The patient may fall to the ground, or merely become suddenly very weak. Consciousness is preserved during the attack, and there is rapid recovery.

Other symptoms include:

- hallucinations—hypnagogic (at the onset of sleep) or hypnopompic (upon waking up);
- sleep paralysis—the inability to move on going to or waking up from sleep;
- sleep talking;
- frequent awakenings whilst asleep;
- nightmares (often violent and terrifying), night terrors, and sleep walking;
- there is an association with obesity.

Narcolepsy interferes with every part of life, and can be very incapacitating. Secondary depression, anxiety, and underachievement at school or work are very common.

Investigations

Narcolepsy is essential a clinical diagnosis, as there is no specific diagnostic test. Patients should be referred to a specialist to undergo investigations which can help confirm a suspected case.

Polysomnography shows a distinctive pattern of a short sleep latency (time to get to sleep), short periods of REM sleep, increased stage 1 NREM sleep, and frequent awakenings.

Human leucocyte antigen (HLA) typing. The HLA-DR2 haplotype is found in 80 to 90 per cent of patients with narcolepsy.

Reduced hypocretin-1 concentration in the CSF is a highly sensitive and specific marker for narcolepsy.

Management

The general measures outlined in Table 28.4 should be followed.

Practical support. Psychoeducation, support at school or work, and participation in support groups for narcolepsy are all very important. This is especially the case if cataplexy limits activities that can be undertaken (e.g. driving).

Scheduled naps. Short 20-minute naps should be built into the daily timetable to reduce the likelihood of irresistible sleeps.

Stimulants are the medications most frequently used to deal with daytime sleepiness. Methyphenidate, methamphetamine, and modafinil are the most commonly used. They are safe and effective, but may cause restlessness, irritability, or GI upset.

Antidepressants such as tricyclics or venlafaxine are used to treat cataplexy, but there is little randomized controlled evidence to prove their efficacy.

Klein–Levin syndrome (recurrent hypersomnia)

This is a rare condition, exclusively affecting adolescent males, which is characterized by recurrent episodes of hypersomnia and binge eating. Periods of excessive sleepiness last for weeks at a time, during which there is rapid weight gain. It may be accompanied by sexual disinhibition, irritability, odd behaviours, and psychotic symptoms. The latter may lead to an erroneous diagnosis of schizophrenia. Between attacks the patient recovers completely. Klein–Levin syndrome is a clinical diagnosis, which usually lasts for the adolescent years and then gradually burns out in the twenties. Treatment is similar to that for narcolepsy, with stimulants and behavioural modification being the first-line approaches. Occasionally, mood stabilizers (carbamazepine, lithium, valproate) may be helpful if there is severe functional disruption during episodes.

Idiopathic hypersomnia (primary hypersomnia)

Idiopathic hypersomnia is a state of daily excessive sleepiness of unknown aetiology. It has three characteristic features:

1 prolonged night-time sleeping (more than 10 hours)—the person sleeps very soundly and cannot be woken by alarms, telephones, etc.;

2 sleep drunkenness on waking—there is often difficulty in waking up, confusion, and irritability for an hour or more;

3 excessive daytime sleepiness with frequent, unrefreshing naps.

Diagnosis is made on exclusion of other hypersomnias, usually by polysomnography. Treatment is as for narcolepsy, but without the scheduled naps, as these are unrefreshing and therefore unhelpful.

Sleep apnoea

Sleep apnoea is a group of conditions in which there are pauses in breathing during sleep. The pause must last at least 10 seconds to meet diagnostic criteria, during which there is a measurable desaturation in blood oxygen levels. Frequent awakenings when breathing resumes lead to unrefreshing sleep and daytime sleepiness. A clinically relevant level of sleep apnoea is thought to be more than five episodes per hour. Obstructive sleep apnoea is very common, whereas central sleep apnoea syndromes are very rare.

Obstructive sleep apnoea (OSA)

Obstruction of the upper airways occurs during sleep if there is a combination of low muscle tone and excessive soft tissue around the airway. The major risk factor is obesity, but it is also more common in certain anatomical neck variants, men, and the elderly. OSA has a prevalence of 4 per cent and 2 per cent in adult men and women, respectively. It usually presents from 40 to 60 years.

Symptoms include:

- snoring;
- apnoeic episodes ending with loud resumption of breathing;
- nocturia;
- severe fatigue upon waking up;
- daytime headaches;
- excessive daytime sleepiness;
- poor concentration, irritability, and loss of libido.

Diagnosis is made by polysomnography, including audio-video recording of a night's sleep.

Treatment of obstructive sleep apnoea

Weight loss. Even loss of only 5 per cent of body weight can reduce symptoms dramatically.

Avoidance of alcohol and sedatives.

Continuous positive airway pressure (CPAP) at night is the most effective treatment. It involves wearing a large, heavy mask in bed, which is difficult to get used to. However, good compliance leads to excellent results and many patients do persevere.

Surgery is occasionally used to reconstruct the nose or upper airways if the cause is an anatomical aberration.

Parasomnias

The word parasomnia literally means *around sleep*, and refers to undesirable, abnormal skeletal muscle activity, behaviours, or emotional–perceptual events that occur during sleep. Parasomnias may happen at sleep onset, during sleep, during transition between stages of sleep, or when going from sleep to wakefulness. There are a number of reasons why a good understanding of parasomnias is important for all clinicians, but especially psychiatrists and primary care physicians.

1 Parasomnias are extremely common; sleep walking alone occurs in 17 per cent of children and 5 per cent of adults.

2 Stress exacerbates parasomnias (e.g. diagnosis of a general medical condition, surgery, or bereavement).

3 Parasomnias often cause psychological distress.

4 The unusual nature of experiences can lead to patients being misdiagnosed with other psychiatric disorders. This has huge consequences in terms of treatment and stigma.

5 Parasomnias may be the presenting feature of a psychiatric disorder (e.g. nocturnal bulimia nervosa).

6 Very rarely, parasomnias may manifest as sleep-related violence, which becomes the domain of forensic psychiatry.

Classification of parasomnias

There are a variety of different approaches to classifying parasomnias. The ICSD-2 uses the stage of sleep in which the experience occurs, but it is much simpler to consider parasomnias in two categories:

1 symptoms due to a primary disorder of sleep itself;

2 symptoms during sleep which are secondary to an underlying medical or psychiatric condition.

The main types of parasomnias are outlined in Table 28.8.

Assessment

Polysomnography with audio-visual recording is the gold standard diagnostic tool. It picks up abnormal motor and brain activity during sleep, which can be linked to motor activities and behaviour seen on the video.

Sleepwalking (somnambulism)

Sleepwalking is characterized by complex, automatic behaviours occurring during sleep. Typical activities include wandering around the house, rearranging objects, eating, and urinating. Very rarely more dangerous activities such as carrying weapons, driving, and homicide have occurred. The person's eyes are usually wide open, and they stare into space. It is not possible to communicate with the person, although they may mumble to themselves. Sleepwalking usually occurs in the first 20 minutes of sleep, and may last anywhere from a few minutes to 2 hours. The person usually returns to bed easily, and the episode is not remembered in the morning,

Sleepwalking occurs in approximately 17 per cent of children, and 2 to 4 per cent of adults. It is found equally

Table 28.8 Classification of parasomnias

Primary sleep phenomena

- Disorders of arousal: *sleepwalking, sleep terrors, confusional arousal*
- *Nightmares* (occur in REM sleep)
- Sleep paralysis
- REM sleep behaviour disorder
- Sleep-related eating disorder
- Restless legs syndrome/periodic limb movements in sleep
- Obstructive sleep apnoea-related parasomnias
- Rarities: sleep bruxism, nocturnal paroxysmal dystonia, sudden unexplained nocturnal death syndrome, infant sleep apnoea

Secondary sleep phenomena

- Seizures
- Headaches
- Nocturnal psychiatric symptoms: dissociative disorders, panic attacks, bulimia nervosa, or PTSD
- Arrhythmias
- Asthma
- Gastro-oesophageal reflux

Malingering (rare)

Conditions shown in italics denote common disorders likely to be seen in everyday practice.

frequently in males and females. The peak is at 4 to 8 years, and it is rare for the condition to start later than early adolescence. Family history is usually positive for sleepwalking and/or other parasomnias. There are a variety of risk factors and associations with sleepwalking, which are shown in Box 28.4.

Treatment

In the majority of cases of sleepwalking, no treatment is necessary. It is important to reassure the family, make sure the patient is safe at night, and ensure good sleep hygiene. Avoidance of sleep deprivation and stressors can also reduce the severity of episodes. For patients with very disruptive behaviours or sleep-related injuries, consider a low-dose medication at night. Options include:

- benzodiazepines (e.g. clonazepam 0.25–2.5 mg at night);
- antidepressants (e.g. low-dose imipramine or paroxetine).

Sleep terrors (parvor nocturnes, incubus)

Sleep terrors are characterized by a sudden awakening in which the patient sits upright, screams loudly, and has marked autonomic activation (sweating, mydriasis, tachycardia, tachypnoea). Occasionally there may be frantic motor activity, which can lead to falling out of bed and injury. The episode occurs early in the night (may be later in small children), and usually lasts 10–15 minutes. The patient soon quietens and goes back to sleep, and is unable to remember the events in the morning.

Sleep terrors have a prevalence of 3 per cent in children, reducing to 1 per cent in adults. They are just as common in males as females, and a family history is often present.

Associations are shown in Box 28.4. Sleep terrors are investigated and managed in the same way as sleepwalking.

Confusional arousal ('sleep drunkenness')

Sleep drunkenness refers to patients who have a long period of confusion, disorientation, and slowness upon awakening from sleep, usually worse when awoken from

 Case study 28.2 Sleepwalking

Sarah, an 8-year-old girl, was taken to see her paediatrician by her mother Claire. Claire said that she had been keen for Sarah to attend a weekend away with her Brownie Pack, but was worried about her going due to Sarah's frequent sleepwalking. From the age of three, Sarah had got up almost every night and wandered about the house in a daze. She sometimes drew pictures in the playroom, and often needed assistance in going back upstairs to bed. Claire was concerned that Sarah would hurt herself at night if she was in an unfamiliar environment, or that the other girls would tease her. She had read on the Internet that sleepwalking can be associated with other psychiatric problems, and was concerned that Sarah might

develop one if it continued. Sarah had no previous medical history or other symptoms, and physical examination was normal. The paediatrician reassured Claire that sleepwalking is extremely common in children, and that Sarah would probably grow out of it. He explained that sleepwalking is *associated* with some medical conditions, but it is not a *causative* factor in these and that Sarah appeared healthy at present. He stressed that Claire should be safety conscious and discuss the problem with the adults supervising the Brownie trip. Claire did so, and Sarah went on the trip as planned. She did sleepwalk, but the hall had been made safe for her, and there were no adverse consequences.

BOX 28.4 Factors associated with sleepwalking and sleep terrors

Sleep deprivation	Febrile illness	Lithium carbonate	'Z-drugs'
Alcohol	Pregnancy	Stress	Anticholinergic drugs
Menstruation	Obstructive sleep apnoea	Family history	Neurological disorders
Periodic limb movements	Nocturnal seizures		

a deep sleep. During the period the person may walk about, get dressed, and undertake normal behaviours, but these are very slow and inaccurate. The phenomenon is extremely common in young children but rare in adults, where it is usually associated with another sleep disorder (narcolepsy, sleep apnoea, idiopathic hypersomnia). There is no specified treatment, but all the supportive and general measures for managing sleep disorders may be helpful.

Nightmares

Nightmares are frightening dreams that cause the patient to wake up, usually feeling slightly confused. The patient may be distressed, and can take time to get back to sleep. They occur during REM sleep, and show a distinctive increase in activity on the EEG. Nightmares frequently occur after a stressful event, high fever, or occasionally after eating certain foods. Nightmares occur occasionally in 50 per cent of adults, but the prevalence of having one or more nightmares per week is approximately 1 per cent. There are a large number of drugs that are associated with bad dreams or nightmares; these are shown in Box 28.5. Treatment is rarely needed, but infrequently sleep will be adversely affected enough for the patient (or their bed partner) to seek medical attention. In that situation, the following may be tried:

- avoid unnecessary stressors;
- avoid alcohol and sedatives in the evening;
- avoid drugs which cause nightmares;
- try low-dose antidepressants: SSRI or tricyclic.

BOX 28.5 Drugs associated with nightmares

Antimuscarinics	Beta-blockers
Clonidine	Digoxin
Indomethacin	Methyldopa
Nicotine patches	Pergolide
Reserpine	Verapamil
Withdrawal from alcohol, benzodiazepines, or opiates	

REM-sleep behaviour disorder (RSBD)

This is a disorder that was not fully characterized until the 1980s, and is usually found in males aged 50–60 years. The patient has vivid, intense, violent dreams combined with furious motor activity. Sleep injury (of both patient and bed partner) is common. Sleep for both the patient and bedroom companion is disrupted, and can lead to relationship problems.

The prevalence of RSBD is 0.3 to 0.5 per cent, but 50 per cent of these cases are associated with neurological disease. Common conditions include narcolepsy, parkinsonism, stroke, and other neurodegenerative disorders. RSBD may be the first manifestation of the condition, which may not develop until several years later. Rarely, RSBD may be triggered by psychotropic medications, or withdrawal from alcohol, or recreational drugs.

Treatment

- Ensure a safe sleeping environment for the patient and their bed partner.
- Eliminate or treat any predisposing or aggravating factors.
- Clomazepam 0.5-1.0 mg at night is very effective at controlling the symptoms in most patients.

Restless legs syndrome (RLS, Ekbom's syndrome)

This is a common condition, affecting 5 to 10 per cent of the general population, that can cause severe sleep disturbance and insomnia. It is characterized by unpleasant, painful sensations in the lower limbs that occur especially at the transition from wakefulness to sleep, and are relieved by movement or stimulation of the legs. Severely affected individuals get the sensations whenever their legs are still (e.g. watching TV, in aeroplanes) and can find it difficult to concentrate because of them. The majority of patients have a family history of RLS, but the symptoms are often triggered or worsened by caffeine, alcohol, fatigue, and stress. RLS is associated with renal failure, diabetes, pregnancy, psychotropic medications, and peripheral neuropathies.

Treatment

Heat, massage, and stretching may provide minimal relief, but usually medication is required. Options include benzodiazepines (e.g. clonazepam), dopaminergics, opiates, and quinine.

Circadian rhythm disorders

Circadian rhythm disorders are **disruptions to the normal sleep–wake cycle**, such that the patient is out of synchrony with the sleep–wake schedule of their society. If left to their own timetables, patients with circadian rhythm disorders usually achieve adequate normal-quality sleep. However, if they are trying to function in line with other people, they often suffer severe insomnia and/or hypersomnia, which can interfere with normal social and occupational activities. The major causes of circadian rhythm disorders are outlined in Table 28.9.

Assessment

This is as for any other sleep disorder, but with greater emphasis on a detailed sleep diary. At least 2 weeks of a sleep diary should be completed. Actigraphy is useful to accurately quantify the sleep–wake cycle.

Treatment

General measures. It is very important to explain the nature of a normal sleep pattern, appropriate sleep hygiene, and the usefulness of a regular daily routine. Shift workers and time-zone travellers should adhere to regular meals and sleep wherever possible.

Chronotherapy. Depending of the nature of the sleep–wake aberration, attempts should be made to retrain the patient into a normal routine, by manipulating bedtime. A regular sleeping and waking time must be established, with no more than 7 to 8 hours' total sleep. If necessary, a phase-delay approach can be used. This involves going to bed 2 or 3 hours later than usual until the desired bedtime is reached, and then staying at this time. These are difficult strategies, and require cooperation from the patient and their family/cohabitants.

Light therapy. Phototherapy is given with a 10 000 lux lamp for 30–90 minutes before the patient's usual spontaneous awakening. The timing of the light can be gradually altered until a satisfactory waking time is reached. Light restriction may be necessary in the evenings, especially during summer. For those with advanced wakening, the light should be used in the evening to delay sleep.

Melatonin is a hormone secreted from the pineal gland during darkness, which links the sleep–wake and light–dark cycles. Many people find taking melatonin 1–2 hours before their usual bedtime can induce sleepiness. It is frequently used by travellers to avoid jetlag, especially if they have been flying eastwards.

Table 28.9 Circadian rhythm disorders

Name of disorder	Essential characteristics
Time-zone change syndrome ('jet lag')	This occurs in people who frequently travel between different time zones. Symptoms include insomnia, daytime fatigue, apathy, depression, reduced daytime alertness, and physical complaints (e.g. diarrhoea, headache).
Shift-work sleep disorder	This condition can affect those who work night shifts, or are on frequently changing rotas. Often patients complain of physical symptoms (e.g. GI upset, headaches, aches) rather than sleep difficulties.
Delayed sleep phase syndrome	The time of naturally feeling ready for sleep is delayed by 3 to 6 hours, typically until about 2 am. Total sleep time and behaviour are normal, but enforced awakening at socially convenient times produces excessive morning sleepiness. It usually presents in adolescents, in whom there is a strong association with mental disorders.
Advanced sleep phase syndrome	This is the opposite of the above, with early sleep onset (6–8 pm) and very early awakening. It is occasionally misdiagnosed as depression, due to the early morning waking.
Non-24-hour sleep–wake disorder (free-running disorder)	A rare condition in which sleeping and waking occur 1–2 hours later each day, continually going around the full 24-hour cycle. It is more common in blind individuals, and those with a history of severe head injury. It is rare that 'free-running' individuals are able to hold down conventional jobs.
Irregular sleep–wake pattern	Sleep occurs at completely irregular times, often more than one per 24 hours and for variable lengths of time. It is associated with Alzheimer's disease, hypothalamic tumours, and developmental disorders.

■ Sleep problems related to psychiatric disorders

Characteristic patterns of sleep disturbance are a part of many psychiatric conditions. It is relatively rare for patients to primarily present with a sleep disorder, but extremely common for sleep disturbance to occur secondary to the disorder or psychotropic medications. The diagnostic criteria of several psychiatric conditions (e.g. depression, mania) include sleep disturbance as an

Science box 28.1 Melatonin and jet lag

Jet lag is a miserable experience, and one increasingly encountered as international travel becomes cheaper and more widely available. Jet lag is the response of the body struggling to adjust to moving across several time zones. Symptoms include sleep disturbance for several days, fatigue, irritability, and poor concentration. This can impact significantly on those travelling for business. Melatonin is a hormone produced by the pineal gland, which is under the influence of the suprachiasmatic nuclei (SCN) of the hypothalamus. Melatonin secretion is switched off by light, so its release is associated with the time for sleep. It was claimed in the early 1990s that short-term use of melatonin could reduce the length and severity of jet lag. Has this claim been substantiated?

Many large randomized controlled trials (RCTs) have been published, the majority reporting that melatonin reduces symptoms of jet lag. In 2003, a Cochrane review was published on this topic.[1] Ten RCTs were included of airline passengers, airline staff, or military personnel given oral melatonin or placebo when crossing five or more time zones. Eight trials found melatonin to significantly reduce jet lag compared with placebo. It was found that doses of 0.5–5 mg taken at night are equally effective, but people report better sleep with 5 mg. The authors calculated the number needed to treat (NNT) as 2 (compare with a NNT of 4 for paracetamol used for acute post-operative pain). For the positive effects, melatonin must be taken in the evening. There appear to be few side effects, but it is contraindicated in those on warfarin or epileptics, and there are no safety data for children or pregnant women.

In 2006, the *British Medical Journal* published another systematic review looking at the efficacy of melatonin in various sleep disorders, including jet lag.[2] This reported no significant reduction in any sleep disturbance with melatonin compared with placebo. It did, however, confirm that melatonin is safe to use. It is clear that further research is needed to firmly establish the efficacy of melatonin in counteracting jet lag.

Melatonin is available over the counter in several countries, including the USA, but at the time of writing is not licensed for use in the UK or much of Europe.[3] It is increasingly prescribed off-licence, despite the conflicting evidence as to its efficacy.

1 Herxheimer, A. & Petrie, K. J. (2002). Melatonin for the prevention and treatment of jet lag. *Cochrane Database Systematic Review* 2: CD001520.

2 Buscemi, N., Vandermeer, B., Hooton, N., *et al.* (2006). Efficacy and safety of exogenous melatonin for secondary sleep disorders and sleep disorders accompanying sleep restriction: meta-analysis. *British Medical Journal* **332**: 385–93.

3 Jackson, G. (2010). Come fly with me: jet lag and melatonin. *International Journal of Clinical Practice* **64**: 135–41.

---

essential component. The general measures for management of sleep disorders (p. 360), are relevant in the treatment of all of the conditions below.

Mood disorders

Sleep disturbance is a central feature of all mood disorders. As sleep deprivation or excess is linked to alterations in mood (specifically irritability and depression), it is important to manage the sleep disturbance effectively. Patients with depression typically suffer from one or more of the following (in order of frequency):

- early-morning waking;
- insomnia;
- frequent awakenings during the night;
- vivid, frightening dreams;
- excessive daytime sleepiness.

Disturbed sleep is also common in manic episodes, and a reduced need for sleep is a common early warning sign of a manic episode. Antidepressants may cause a variety of disturbances of sleep, including insomnia, sleepiness, restless leg syndrome, and REM sleep behaviour disorder.

Treatment

The most important aspect of management is aggressive treatment of the underlying mood disorder, along usual guidelines. Alongside this the following may be helpful.

- Ensure a strict daily timetable of activities, good sleep hygiene, and set bedtimes. Depressed individuals often lack motivation, and will rest for excessive periods (which worsen insomnia) if not engaged in structured activities.

- Choose sedating antidepressants for insomnia; for example, mirtazapine, tricyclics, trazodone.

- Choose stimulating antidepressants for hypersomnia; for example, SSRIs, bupropion, MAOIs.

- Treat mania aggressively with antipsychotics and mood stabilizers. Try to avoid sedatives wherever possible, as they are rarely effective.

Anxiety disorders

Insomnia is a characteristic feature of all anxiety disorders, especially if they have been triggered by a stressful event. Patients also present with disrupted, poor-quality sleep, frequent awakenings, early-morning waking, and reduced total sleep time. In post-traumatic stress disorder nightmares relating to the traumatic event are common, and nocturnal panic attacks occasionally occur in panic disorder.

Treatment

The key to managing the sleep disorders is treatment of the primary anxiety disorder.

- Psychoeducation, support, and reassurance can help to reduce worrying thoughts at night. Self-help materials can be useful.
- Teach relaxation techniques, mindfulness, or yoga.
- Choose sedating antidepressants where possible.
- Short-term benzodiazepines may be used to cover the period it takes antidepressants to start working, but should not be used long term.

Eating disorders

Sleep disturbance is common in all eating disorders, but especially in anorexia nervosa. The majority of patients with anorexia nervosa suffer from insomnia, with frequent night-time awakenings and early morning waking. Some individuals wake at night to eat or to exercise in secret, and sleep may be further disturbed by anxious thoughts. Bulimia nervosa is associated with fewer sleep disturbances, but some patients complain of excessive daytime sleepiness, and others wake at night to binge.

Treatment

Appropriate management of the underlying eating disorder is the best treatment for sleep disturbance.

- Anorexia nervosa:
  - Restoration of weight to within the healthy range usually leads to a dramatic improvement in insomnia.
  - Adequate food intake in the evening and a daily planned breakfast can reduce the night-time awakenings to eat.
  - Choose sedating antidepressants where possible (e.g. mirtazapine is particularly good in eating disorders).
- Bulimia nervosa:
  - Tackling the binge–purge cycle is the key to improving sleep.
  - Adequate food intake in the evening can reduce night-time binges. Members of the household (especially the patient's bed partner) can help to reduce binges by discouraging getting up during the night.
  - SSRIs can be activating and help to decrease excessive daytime sleepiness.

Schizophrenia

Patients with schizophrenia often have insomnia, nocturnal wakefulness, or occasionally daytime sleepiness. Sleep disturbance is more common in those with persecutory symptoms. Unfortunately, it is frequently difficult to disentangle the effects of medications, psychotic symptoms, and disorganized behaviour from more fundamental sleep problems.

Treatment

- Promote good sleep hygiene.
- Behavioural approaches are often useful if the patient displays very disorganized activities and behaviour.
- Most antipsychotics promote sleep, so aggressive treatment of the underlying psychosis often helps to improve sleep patterns.
- Short-term prescription of hypnotics may be necessary when psychosis is florid, or while waiting for antipsychotics to take effect.

Dementia

All the dementia syndromes characteristically reduce total sleep time and cause poor sleep quality. Daytime napping is frequent, and often the sleep–wake cycle becomes disrupted. Night–day reversal is common in the later stages of Alzheimer's disease, which can be very difficult for carers to manage. Increased disorientation and confusion may occur in the evenings, with agitation at bedtime.

Treatment

- General principles of treating sleep disorders should be followed.
- It is important to reinforce the 24-hour cycle using environmental cues, strict daily routines, and avoidance of daytime naps.
- Evening confusion and agitation may respond to low-dose sedating antidepressants (e.g. trazodone).
- Avoid the use of hypnotics.

Alcohol and substance misuse

Both use of and withdrawal from substances can cause disturbances in sleep. Typically there is insomnia, with poor quality of sleep and a disrupted sleep–wake cycle. Symptoms of withdrawal from alcohol, opiates, or benzodiazepines cause agitation, which prevents sleep from occurring.

Treatment

- Manage the chemical dependency issues along usual guidelines. If in hospital, treat alcohol withdrawal with a reducing regime of chlordiazepoxide and regular thiamine (Pabrinex®).
- Promote good sleep hygiene measures.
- Avoid use of sedatives and hypnotics.

■ Sleep problems related to general medical conditions

It is impossible to cover the sleep disturbance related to every medical condition; therefore this section aims to highlight general principles, and the more common and/or important conditions. It is important to ask all patients—especially those in hospital—about their sleep, as poor sleep has negative effects on almost every organ system (Table 28.2) Simple measures can often improve the situation, and can have a big impact on the patient's ability to cope with their other problems. The following points should be borne in mind.

- Treatment of the underlying medical condition should be the first priority.
- Where necessary, additional treatment for the sleep disorder should be considered, and advice sought as to what is appropriate given other medications/treatments the patient is having.
- Always screen for anxiety and depression and treat along usual guidelines.
- Take a full drug history, asking specifically about over-the-counter medications. Some off-prescription drugs affect sleep adversely (e.g. nasal decongestants, slimming pills) or the patient may have tried sleeping aids. Caffeine intake in the afternoon/evenings may also be relevant.
- Avoid hypnotics wherever possible, especially in respiratory disorders, due to the risk of respiratory depression.

Table 28.10 shows a variety of sleep disorders caused by common medical conditions.

■ Drugs and sleep

Drugs, be they prescription, over-the-counter, or recreational, are a common cause of sleep disturbance. It is

Table 28.10 Sleep disorders related to general medical conditions

Medical condition	Sleep disturbance	Specific treatment strategies
Respiratory disease	Paroxysmal nocturnal dyspnoea	Tackle anxiety
• COPD	Nocturnal awakenings	Avoid hypnotics
• Asthma	Insomnia due to anxiety related to dyspnoea	Theophylline and excessive salbutamol can cause insomnia
Cardiovascular disease	Orthopnoea	Review antihypertensives, as some cause insomnia
• Cardiac failure	Nocturnal angina	
• Angina		Beta-blockers cause nightmares
Gastro-oesophageal reflux disease, peptic ulcers, oesophagitis	Nocturnal awakenings related to reflux	
Iron deficiency	Restless leg syndrome	Iron supplements; treat underlying condition
	Periodic limb movements in sleep	
Endocrine disease	Awakenings, OSA	
• Diabetes	Insomnia	
• Hyperthyroidism	OSA	
• Hypothyroidism		

Table 28.10 Sleep disorders related to general medical conditions (*Continued*)

Medical condition	Sleep disturbance	Specific treatment strategies
Parkinson's disease	Progressive insomnia	Review antiparkinson medication
	Parasomnias	Behavioural modifications
	Hypersomnia	Clonazepam is very effective
	Periodic limb movements in sleep	
Epilepsy	Disrupted night-time sleep combined with hypersomnia	Control seizures
		Sedating anti-epileptic drugs
Conditions causing chronic pain (including rheumatological conditions and cancer)	Insomnia, disrupted sleep	Corticosteroids and NSAIDs disrupt sleep
		Optimize pain relief; many strong analgesics are sedatives
Chronic renal failure	Disrupted sleep, OSA, restless leg syndrome	Improves with dialysis

OSA, obstructive sleep apnoea.

Reproduced (with alterations) from Gelder, M., Andreasen, N., Lopez-Ibor, J, & Geddes, J. (eds). *New Oxford Textbook of Psychiatry*, 2nd edn (2009), p. 92. Oxford University Press, Oxford.

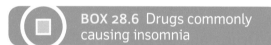

BOX 28.6 Drugs commonly causing insomnia

Antidepressants (SSRIs, MAOIs, venlafaxine)
Antiparkinsonian medication
Bronchodilators
Cardiovascular medication (beta-blockers, digoxin, verapamil)
Chemotherapy drugs
Corticosteroids
NSAIDs
Stimulants (methylphenidate, metamphetamine, dexamphetamine, cocaine, caffeine, nicotine)
Thyroxine
Withdrawal (hypnotics, opiates, alcohol, cannabis)

BOX 28.7 Drugs commonly causing hypersomnia

Antidepressants	Anti-epileptic drugs
Anti-emetics	Antihistamines
Antipsychotics	Antiparkinson drugs
Anxiolytics	Hypnotics
Progestogens	Methyldopa

imperative always to take a full drug history (including all three categories, and alcohol, caffeine, and nicotine) in all patients you see. Boxes 28.6 and 28.7 show some of the more common culprits causing insomnia and hypersomnia, respectively, but these are not comprehensive lists and it is worth always looking up individual drugs.

Alcohol is a highly effective sedative, and is commonly used by those with anxiety and mood disorders to self-medicate insomnia. Acute use of alcohol causes an increased total sleep time, but also vivid dreams and nightmares. However, chronic alcoholism or withdrawal from alcohol can cause insomnia.

Nicotine is a stimulant, and smoking in the evenings can disrupt sleep patterns or cause insomnia. High-dose nicotine patches may have the same effect, so the 16-hour (rather than 24-hour) patches may be preferred by patients.

Opiates tend to cause sedation and improved sleep quality when used in therapeutic doses, but produce profound insomnia when associated with misuse. Insomnia and increased alertness are important features of withdrawal, and are often difficult for patients to manage.

Further reading

National Institute of Clinical Excellence (2004). *Guidance on the Use of Zoleplon, Zolpidem and Zopiclone for the Short-Term Management of Insomnia.* http://guidance.nice.org.uk/TA77/Guidance/pdf/English.

National Institute of Clinical Excellence (2008). *Continuous Positive Airway Pressure for the Treatment of Obstructive Sleep Apnoea/Hypoapnoea.* http://guidance.nice.org.uk/TA139/

American Academy of Sleep Disorders (2001). *The International Classification of Sleep Disorders, Revised. A Diagnostic and Coding Manual.* American Academy of Sleep Disorders, Darien, IL.

Arroll, B., Fernando III, A. & Falloon, K. (2008). 10 minute consultation: sleep disorder (insomnia). *British Medical Journal* **337**: a1245.

Smith, M. T., Perlis, M. L., Park, A., *et al.* (2002) Comparative meta-analysis of pharmacotherapy and behavior therapy for persistent insomnia. *American Journal of Psychiatry* **159**: 5–11.

Schwartz, J. R. & Roth, T. (2008). Neurophysiology of sleep and wakefulness: basic science and clinical implications. *Current Neuropharmacology* **6**: 367–78.

CHAPTER 29

Problems due to use of alcohol and other psychoactive substances

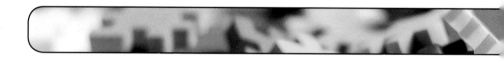

■ Overview of issues relating to psychoactive substance misuse

The use of alcohol and other psychoactive substances has been recorded throughout history, often with the primary aim of changing an individual's mood or relieving the distress of harsh circumstances. Early examples include the chewing of tobacco leaves or coca (cocaine) in North America and Peru, respectively. Humans are clearly vulnerable to the desire to use substances; this is illustrated by the fact that alcohol and other psychoactive substances remain a leading cause of medical and social problems worldwide. World Health Organization (WHO) statistics report that alcohol is the primary causative factor in 4 per cent of the global burden of disease. Although there are a vast number of different substances available, only a few are commonly used, and all produce similar harms upon the individual and society. This chapter will cover the following, focusing on providing a general approach to managing a patient presenting with a problem stemming from substance misuse:

- epidemiology of substance use and misuse;
- terminology (which is often confusing);
- problems associated with alcohol and their management;
- problems associated with the use of substances other than alcohol, and the generic principles of assessment and treatment;
- a brief overview of the characteristics of some commonly used substances;
- principles of prevention of drug misuse.

Epidemiology

It is extremely difficult to gather accurate data on the use of substances in the general population, especially if they are illegal. It is therefore likely that most figures are under-estimations of the true incidence. The WHO estimates that tobacco, alcohol, and illicit drugs are a factor in 12.4 per cent of all deaths worldwide. This is a stark reminder of the severity that problems associated with substance usage can reach, but the morbidity surrounding them affects a much wider section of society. In the UK, 90 per cent of adults drink alcohol, a quarter smoke tobacco, and 10 per cent admit to having used an illegal drug at least once in their lifetime. Worldwide, the highest prevalence of drug misuse is found in the 16- to 30-year age group, with males outnumbering females at a ratio of 4 to 1. Table 29.1 shows a selection of epidemiological figures associated with commonly used substances.

Terminology related to the use of psychoactive substances

Substance misuse is associated with an array of confusing terminology, the majority describing different disorders that may occur due to use of any substance. The terms used are common to the DSM-IV and ICD-10 classifications, and are internationally agreed.

- **Intoxication** is the direct psychological and physical effects of the substance that are dose dependent and time limited. They are individual to the substance and typically include both pleasurable and unpleasant symptoms.

- **Harmful use.** A pattern of psychoactive substance use that is causing damage to health. The damage may be

Table 29.1 Epidemiology of psychoactive substance misuse

Substance	Prevalence
Alcohol	2 billion users worldwide
	26% of UK adults have alcohol use disorder
	6% of UK adults have alcohol dependency
Tobacco	26% of UK adults, 28% in the USA
Cocaine	2–5% lifetime prevalence in Europe
Opioids	Estimated 3 million IV users worldwide; UK cost £1 billion per year
Hallucinogens	3% aged 16–30 years report lifetime use
Benzodiazepines	15% lifetime risk in developed countries
Ecstasy	15% of young people report lifetime use

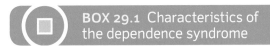

BOX 29.1 Characteristics of the dependence syndrome

1 A **strong desire** or sense of compulsion to take the substance.

2 **Difficulties in refraining** from using the substance.

3 A physiological **withdrawal state** when substance use has stopped or been reduced. Withdrawal symptoms may be avoided by further use of the substance.

4 Evidence of **tolerance**.

5 Progressive **neglect of alternative pleasures or interests** due to the use of the psychoactive substance and the time needed to obtain supplies, or to recover from its effects.

6 **Persistent use of the substance despite clear evidence of harm.**

physical (for example, abscesses due to the self-administration of injected substances) or mental (e.g. memory loss secondary to heavy consumption of alcohol).

- **Dependence.** A syndrome that includes withdrawal states, tolerance, and other features such as persistent use despite harmful effects (Box 29.1). Dependence may be both *physical* (when physiological tolerance occurs) and *psychological*.

- **Tolerance** is the state in which repeated administration leads to decreasing effect.

- **Withdrawal** is a set of symptoms and signs occurring when a substance is reduced or stopped after persistent usage. The nature, time to onset, and course of the symptoms vary for different substances and may include convulsions or delirium.

- **Substance-induced psychosis.** Hallucinations and/or delusions directly due to substance misuse. Psychosis may occur during intoxication or withdrawal, or as a chronic aspect of dependency.

- **Amnesic syndrome** is the chronic prominent impairment of recent and remote memory. Immediate recall is usually preserved and recent memory is characteristically more disturbed than remote memory. Disturbances of time sense and ordering of events are usually evident, as are difficulties in learning new material. Confabulation may be marked but is not invariably present. Other cognitive functions are usually relatively well preserved and amnesic defects are out of proportion to other disturbances. It may be caused by intoxication or chronic use of alcohol, solvents, benzodiazepines, and possibly cannabis.

Why do people use substances?

There are a myriad of reasons why someone might take a substance at a given time; however, some general reasons apply and are listed below. The initial reason for taking a substance is often straightforward, but may become more complex and change over time.

Pleasurable experiences. About one-fifth of drug use is primarily to gain pleasure, usually in the form of a buzz or high, numbness, drowsiness, or comfort. Those who experience energy and confidence will often use to try and relive the initial experience they encountered. In the 1960s, when drug taking was especially prevalent, the 'search for meaning' or 'mystical experiences' was a frequent reason for usage, but this has declined since.

Availability. The availability of most psychoactive substances is limited in one way or another. If a substance is easily available people are more likely to use it; however, illegal substances also hold a particular fascination to some individuals. Psychoactive substances are usually obtained in one of three ways:

- prescribed by doctors (e.g. benzodiazepines);
- purchased legally (e.g. nicotine, alcohol, and, for adults, solvents);
- purchased illegally: this category includes most of the other substances discussed in this chapter plus nicotine, alcohol, and solvents under certain age limits. Control of the availability of such drugs depends on political action and requires extensive activity by the police and other enforcement agencies to detect and control the importation and distribution of drugs.

Anxiety disorders are the commonest form of psychiatric disorder and many people take drugs (especially alcohol and benzodiazepines) to reduce anxiety. Those with undiagnosed social anxiety disorder are the most likely to do so.

Self-medication for psychiatric co-morbidities is extremely common, with the aim of reducing unwanted symptoms. Alcohol is used in anxiety, depression, and stress-related disorders. Stimulants and cannabis are commonly taken by schizophrenics and those with bipolar disorder.

Relieving physical symptoms such as pain is a relatively common reason for substance use. People with chronic pain syndromes or neurological conditions such as multiple sclerosis are the frequent users.

Boredom is occasionally cited as a reason to take drugs, especially amongst young men in difficult social circumstances.

Peer pressure may be prevalent amongst teenagers and university students. Personal vulnerability (a lack of personal resources needed to cope with the challenges of life) is a cause of the success of peer pressure.

Attitudes of the community. Some social, cultural, and religious groups disapprove of drug taking, and this shared value helps to restrain its members. In other groups, drug taking is condoned or even encouraged and it gives a person status among his peers.

Dependence and tolerance develop as time progresses, and a physical and psychological 'need' for the drug will take over from previous reasons for use.

The law

In the UK, the legal framework for managing people who take psychoactive substances is defined by the **Misuse of Drugs Act of 1971** and its subsequent amendments. The allied laws within the USA are under the **Controlled Drugs Act,** and most other countries have relevant legislation. The Misuse of Drugs Act segregates illegal drugs into three classes (A, B, and C) according to the relative dangers of each drug to both an individual and society as a whole. Some of the drugs in each category are shown in Box 29.2. The current law was not created from a scientific evidence base pertaining to individual risks, but on socio-economic damage to society. There is therefore some debate as to the validity of the current system. The classification of a particular substance is not set in stone; for example, cannabis was changed from a class B to a class C drug in 2004, and then back to class B in 2009. It is notable that as non-controlled legal drugs, alcohol and tobacco do not feature at all in the classification system. Punishable offences include:

- possession of a controlled substance unlawfully;
- possession of a controlled substance with intent to supply it;
- supplying or offering to supply a controlled drug;
- allowing premises you occupy or manage to be used unlawfully for the purpose of producing or supplying controlled drugs.

The penalties do not relate to individuals holding a valid prescription or licence for the drug (e.g. heroin as diamorphine may be prescribed by a doctor). In the UK it is the patient's responsibility to inform the Driver and Vehicle Licensing Agency (DVLA) of 'any disability likely to affect safe driving', which includes drug misuse. In 2000, a new piece of legislation called Drug Testing and Treatment Orders was introduced. A court may order a person with a drug problem to undergo treatment and follow-up in the community for up to 3 years. This includes urine drug toxicology.

BOX 29.2 Classification of illegal drugs under the UK Misuse of Drugs Act 1971

Class A

- Ecstasy
- LSD
- Heroin
- Cocaine and crack
- Magic mushrooms (whether prepared or fresh)
- Methylamphetamine and other amphetamines if prepared for injection

Possession—up to 7 years' imprisonment and/or an unlimited fine
Supply—up to life imprisonment and/or an unlimited fine

Class B

- Cannabis
- Amphetamines

- Methylphenidate (Ritalin)
- Pholcodine

Possession—up to 5 years' imprisonment and/or an unlimited fine

Supply—up to 14 years' imprisonment and/or an unlimited fine

Class C

- Tranquillizers
- GHB (gamma hydroxybutyrate)
- Ketamine
- Benzodiazepines
- Anabolic steroids

Possession—up to 2 years' imprisonment and/or an unlimited fine

Supply—up to 14 years' imprisonment and/or an unlimited fine

The harms associated with taking psychoactive substances

There are a variety of potential problems associated with taking substances. These are discussed in further detail under the specific sections for each substance, but Table 29.2 shows the general types of problems that commonly occur. It is rare for one negative effect of a drug to occur in isolation; frequently if the person is being physically affected by their drug usage, it is likely they will be dependent upon the substance and that it will be having social consequences too.

The stages of change model in relation to substance misuse

Much of the way in which we approach the treatment of problems relating to drug usage is based upon the concept

Table 29.2 Categories of harm associated with taking substances

Physical damage	Relating to dependence	Social harm
Acute: harms following a single dose of the drug (e.g. respiratory depression from opioids).	**Intensity of pleasure:** highly pleasurable drugs tend to fetch a higher street value. Smoking or IV injection of drugs creates the fastest effects but requires stronger, more dangerous formulations.	**Intoxication:** harm or damage to property and people due to a single drug use (e.g. violence or car accidents due to alcohol).
Chronic: harms due to long-term or regular drug use (e.g. lung cancer caused by tobacco).		**Social harms:** destruction of the individual's social circle, family, and personal achievements.
Intravenous drug use: highest risk of acute toxicity and secondary harms; for example, blood-borne viruses (HIV, hepatitis) or abscesses.	**Physical dependence and tolerance:** needing drugs in ever higher doses to avoid withdrawal.	**Cost to the economy:** unemployment or poor productivity, the police, and the cost to health service providers can be very high.
	Psychological dependence: intense cravings.	

that there are stages of change. It is therefore helpful to understand this idea before moving on to the descriptions of managing specific substance problems. The stages of change model was developed in the late 1970s by DiClemente and Prochaska and was based on work studying how cigarette smokers could give up the habit. It relates to all drugs on which humans become dependent, but is most commonly used in alcohol and opioid misuse or weight loss/eating disorder programmes. The premise is that deciding to stop using the substance is a behavioural change, and that behavioural change only occurs via a series of steps rather than one leap. Each person progresses through these steps (or stages) at their own pace. The five stages of change (shown in Figure 29.1) are:

- **Precontemplation.** Not yet acknowledging that there is a problem behaviour that needs to be changed. At this stage the person is not interested in any form of help, and any imposed treatment will not be successful.

- **Contemplation.** Acknowledging that there is a problem but not yet ready or sure of wanting to make a change. These individuals are usually open to receiving more education about the risks of their behaviour, and will consider the advantages and disadvantages of making a change.

- **Preparation.** Getting ready to change. The person has made a commitment to change, and will research methods of doing so.

- **Action.** Changing behaviour. This is the time when people are usually open to receiving help, and may seek support in doing so.

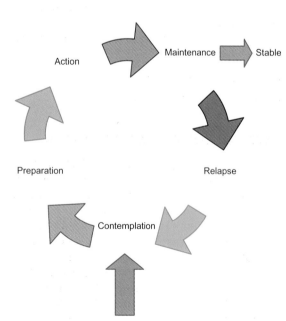

Fig. 29.1 The stages of change model.

- **Maintenance.** Maintaining the behaviour change, and successfully avoiding any temptation to return to old habits.

- **Relapse.** Returning to older behaviours and abandoning the new changes. This may then link back into precontemplation to complete the cycle.

The majority of individuals with a substance misuse problem will go around the cycle many times before entering a stable state. They may learn to recognize the pitfalls that led them to relapse on a previous occasion, and reduce their chance of doing so again. Understanding what stage your patient is at is essential for determining if they are likely to engage with treatment, deciding what support is appropriate, and having realistic expectations of the outcome.

■ Alcohol-related problems

There are at least two billion users of alcohol worldwide, and alcohol is a major public health concern in most countries. Remembering to screen for alcohol misuse, recognizing the physical and psychological complications, and having the ability to offer basic advice and treatment are essential for all clinicians.

Terminology

Although the term **alcoholism** is widely used in everyday speech, it has too broad a meaning to be clinically useful. It can refer to excessive consumption of alcohol, to dependence on alcohol, or to the damage caused by excessive use. The following terms constitute more useful categories.

- **Hazardous drinking** is a level or pattern of drinking that will eventually cause harm. It applies to anyone drinking above the recommended limits, but without current alcohol-related problems. It is not a diagnostic term in ICD-10/DSM-IV.

- **Harmful drinking** refers to a pattern of use that has already caused physical, mental, or social damage to the user. It excludes those with dependence syndrome. Damage may be acute or chronic. It is a term used in the ICD-10 but not the DSM-IV.

- **Alcohol abuse** is the term used in the DSM-IV that is most similar to harmful drinking. It involves the continued drinking of alcohol despite significant employment, social, legal, or dangerous problems resulting from it.

- **Dependent drinking (ICD-10) or alcohol dependency (DSM-IV).** There are seven characteristics of dependence upon alcohol, three of which must have been present in the previous year to make a diagnosis:

1 Tolerance, as defined by either of the following:

   a a need for markedly increased amounts of alcohol to achieve intoxication or the desired effect;

   b a markedly diminished effect with continued use of the same amount of alcohol.

2 Withdrawal, as defined by either of the following:

   a the characteristic withdrawal syndrome for alcohol;

   b alcohol is taken to relieve or avoid withdrawal symptoms.

3 Alcohol is often taken in larger amounts or over a longer period than was intended.

4 There is a persistent desire for or there are unsuccessful efforts to cut down or control alcohol use.

5 A great deal of time is spent in activities necessary to obtain alcohol, use alcohol, or recover from its effects.

6 Important social, occupational, or recreational activities are given up or reduced because of alcohol use.

7 Alcohol use is continued despite knowledge of having a persistent or recurrent physical or psychological problem that is likely to have been caused or exacerbated by the alcohol.

Collectively, all of these categories of disorder are best described as **alcohol problems.**

Alcohol dependence syndrome

Heavy drinking can lead to an alcohol dependence syndrome. The specific features of alcohol dependence are that in the late stages of dependence, due to liver damage, tolerance falls and the dependent drinker becomes incapacitated after only a few drinks. Since they can stave off withdrawal symptoms only by further drinking (**relief drinking**), many dependent drinkers take a drink on waking. In most cultures, early-morning drinking is diagnostic of dependency. With an increasing need to stave off withdrawal symptoms during the day, the drinker typically becomes secretive about the amount consumed, hides bottles, or carries them in a pocket or handbag. Rough cider and cheap wines may be drunk regularly to obtain the most alcohol for the least money. A person dependent on alcohol develops a **stereotyped pattern of drinking.** Whereas the ordinary drinker varies his intake from day to day, the dependent person drinks at regular intervals to relieve or avoid withdrawal symptoms. Once established, the syndrome usually progresses steadily and destructively, unless the patient stops drinking or manages to bring it under control. A severely dependent person who achieves abstinence but then drinks again is likely to relapse quickly and totally, returning to his old drinking pattern within a few days (**reinstatement after abstinence**).

What is a safe level of alcohol consumption?

The relation between alcohol consumption and harm is not straightforward. Low levels of alcohol consumption may protect older people against coronary heart disease. Very high levels clearly do harm, but where is the dividing line between safe and unsafe consumption? A widely accepted measure is in terms of **units of alcohol**; one unit is 8 g of ethanol, and corresponds to the following measures in which alcohol is usually consumed:

- half a pint of beer (3–4 per cent);
- a wine glass of wine (125 ml);
- a sherry glass of sherry or other fortified wine (50 ml);
- a standard measure of spirits (25 ml).

These measures are clinically useful but should not be regarded as precise because the strengths of different beers and wines vary. Although it is difficult to assess the exact relationship between intake and harm, it is generally agreed that the 'safe level' of alcohol consumption is:

- men: up to **21 units** per week;
- women: up to **14 units** per week (lower because of the lower average body weight of females).

These levels assume that the whole amount is not taken on one occasion and that there are occasional drink-free days. This level is equivalent, for example, to an average of three half pints of beer a day for a man. These limits should be modified in some patients; for example, pregnant women should be advised to abstain from alcohol.

Dangerous levels of drinking (i.e. levels of consumption at which harm is likely) are:

- men: over **50 units** per week;
- women: over **35 units** per week.

Alcohol consumption in the population

Reliable epidemiological data are difficult to obtain because people tend to underestimate both the amount they drink and the consequences of their drinking. Since 1945, the absolute quantity of alcohol consumed in Britain has increased threefold. UK National Statistics report that 93 per cent of men and 87 per cent of women drink alcohol, and one-quarter (women) to one-third (men) of these individuals have an alcohol problem. Alcohol dependence is not particularly common (6 per cent of males and 2 per cent of females in the general population). The lifetime risk of an alcohol use disorder for a British male is 20 per cent. Overall problems relating to alcohol are more common in men than in women, although the gap is gradually closing. Excessive binge-drinking is most likely in young males, but alcohol problems are most common in those aged 30–50 years. Whereas men in lower socio-economic classes are the highest consumers of alcohol amongst their peers, women in professional and managerial employment are the most at risk.

The rates of dangerous consumption of alcohol are much increased among people working in occupations that provide easy access to alcohol; for example, barmen, brewery workers, and kitchen porters. They are also higher among executives, salesmen, journalists, actors, and others whose work is associated with social drinking. Doctors also have high rates of dangerous consumption.

There is marked international variation in alcohol consumption per capita. European countries such as France and Italy have higher levels of consumption than countries such as the USA and UK—although the differences are decreasing with time. The higher the average consumption in a community, the greater the percentage of people who drink dangerous amounts of alcohol. This is because the consumption of alcohol in the general population is normally distributed; thus the higher average is not due to an outlying group of very heavy drinkers. This has an important practical implication. It means that population-based methods aimed at reducing everyone's level of alcohol consumption will reduce the number of people who drink dangerous amounts of alcohol.

Alcohol-related harm

Consumption of alcohol can lead to three types of harm: physical, neuropsychiatric, and social. This harm can occur whether or not the person has become dependent on alcohol, although very high levels of consumption are likely to cause dependency.

Alcohol intoxication. Clinical symptoms of alcohol intoxication relate jointly to the level of alcohol in the blood and the tolerance of the individual. Increasing blood alcohol levels lead to elated or unstable mood, impaired judgement, disinhibition, impaired social and occupational functioning, cognitive impairment, ataxia, slurred speech, incoordination, nystagmus, and eventually coma. This state leads to an increased risk of accidents (especially road traffic accidents), violence, and public order offences.

Physical effects of alcohol abuse

The main physical consequences of dangerous use of alcohol (Table 29.3) are as follows.

- **Gastrointestinal disorders.** These are common, notably gastritis and peptic ulcer, damage to the liver, oesoph-

Table 29.3 Physical effects of the excessive use of alcohol

Gastrointestinal	Malnutrition and vitamin deficiencies (A, B, D, E, and folate)
	Carcinoma of the lip, tongue, pharynx, and larynx
	Gastritis and peptic ulcer
	Oesophageal varices
	Oesophageal carcinoma
	Acute and chronic pancreatitis
	Fatty liver, hepatitis, cirrhosis, and primary liver carcinoma
Neurological	Peripheral neuropathy
	Dementia
	Wernicke's encephalopathy
	Korsakoff's syndrome
	Cerebellar degeneration
	Epilepsy
	Fetal alcohol syndrome
Other	Anaemia, thrombocytopenia, and leukopenia
	Episodic hypoglycaemia
	Haemochromatosis
	Hypertension
	Cardiomyopathy
	Myopathy
	Osteoporosis and osteomalacia
	Obesity or emaciation
	Facial erythema (plethora)
	Exacerbation of psoriasis
	Gout

ageal varices and carcinoma, and acute or chronic pancreatitis. The ratio of acute pancreatitis caused by gallstones compared with alcohol is decreasing in the Western world. About 5 per cent of those with alcohol dependence develop chronic pancreatitis, and present with weight loss, steatorrhoea, and diabetes mellitus. Damage to the liver includes fatty infiltration, hepatitis, cirrhosis, and hepatocellular carcinoma. A person dependent on alcohol has a tenfold greater risk than average of dying of cirrhosis of the liver. Eighty per cent of cirrhosis deaths are due to alcohol.

- **Malnutrition and vitamin deficiency** are due to a combination of poor food intake and malabsorption caused directly by alcohol. Alcoholics almost universally have deficiencies in vitamins B_1 (thiamine), A, D, B_6, E, and folate. The latter causes a macrocytic anaemia, which adds to the direct toxic effect of alcohol upon the bone marrow.

- **Disorders of the nervous system.** These include peripheral neuropathy, dementia, cerebellar degeneration, and epilepsy, as well as several less common effects on the optic nerve, pons, and corpus callosum. Neuropsychiatric disorders are described below.

- **Cardiovascular disorders.** Alcohol increases blood pressure, thereby increasing the risk of stroke. Modest amounts of alcohol have been shown to actually reduce the level of coronary artery disease, but this association does not continue above safe drinking limits. A dilated cardiomyopathy is common. Thiamine deficiency can lead to beriberi, which in turn can produce a high-output cardiac failure. This is now rare.

- **Musculoskeletal disorders** secondary to alcohol misuse are an under-recognized phenomenon. Chronic myopathy, which can include severe wasting, is seen in 60 per cent of those with a long history of alcohol dependency, as alcohol is toxic to skeletal muscles. Patients complain of pain and weakness, and immobility can become a problem, predisposing to infection. Osteoporosis and osteomalacia may also occur, and are a combination of dietary insufficiencies and direct toxicity of alcohol upon bone.

From these and other causes, the overall **mortality rate** of subjects consuming dangerous levels of alcohol is estimated to be about twice the expected level.

Effects on the fetus

It was recognized that alcohol could adversely affect the developing fetus in the mid-1960s. Heavy drinking during pregnancy may cause a syndrome of facial abnormality, growth retardation, muscular incoordination, low intelligence, and hyperactivity known as **fetal alcohol syndrome**. It is uncertain whether such effects are seen only after very heavy drinking by the mother or whether lesser degrees of damage are seen after less heavy drinking. Nevertheless, it is prudent to advise pregnant women to abstain from alcohol throughout pregnancy. If they will not accept this advice, they should be counselled strongly to avoid drinking in the first trimester, and to avoid heavy drinking.

Neuropsychiatric disorders due to alcohol abuse

Alcohol-related psychiatric disabilities fall into several groups (Table 29.4).

Abnormal forms of intoxication

As well as the familiar picture of drunkenness described previously, people who consume dangerous amounts of alcohol persistently may develop two syndromes.

Table 29.4 Neuropsychiatric effects of the excessive use of alcohol

Intoxication states	Memory blackouts
	Idiosyncratic intoxication
Withdrawal states	Simple and complex withdrawal
	Delirium tremens
Toxic and nutritional states	Korsakov's syndrome
	Wernicke's encephalopathy
	Alcoholic dementia
Perceptual disturbances	Transient hallucinations
	Alcoholic hallucinosis
Neurological conditions	Cerebellar degeneration
	Marchiafava–Bignami syndrome
Associated states	Depressive disorder
	Anxiety symptoms
	Suicide and deliberate self-harm
	Personality change
	Pathological jealousy
	Sexual dysfunction

- **Memory blackouts (alcohol-induced amnesia)** are losses of memory for events that occurred during a period of intoxication. Such episodes can occur after a single episode of heavy drinking in people who do not habitually abuse alcohol. When they occur regularly they indicate frequent heavy drinking; when they are prolonged, affecting the greater part of a day or whole days, they indicate sustained excessive drinking.

- **Idiosyncratic intoxication** (or pathological drunkenness) is a marked change of behaviour occurring within minutes of taking alcohol in amounts that would not induce drunkenness in most people. Often, the behaviour is aggressive.

Withdrawal phenomena

Alcohol withdrawal syndrome

Withdrawal symptoms appear characteristically on waking, after the fall in blood alcohol concentration during sleep. The earliest and commonest feature is acute tremulousness affecting the hands, legs, and trunk ('the shakes'). The sufferer may be agitated and easily startled, and often dreads facing people or crossing the road. Nausea, retching, and sweating are frequent. If more alcohol is drunk, these symptoms are usually relieved quickly; if not, they may last for several days. As withdrawal progresses, misperceptions and hallucinations may briefly occur. Objects appear distorted in shape, or shadows seem to move; disorganized voices, shouting, or snatches of music may be heard. Later there may be epileptic seizures, and finally, after about 48 hours, **delirium tremens** may develop.

Delirium tremens

This is a severe form of withdrawal syndrome that occurs when the patient is physically dependent on alcohol. The features are as follows.

- **Delirium**: clouding of consciousness, disorientation in time and place, impairment of recent memory, illusions and hallucinations, fearfulness, and agitation.

- Special features of gross **tremor** of the hands (which gives the condition its name), ataxia, **autonomic disturbance** (sweating, tachycardia, raised blood pressure, dilation of the pupils), and marked **insomnia**. There may also be fever.

- **Hallucinations** are characteristically visual and often frightening, involving Lilliputian people or animals. Auditory and tactile hallucinations also occur.

- **Dehydration and electrolyte disturbance** are characteristic. Blood testing shows leucocytosis, raised erythrocyte sedimentation rate (ESR), and impaired liver function.

Delirium tremens usually lasts 3–4 days. As in other kinds of delirium, the symptoms are characteristically worse at night. The condition often ends in deep and prolonged sleep from which the person awakes with no symptoms and little or no memory of the period of delirium. It has a mortality rate of up to 5 per cent. The treatment of delirium tremens (p. 391) is described for withdrawal plus the general measures for treating delirium on p. 317.

Toxic and nutritional conditions

There are three neuropsychiatric disorders of this kind: (i) **Wernicke's encephalopathy,** (ii) **Korsakoff's syndrome,** and (iii) **alcoholic dementia**.

Wernicke's encephalopathy

Wernicke's encephalopathy is an acute-onset degenerative encephalopathy due to thiamine deficiency. The deficiency results from a combination of poor nutritional intake, reduced absorption, decreased hepatic storage, and impaired usage. It is occasionally seen in non-alcoholics; for example, anorexia nervosa, hyperemesis gravidarum, starvation, or post-gastric resection. Wernicke's is characterized by haemorrhages and secondary gliosis in the periventricular and periaqueductal grey matter, which causes damage to the structures surrounding them. The worst affected areas are the hypothalamus, midbrain, and cerebellar peduncles. Clinically,

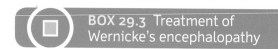

BOX 29.3 Treatment of Wernicke's encephalopathy

- Admit as an inpatient to a general hospital setting with resuscitation facilities.

- Give high-dose parenteral B vitamins for 3–7 days. Typically two ampoules of Pabrinex® (500 mg thiamine) are given IV three times daily.

- There is a high risk of anaphylaxis with Pabrinex® IV, reduced by giving IM. The patient should be closely monitored.

- Treat withdrawal with a benzodiazepine reducing regimen.

- If the patient responds, continue Pabrinex® until the improvement ceases. If there is no response, stop the treatment.

- Continue oral thiamine 100 mg three times daily for at least a month.

Wernicke's presents as a tetrad of **acute confusion, ophthalmoplegia, nystagmus,** and **ataxia**. The patient may also develop an acute peripheral neuropathy and tachycardia. This is an emergency presentation, the treatment of which is shown in Box 29.3. Prevention of Wernicke's is simple—adequate provision of thiamine. Patients with an alcohol problem should be advised to take vitamin B supplements, and those undergoing detoxification prescribed high-dose prophylaxis.

Korsakoff's syndrome (amnesic syndrome)

About 80 per cent of people who have Wernicke's encephalopathy go on to develop Korsakoff's syndrome, but it may also occur independently. The central features of Korsakoff's syndrome are retrograde and anterograde amnesia, especially a profound impairment of recent memory. The patient can recall events immediately after they have occurred, but cannot do so even a few minutes afterwards. Thus, on the standard clinical test of remembering an address, immediate recall is good, but grossly impaired 10 minutes later. One consequence of the profound disorder of memory is an associated disorientation in time. Gaps in memory are often filled by confabulation.

The patient may give a vivid and detailed account of recent activities that, on checking, turn out to be inaccurate. Such a patient is often suggestible and therefore vulnerable. Other cognitive functions are relatively well preserved. Unlike the patient with dementia, the patient with an amnesic syndrome seems alert and able to reason or hold an ordinary conversation, so that the interviewer may at first be unaware of the extent of the memory disorder. The aetiology is not clear, but may be partly due to thiamine deficiency. Long-term thiamine replacement is therefore recommended. About 75 per cent of patients will have static memory impairment, whilst the other quarter are split equally into those who slightly improve and those who decline in a step-wise process.

Alcoholic dementia

Alcoholic dementia can arise after prolonged, heavy intake of alcohol. Intellectual impairment is often associated with enlarged ventricles and widened cerebral sulci, as seen on a computed tomography (CT) scan. After prolonged abstinence, some gradual improvement occurs in these changes, suggesting that the shrinkage is not wholly due to the loss of the brain cells. The causes of the dementia are uncertain but probably include a direct toxic effect of alcohol on the brain, and secondary effects of liver disease.

Perceptual disturbances

Transient hallucinations of vision or hearing are reported by some heavy drinkers, generally during withdrawal, but without all the features of delirium tremens or alcoholic hallucinosis.

Alcoholic hallucinosis is a rare condition characterized by distressing auditory hallucinations (usually of voices uttering threats) occurring in clear consciousness. Some patients argue aloud with the voices, others feel compelled to follow instructions from them. Delusional misinterpretations may follow, often of a persecutory kind, so that the clinical picture can resemble schizophrenia. The condition can arise while the person is still drinking heavily, or when intake has been reduced. It is of variable duration and when chronic needs to be distinguished from a primary schizophrenic disorder. It usually responds to antipsychotics and has a good prognosis. The symptoms may reoccur if drinking resumes.

Cerebellar degeneration

Alcohol is directly toxic to the Purkinje cells of the cerebellar cortex. Destruction of these cells leads to a chronic cerebellar atrophy in about 40 per cent of chronic alcoholics. Patients present with severe limb ataxia, dysarthria, poor coordination, slurred speech, and occasionally nystagmus.

Associated psychiatric disorders

- **Depressive disorder** may be induced by drinking as alcohol is a central nervous system depressant. However, depressed patients sometimes drink heavily to relieve their symptoms, so care needs to be taken to find out the sequence of changes. In alcohol dependence, 80 per cent of patients fit diagnostic criteria for depression. Many will recover without treatment if they remain abstinent, otherwise an antidepressant may be beneficial.

- **Anxiety symptoms** occur frequently, especially during periods of partial withdrawal. The most common are phobias, generalized anxiety, and panic attacks. The latter may occur during intoxification, withdrawal, or up to 4 weeks after cessation of drinking. Also, some patients with a primary anxiety disorder use alcohol to relieve their symptoms. So, as with depression, care is needed to determine the sequence.

- **Suicidal behaviour and deliberate self-harm** are more frequent among people who use alcohol heavily than among other people of the same age. Estimates of the proportion of harmful users of alcohol who eventually kill themselves vary from 6 to 20 per cent.

- **Personality change** in heavy users of alcohol often includes self-centredness, lack of concern for others, and a decline in standards of conduct (particularly honesty and responsibility).

- **Pathological jealousy (Othello's syndrome)** is an infrequent but serious complication of heavy alcohol use.

- **Sexual dysfunction** is common, usually as erectile dysfunction or delayed ejaculation. The causes include the direct effects of alcohol and a generally impaired relationship with the sexual partner as a result of heavy drinking.

Social damage due to alcohol

Excessive drinking can cause serious social damage, including:

- poor work performance and sickness absence;
- unemployment;
- violence and aggressive behaviour towards the family or general public;
- accidental damage;
- road accidents: in the UK about a third of drivers killed on the road have blood alcohol levels above the statutory limit, and among those killed on a Saturday night the figure is estimated to be three-quarters;
- crime, mainly social disorder and petty offences, but also fraud, sexual offences, and crimes of violence including murder;
- emotional and conduct problems in the patient's children;
- healthcare costs tend to be extremely high; alcohol is implicated in 50–70 per cent of emergency room admissions and 16 per cent of total hospital admissions.

Co-morbidities

The majority of psychiatric disorders are more common in patients with alcohol problems, and the issue is clouded by alcohol being a causative factor in many of them too. Frequent co-morbidities include:

- depression;
- anxiety disorders;
- suicide (4 per cent lifetime risk) and deliberate self-harm;
- schizophrenia (20 per cent of those with schizophrenia have an alcohol problem);
- substance misuse: people may take substances either to enhance the positive aspects of alcohol or reduce the unpleasant side effects; benzodiazepines are a particular risk, especially given the relative ease of obtaining them on prescription to avoid withdrawal;
- eating disorders: up to half of patients with an eating disorder misuse alcohol, especially those with bulimia nervosa.

Aetiology

As with most psychiatric conditions, the cause of an alcohol problem in a given individual is likely to be multifactorial and highly related to the time and context. Some of the simple social reasons why people may drink alcohol were discussed in the introductory section on p. 378. The best way to consider the aetiology of alcoholism is via the biopsychosocial model (Table 29.5).

Genetics

The heritability of alcohol problems is estimated to be 40–60 per cent. Twin studies have shown a concordance between monozygotic twins of 48 per cent, and dizygotic twins of 32 per cent. A family history of alcoholism is a strong risk factor, as is the onset of drinking before age 15. Gene linkage studies have found a number of genes that appear to be associated with alcohol problems. These include alcohol dehydrogenase, monoamine oxidase, the serotonin transporter, and GABA-A. Polymorphisms in genes that metabolize alcohol (e.g. aldehyde dehydrogenase, *ALDH2*) tend to carry a lower risk of alcohol problems than the wild type.

Alcohol metabolism

Up to 10 per cent of alcohol ingested is excreted directly through the lungs, skin, and urine, whilst the other 90 per cent is metabolized. Levels of the enzymes that metabolize alcohol may be important in determining the physical and psychological response. Alcohol is initially metabolized to acetaldehyde by alcohol dehydrogenase (ADH), and then converted to carbon dioxide and water

Table 29.5 Aetiology of alcohol use problems

Biological
- Heritable genetic factors
- Variations in alcohol metabolism
- Individual responses to alcohol
- Family history of substance abuse
- Intrauterine exposure to drugs and alcohol

Psychological
- Risk taking and other personality traits
- Psychiatric problems in childhood (e.g. conduct disorder, abuse)
- Co-morbid psychiatric disorders

Social
- Laws affecting availability and price of alcohol
- Cultural attitudes and practices
- Peer pressure and/or role models
- Economic situation and employment
- Level of education
- Behaviour within the family unit
- Divorce or relationship problems

by aldehyde dehydrogenase (ALDH). There are a variety of variations of ADH which produce slightly quicker breakdown of alcohol. An inactive form of ALDH (*ALDH*2*) is carried by about half of Asian people; this leads to a build-up of aldehyde on ingestion of alcohol. Vomiting, flushing, and tachycardia ensue, which tend to cause homozygous individuals to avoid alcohol.

Individual responses to alcohol

There is great variation in sensitivity to alcohol between individuals, with those who are more sensitive tending to drink less. This provides them with a lower risk of alcoholism. Alcohol enhances inhibitory GABA systems throughout the brain causing relaxation, sleepiness and intoxication. Alcohol also releases dopamine and activates the reward pathways, which may well lead to the cravings seen in dependent individuals. There appears to be an association between alcohol dependence and the dopamine D2 receptor, but this is not completely characterized.

Psychological factors

Personality traits play a distinct role in the aetiology of alcohol problems, especially in the early stages. Some individuals are willing to take higher risks to achieve pleasure or excitement, and are less concerned about the harmful consequences. In young males with a high alcohol intake, these are the prevailing features. Anxious–

avoidant personalities are also at risk, as their personality traits cause them significant problems in social situations, which can be somewhat alleviated by alcohol. Those who had a conduct disorder in childhood, or have antisocial personality disorder/traits have the highest risk of alcohol-related problems.

Psychiatric co-morbidities almost inevitably make a patient at higher risk of developing an alcohol problem. The most commonly associated are conduct disorder, ADHD, social phobia, and depression. It can be quite difficult to work out if a mood or anxiety disorder is the primary condition or a secondary consequence of alcohol misuse. These associations make sense; either the alcohol helps to reduce symptoms or dull feelings, or it is a manifestation of thrill-seeking behaviour. There is a lesser association with schizophrenia and bipolar disorder, which has yet to be explained.

■ Assessment and treatment of people with alcohol problems

Screening for alcohol use problems

In the UK, 20 per cent of patients attending primary care appointments and up to 30 per cent of hospital inpatients drink more than the recommended weekly limits of alcohol. The simplest method of screening is to ask the patient how much alcohol they drink per week, and try to calculate the units consumed from this. Given the answer to this question, and considering the high-risk groups for alcohol misuse (Box 29.4), further screening questionnaires can then be used.

Questionnaires are the standard method for identifying alcohol use disorders. In primary care, the **Alcohol Use Disorders Identification Test** (AUDIT) can be used (Box 29.5). A cut-off score of five on this questionnaire has a sensitivity of 84 per cent, a specificity of 90 per cent, and a likelihood ratio for a positive result of 8.4. The briefer **CAGE Questionnaire** is probably less sensitive but more specific; a score of three or more has a specificity of almost 100 per cent (Box 29.6). If the screening questions raise the possibility of an alcohol problem, a full assessment of the patient should be made. This can usually be managed in primary care if there are no physical or significant psychiatric complications arising at that time.

Assessment

A full psychiatric history should be taken, including information from the patient, a third-party informant, primary care physician, and old hospital notes. Specific areas to cover include:

BOX 29.4 High-risk groups for alcohol problems

- Patients with psychiatric co-morbidities
- Personal or family history of alcohol misuse
- History of conduct disorder, ADHD, or antisocial personality disorder
- Relationship or sexual problems
- Legal difficulties
- Unemployment, repeated absences from work
- Emotional or behavioural issues with the patient's children
- Patients presenting with gastritis, peptic ulcer, liver disease, peripheral neuropathy, seizures (especially those starting in middle life), and repeated falls among the elderly

---

- How much alcohol does the patient drink on a typical 'drinking day'?
- What is the pattern of drinking?
- Is the intake stereotyped?
- How does the patient feel after going without alcohol for a day or two?
- How does the patient feel on waking?
- Questions should be asked about performance at work and in family life, and about any legal problems. Relevant questions about work include extended meal breaks, lateness, absences, declining efficiency, missed promotions, and accidents. Current accommodation and finances should be covered. It is important to find out about dependent children.
- In appropriate cases, systematic enquiry should be made about features of the alcohol dependence syndrome and all the physical, psychological, and social disabilities described above.
- Physical symptoms, and any alcohol-related problems.
- Personal history of alcohol and other psychiatric problems.
- Previous treatments and how successful they were.
- Current medications (prescribed, illicit, over-the-counter, caffeine, nicotine).
- Premorbid personality traits.
- Assess what stage of change the patient is at. Do they accept there is a problem? Are they willing to listen to advice and consider the options? This will help to plan further interventions.
- Screen for depression and anxiety disorders.

BOX 29.5 Alcohol Use Disorders Identification Test (AUDIT)

1 How often do you have a drink containing alcohol?
(0) Never
(1) Monthly or less
(2) 2–4 times a month
(3) 2 or 3 times a week
(4) 4 or more times a week

2 How many drinks containing alcohol do you have on a typical day when you are drinking?
(0) 1 or 2
(1) 3 or 4
(2) 5 or 6
(3) 7 to 9
(4) 10 or more

3 How often do you have six or more drinks on one occasion?
(0) Never
(1) Less than monthly
(2) Monthly
(3) Weekly
(4) Daily or almost daily

4 How often during the past year have you found that you were not able to stop drinking once you had started?
(0) Never
(1) Less than monthly
(2) Monthly
(3) Weekly
(4) Daily or almost daily

5 How often during the past year have you failed to do what was normally expected of you because of drinking?
(0) Never
(1) Less than monthly
(2) Monthly
(3) Weekly
(4) Daily or almost daily

6 How often during the past year have you needed a first drink in the morning to get yourself going after a heavy drinking session?
(0) Never
(1) Less than monthly
(2) Monthly
(3) Weekly
(4) Daily or almost daily

7 How often during the past year have you had a feeling of guilt or remorse after drinking?
(0) Never
(1) Less than monthly
(2) Monthly
(3) Weekly
(4) Daily or almost daily

8 How often during the past year have you been unable to remember what happened the night before because you had been drinking?
(0) Never
(1) Less than monthly
(2) Monthly
(3) Weekly
(4) Daily or almost daily

9 Have you or has someone else been injured as a result of your drinking?
(0) No
(2) Yes, but not in the past year
(4) Yes, during the last year

10 Has a relative or friend or a doctor or other health worker been concerned about your drinking or suggested that you cut down?
(0) No
(2) Yes, but not in the past year
(4) Yes, during the last year

Score in the number in brackets for each answer; more than 5 suggests an alcohol use disorder, and more than 8 alcohol dependence.

From Piccinelli, M., Tessari, E., Bortolomasi, M., *et al.* (1997). Efficacy of the Alcohol Use Disorders Identification Test as a screening tool for hazardous alcohol intake and related disorders in primary care: a validity study. *British Medical Journal* **314**, 420–4.

A detailed physical examination is essential, both to identify harm already caused by alcohol and to predict future problems. It should concentrate on looking for signs of liver disease, malnutrition, neurological signs, and problems with cognition.

Appropriate basic investigations should be carried out. The most simple and useful are blood tests for markers that change in the context of heavy alcohol intake. They are not as sensitive as questionnaires, but add evidence to the diagnosis and may help the patient to understand that alcohol is affecting their health. Markers may also be used to monitor response to treatment. In addition, it is worth checking an FBC, U&Es, creatinine, haematinics, and lipid profile.

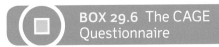

BOX 29.6 The CAGE Questionnaire

1 Have you ever felt you ought to Cut down your drinking?

2 Have people ever Annoyed you by criticizing your drinking?

3 Have you ever felt Guilty about your drinking?

4 Have you ever had a drink first thing in the morning as an 'Eye-opener'?

Two or more positive replies identify problem drinkers; one is an indication for further enquiry about the person's drinking.

From Mayfield, D., McLeod, G., Hall, P., *et al.* (1974). The CAGE questionnaire: validation of a new alcoholism screening instrument. *American Journal of Psychiatry* **131**, 1121–3.

1 **Blood alcohol** concentration estimation using a breathalyzer is the most direct measure, although this does not distinguish between a single recent episode of heavy drinking and chronic abuse.

2 **Gamma-glutamyltranspeptidase (GGT)** levels are raised in about 80 per cent of people with drinking problems. It has a sensitivity and specificity of about 60 per cent.

3 **Mean corpuscular volume (MCV)** is increased in about 60 per cent of people with drinking problems.

4 **Carbohydrate-deficient transferrin.** Transferrin is a glycoprotein that binds iron tightly for transportation. The proportion of carbohydrate on the transferrin structure varies with alcohol intake. A value of > 20 units per litre indicates heavy drinking, and has a sensitivity of 75 per cent and a specificity of 90 per cent.

5 **Urate levels** are raised in about half of all people with drinking problems, but they are only useful as screening tests for men as they are poor discriminators in women.

6 **Liver function tests.** Alanine and aspartate aminotransferases increase in heavy drinking, and represent hepatocellular damage. They are useful in gauging the level of liver damage that has already been caused.

Treatment of people with alcohol problems

Managing patients with alcohol problems can be quite difficult, partly because there is a confusing array of treatments available. Alcohol use disorders should be viewed as a chronic relapsing and remitting condition; success may not come first time around. An initial first step for all is a thorough enquiry into drinking habits and related problems. This is not only a way of detecting the harmful user of alcohol, but also a first step in treatment because it helps the patient to recognize the extent and seriousness of his problem. This recognition is needed as a means of motivating the patient to control his drinking. Without such motivation, treatment will fail.

There are four steps in the basic approach to managing alcohol problems (Table 29.6):

1 assessment (as described previously);

2 psychoeducation and motivational therapy;

3 safe withdrawal from alcohol;

4 relapse prevention and treatment of underlying issues.

When to obtain specialist help

Most problem drinkers can be treated in primary care. The general practitioner knows the patient and the

Table 29.6 Treatment options for a patient with an alcohol problem

Assessment

- Extent of drinking, evidence for dependence, alcohol-related disabilities, and co-morbidities
- Arrange medical treatment for physical complications
- Arrange psychiatric treatment for mental health problems

Psychoeducation

- Safe drinking advice
- Education for patient and family
- Self-help materials

Motivation for change

- Brief interventions
- Motivational interviewing (extended brief interventions)
- Self-help materials

Safe withdrawal

- Community based: benzodiazepines and oral thiamine
- Inpatient based: benzodiazepines and parenteral thiamine, management of complications

Relapse prevention and treatment of underlying issues

- Outpatient follow-up or CBT
- Residential or day-patient programmes
- 12-step programmes (e.g. Alcoholics Anonymous)
- Marital or family therapy
- Medications: disulfiram, acamprosate, and naltrexone
- Ongoing vitamin supplementation
- Antidepressants for depression or anxiety disorders
- Assistance with employment, accommodation, and legal issues

family, and can carry out the treatment of the problem drinking in the context of the patient's general health, an approach that is often acceptable to the patient.

The main reasons for referral to a specialist are:

1 severe withdrawal symptoms, especially fits or delirium tremens, which should be treated as emergencies;

2 planned withdrawal from alcohol when home withdrawal is inappropriate;

3 medical or psychiatric complications requiring specialist assessment;

4 complex personal or interpersonal problems requiring more intensive psychological treatment than simple counselling.

Initial goals

Treatment begins with a review of the extent of the drinking, the evidence for dependence, the effects of the patient's heavy drinking, and the likely consequences if it continues. Any urgently needed medical or psychiatric treatment is arranged and a decision is made about withdrawal. The patient should be involved in formulating the treatment plan, and if possible their partner should take part. Specific and attainable goals should be set and the patient given responsibility for reaching them. These goals should include control of drinking, collaboration with treatment for any associated medical condition, and resolution of problems in the family, at work, and with the law. These initial goals should be short term and achievable. For example, if the amount drunk is not too great, the aim should be to reduce consumption to the safe limit in the first 2 weeks. Unrealistic goals, especially in the early stages, will lead to failure, demoralization, and a return to drinking.

Abstinence versus controlled drinking

It is important to decide whether to aim for total abstinence from alcohol or for controlled drinking. Abstinence is the most appropriate goal for people with harmful use of alcohol, including dependence. However, not all such patients will accept this goal; they either refuse treatment or report abstinence while continuing to drink alcohol. Controlled drinking is **not** a suitable goal for those patients who:

- have previously been alcohol dependent;
- had a previous failure of controlled drinking;
- have serious psychiatric co-morbidity;
- have incurred serious physical consequences of drinking that require abstinence;
- are in a job (such as heavy goods vehicle driving) that carries a risk to others;
- are pregnant.

The target can be the usual safe limit of 21 units per week for men and 14 for women. Reduction to these limits should be in achievable stages, say 5 or 10 units a week, but the process should not be so prolonged that motivation is lost. If it becomes obvious that this technique is not working, abstinence should be aimed for immediately.

Psychoeducation for the patient and family

The patient and their partner should be fully informed of the dangers of alcohol and what is a safe amount to drink. They should understand the impact that alcohol has already had on the patient and family. Options for treatment should be explained, and where possible, choices given. Family members (this can include older children) should be asked to encourage and reward changes in the patient's drinking pattern, but not to punish slips or relapses. It is important to avoid confrontation and aggression, so some interpersonal skills may need to be taught. Occasionally family members are unable to help in the patient's recovery; in this case, it may be necessary to ask the family to step back and allow other people to help in the short term. Self-help materials based on motivational techniques, CBT, and 12-step programmes are frequently helpful for all concerned.

Motivation for change

There are a variety of techniques for helping to move a precontemplative or contemplative patient into the next part of the cycle of change. It may be that the discussion in the sections above is adequate to motivate change, but frequently another intervention is needed. In systematic reviews, motivation enhancement techniques alone have similar outcomes to CBT and Alcoholics Anonymous programmes.

The simplest intervention is called a **brief intervention** and can be delivered easily by any trained health professional in a few minutes. It involves giving simple, structured advice that aims to reduce alcohol intake to less dangerous levels. This can be done in a primary care setting, the emergency room, or during an internal medical ward round.

Extended brief interventions take approximately 30 minutes, and are based on motivational interviewing. They use the FRAMES acronym to provide the tools for change and strategies for making changes dealing with underlying issues (Box 29.7). They are best administered by a trained alcohol support worker.

Withdrawal from alcohol: detoxification

When the patient is dependent on alcohol a sudden cessation of drinking may cause severe withdrawal symptoms, including delirium tremens or seizures. Since these complications may be dangerous, withdrawal (detoxification) should be carried out under medical supervision.

BOX 29.7 FRAMES: a brief intervention for alcohol use disorders

- Structured **feedback** about personal risks
- Emphasis on it being the patient's **responsibility** to make changes
- **Advice** to cut down or cease drinking
- **Menu** of options for making changes to the drinking pattern

- Being **empathetic** in interviewing
- Reinforcing a patient's **self-efficacy** for change

Reproduced with permission from Bein T. H. *et al.* (1993). Motivational interviewing with alcoholic outpatients. *Behavioural and Cognitive Psychotherapy* **21**: 347–56.

In both contexts, the treatment is a combination of long-acting benzodiazepines and B vitamins. Benzodiazepines work in two ways: firstly by reducing the risk of seizures and delirium tremens, and secondly by decreasing the cravings, tremor, anxiety, insomnia, and nausea that occur during withdrawal. Chlordiazepoxide is the drug of choice, because it has a long half-life and less ability to be abused than diazepam.

Withdrawal in the community

Randomized controlled trials have shown that in less severe cases, and where there is no significant physical illness or history of previous withdrawal seizures, withdrawal can be done safely at home provided that there is someone to look after the patient. It is important that daily support is available at home to monitor the withdrawal, and that they understand the complications of withdrawal and call for help quickly if they occur. The GP should supply benzodiazepines according to a reducing regimen (see below) and oral thiamine plus a multivitamin. They should tell the patient and family that the benzodiazepines must be stopped and returned to the pharmacy should drinking resume. The patient should be advised to drink water and fruit juices to quench thirst, and be offered three balanced meals per day. Caffeine should be avoided.

Withdrawal in hospital

Patients with severe dependence, previous withdrawal seizures or delirium tremens, failed outpatient detoxification, or no social support need hospital admission for detoxification. They should be treated with a reducing regimen of chlordiazepoxide, for example:

- day 1: 20 mg chlordiazepoxide four times daily;
- day 2: 15 mg chlordiazepoxide four times daily;
- day 3: 10 mg chlordiazepoxide four times daily;
- day 4: 5 mg chlordiazepoxide four times daily;
- day 5: 5 mg chlordiazepoxide twice daily;
- as needed doses may be added up to a maximum of 200 mg per day.

Patients with seizures or delirium tremens may need higher doses for longer, with a course of about 2 weeks in total. Metoclopramide is the most effective anti-emetic in withdrawal. All patients should receive high-dose B vitamins, following local guidelines, either oral thiamine or parenteral Pabrinex®. Seizures are best treated by giving 10 mg diazepam, which may need to be doubled in those who are already taking benzodiazepines. Starting an anticonvulsant is not recommended. Patients with delirium tremens may need parenteral benzodiazepine and an antipsychotic.

Relapse prevention and treatment of underlying problems

There is little point in detoxification if it is not followed up with support to maintain abstinence and work upon the reasons behind the alcohol problem. The options available for further treatment divide into two main groups:

1 **Psychological treatments:**
   (i) outpatient follow-up or CBT;
   (ii) residential or day-patient programmes;
   (iii) 12-step programmes (e.g. Alcoholics Anonymous);
   (iv) marital or family therapy.

2 **Pharmacological treatments:**
   (i) medications to prevent relapse: disulfiram, acamprosate, and naltrexone;
   (ii) ongoing vitamin supplementation;
   (iii) antidepressants (and other medications) for psychiatric co-morbidities.

Psychological treatments

A range of different psychological therapies and interventions are available; there is no evidence that one is consistently superior in efficacy. Individual cognitive behavioural therapy (CBT) can be effective in maintaining changes in behaviour. CBT can teach the patient to understand what led to the urges to drink, and how to avoid alcohol should the temptation reoccur. It can reverse abnormal beliefs surrounding drinking, and develop problem-solving skills. It tends to improve the coping skills of patients, especially if combined with aspects of communication skills, assertiveness, or social skills training. Anger management and relaxation therapy can also be beneficial. All of these types of therapy can also be administered in a group setting, as this provides the opportunity to learn through role play and role models.

If a more intensive form of treatment is required to prevent relapse, then a day-patient or residential rehabilitation programme may be indicated. In the UK, such treatment is rarely available in the National Health Service because residential (or inpatient) programmes have not been shown to be cost-effective, or to have a higher success rate at maintaining long-term abstinence than community-based programmes. In other countries, and in the private sector, these therapeutic programmes and communities are readily available. The advantage of this treatment is that it removes the opportunity to drink in the early stages, and provides intensive individual and group therapy. Often working with a peer group who support one another to work through problems can be very helpful. Residential treatment may also be indicated if the patient has complex psychiatric co-morbidities (e.g. severe anorexia nervosa or depression).

There are a variety of self-help groups for people with alcohol-related problems, which can be very useful in helping to maintain motivation. They also provide a valuable means of support. Patients with alcohol problems often find it easier to talk to others who have had similar problems. **Alcoholics Anonymous (AA)** is the largest organization, with 90 000 groups worldwide, and holds group meetings based on a 12-step programme. The programme views alcoholism as a chronic condition only cured by total abstinence. At the meetings members will introduce themselves to one another, talk about their problems, and gain support from other members. Individuals work through the 12 steps at their own pace, discussing their progress with the group each week. Not all problem drinkers are willing to join the organization because it requires total abstinence and because the meetings involve repeated confession of each person's faults and problems. Those who remain in the organization are usually helped, and anyone with a drink problem should be encouraged to try it. Local AA groups widely publicize their contact details, and are usually happy to receive new members. Doctors are welcome to sit in on a meeting to see how it works.

Help for the family should always be offered. Marital therapy may be helpful in realigning a couple, essential in promoting an individual's recovery. The partner or teenage children may need counselling about problems of their own that are consequent on the patient's heavy drinking. They may also need help in supporting the patient's efforts to reduce his drinking.

Doctors have higher than average rates of alcohol problems, and they too often have difficulty in admitting their problems and seeking help, especially from colleagues working in the same area. In some countries, including the UK, arrangements exist for doctors to obtain help outside their area of work, through a national scheme for sick doctors. Their website is www.sick-doctors-trust.co.uk.

Pharmacological treatments

Disulfiram (Antabuse: 100–200 mg/day) is used, usually in specialist practice, as a deterrent to impulsive drinking. It interferes with the metabolism of alcohol by irreversibly blocking acetaldehyde dehydrogenase. As a result, when alcohol is taken acetaldehyde accumulates with consequent flushing, headache, choking sensations, rapid pulse, and anxiety. These unpleasant effects discourage the patient from drinking alcohol while taking the drug. Treatment with disulfiram carries the occasional risks of cardiac irregularities or, rarely, cardiovascular collapse. Therefore, the drug should not be started until at least 12 hours after the last ingestion of alcohol. Disulfiram has unpleasant side effects, including a persistent metallic taste in the mouth, gastrointestinal symptoms, dermatitis, urinary frequency, impotence, peripheral neuropathy, and toxic confusional states (extremely rare). It should *not* be used in patients with recent heart disease, severe liver disease, or significant suicidal ideation. The main use of disulfiram is to provide the patient with time to recover confidence that they can manage life without alcohol; 6 months is the recommended prescription time. Single-blind studies (the patient must know they have taken the drug for it to work) show disulfiram to be effective in preventing relapse, and more so than acamprosate or naltrexone.

Acamprosate is a drug that enhances GABA transmission in the central nervous system. In animals, acamprosate reduces drinking in dependent animals and reduces relapse in animals offered alcohol after a period of abstinence. RCTs have shown it to reduce cravings for alcohol in patients with alcohol dependence. The usual dose is 666 mg three times daily, and is started 2–7 days after cessation of drinking. Patients who benefit from it should continue for 6 months to a year.

Naltrexone is an opiate antagonist, which inhibits the action of endogenous endorphins released when alcohol is drunk. It reduces the urge to drink, reduces the pleasurable 'high' produced by alcohol, and reduces the loss of control it causes. Short-term usage seems to reduce the risk of relapse, but is less effective than disulfiram. It is started once abstinence is achieved at 50 mg once daily.

Patients recovering from an alcohol problem should be advised to continue taking vitamin supplements for at least 3 months after cessation of drinking. At the very least, 100 mg of thiamine should be taken daily. Dietetic advice may also be valuable.

Anxiety and depression caused by alcohol usually spontaneously improve with abstinence. Underlying co-morbidities may benefit from treatment with antidepressants along standard guidelines.

Prognosis and the results of treatment

Alcohol misuse is associated with a 3.6-fold increased all-cause mortality when compared with age-matched controls. The risk of suicide is 10–15 per cent in patients with alcohol dependency for more than 5 years. For the majority of problem drinkers, brief interventions are as effective as more intensive treatments and a good proportion of patients improve or are cured. The results of treatment for patients with serious drinking problems are poor and the aim should therefore be the early detection and treatment of alcohol problems. It is important to maintain a helpful and non-judgmental attitude. Relapses should be viewed constructively and further help offered.

In the early stages of dangerous drinking, the patient is more likely to have the *characteristics related to good outcome*:

- good insight;
- strong motivation;
- a supportive family;
- a stable job;
- the ability to form good relationships;
- control of impulsivity;
- the ability to defer gratification.

■ Preventing alcohol-related harm

As described in the sections on epidemiology, the public health implications of alcohol use disorders are vast. In most Western populations, approximately 90 per cent of adults drink alcohol, and many occasionally get intoxicated. Whilst the majority of individuals are well aware of the general risks of alcohol, a complicating factor is the marginal benefit that small amounts have on cardiovascular health. There are seven main ways in which alcohol problems in society may be reduced.

1 **Educate people,** effectively persuading them not to misuse alcohol. Talking in schools, harnessing community groups, and television advertisements are all effective delivery methods. School-age education programmes are particularly important. Television and billboard adverts showing the harm alcohol may cause can deliver a striking message.

2 **Deter** harmful drinking with penalties. Laws on driving whilst intoxicated have massively reduced the number of road traffic accidents due to alcohol.

3 **Provide alternatives** to drinking alcohol and engaging in drink-related activities.

4 **Instigate harm-reduction strategies.** For example, the mandatory use of seatbelts, airbags, and low speed limits has reduced driving-related morbidity and mortality.

5 **Regulate the availability** of alcohol and its price. Increasing taxation on alcohol, limiting the hours it may be sold, and having a minimum age for purchase are all effective methods.

6 **Promote social, cultural, and religious movements** to reduce alcohol consumption.

7 **Treat individuals** who have alcohol-related problems.

■ Problems due to the use of psychoactive substances

The term **psychoactive substance** is used instead of the term **drug** because some people use substances that are not generally regarded as drugs; for example, organic solvents or mushrooms with psychedelic properties. This chapter uses 'psychoactive substance' when the broad meaning is required, while retaining the word 'drug' for specific purposes. The general information at the start of this chapter (p. 377) is relevant to all the substances discussed below. The initial section will cover some basic principles surrounding psychoactive substance misuse, including a generic plan for assessment and treatment, and the latter part will discuss specific substances in detail. It will also be useful to refer back to the introductory information at the beginning of this chapter.

The substances that are commonly misused fall into six groups:

1 **opioids:** heroin (diamorphine), morphine, dihydrocodeine, methadone, codeine, buprenorphine, pethidine;

2 **anxiolytics and hypnotics (depressants):** benzodiazepines, barbiturates, GHB, alcohol;

3 **stimulants:** amphetamine, cocaine, ecstasy, MDMA;

4 **hallucinogens:** LSD, PCP, magic mushrooms, ketamine;

5 **cannabis;**

6 **organic solvents.**

In this chapter, we focus on the harmful effects of these substances to the user's health. The use of many of these substances is illegal in many countries. The use of others (e.g. nicotine) is legal despite the harmful medical consequences of smoking. It is important to distinguish between **harmful** use and **illegal** use of substances. The clinician's role should be directed at the former—to help the user overcome dependence and to avoid the adverse health consequences of psychoactive substance use. An explanation of the UK law surrounding illegal substance use is given on p. 379.

Epidemiology of psychoactive substance use

The extent of supply and consumption of drugs is often concealed because the possession of many drugs is illegal or socially unacceptable. Therefore, there are no reliable estimates of the extent of drug consumption in the population. In the UK, indirect information has been collected about drug-related offences, hospital treatment, and cases reported to government agencies but none of these sources are reliable. Similar difficulties are encountered in different countries, so that no accurate international comparison can be made. Some statistics are shown in Table 29.1 on p. 377.

In the UK, surveys of the general public suggest one-third of adults have used an illegal substance at least once in their lifetime. By the age of 16 years, at least

 Science box 29.1 HIV amongst injecting drug users—a growing problem

It is undeniable that both HIV and injecting drug use (IDU) are global public health problems, and unfortunately there is a strong link between them. In 2009, there were an estimated 40 million HIV-positive individuals worldwide, 90 per cent of whom live in developing or transitional countries.[1] Of these, 10 per cent of infections are directly attributable to IDU.

In 2008, Mathers and colleagues published a systematic review, summarizing the prevalence of IDUs and HIV-positive IDUs in 200 countries.[2] It is a difficult area in which to conduct primary research, as there is no universal definition of 'injecting drug use', it is often difficult to access IUDs and obtain reliable information, and within countries there is great heterogeneity. The study reports that 148 countries had evidence of IDU within them. The prevalence of IDU was hugely variable, from 0.02 per cent in Cambodia to 5.2 per cent in Azerbajan. The global median was 0.36 per cent, representing approximately 16 million people. The majority of countries reported that less than 5 per cent of their IDUs were HIV positive. However, in five countries 20–40 per cent were HIV positive, and in nine countries the figure was greater than 40 per cent. The areas with the highest burden of co-morbid HIV and IDU were Eastern Europe, South East Asia, and Latin America. In the UK, an estimated 1 per cent of IDUs were infected with HIV. Similar figures were published by a 2009 review, which also suggested that many of the extra cases seen in the last decade can be accounted for in a few geographical areas.[3]

One area of particular concern is prisons, which are well known to have a high level of drug dependency. In Russia, 4 per cent of the prison population admit to IDU—there are probably 9 million individuals worldwide in this situation.[4] Epidemiological studies of HIV consistently report imprisonment as a strong risk factor for HIV-positive status.

Why is IDU so strongly associated with HIV? The answer to this appears to be threefold. The first reason is that sharing of infected needles is a very efficient way of transmitting the virus. Secondly, IDUs tend to be young, sexually active risk takers. They frequently have multiple partners, and do not use condoms. One study showed 80 per cent of IDUs reported having unprotected sex regularly.[3] Thirdly, there is an association between IDU and the sex industry—infection of non-IDU individuals occurs and can then spread into the general population.

A variety of measures have been implemented to try and prevent further epidemics of HIV amongst IDUs, and to stop further growth of those that have already occurred. Needle exchange programmes, especially those including education, addictions treatment, and access to health services are effective. In the mid-1980s, the prevalence of HIV amongst IDUs in New York was 50 per cent. The introduction of needle exchange and community outreach programmes in 1992 had cut this figure to 15 per cent by 2008. HIV infection in IDU is a problem of global significance currently; however, we do now have multiple strategies which can effectively reduce this in the future.

1 Aceijas, C., Stimson, G. V., Hickman, M. *et al.* (2004). Global overview of injecting drug use and HIV infection among injecting drug users. *AIDS* **18** :2295–303.

2 Mathers, B. M., Degenhardt, L., Phillips, B. *et al.* (2008). Global epidemiology of injecting drug use and HIV among people who inject drugs: a systematic review. *Lancet* **372**: 1733–45.

3 Des Jarlais, D. C., Arasteh, K., Semaan, S. *et al.* (2009). HIV among injecting drug users: current epidemiology, biologic markers, respondent-driven sampling, and supervised-injection facilities. *Current Opinion in HIV and AIDS* **4**: 308–13.

4 Jurgens, R., Ball, A., & Verster, A. (2009). Interventions to reduce HIV transmission related to injecting drug use in prison. *Lancet Infectious Diseases* **9**: 57–66.

25 per cent of schoolchildren have used an illicit substance. Cannabis is the most commonly used illegal substance, accounting for about 80 per cent of those who admit to having used substances. Apart from alcohol, tobacco (nicotine) is the most frequently used legal substance. In the UK and USA, approximately 25 to 30 per cent of adults smoke. In most developed countries, the extent of psychoactive substance use seems to be increasing. The ratio of males to females using all substances is 3–4:1.

Patterns of substance misuse

There are a variety of different patterns of substance misuse seen in society.

- **Experimentation** is common amongst teenagers and students. Accessibility to substances and peer pressure promote usage, which aims to discover how the substances makes one feel. Cannabis, stimulants, and mushrooms are commonly taken, opioids and other 'harder' substances more rarely.

- **Use limited to particular situations.** Cannabis is frequently taken at house parties and as part of experimental sexual experiences, ecstasy and LSD at nightclubs and raves.

- **Recreational use.** These groups of individuals regularly use substances, but are not dependent upon them. Typically, they will contain to use for a defined period, and then stop without any difficulties. A variety of substances may be used, and rarely they may progress to dependent usage. A classical example would be the use of cannabis during university, which ceases once a career is begun and a family obtained.

- **Dependence.** A dependence syndrome (p. 377) develops, and substance use continues more to avoid the withdrawals than for the positive effects of the substance. The majority of the time only the dependent substance will be taken, but others may be substituted if the primary one is unavailable or the user is looking for a new experience or to make a change. Opioids and benzodiazepines typically fall into this category.

- **Substance misuse combined with mental illness.** There are a group of individuals with substance problems who have a co-morbid psychiatric disorder. They may be using the substance to reduce their unwanted psychiatric symptoms, or may be highly vulnerable to suggestion or pressure from their peers.

Causes of the harmful use of psychoactive substances

The reasons why people may use substances are described on p. 378.

Types of dependence

Not all people who use psychoactive substances become dependent on them. Dependence may be pharmacological or psychological, and the two may be mutually exclusive.

1 **Pharmacological dependence** is caused by changes in the receptors and other cellular mechanisms affected by the substance. Substances vary in the degree to which they cause pharmacological dependence: opioids and nicotine readily cause it; cannabis and hallucinogens are less likely to do so.

2 **Psychological dependence** operates partly through conditioning. Some of the symptoms experienced as a substance is withdrawn (e.g. anxiety) become conditioned responses that reappear when withdrawal takes place again. Cognitive factors are also important—patients expect unpleasant symptoms and are distressed by the prospect. For this reason, reassurance is an important part of the treatment of patients who are withdrawing from drugs. Drugs such as hallucinogens and stimulants frequently cause psychological dependence.

Harm related to the use of substances

Substance-related harm (Table 29.2) may be due to:

1 the toxic properties of the substances themselves (see individual substances below);

2 the method of administration (e.g. problems due to the intravenous use of substances; see Box 29.8);

3 the social consequences of regular use of substances (Box 29.9).

How do patients with substance use problems present?

Dependent people may come to medical attention in several ways.

1 They may declare that they are dependent on or using a substance during a consultation, at health screening, or whilst in hospital for another reason.

2 They may request drugs for medical reasons. Some patients conceal their dependency, asking instead for opioids to relieve pain or for hypnotics to improve sleep. General practitioners and emergency department staff should be wary of such requests from patients whom they have not met before, and if possible should obtain information about previous treatment (if necessary by telephone) before prescribing.

3 They may ask for help with the complications of substance use such as cellulitis, pneumonia, hepatitis, HIV/AIDS, or

BOX 29.8 The harmful effects of intravenous drug taking

Some drug abusers administer drugs intravenously in order to obtain an intense and rapid effect. The practice is particularly common with opioids, but barbiturates, benzodiazepines, and amphetamines are among other drugs that may be taken in this way. Intravenous drug use has important consequences—some local, some systemic.

Local complications include:

- thrombosis of veins;
- wound infection or abscesses at the injection site;
- cellulitis;
- deep venous thrombosis (DVT)—repeated injection into the femoral veins damages the valves and reduces venous return, which promotes clotting;

- damage to arteries;
- emboli—these may cause gangrene if within arteries, or a pulmonary embolus if from the veins.

Systemic effects are due to transmission of infection, especially when needles are shared. They include:

- sepsis;
- bacterial endocarditis;
- blood-borne infections: hepatitis B and C, HIV, syphilis;
- increased risk of overdose.

accidents, or for the treatment of a drug overdose, withdrawal symptoms, or an adverse reaction to a hallucinogenic drug.

4 Their dependence might be detected during treatment of an unrelated illness. A common scenario is the patient admitted to hospital for another reason, who then develops withdrawal symptoms.

■ Assessment and treatment of problems due to psychoactive substance misuse

Assessment

Accurate, detailed assessment is essential to provide the appropriate support for the patient. It is important to diagnose dependence early, at a stage when tolerance is less established, behaviour patterns are less fixed, and the complications of intravenous use have not developed. A doctor who is not used to treating substance-dependent people should remember that the patient may be trying to deceive him, and may not volunteer information unless specifically asked. Some patients overstate the dosage in the hope of obtaining extra supplies to use themselves, give to friends, or sell. Others take more than one substance but do not admit it. It is important to check the patient's account for internal inconsistencies and to seek external verification whenever possible (e.g. by obtaining permission to contact another doctor who has treated the same patient).

History taking

A full psychiatric history should be taken, including information from the patient, a third-party informant, primary

BOX 29.9 Social harm due to the use of psychoactive substances

There are various reasons why drug abuse has undesirable social effects.

1 Acute intoxication can lead to harm or damage to people or property. Violence and aggression may be a particular problem.

2 Chronic intoxication may affect behaviour adversely, leading to a poor work record, unemployment, motoring offences, failures in social relationships, and family problems including the neglect of children.

3 The need to finance the habit. Most illicit drugs are expensive and the abuser may cheat or steal to obtain

money. Women may adopt prostitution, putting themselves at risk of sexually transmitted diseases and other problems.

4 The creation of a drug subculture. Drug users often keep company with one another, and those with previously stable social behaviour may be under pressure to conform to a group ethos of antisocial or criminal activity.

5 Stigmatization. Many social communities do not welcome those who have had substance problems, even after successful treatment. The individual may find it hard to reintegrate into society.

care physician, and old hospital notes. Then a focused substance misuse history, covering current, past, and future usage, should be taken.

1 **Current use: TRAP (Type, Route, Amount, Pattern)**

- What type of drug(s) do you use? Always clarify any street names used. Include alcohol, tobacco, and cannabis. Then work through the questions below for each substance.

- How do you use it? Smoking, snorting, intravenous (IV), intranasal, orally, etc. Ask about needle sharing in IV use.

- How much do you use? Ask how much of each drug they buy (e.g. heroin is sold in grams, cannabis in eighths of an ounce).

- How often do you use it? Get them to describe a typical daily usage.

2 **Evidence of dependency and harms**

- Do you feel you need more of the substance than you used to, to get the same effects from it? Tolerance.

- How do you feel before your first dose/hit/drink/smoke of the day? How do you feel if the substance is unavailable? What happens if you stop taking the substance? Withdrawal.

- Do you ever crave the substance?

- Once you have had one dose/smoke/drink/hit, is it hard to stop taking another? Do you feel your usage is out of control?

- Do you have a typical daily pattern of usage?

- Why do you use (the substance)?

- Ask about normal activities: employment, studying, family life, hobbies, etc. Try to decide if the substance taking has taken over from all other activities. Problem use is suggested by repeated absence from school or work, occupational decline, self-neglect, loss of former friends, petty theft, prostitution, and joining the 'drug culture'.

- Has the substance affected your health? Ask about physical symptoms, and any previous medical treatment for complications.

- Complications of drug use: overdoses (deliberate or accidental), history of cellulitis, abscesses, DVT, blood-borne virus. Always ask about HIV status.

3 **Past use and general history**

- When was the first time you used (a substance)? What has happened between then and now? Ask specifically about how usage has changed over time, if different substances have been tried, and why they were stopped.

- Have you ever tried to stop taking substances and get help? Determine what treatments were tried, what happened during withdrawal, how long they were 'clean' for, and what the triggers for relapse were.

- Personal history of other psychiatric problems.
- Premorbid personality traits.
- Family history of psychiatric disorders and substance abuse.
- Current accommodation and finances should be covered. It is important to find out about dependent children. Ask about legal difficulties and debts.
- Sexual orientation and relationships.

4 **Future usage**

- Assess what stage of change the patient is in. Do they accept there is a problem? Are they willing to listen to advice and consider the options? What type of help would they like? This will help to plan further interventions.

A standard MSE should be undertaken. Look specifically for signs of depression, suicidal ideation, and anxiety disorders. Ask about perceptual disturbances and their relationship to drug usage, as many substances can cause or precipitate psychosis. Insight into current problems should be covered in detail. A clear risk assessment should be made as to mood state, risk of violence, risk of suicide, and dependent others.

A full physical examination should be done. Include weight, height, BMI, and dentition. Feel for hepatomegaly. Clinical signs that suggest that drugs are being injected include:

- needle tracks and thrombosis of veins, especially in the antecubital fossa;
- scars of previous abscesses;
- concealing the forearms with long sleeves even in hot weather.

Intravenous drug use should be considered in any patient who presents with subcutaneous abscesses, hepatitis, or HIV/AIDS, whether or not the person is asking for help with substance use.

Investigations should be used whenever possible to confirm the diagnosis, and assess physical health.

- **Urine drug screening.** Most substances can be detected in the urine, the notable exception being lysergic acid diethylamide (LSD). Specimens should be examined as quickly as possible, with an indication of the interval between the last admitted drug dose and the collection of the urine sample. Amphetamines and heroin can be detected up to 48 hours after last usage, cocaine and methadone for 7 days, and cannabis for up to a month. The laboratory should be provided with as complete a list as possible of drugs likely to have been taken, including those prescribed, as well as those obtained in other ways. Serial urine toxicology over a few days will usually provide a definite diagnosis as to substance dependence.

- **Blood tests:** full blood count, including mean cell volume, urea and electrolytes, liver function tests, gamma-glutamyl transferase. Hepatitis and HIV screening.

Principles of treatment and rehabilitation

Ideally, the long-term aim of treatment will be to achieve complete abstinence and a return to normal living. This goal may need to be reached via a step-wise process in many individuals, and therefore an individual plan of treatment needs to be designed. The aims of any treatment plan should be:

- to motivate the patient towards change, and involve them in treatment planning;
- to minimize harms related to taking substances (physical, psychological, and social);
- to improve physical and mental health;
- to reduce criminal activity;
- to reduce the rates of blood-borne infections in the community;
- to stop substance use, or to substitute a safer alternative to provide maintenance in the short to medium term.

An outline of the treatment options is shown in Table 29.7. The majority of dependent substance users (except for nicotine and sometimes cannabis users) will need referral to a specialist addictions service.

Psychoeducation

Providing accurate information about the harms and consequences of substance misuse to the patient and their family is the first step in enhancing motivation to change. An empathetic, non-patronizing, and non-judgmental approach should be taken to interviewing and delivering information. It is important to cover the basics of pharmacological and psychological dependence, and help the patient to understand why they have become 'addicted' to the substance. This can also help family members to understand that the patient is not to blame for their dependency. Written information and self-help materials should be offered.

Treatment plan

The various options for treatment should be discussed with the patient, and a plan of action agreed. It is helpful to provide this to all involved in treatment (patient, family members, yourself, colleagues, GP, other hospital specialists). Urgent physical or psychiatric problems should be treated.

Table 29.7 Treatment plan for a person using substances harmfully

Assessment
- Type of drug(s) and amounts taken, intravenous usage and its dangers, evidence of dependence, and consequences of drug taking
Psychoeducation of patient and family
- Pharmacology and psychology of dependence
- Harms related to substance misuse
- Self-help strategies and materials
Clarification of treatment goals
- Production of a written treatment plan
Treat urgent medical or psychiatric complications
Harm reduction strategies
Arrange withdrawal of the substance(s)
- Unsupported in the community
- Supported in the community with or without symptomatic medications
- Supported in the community with substitute medications
- In-hospital or residential detoxification
Substitute prescribing for maintenance
Address underlying needs
- Individual counselling, CBT, or other therapies
- Treatment of depression or anxiety
- Marital or family therapy
- Help dealing with social issues: accommodation, employment, legal problems
- Help establishing new interests
Relapse prevention and longer-term support

Harm reduction strategies

In the short term, promoting safer substance use habits may reduce harm until abstinence can be achieved. Examples include using oral rather than IV drug preparations, providing clean needles in a needle exchange programme, and offering free contraception and access to sexual health services.

Withdrawal

Withdrawal of a substance can be done in several different ways, depending on the substance involved and the wishes of the patient. For most substances, withdrawal is achieved by reducing the dose progressively over a period of 1–3 weeks, depending on the initial dose. For opioids and benzodiazepines it is usual to begin by replacing the substance with an equivalent dose of a longer-acting compound of the same type (which has less acute withdrawal effects), and then withdrawing that substance. As noted above, psychological factors contribute to dependence, and strong and repeated reassurance is an important part of treatment. In most situations, withdrawal can be done at home under close supervision. Patients who have a need for urgent medical attention, severe psychiatric co-morbidities, or a history of complex withdrawals may need to be admitted to hospital for detoxification. There are a number of different options for how detoxification can take place.

- **Unsupported.** Some patients decide they would like to manage by themselves, and withdraw unsupported in the community. There are many cases of this method which are never recognized by medical services.

- **Supported without medication.** In this scenario the patient undergoes a planned detox, without the use of any further drugs but with support from some form of medical services.

- **Supported with symptomatic medication.** In this case, withdrawal is assisted by prescribed medications to reduce the symptoms of withdrawal. For example, antidiarrhoeals, anti-emetics, antipyretics, or lofexidine are helpful in opiate withdrawal.

- **Supported with substitute prescribing.** The patient is changed from the dangerous illegal substance (e.g. heroin) to a safer prescribed version (e.g. methadone). Then the substitute is gradually reduced.

Maintenance programmes

Maintenance refers to the continued prescribing of a substance, usually an opioid or benzodiazepine, for a person who is unwilling to withdraw, combined with help with social problems and a continuing effort to bring the person to accept withdrawal. Maintenance is therefore more than merely providing drugs. The rationale for this procedure is to minimize harm in the following ways:

1 **to remove the need to obtain 'street' drugs,** and thereby reduce the need to steal, engage in prostitution, or associate with other drug users;

2 **to stop intravenous use,** thus reducing the spread of blood-borne viruses;

3 **to provide social and psychological help** to bring the person to the point at which he will be willing to give up drugs;

4 **to provide an incentive** for the patient to remain in contact with addiction services.

Unfortunately, the available evidence does not suggest that these aims are achieved regularly; many patients continue in their previous way of life, many continue to take street drugs as well as prescribed methadone, and few become willing to give up drugs. Despite these drawbacks, this treatment is in use in the hope that it may have some effect in reducing intravenous usage, thereby limiting the spread of blood-borne viruses.

In the UK, any doctor can prescribe continuing scripts for methadone or buprenorphine for the treatment of opiate dependence, but it should be initiated by a specialist. Substitute prescribing should only be considered for patients who are actively trying to change their behaviour, and who the doctor thinks are likely to comply with the treatment plan. Prescriptions are dispensed daily by a general practitioner, and the patient must visit the pharmacy daily to receive them. Most patients have supervised doses, meaning a registered person at the pharmacy watches them take the substance. Some patients on maintenance therapy attend a succession of general practitioners in search of supplementary supplies of drugs, posing as temporary residents. The doctor should not prescribe but should help the patient to return to the clinic where they are in treatment.

Longer-term treatments

After a successful detoxification, it is important to provide support to prevent relapse, tackle the issues underlying the substance misuse, and mend or minimize problems related to harm caused by the substance use. Individual counselling or CBT is helpful for addressing issues such as poor self-esteem, depression, anxiety, vulnerability, marital or sexual problems, and anger management. Group therapies teaching social skills, communication skills, relaxation, and assertiveness can be useful. Patients often find great support from discussing their substance problems with others in similar positions. Marital or family therapy can be essential in teaching the family how to cope with withdrawal and in building a new life for the patient. There may be emotional or behavioural issues in children or the partner relating to the effects of substance misuse.

Psychiatric follow-up should be arranged for patients with a co-morbid disorder such as depression or anxiety. Antidepressants or specialized therapy may be indicated. A community psychiatric nurse can be a valuable aid in monitoring the patient's progress. They can also help to arrange new activities to fill their time.

A social worker should be assigned to the patient to provide help in finding suitable accommodation and employment, and in managing money. There may be legal problems to contend with. There are a range of special forms of accommodation, back-to-work schemes, and educational courses designed for those recovering from substance misuse.

Rehabilitation

People who have abused drugs for a long time may need considerable help in making social relationships and in obtaining and retaining a job. When these problems are severe, treatment in a therapeutic community for a prolonged period can be helpful.

Principles of prevention

There are two main strategies for prevention of harm related to the use of psychoactive substances.

1 **Reducing use.** This includes:

- limiting availability;
- penalties for usage;
- health education, particularly in schools, but also centred on locations with widespread drug use, such as certain clubs;
- media campaigns;
- tackling social causes such as poor social conditions, unemployment among young people, and lack of leisure facilities.

However, there is little evidence that any of these measures are effective. Indeed, some health education and media campaigns may actually increase the extent of use.

2 **Reducing harm** associated with use of substances. The harm reduction approach became more accepted in the 1980s in response to the spread of HIV/AIDS through intravenous drug use and sexual intercourse. The main features of this approach include:

- the *education* of drug users about the dangers of intravenous use; such advice is often more effective when given by ex-drug users than by doctors;
- schemes for *providing clean syringes and needles* in exchange for used ones in the hope of reducing the sharing of contaminated ones;
- the prescription of *oral maintenance drugs* to avoid the use of intravenous drugs;
- free supply of *condoms* to reduce sexual transmission.

These approaches are controversial since some of the measures can be seen to condone drug taking, but the danger of HIV infection is now generally considered to be greater than that of increasing drug abuse.

■ Effects and harmful use of specific substances

Opioids

This group of drugs includes morphine, diamorphine (heroin), codeine, dihydrocodeine, and synthetic analgesics such as pethidine and methadone. Opioids are substances that mimic the effects of endogenous opioids (endorphins and enkephalins) by acting as agonists at the opioid receptors. The first record of opioid use by humans was in Mesopotamia in around 3400 BC, when people extracted the natural opioids from poppies and smoked them. An English chemist, C. R. Wright, was the first to synthesize diamorphine, doing so in 1874. Originally it was marketed as a less addictive form of morphine, but unfortunately this turned out to be completely wrong. Diamorphine is the mostly widely used opioid, as it produces the most powerful euphoria. The UN estimates that 15–20 million people worldwide are dependent upon diamorphine at any one time.

As well as the desired euphoric effect of opioids, they also have a wide range of other effects upon the body. These are shown in Table 29.8, with the most commonly experienced being analgesia, constipation, anorexia, and loss of libido. The high risk of respiratory depression makes the uncontrolled use of opioids very dangerous.

Route of administration

Opioids can be taken by mouth, intravenously, by inhaling, or by smoking. When diamorphine is taken orally it undergoes extensive first-pass metabolism, converting it to morphine and reducing the euphoric effects. Intravenous (IV) use avoids this metabolism, and diamorphine crosses the blood–brain barrier quickly and produces a rapid powerful euphoria. IV use of heroin carries all of the risks discussed earlier in the chapter. The antecubital fossa is usually the site first used for injecting, but eventually the veins become damaged and the user moves elsewhere. When venous access becomes extremely difficult, users may inject either subcutaneously (**skin popping**) or intramuscularly. The form of heroin most commonly used in the UK will only dissolve if mixed with an acid and heated. The use of citric acid powder and lemon juice is typical, with heating occurring on a spoon over a heat source. The use of acids is particularly troublesome because it causes immense damage to the veins.

Tolerance and dependence

Although some people take heroin intermittently without becoming dependent, with regular usage dependence

Table 29.8 Physiological effects of opioids

Psychological and neurological

- Tolerance and dependence
- Anxiolysis
- Confusion or delirium
- Euphoria
- Drowsiness
- Analgesia

Cardiovascular

- Bradycardia
- Hypotension

Respiratory

- Respiratory depression
- Hypoventilation

Gastrointestinal

- Nausea and vomiting
- Constipation
- Dyspepsia

Miscellaneous

- Dry mouth
- Pupil constriction
- Urinary retention
- Muscle spasticity
- Itching

Table 29.9 Symptoms of the opioid withdrawal syndrome

- Intense craving for the drug
- Restlessness and insomnia
- Muscle and joint pain
- Running nose and eyes
- Sweating
- Abdominal cramps
- Vomiting and diarrhoea
- Piloerection
- Dilated pupils
- Raised pulse rate
- Instability of temperature control

develops rapidly, especially when the drug is taken intravenously.

Tolerance develops rapidly, leading to ever increasing usage. When the drug is stopped, tolerance diminishes so that a dose taken after an interval of abstinence has a greater effect than it would have had before the interval. This loss of tolerance can result in dangerous—sometimes fatal—respiratory depression when a previously tolerated dose is resumed after a drug-free interval; for example, after a stay in hospital or prison.

Withdrawal. The symptoms due to withdrawal from opioids are shown in Table 29.9. With heroin, these features usually begin about 6 hours after the last dose, reach a peak after 36–48 hours, and then wane. These symptoms cause great distress, which drives the person to seek further supplies but seldom threatens the life of a person in reasonable health.

Complications of opioid use

These are shown in Table 29.10. The most common cause of death amongst opioid users is opioid overdose, which most frequently occurs after a period of abstinence

during which tolerance has decreased. However, the rate of suicide amongst those dependent upon opioids is 14 times the rate of the general population, usually because of co-morbid depression.

The babies of opioid-dependent women are more likely than other babies to be premature and of low birth weight. Also, they may show withdrawal symptoms after birth, including irritability, restlessness, tremor, and a high-pitched cry. These signs appear within a few days of birth if the mother was taking heroin, but are delayed if she was taking methadone, which has a longer half-life. Later effects have been reported, these children being more likely as toddlers to be overactive and to show poor persistence. It is uncertain whether these late effects result from the unsuitable family environment provided by these mothers, or from a lasting effect of the exposure to the drug.

In those who use heroin for a long time, there is a small risk of developing a toxic leukoencephalopathy. It is unknown if this is a direct effect of the opioid itself, or caused by a contaminant (or 'cutting' agent) added to the drug during production. Symptoms include confusion, ataxia, and deteriorating neurological function over some weeks.

Treatment of opioid dependence

The general principles of assessment and management should be carried out as described on pp. 396–400.

Treatment of an opioid overdose

The key clinical findings in a patient who has taken an overdose of opioids are:

1 respiratory depression (rate less than eight breaths per minute), possibly leading to respiratory arrest;

2 unreactive pinpoint pupils;

Table 29.10 Complications of opioid use

Biological	Psychological	Social
Infections	• Depression	• Unemployment
• Abscesses and cellulitis	• Anxiety disorders	• Loss of accommodation
• Sepsis	• Deliberate self-harm	• Breakdown of relationships
• HIV	• Suicide	• Loss of friends
• Hepatitis B or C		• Criminal record
• Bacterial endocarditis		
Cardiorespiratory		
• Deep vein thrombosis or pulmonary embolism		
• Aspiration		
• Respiratory depression		
• Cardiac arrhythmias		
Complications of pregnancy		
Death from overdose		

3 bradycardia;

4 hypotension;

5 snoring or other upper airway sounds;

6 reduced level of consciousness.

Patients should be approached using the principles of *airway*, *breathing*, and *circulation* and treated with oxygen, respiratory support, fluids, and inotropes if necessary. The antidote to opioids is **naloxone**, which may be given IV (preferably) or IM. The usual dose is 400 µg IV. Naloxone has a short half-life and repeated doses will need to be given every few minutes. Once the acute effect of the opioids has been reversed, supportive management is given.

Planned withdrawal of opioids (detoxification)

The general principles of drug withdrawal have been outlined above. When heroin is withdrawn, psychological support is particularly important to avoid immediate relapse. Withdrawal is usually undertaken by substituting methadone (a longer-acting drug) for heroin. The main steps are shown in Box 29.10. Buprenorphine (Subutex) or alpha-2 agonists (clonidine or lofexidine) may also be used, and are equally effective.

Continued prescribing (maintenance)

The principles of maintenance treatment for opiate dependence have been discussed. Methadone is a synthetic opioid agonist which is active when given orally, and has a long half-life (36 hours), making it suitable for once-daily dosing. Methadone is prescribed and dispensed daily, usually in a liquid preparation formulated to discourage efforts to inject it. The equivalent dosage is difficult to determine since street drugs are adulterated to a varying degree, but 60–120 mg per day is the usual

---

BOX 29.10 The planned withdrawal of opioids (detoxification)

• When the starting dose is very high, or there have been previously complicated or failed withdrawals, withdrawal should occur in hospital.

• It is often difficult to judge the starting dose because patients often take adulterated preparations of heroin (and may lie about the amount taken). For this reason treatment should be discussed with, and often carried out by, a specialist in drug dependence.

• The starting dose of methadone is usually 10–20 mg daily, which is increased in 10- to 20-mg steps until

there are no signs of intoxication or withdrawal. The usual daily dose is 60–120 mg.

• The initial dose is reduced by about a quarter every 2 or 3 days, but a slower rate may be needed.

• The regimen should be agreed with the patient as a contract that he will accept throughout the treatment.

• Urine tests for drugs should be carried out weekly after withdrawal until the doctor is confident that the patient is remaining drug free.

range. There is good evidence that patients treated with doses higher in that range (80–120 mg) are less likely to restart using illicit opioids. The treatment should be initiated by a specialist, although care can be shared with the primary care physician.

In some European countries, there have been trials using supervised injection of methadone or diamorphine for maintenance therapy. The two drugs appear to be equally effective, and there is a higher chance of preventing the illicit use of IV heroin than when using oral methadone. This treatment is available in a few countries at present, in programmes run by specialists in addictions.

Psychological treatments

All of the forms of therapy and treatment described previously are applicable to opioid misuse. The most successful programmes are those which combine withdrawal/ maintenance with psychological and social support. Motivational interviewing and relapse prevention are useful, and for those patients with psychiatric co-morbidities, CBT is an effective intervention. Narcotics Anonymous is a similar group programme to Alcoholics Anonymous, based on a 12-step mantra. It is growing in popularity in Europe and can provide support for patients, especially those with a complete breakdown of social structure.

Prognosis

Opioid dependence is a chronic relapsing–remitting condition, and the outcomes of treatment are allied to those seen for other chronic diseases. Although about 90 per cent of opioid-dependent patients can withdraw successfully, about 50 per cent will recommence use by 6 months following withdrawal. After 7 years, only one-quarter to one-third of opioid-dependent people will have become abstinent, and between 10 and 20 per cent will have died from causes related to drug taking. Deaths are from accidental overdose—often related to loss of tolerance after a period of enforced abstinence—and from medical complications such as infection with HIV. When abstinence is achieved, it is often related to changed circumstances of life, such as a new relationship with a caring person.

Anxiolytic and hypnotic drugs

The most frequently used drugs in this group are now benzodiazepines. The most serious health problems are presented by barbiturates, which, although seldom used therapeutically, are available as street drugs.

Barbiturates

Barbiturates are taken by mouth and intravenously. Some elderly people are dependent on barbiturates prescribed originally many years ago as prescribed hypnotics.

Younger dependent people use illegal supplies of barbiturates, and some dissolve capsules and inject intravenously—a particularly dangerous practice leading to phlebitis, ulcers, abscesses, and gangrene. The symptoms of barbiturate intoxication resemble those of alcohol: slurred speech, incoherence, drowsiness, and low mood. Younger intravenous users are often unkempt, dirty, and malnourished. **Nystagmus**, a useful diagnostic sign, may be present. Urine should be examined to investigate the possible simultaneous abuse of other drugs. Blood levels are generally useful only in acute poisoning.

Tolerance develops to barbiturates, although less quickly than to opioids. Tolerance of the psychological effects of barbiturates is greater than tolerance of their depressant effects on respiration, so increasing the risks of unintentional fatal overdosage.

Withdrawal. The abrupt withdrawal of barbiturates from a dependent person can be followed by a withdrawal syndrome resembling that occurring with alcohol, with a *high risk of seizures*. With longer-acting drugs, the withdrawal syndrome may be delayed for several days after the drug has been stopped; for this reason observation should be prolonged if dangerous consequences are to be avoided. The syndrome of barbiturate withdrawal begins with anxiety, restlessness, disturbed sleep, anorexia, and nausea. It may progress to tremulousness, disorientation, hallucinations, vomiting, hypotension, pyrexia, and major seizures. If the withdrawal syndrome is not treated, some patients die.

When drugs are withdrawn as part of treatment, the patient should be supervised closely in hospital, unless (i) the starting dose is small and (ii) there is no history of epilepsy. Phenothiazines should be avoided because they may lower the seizure threshold. Unless it is certain that the dosage is small, the advice of a specialist should be obtained.

Benzodiazepines

The benzodiazepines were developed in the 1950s as a response to concerns surrounding the safety of barbiturates, but did not become widely used until the mid-1960s. They have completely replaced the use of barbiturates now as they do not have the same risks of respiratory depression. Benzodiazepines are effective anxiolytics, hypnotics, anticonvulsants, and muscle relaxants, acting via the enhancement of GABA transmission in the CNS. Initially, it was not recognized that they carried a risk of dependence, so they were freely prescribed. By the 1980s, it became evident that many people had started abusing the drugs and were easily becoming addicted to them. It is now known that tolerance develops quickly, and crosses between all drugs in the group. Therapeutic use of benzodiazepines should initially be for 2 weeks, with an absolute maximum of 4–6 weeks.

There are no reliable epidemiological statistics available, but one large study in the USA reported 15 per cent of teenagers having used benzodiazepines more than once.

A variety of different benzodiazepines are available, varying in their length of action. Temazepam and oxazepam are short-acting, lorazepam and alprazolam medium-acting, and nitrazepam, chlordiazepoxide, and diazepam long-acting. Flunitrazepam, a particularly short-acting and potent benzodiazepine, is no longer available legally in many countries. It is also known as Rohypnol, and has been used as a 'date-rape' drug.

Benzodiazepines are usually taken orally, but occasionally intravenously. IV use carries the usual risks of injecting, but also a high risk of acute limb ischaemia secondary to the use of melted tablets. Availability of forms of the drugs which may be taken IV appears to be the main factor in determining the rate of IV use. In the 1980s, a liquid-filled capsule version of temazepam became available. This led to a surge in IV-use-related deaths, and it was quickly withdrawn.

The **benzodiazepine withdrawal syndrome** is characterized by irritability and anxiety, disturbed sleep, nausea, tremor, sweating, palpitations, headache, and seizures.

Management of benzodiazepine misuse

At the time of writing, there is no evidence base to guide the treatment of illicit benzodiazepine misuse. However, there is evidence of managing those patients who become dependent on prescribed benzodiazepines.

Planned withdrawal of benzodiazepines

The withdrawal symptoms are less pronounced with long-acting (e.g. diazepam) than with short-acting benzodiazepines (e.g. lorazepam), so a short-acting drug should be replaced with a long-acting drug in the equivalent dose before starting withdrawal. Where possible, if large doses are involved then these should be dispensed daily by a specified pharmacist. When benzodiazepines are withdrawn therapeutically, the dose should be reduced very gradually, by about 10 per cent every 2 weeks. This plan should be agreed in writing at the start of the withdrawal. If withdrawal symptoms appear during withdrawal, the dose can be increased slightly, and then reduced again by a smaller amount than before. As the dose decreases, it may not be possible to achieve the required dose reduction with the strengths of tablets available. At this stage the drug can be taken on alternate days or a liquid preparation (e.g. diazepam elixir or nitrazepam syrup) can be used. Occasionally, inpatient detoxification may be needed, especially if there are acute psychiatric or physical co-morbidities to be treated. If the patient has previously had seizures during withdrawal, they should be admitted to a general hospital environment and carbamazepine given alongside the withdrawal.

Psychological treatments

A full psychiatric assessment is needed to identify co-morbidities and the reasons behind substance misuse. Appropriate management should then be initiated; for example, antidepressants, individual or group CBT, or relaxation therapy.

Prescribing benzodiazepines

All doctors should follow the guidance below to avoid their patient becoming dependent on benzodiazepines.

- Be very cautious about initiating a prescription for benzodiazepines.
- Prescribe the lowest dose possible.
- Limit the prescription to 2–3 weeks.
- Do not have prescriptions available for routine repeat refills.
- Never re-prescribe if the patient reports losing or forgetting their tablets.
- Do not prescribe benzodiazepines for another doctor's patients; tell them to go to their usual prescriber.

Stimulant drugs

Stimulant drugs potentiate the effects of neurotransmitters (including serotonin, dopamine, and norepinephrine (noradrenaline)), causing increased energy, a state of alertness, and euphoria. At the same time there is an increase in confidence and impulsivity and a decrease in judgement. This can lead to risky behaviour. The stimulant drugs abused most often are amphetamines and cocaine.

- **Amphetamine sulphate** is taken by mouth or by intravenous injection.
- **Free-base amphetamine** (made by heating amphetamine sulphate) is usually smoked and absorbed through the lungs, from which it is absorbed rapidly.
- **Cocaine hydrochloride** is taken by sniffing into the nose (where it is absorbed through the nasal mucosa) or by injecting.
- **Free-base cocaine** ('crack') is usually smoked to give a rapid and intense effect.

Stimulants are most commonly used by young people, especially males from lower socio-economic backgrounds. Cocaine has a secondary following in the upper middle classes, often young professionals aged 25–35 years. The USA has the highest level of cocaine usage—10 per cent of adults admit to usage in their life-time—whilst most European statistics are in single figures.

Clinical features

Stimulants produce an elevation of mood, overactivity, overtalkativeness, insomnia, anorexia, and dryness of the mouth and nose. The pupils dilate, the pulse rate and blood pressure increase, and with large doses there may be cardiac arrhythmia and circulatory collapse. The over-activity can cause dehydration; overhydration can occur if the user drinks large amounts of water to overcome the dehydration. Occasionally, patients complain of an unu-sual feeling under the skin, as if insects were there ('formication').

The *prolonged use* of large quantities of these drugs may result in disturbances of perception and thinking. Particularly with amphetamines, a **paranoid psychosis** may occur closely resembling the paranoid form of schiz-ophrenia, with persecutory delusions, auditory and vis-ual hallucinations, and sometimes aggressive behaviour. Usually, the condition subsides within a week or two of stopping the drug, but occasionally persists for months. In some of these prolonged cases the diagnosis proves to be schizophrenia, not drug-induced psychosis. **Depression** may also follow long-term use of stimulants.

Stimulant drugs do not readily induce *tolerance*. On stopping the drugs there is low mood, reduced energy, and increased appetite but it is unclear if this is a with-drawal syndrome or merely rebound symptoms. There is an ongoing debate as to whether these drugs induce a psychological dependence or physical dependence.

Complications of stimulants

The complications of stimulants are mostly general; for example, the risks of injecting substances. Regular use tends to lead to a decline in physical health, including weight loss, poor dentition, malnutrition, mood distur-bances, and social problems. It can also lead to hyperten-sion and arrhythmias, which occasionally cause a myocardial infarction. Pregnant females may miscarry or go into premature labour. Frequent snorting of cocaine can lead to perforation of the nasal septum.

Treatment of misuse of stimulants

There is no specific management for stimulant misuse; the general principles of treating any substance problem apply. There is evidence that education, harm-reduction measures, and targeting treatments at high-risk groups are all effective. For individuals with a long-term cocaine problem, more intensive programmes are often needed. Inpatient rehabilitation is frequently undertaken, with a comprehensive detoxification and therapy programme over several months. This can be very effective if the patient is motivated to change. For emergency situations

(e.g. psychosis) the usual forms of treatment should be used. Antipsychotics are effective for psychosis induced by stimulants, and fluoxetine has the best evidence base if an antidepressant is needed.

Prognosis

Unlike opioid and benzodiazepine misuse, the majority of individuals using stimulants do so for recreation and not on a regular basis. Very few continue to do so in the long term, and less than 1 per cent suffers a complication of usage. Heavy use of cocaine has a less good prognosis, but if treatment is sought it is usually effective.

Ecstasy (3, 4-methylenedioxymetham-phetamine, MDMA)

Ecstasy is a substance available in tablet form which has been used increasingly since the 1980s, especially at dances ('raves') and clubs. It produces an intense feeling of well-being and increased energy. It is similar to a stim-ulant, but has some hallucinogenic properties as well.

Ecstasy is usually taken at the weekends in nightclubs, mostly by teenagers and students. Studies in the UK have reported approximately 50 per cent of 20- to 22-year-old have been offered ecstasy at some point, and 15 per cent have tried it at least once. Most individuals might take one or two tablets in a night, with regular users taking four to six tablets every few days. It is associated with spe-cial events, such as a holiday or birthday night out, and is usually used together with alcohol or other stimulants.

Ecstasy causes increased energy, tachycardia, hyper-tension, dilated pupils, increased sweating, weight loss, and anorexia. Frequently, people experience some nau-sea and vomiting, diarrhoea, or dehydration after usage. Rarely, there may be life-threatening arrhythmias, sei-zures, dehydration, renal failure, rhabdomyolysis, or liver failure. Ecstasy reduces the body's ability to thermoregu-late, inducing hyperthermia. Coupled with the drinking of hypotonic fluids to counter dehydration (e.g. water, beer) this can lead to lethal hyponatraemia.

Treatment is rarely needed for individuals misusing ecstasy, unless there are co-morbid psychiatric or other substance misuse problems. The majority of users 'grow out of it' and suffer no long-term complications of usage.

Hallucinogens

This group of drugs includes synthetic compounds such as **lysergic acid diethylamide (LSD)** and naturally occur-ring substances found in species of mushroom (e.g. *Psilocybe semilanceata*). Phenylcyclidine (PCP) and keta-mine are becoming increasingly popular. Synthetic and naturally occurring **anticholinergic drugs** are also abused for their hallucinogenic effects. The use of LSD is thought to have reduced markedly in the last 10 years, while that of mushrooms has increased. This is thought to be due to reduced availability, and a better appreciation of the risks of LSD.

LSD becomes psychoactive in a drop of solvent, and dissolved into an aqueous solution. It is then placed on to small pieces of blotting paper with pictures on ('tabs') or on to sugar cubes. These are then eaten, and the drug induces a 'trip', which may last for up to 12 hours. Mushrooms may be eaten or drunk as a broth.

The drugs produce distortions or intensifications of sensory perception, sometimes with 'cross-over' between sensory modalities so that, for example, sounds are experienced as visual sensations. Objects may seem to merge or move rhythmically, time appears to pass slowly, and ordinary experiences may seem to have a profound meaning. The body image may be distorted or the person may feel as if outside his body. These experiences can be pleasurable, but at times they are profoundly distressing and lead to unpredictable and dangerous behaviour. The physical effects of hallucinogens are variable; LSD can cause a rise in heart rate and dilation of the pupils.

Complications of hallucinogen use tend to relate to the user experiencing terrifying experiences. This can lead to panic attacks, outbursts of aggression, and violence. In the acute situation, a dose of benzodiazepine will stop these effects within minutes but usually only strong reassurance is necessary. Occasionally, regular users of hallucinogens can develop a persistent perceptual disorder, in which hallucinations occur days or weeks after the last dose. These may be new experiences, or 'flashbacks' of experiences occurring originally during intoxication. These can intermittently occur for years afterwards even if no more drugs are taken, but they do usually eventually cease. Individuals may need some form of psychotherapy to help them live with these experiences long term.

PCP or 'angel dust' is a synthetic hallucinogen with particularly dangerous effects. It is occasionally used as a pure drug, but is frequently mixed with either cocaine or cannabis and may be taken orally, smoked, snorted, or injected. Intoxication with this drug can be prolonged and hazardous, with agitation, aggressive behaviour, and hallucinations together with nystagmus and raised blood pressure. With high doses, there may be ataxia, muscle rigidity, and convulsions, and in severe cases, an adrenergic crisis with heart failure, cerebrovascular accident, or malignant hypothermia. Treatment is supportive, but should include antihypertensives, diuretics, and neuroleptics.

Cannabis

Cannabis, which derives from the plant *Cannabis sativa* and is the most commonly used illicit substance, is consumed in two forms. The dried vegetative parts of the plant form marijuana ('grass'); the resin secreted by the flowering tops of the female plant forms cannabis resin ('hashish'). The active constituent is delta-9-tetrahydrocannabinol (THC). In many parts of the world cannabis is consumed widely, much as alcohol is consumed in the West. In most Western societies the use of cannabis, although illegal, is widespread. Cannabis is currently being investigated as a therapeutic agent for multiple sclerosis and other chronic and painful disorders. Cannabis has been tried, or is used regularly, by most young adults in Western countries. The typical age of onset is late teens, and most users have given it up by age 30. Heavy cannabis use implies daily usage and is much less common.

The effects of cannabis vary with the dose, the user's expectations, and the social setting. Like alcohol, cannabis seems to exaggerate the pre-existing mood, whether euphoria or dysphoria. It produces a feeling of enhanced enjoyment of aesthetic experiences, and distorts experiences of time and space. Cannabis intoxication can lead to dangerous driving. The physical effects of cannabis include reddening of the conjunctiva, dry mouth, and tachycardia.

Cannabis does not produce a *withdrawal syndrome*, and although *psychological dependence* can develop, physical dependence does not seem to occur. Occasionally people will present asking for help in reducing their cannabis usage.

It is not certain whether cannabis causes a *psychosis*. Some patients develop an acute psychosis while consuming large amounts of cannabis, recovering quickly when the drug is stopped. In these cases it is uncertain whether cannabis caused the psychosis, or the increased use of cannabis was a response to the early symptoms of a psychosis with a different cause. There is also an association between schizophrenia and cannabis. There is a consistent body of evidence suggesting that in genetically vulnerable individuals, cannabis can precipitate the onset of schizophrenia. Fortunately, this uncertainty seldom causes practical problems since the clinical management is unaffected: the drug should be stopped, the progress of the symptoms observed, and an antipsychotic drug prescribed if symptoms do not subside within a week.

There have been reports suggesting that consistent use of cannabis could cause cognitive impairment. Acutely, memory and concentration are affected, but for occasional recreational use there is no evidence of long-term harm. For heavy users, a decline in memory, organization, and attention is seen over time. More relevant is the **amotivational syndrome**. Societies in which cannabis use is integrated into the culture report high levels of impaired motivation and poor performance at work and in the home. This is also seen amongst heavy cannabis

Table 29.11 Clinical features of solvent intoxication

- Slurring of speech
- Disorientation
- Incoordination of gait
- Nausea and vomiting
- Coma
- Visual hallucinations (often frightening)

users in Western countries, notably with once high-achieving children deciding not to go to university as it is 'too much effort'.

Good-quality public education about the harms of cannabis smoking may have an important impact on use trends in the future.

Organic solvents

The use of volatile solvents occurs mainly among teenagers, usually as occasional experimentation. Data from the 2003 European Schools Project on Alcohol and Other Drugs reported 12 per cent of teenagers as having used solvents. Males and females were equally represented. Serious problems arise in a minority who use solvents regularly, and any user may take an accidental overdose or become asphyxiated while taking the substance.

The solvents used most often are cleaning fluids, adhesives, and aerosols. Petrol, butane, and fire extinguishers may also be used. The substance is inhaled from a partially closed container in which the concentration can build up, or from an impregnated cloth, or plastic bag. The main features of solvent intoxication are similar to those of alcohol, and are shown in Table 29.11.

Acute harmful effects include overdose on the solvent, irritation of the airways, headache, or cardiac arrhythmias. Rarely, the individual may accidentally suffocate, or aspirate causing a chemical pneumonitis. Longer-term effects of solvent usage include fatigue, anorexia, memory loss, and a change in mood. There are some reports of liver or kidney failure. Psychological dependence occurs but physical dependence is unusual. Chronic heavy users may develop a transient psychosis. Some of these substances have neurotoxic effects with resultant peripheral neuropathy and cerebellar dysfunction. There is the added risk of fire when dealing with flammable agents.

In an emergency situation, the harmful substance should be removed and the intoxicated individual approached calmly and reassured. Usually, they will return to normal within 20–30 minutes. Treatment is along the general lines of that for the harmful use of drugs described on p. 396.

Further reading

Gelder, M., Andreasen, N., Lopez-Ibor, J, & Geddes, J. (2009). *New Oxford Textbook of Psychiatry*, 2nd edn. Section 4.2. Substance use disorders, pp. 426–520. Oxford University Press, Oxford.

Latt, N. *et al.* (2009). *Addiction Medicine*, 1st edn. Oxford University Press, Oxford.

Parker, A. J. R, Marshall, E. J & Ball, D. M. (2008). Diagnosis and management of alcohol use disorders. *British Medical Journal* **336**: 496–501.

Schuckit, M. A. (2009). Alcohol-use disorders. *Lancet* **373**: 492–501.

Alcoholics Anonymous. Northern American website: www.aa.org/. United Kingdom website: www.alcoholics-anonymous.org.uk/.

Fergusson, D. M. *et al.* (2006). Cannabis and psychosis. *British Medical Journal* **332**: 172–6.

Robson, P. (1999). *Forbidden Drugs*, 2nd edn. Oxford University Press, Oxford.

CHAPTER 30

Problems of sexuality and gender

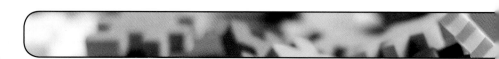

Chapter contents

Sexual problems are included in this book because human sexuality involves complex psychological and neurobiological mechanisms, and sexual problems commonly accompany other mental disorders. There are four types of problem that commonly present to doctors:

1 sexual dysfunction—impaired or dissatisfying sexual enjoyment or performance;

2 abnormalities of sexual preference—unusual sexual interests and activities that are preferred to heterosexual intercourse;

3 disorders of gender identity—in which the patient feels as if they are of the opposite sex to their biological sex;

4 psychological problems encountered by homosexual people.

Of these, the first group are the most common. In this chapter, we describe the common sexual disorders and outline their treatment. After studying the chapter, the reader should:

- know the clinical features of the most common sexual problems;

- be able to take a history of a sexual problem;

- understand how to formulate a sexual problem.

We assume that readers will have learnt about the physiology of the sexual response elsewhere—if not, we recommend reading the appropriate chapters of Bancroft's *Human Sexuality and its Problems*, 3rd edition, Churchill Livingstone, 2009. The main stages of the physiology of the sexual response are summarized in Tables 30.1 and 30.2.

Table 30.1 Male sexual response

	Excitement	Plateau	Orgasm	Resolution
Penis	Erection	Erection maintained	Urethra contracts repeatedly	Gradual detumescence
Scrotum	Skin thickens, testes raised	Testes raised further	No change	Return to normal
Prostate, seminal vesicles	Contract with emission of seminal fluid to urethra	Return to normal		
Pulse and blood pressure	Increase	Further increase	Further increase	Return to normal
Respiration		Rate increases	Rate increases further	Return to normal

■ Sexual behaviour in the population

Some knowledge of normal sexual behaviour will help a doctor to assess a patient's presenting problem.

The age of first intercourse is dropping over time. This is probably due to a combination of a trend to earlier sexual maturity and a relaxation of social attitudes towards sexuality. At present, about 20 per cent of females and about 30 per cent of males experience heterosexual intercourse before the age of 16 years. More than 80 per cent of both sexes have experienced sexual intercourse by the age of 20 years. Earlier age of first intercourse is associated with lower social class, lower levels of education, and lack of religious affiliation.

The earlier first intercourse occurs, the less likely it is to be accompanied by adequate contraceptive use and the more it is felt by the subject, in retrospect, to have been too early. When surveyed, over half of adults report having engaged in vaginal intercourse in the preceding week and more than half report having experienced oral sex in the preceding year. Ninety-six per cent of men and 97 per cent of women report mostly or exclusively **heterosexual** (erotic thoughts and feelings are directed towards a person of the opposite sex) experience and attraction. One per cent of men and 0.25 per cent of women report mostly or exclusively **homosexual** (erotic thoughts and feelings are directed towards a person of the same sex) experience and attraction. However, 6 per cent of males and 3 per cent of females report some homosexual experience in addition to their mainly heterosexual orientation. Homophobic attitudes are widespread—a survey in 1994 suggested about two-thirds of the population believe that homosexuality is always or mostly wrong.

Table 30.2 Female sexual response

	Excitement	Plateau	Orgasm	Resolution
Breasts	Nipple erection in some	Enlargement, areolar engorgement	No change	Return to normal
Labia		Engorgement	No change	Return to normal
Clitoris	Head swells	Head withdraws	No change	Return to normal
Vagina	Lubrication, expansion, distension of inner two-thirds	Outer third swells, inner two-thirds distend further	Contractions of outer third	Return to normal
Uterus	Body and cervix raised	Further elevation	Contractions	Position returns to normal; os gapes open
Pulse and blood pressure	Slight elevation	Further increase	Increase continues	Return to normal
Respiration		Rate increases	Rate increases further	Return to normal

■ Sexual dysfunction

It is difficult to establish the prevalence of sexual problems in the population because of the difficulties involved in carrying out surveys of people's sexual behaviour. The commonest kinds of problems presenting to a sexual dysfunction clinic are shown in Table 30.3; the terms are explained below.

The assessment of sexual dysfunction

Patients with sexual problems initially often complain about other symptoms because they feel too embarrassed to reveal a sexual problem directly. For example, a patient may ask for help with anxiety, depression, poor sleep, or gynaecological symptoms. It is therefore important to ask routinely a few questions about sexual functioning when assessing patients with non-specific psychological or physical symptoms.

In a full assessment, the interviewer should begin by explaining why it will be necessary to ask about intimate details of the patient's sexual life, and should then ask questions in a sympathetic, matter-of-fact way (Box 30.1). Whenever possible both sexual partners should be interviewed, at first separately and then together.

The assessment should cover the following issues.

- Has the problem been present from the first intercourse, or did it start after a period of normal sexual functioning? Each partner should be asked, separately, whether the same problem has occurred with another partner, or during masturbation.

- The *strength of sexual drive* should be assessed in terms of the frequency of sexual arousal, intercourse, and masturbation. *Motivation* for treatment should be assessed,

Table 30.3 Relative frequency of sexual problems presenting to a sexual dysfunction clinic

Women	
Low sexual desire	50%
Orgasmic dysfunction	20%
Vaginismus	20%
Dyspareunia	5%
Men	
Erectile dysfunction	60%
Premature ejaculation	15%
Delayed ejaculation	5%
Low sexual desire	5%

Adapted from: Hawton, K. (1985). *Sex Therapy: A Practical Guide.* Oxford Medical Publications, Oxford University Press.

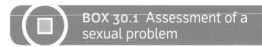

BOX 30.1 Assessment of a sexual problem

- Define the problem:
  - its nature;
  - recent or long-standing;
  - whether with this partner only.
- Assess sexual drives of both partners.
- Enquire about the marital relationship and social relationships in general.
- Sexual development including traumatic experiences.
- Previous and present psychiatric and medical illness and treatment; pregnancy, childbirth and abortion(s); alcohol and drug use.
- Assess the mental state, especially for depressive disorder.
- Assess motivation for treatment.
- Physical examination and any relevant laboratory tests.

starting with questions about who took the initiative in seeking treatment and for what reason.

- Assess each partner's *social relationships* with the other sex, with particular reference to shyness and social inhibition.

- Enquiries should be made about the partners' *feelings for one another*: partners who lack a mutual caring relationship are unlikely to achieve a fully satisfactory sexual relationship. Many couples say that their relationship problems result from their sexual problems, when the causal connection is really the reverse. Tactful questions should be asked about commitment to the partner and, when appropriate, about infidelity and fears of sexually transmitted disease, including HIV.

- Assess *sexual development* and *sexual experience*, paying particular attention to experiences such as child abuse, incest, or sexual assault that may have caused lasting anxiety or disgust about sex.

- Enquiry should be made about homosexual as well as heterosexual feelings.

- In the *medical history*, the most relevant things to look for are previous and present psychiatric and chronic physical disorders and their treatment, pregnancy, childbirth, and abortion(s), and use of alcohol or drugs, such as selective serotonin reuptake inhibitors (SSRIs).

- In the *mental state examination* look especially for evidence of depressive disorder.

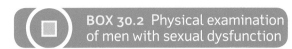

BOX 30.2 Physical examination of men with sexual dysfunction

1   Is there evidence of diabetes mellitus or adrenal disorder?
    Hair distribution, gynaecomastia
    Blood pressure, peripheral pulses
    Fundi for retinopathy
    Reflexes, especially ankle
    Peripheral sensation

2   Are there any abnormalities of the genitalia?
    Penis: congenital abnormalities, foreskin, pulses, tenderness, plaques, infection, urethral discharge
    Testicles: size, symmetry, texture, sensation

- *Physical examination* is important because physical illness often causes sexual problems (see Box 30.2 and Table 30.4). Physical examination of women may require specialist gynaecological help. Further investigations may be necessary depending on the findings from the history and examination (e.g. if diabetes is suspected as a cause of sexual disorder).

■ Specific sexual disorders

Low sexual desire

This problem may occur in both sexes but is commoner in women. In some cases, sexual desire has always been low (**primary low sexual desire**); this may be the extreme of the range of biological variation, or it may be due to fears originating from adverse experiences in childhood, such as sexual abuse. In other cases, sexual desire has been normal in the past but has become impaired (**secondary low sexual desire**); the causes then include general problems in the relationship between the partners, physical disorders (Table 30.4), and depressive disorder (in which lack of sexual desire may continue for some weeks after other symptoms have resolved).

Treatment

Treatment is of the cause if one can be identified. The relationship between the partners may improve with couple therapy (p. 142), a depressive disorder should be treated in the usual way (see p. 232), and fear or guilt caused by adverse experiences in early life may respond to psychotherapy (p. 140). Low sexual drive cannot be increased by giving hormones.

Male erectile dysfunction

Erectile dysfunction is the inability to reach erection or sustain it long enough for satisfactory coitus. Primary erectile dysfunction is rare and usually has a physical basis, such as neurological damage or leakage from the penile cavernous bodies.

The common causes of secondary erectile dysfunction are:

- anxiety about sexual performance;
- alcohol abuse;
- drug side effects (see Table 30.5);
- diabetes;
- arteriosclerosis;
- age-related diminution of sexual function.

Assessment of erectile dysfunction should identify whether it is invariable (suggesting a physical or drug cause) or present only in some circumstances (suggesting a psychological cause). Questions should be asked about erections on waking from sleep, and during masturbation; if they are present, a physical cause is unlikely.

Table 30.4 Physical disorders and drugs causing low sexual desire

Physical disorders	Drugs
Hypogonadism	Hypnotics
Angina and previous myocardial infarction	Anxiolytics
Epilepsy	Antipsychotics
Renal failure and dialysis	
Hypothyroidism	
Mastectomy	
Oophorectomy	
Colostomy	
Ileostomy	

Table 30.5 Physical disorders and drugs causing erectile dysfunction

Physical disorders	Drugs
Diabetes mellitus	Antihypertensives
Arteriosclerosis	Beta-blockers
Hyperprolactinaemia	Diuretics
Pelvic autonomic neuropathy	Cimetidine
Rectal surgery	Tricyclic antidepressants
	Monoamine oxidase inhibitors
	Antipsychotics

Treatment

Treatment of erectile dysfunction should combine psychological approaches with physical approaches as appropriate. If the disorder is caused by a drug or other physical cause, these should be stopped or treated if possible. Psychological treatment includes the use of sexual therapy techniques (see below) and anxiety management. Physical treatments of erectile dysfunction include drug treatment with sildenafil (a potent inhibitor of phosphodiesterase type V), intracavernosal injections of smooth muscle relaxants (e.g. papaverine or prostaglandin E_1), vacuum devices, and, occasionally, surgical insertion of semi-rigid rods.

Conditions with discomfort or pain

Pain on intercourse occurs mainly among women, either as vaginismus or as dyspareunia.

Vaginismus

Vaginismus is painful spasm of the vaginal muscles during intercourse. This spasm may be due to aversion to intercourse or may result from painful scarring after episiotomy or other procedures. The condition may be made worse by an inexperienced or inconsiderate partner. Generally, the spasm begins when the man attempts penetration, but in severe cases it occurs even if the woman attempts to insert her own finger into the vagina. In such severe cases no intercourse can take place.

Treatment

It should be explained to the patient that vaginismus is a form of muscle spasm which can be overcome by relaxation exercises. A graduated behavioural approach to treatment is used. At first, diagrams and mirrors are used to improve the patient's understanding of sexual anatomy and response. Once the woman is familiar and comfortable with her genitals, she is encouraged to introduce the tip of her finger into the vagina. She gradually inserts the whole of her finger and, once she can do this without discomfort, she should try inserting two fingers. In many women, this process will allow the woman to overcome the vaginismus. In situations where the woman finds it difficult to transfer from finger to penile penetration, graduated dilators can be used.

Vaginismus should be distinguished from lack of vaginal lubrication which is usually due to lack of sexual arousal, but may also be due to drug side effects and physical disorders (e.g. diabetes). It is more common following the menopause. Treatment consists of removing the cause or using additional lubrication.

Dyspareunia

Dyspareunia is pain on intercourse (Table 30.6). When the pain arises after even partial penetration of the vagina, it may result from impaired lubrication with vaginal secretions (due to aversion to intercourse or inadequate foreplay) or from painful scarring. When pain is felt only during deep penetration, it may be due to pelvic pathology such as endometriosis, pelvic inflammatory disease, ovarian cyst, or tumour. Pain on deep penetration may also result from diminished lubrication in the later stages of prolonged intercourse.

Treatment

Treatment of dyspareunia depends on the cause. When it is the result of psychological factors causing impaired sexual arousal, sexual therapy techniques can be used. Referral to a gynaecologist should be made if simple measures are ineffective.

The few cases of dyspareunia among men involve **painful ejaculation**, an uncommon disorder usually caused by urethritis or prostatitis, but occasionally without detectable cause.

Orgasmic dysfunction

In men, orgasmic dysfunction is premature ejaculation or retarded ejaculation; in women it is inhibited orgasm.

Premature ejaculation

Premature ejaculation is habitual ejaculation before penetration or shortly afterwards, so that the woman gains no

Table 30.6 Physical disorders and drugs causing pain and orgasmic dysfunction

Pain
Dyspareunia
Episiotomy
Endometriosis
Pelvic inflammatory disease
Pelvic cysts or tumours
Painful ejaculation
Urethritis
Prostatitis
Orgasmic dysfunction
Spinal cord injury
Drugs
Antipsychotics
MAOIs

pleasure. It is common among young men during first sexual encounters, and usually improves with increasing sexual experience. The partner can assist by interrupting foreplay whenever the man feels himself becoming highly aroused (**stop–start technique**). This process prolongs the period during which the man can be highly aroused, but not ejaculate.

Retarded ejaculation

Retarded ejaculation may be part of a general psychological inhibition about relations with women. It can also be caused by drugs, notably antipsychotic drugs, SSRIs, and monoamine oxidase inhibitors. If the condition is caused by drugs, the dose should be reduced if practicable. When the causes are psychological, psychotherapy can be tried although its results are uncertain.

Inhibited female orgasm

Inhibited female orgasm during intercourse is frequent although most women can achieve it through clitoral stimulation. In one survey, a quarter of women said they had not experienced orgasm during the first year of marriage. Whether treatment is requested depends on what the couple regards as abnormal. Failure of female orgasm may be due to the man's incapacity to arouse his partner or show her affection and is a likely cause if the woman can experience orgasm by masturbation. Other causes are tiredness, depressive disorder, physical illness, and the effects of medication.

Treatment

Treatment begins by dealing with any remediable cause. If no such cause is found, the woman is helped to express her sexual needs to the partner, and he is encouraged to respond to them (using sex therapy if necessary, see below). If the relationship between the couple is poor, marital therapy may be used (p. 142).

Sexual dysfunction among people with physical handicaps

Physically handicapped people have sexual problems arising from several sources, including direct effects of the handicap on sexual function (e.g. impairment of the autonomic nerves to the genitalia in disease of the spinal cord), general effects such as tiredness and pain, fears about the deleterious effects of intercourse on the handicapping condition, and lack of information about the sexual activities that are possible for people with the disability. It is helpful if the general practitioner can provide disabled individuals with an opportunity to raise any sexual difficulties. When necessary, treatment is provided by adapting methods already described for treating sexual dysfunction in non-handicapped people.

Psychological treatment of sexual dysfunction

Specific treatment recommendations are given above in the sections on the individual disorders. Many disorders will respond to the steps outlined. However, treatment of a broad range of sexual dysfunction may need more structured psychological treatment. In this form of treatment the couple is seen together whenever possible. There are three stages: (i) improving communication, (ii) education, and (iii) 'graded activities'.

1 **Improving communication** has two main aims: (i) to help the couple to talk more freely about their problems and (ii) to increase each partner's understanding of the wishes and feelings of the other. These aims may be appropriate to various kinds of problems. For example, a woman may believe that her partner should know instinctively how to please her during intercourse; she may then interpret his failure to please as lack of affection rather than as the result of her not communicating her wishes to him. Alternatively, the man may wish the woman to take a more active role in intercourse but be unable to say this to her. A further aim of this stage of treatment is to enable the couple to achieve a general relationship that is more affectionate and satisfying.

2 **Education** focuses on important aspects of the male and female sexual responses; examples are the longer time needed for a woman to reach sexual arousal, and the importance of foreplay, including clitoral stimulation, in bringing about vaginal lubrication. Suitably chosen books on sex education can reinforce the therapist's advice. Educational counselling is often the most important part of the treatment of sexual dysfunction, and it may need to be repeated when the couple have made some progress with the graded activities described next.

3 **Graded activities** begin by negotiating with the couple a mutually agreed ban on full sexual intercourse. The couple are encouraged instead to explore the pleasure that each can give the other by tender physical contact. The partners are encouraged to caress each other but not to touch the genitalia at this stage. When they can achieve caressing in a relaxed way that gives enjoyment to each partner, the next stage is genital foreplay without penetration. When genital foreplay can be enjoyed by both partners, the next stage is the resumption of full intercourse in

a gradual and relaxed way, in which the partner with the greater problem sets the pace. In this stage a graduated approach starts with 'vaginal containment', in which the penis is inserted gradually into the vagina without thrusting movements. When this graded insertion is pleasurable for both partners, movement is introduced, usually by the woman at first. At each stage, each partner is encouraged to find out and provide what the other enjoys. The couple are advised to avoid checking their own state of sexual arousal. Such checking is common among people with sexual disorder, and has the effect of inhibiting the natural progression of sexual arousal to orgasm. Each partner should be encouraged to allow feelings and physical responses to develop spontaneously whilst thinking of the other person.

Hormones have *no place* in the treatment of sexual dysfunction except in cases where there is a primary hormonal disorder. The overall results of sex therapy are that about a third of cases have a successful outcome and another third have worthwhile improvement. Patients with low sexual drive generally have a poor outcome.

■ Disorders of sexual preference

Disorders of sexual preference are sometimes known as **paraphilias**. A sexual preference can be said to be abnormal by three criteria.

1 Most people in a society regard the sexual preference as abnormal.

2 The sexual preference can be harmful to other people (e.g. sadistic sexual practices).

3 The person with the preference suffers from its consequences (e.g. from a conflict between sexual preferences and moral standards).

Doctors may be concerned with these conditions in three circumstances: they may be asked for help by the person with the abnormal sexual preference; they may be approached by the sexual partner; or they may be asked for an opinion when a person has been charged with an offence against the law—for example, exhibitionism or a sexual act with a child. (These offences, and others unrelated to abnormal sexual preference, are considered in Chapter 12.)

Disorders of sexual preference are divided into (i) abnormalities of the sexual 'object' and (ii) disorders of the sexual act (Table 30.7). The aetiology of these conditions is not known, and the various theories will not be discussed. They may, however, be associated with the presence of other disorders, including depression, alcohol abuse, and dementia. Treatment is described after the descriptions of the disorders, on p. 415.

Table 30.7 Abnormalities of sexual preference

1. Abnormalities of the sexual object
• Sexual fetishism
• Transvestism
• Paedophilia
2. Abnormalities of the sexual act
• Exhibitionism
• Voyeurism
• Sexual sadism
• Sexual masochism

Disorders of preference of the sexual object

Fetishism

In this condition, an inanimate object is the preferred or only means of achieving sexual excitement. Almost all fetishists are men and most are heterosexual. Among the many objects that can evoke arousal in different people, common examples are rubber garments, women's underclothes, and high-heeled shoes. The smell and texture of these objects is often as important as their appearance in evoking sexual arousal. Some fetishists buy the objects, but others steal them and so come to the notice of the police. Sometimes the behaviour is carried out with a willing partner or with a paid prostitute, but often it is a solitary accompaniment of masturbation.

Fetishistic transvestism

In this condition, the person repeatedly wears clothes of the opposite sex as the preferred or only means of sexual arousal. It can be thought of as a special kind of fetishism. Nearly all transvestites are men. The clothing varies from a single garment to a complete set of clothing. Cross-dressing nearly always begins after puberty. At first, the clothes are worn only in private; a few people, however, go on to wear the clothes in public, usually hidden under male outer garments, but occasionally without precautions against discovery. A few transvestites wear a complete set of female garments; the condition then has to be distinguished from transsexualism (see p. 416). The essential difference is that transvestites are sexually aroused by wearing the clothing, while transsexuals are not.

Paedophilia

Paedophilia is repeated sexual activity or fantasy of such activity with prepubertal children as the preferred or only means of sexual excitement. Most paedophiles are men. Few paedophiles seek the help of doctors; those who do are mostly of middle age although the behaviour has often started earlier. From the ready sale of pornographic material depicting sex with children, it is likely that paedophilic fantasies are not rare, although paedophilia as an exclusive form of sexual behaviour is infrequent.

The child is usually above the age of 9 years but pre-pubertal, and may be of the same or opposite sex to the paedophile. The sexual contact may involve fondling, masturbation, or full coitus with consequent injury to the child.

Disorders of preference of the sexual act

The second group of disorders of sexual preference involves variations in the behaviour carried out to obtain sexual arousal. Generally, the acts are directed towards other adults but sometimes towards children (e.g. by some exhibitionists or sadists).

Exhibitionism

In this condition, sexual arousal is obtained repeatedly by exposure of the genitalia to an unprepared stranger. Nearly all exhibitionists are men. The act of exposure is usually preceded by a period of mounting tension which is released by the act. Usually, the exhibitionist seeks to shock or surprise a female. Most exhibitionists fall into two groups. The first consists of men with inhibited temperament who generally expose a flaccid penis and feel much guilt after the act. The second consists of men with aggressive personality traits who expose an erect penis while masturbating, and feel little guilt afterwards. In Britain, exhibitionists who are arrested are charged with the offence of **indecent exposure**.

When exhibitionism begins in middle or late life the possibility of organic brain disorder, depressive disorder, or alcoholism should be considered since these conditions occasionally 'release' this pattern of behaviour. In other people, the exhibitionism may start during a period of temporary stress.

Voyeurism

Voyeurism is observing others as the preferred and repeated way of obtaining sexual arousal. Most voyeurs are inhibited heterosexual men. Some voyeurs spy on couples who are having intercourse, others on women who are undressing or naked.

Sexual sadomasochism

Sadomasochism is a preference for sexual activity that involves bondage or inflicting pain on another person. If the individual prefers to receive such stimulation, the disorder is called **masochism**. If the individual prefers to administer such stimulation, the disorder is called **sadism**. Beating, whipping, and tying are common forms of such activity. Sometimes the acts are symbolic and cause

little actual damage, but occasionally the acts cause serious injuries from which the partner may die.

Mild sadomasochistic behaviour is common and is considered to be part of the range of normal sexual activity. The disorder should be diagnosed only if sado-masochistic activity is the most important source of gratification or necessary for sexual stimulation.

Management of disorders of sexual preference

All cases of this kind should be referred to a specialist if possible, although the referring clinician should first assess the problem as follows.

Assessment

The first step is to identify the problem and record its course (Table 30.8). The second step is to *exclude any mental disorder* which may have released the sexual behaviour in a person who previously experienced sexual fantasies but did not act on them. It is particularly important to seek these causes when the abnormal sexual behaviour appears for the first time in middle or late life.

The third requirement is to *assess normal sexual functioning* since one of the main aims of treatment is to strengthen this. Whenever possible the patient's sexual partner should be interviewed. If normal sexual behaviour is inadequate, appropriate treatment is given (see p. 106).

Next, an assessment is made of the *role of the abnormal behaviour* in the patient's life. As well as providing sexual arousal such behaviour may be used as a way of coping with loneliness, depression, or anxiety. If so, the patient should be helped to find adaptive ways of coping with these states.

Finally, *motivation for treatment* is assessed. Often the patient has been urged to attend by another person, usually the partner or the police. In such cases the patient may have no wish to change. Other patients seek help when they become temporarily depressed or guilty, either because the sexual behaviour has caused a problem, or because of some other reason. Such people may lose their motivation quickly when their mood returns to normal.

Table 30.8 Assessment of abnormalities of sexual preference

1. Identify the problem and its course

2. Exclude associated mental disorder (especially depressive disorder, alcoholism, and dementia)

3. Assess normal sexual functioning

4. Consider the 'role' of the abnormal sexual behaviour

5. Assess motivation for treatment

Treatment

Sexual counselling may help with any problems in forming relationships with the opposite sex. Any sexual dysfunction should be treated, using the methods described on pp. 411–413.

The patient should be encouraged to use distraction to control any fantasies of the abnormal sexual behaviour during masturbation, since such fantasies are likely to reinforce and maintain the sexual disorder. He should also stop the use of any pornographic materials to stimulate these fantasies.

Counselling should be used to help with any problems consequent to giving up the deviant sexual behaviour. Often, leisure time has been spent seeking out abnormal sexual stimuli, and new interests may need to be developed. When the sexual behaviour has been used to cope with depression or anxiety, the patient should be helped to develop more adaptive ways of coping.

Anti-androgens and oestrogen have been used to reduce sexual drive, especially in patients whose abnormal sexual behaviour is potentially dangerous to other people. The benefits of such treatment have not been clearly established.

Some people with abnormal sexual preferences appear before the courts. Sanctions such as a suspended sentence or probation order sometimes help a patient to control his behaviour, provided that he is motivated to help himself.

■ Disorders of gender identity: transsexualism

In this rare disorder, the person has the conviction of being of the opposite sex to that indicated by the external genitalia. The person wishes to alter the external genitalia to resemble those of the opposite sex, and to live as a member of that sex. Most transsexuals are men; most women who cross-dress and imitate men are homosexual, not transsexual. In transsexuals, the conviction of being a woman usually dates from before puberty, but medical help is not requested until early adult life, when most transsexuals have begun to dress as women. Unlike transvestites, they report no sexual arousal from cross-dressing, and unlike the homosexuals who dress as women, they do not seek to attract people into a homosexual relationship.

Transsexual men may take a series of steps to become more like women. They practise female styles of speaking, gesturing, and walking, they remove body hair by electrolysis, they attempt to increase breast tissue by taking oestrogen or by obtaining a surgical implant, and they

may seek an operation to remove the male external genitalia and form an artificial 'vagina'. Requests for such operations are often made in a determined and persistent way reflecting the person's great distress, and may be accompanied by threats of suicide or self-mutilation if surgery is not provided. Since such threats are carried out occasionally with serious consequences, a specialist opinion should be obtained.

It might be thought that a logical treatment of transsexualism would be a psychological procedure to alter the person's beliefs about his gender identity. No form of psychotherapy, however, has been shown to succeed in this aim. In any case, most transsexual patients reject this approach, hoping instead to alter their body to conform more closely with the gender they feel is theirs. In a few specialist centres operations with this purpose are carried out on selected patients (gender reassignment), and good results have been reported. However, there is no high-quality evidence of the long-term effectiveness of the procedure. Decisions about such treatment are therefore taken on an individual patient basis with thorough assessment, and are made jointly by an experienced psychiatrist and surgeon, in consultation with the general practitioner.

■ Psychological problems of homosexual people

As described earlier (p. 409), there is no sharp dividing line between homosexual and heterosexual people. About 1 per cent of men and 0.25 per cent of women are exclusively homosexual throughout their lives, while a further proportion are overtly homosexual or bisexual for a few years but subsequently are predominantly heterosexual. This bisexual potential is greatest in adolescence, after which most people settle permanently into one or other sexual role. Homosexuality is not a psychiatric disorder, but some homosexual people experience sexual and emotional problems for which they seek medical help. These problems are the subject of this section.

Helping homosexual people

Homosexual men consult doctors with four kinds of problem.

1 A sexually inexperienced young man who has homosexual thoughts and feelings may ask for advice on whether he is homosexual. The doctor should find out whether the young man has heterosexual as well as homosexual thoughts and feelings, and whether he has decided how

he would prefer to develop. If the man has heterosexual feelings and wishes to develop them, he should be advised to avoid situations that stimulate homosexual feelings, and should be helped to develop social skills with women.

2 The second kind of problem is presented by young men who have realized correctly that they are predominantly homosexual and who ask for counselling about the implications for their lives. Such young men should be helped to think out the implications themselves, and may be put in touch with a self-help group of homosexuals.

3 The third problem is presented by the established homosexual who becomes depressed or anxious because of difficulties in his sexual relationships. Again, counselling is appropriate as for problems in heterosexual relationships.

4 The fourth problem is presented by the homosexual who is concerned about HIV and AIDS. Such a patient requires appropriate medical investigation, treatment, and counselling.

Homosexual women ask for advice less often than homosexual men; when they do seek help, it is usually about problems in their relationship with the partner—often jealousy or depression. Married homosexual women may ask for advice about their relationship with the husband and family, or about dysfunction in heterosexual intercourse. Counselling is the appropriate treatment (p. 132).

 ## Further reading

Bancroft, J. H. J. (2009). *Human Sexuality and its Problems*, 3rd edn. Churchill Livingstone, Edinburgh. A comprehensive account of normal and abnormal sexual behaviour.

Hawton, K. (1985). *Sex Therapy: A Practical Guide*. Oxford University Press, Oxford. Although dated, this still provides a clear and practical account of simple kinds of therapy suitable for use by the non-specialist.

Johnson, A.E., Wadsworth, J., & Field, J. (1994). *Sexual Attitudes and Lifestyles*. Blackwell, Oxford University, Oxford. A large UK survey of sexual experience and attitudes in the general population.

Personality and its disorders

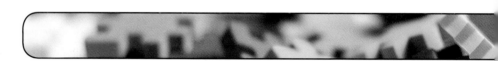

■ Personality and personality disorder

Personality

The term **personality** refers to the enduring patterns of thoughts, attitudes, moods, and behaviours which help to define us as individuals. Every personality is unique but there are common features, called **traits**, which are observed in variable degrees in different people. These traits provide a useful structure in which to describe personality; for example, sociability, aggressiveness, and impulsivity. As these examples indicate, personalities have both favourable and unfavourable features. Although unfavourable personality features are invariably those that precipitate presentation to medical care, in clinical practice it is important to explore the favourable features of the personality as thoroughly as the unfavourable ones. It is often easier to encourage the former than it is to discourage the latter.

Clinicians need to understand personality because it helps to predict their patients' response to illness and its treatment. Clinicians also need to understand the minority of patients who have a **disorder** of personality, that is, a personality that causes problems (either disability or distress) for the patient or for those around them. People with a personality disorder may:

- react in unusual ways to illness or to treatment; for example, by becoming overdependent or aggressive;
- behave in unusual ways when mentally ill, so that diagnosis is difficult;

- react unusually to stressful events; for example, by becoming aggressive or histrionic instead of anxious; sometimes these reactions are so unusual that they may be mistaken for a psychiatric disorder;

- behave in ways that are stressful or dangerous to themselves or other people;

- develop other psychiatric disorders more often than other people.

Personality disorder

It is not difficult to agree that extreme deviations of personality should be classified as disorders, but it is difficult to draw a line between normal personality and personality disorder. If personality could be measured like intelligence, a statistical cut-off could be used (e.g. two standard deviations from the population mean). However, although psychologists have devised measures of some traits, there are no reliable and valid measures of the aspects of personality that are most important in clinical practice. In the absence of such measures, a simple pragmatic criterion is used: *a personality is disordered when it causes suffering to the person or to other people.* This definition may appear simplistic and it is certainly subjective, but it is nevertheless useful in clinical practice and no better alternative has been devised.

Personality disorder versus mental illness

Personality disorder, like other kinds of personality, develops gradually from the early years through adolescence—there is no clear time of onset. Mental illness usually has a definable onset. Differential diagnosis therefore depends on a reliable history of the onset and course of the disorder, and on evidence of the presence or absence of the characteristic features of the various mental illnesses. Difficulties arise occasionally when a schizophrenic prodrome develops slowly in adolescence, when it is difficult to distinguish it from personality disorder (see p. 255).

Personality change

By definition, personality is enduring and stable. Small changes often take place very gradually over many years; for example, a person may become less impulsive and aggressive in middle or late life, or a person who is socially anxious and lacking in confidence in their 20s becomes socially and occupationally adept in their 30s and 40s. The term personality change does not refer to these gradual modifications but to the more abrupt, step-like changes that result sometimes from:

- injury to, or organic disease of, the brain;

- residual effects of severe mental disorder, usually schizophrenia;

- exceptionally severe stressful experiences such as those experienced by hostages or victims of severe torture.

■ Assessment of personality

Sources of information

In everyday life we learn about the personalities of people we know by observing how they respond in various circumstances over the time that we have known them. Clinicians get to know some patients in this way, but they must also assess the personality of patients whom they have just met. They can draw on four sources of information:

1 A description by someone who knows the patient well, a corroborant. If that person is observant and reliable, this is usually the best source.

2 A patient's own account of their past behaviour in a variety of circumstances. This is less objective but potentially more complete.

3 A patient's own account of their personality. This is also subjective and sometimes influenced by the wish to create a good impression, or by depression or elation.

4 The patient's behaviour in the interview. This is often unreliable because it reflects their current mood and the context of the interview.

The evaluation of personality formed from the last two of these items should be checked by comparing it with an objective record of past achievements and difficulties and, whenever possible, with the accounts of people who know the patient well.

Describing personality

Unless there is a personality disorder, personality can be described without using technical terms by listing relevant attributes, for example:

- meticulous, but overcautious, and prone to worry excessively;

- precise and reliable, but irritable and easily offended;

- outgoing and generous, but highly emotional.

Note that these short descriptions include both 'favourable' and 'unfavourable' characteristics. Such brief descriptions are sufficient in most clinical situations, and some useful words are listed in Table 31.1.

Table 31.1 Common personality traits (for brevity, only negative attributes are listed; corresponding positive features should also be noted)

- Prone to worry
- Strict, fussy, rigid
- Lacking self-confidence
- Sensitive
- Suspicious, jealous
- Untrusting, resentful
- Impulsive
- Attention seeking
- Dependent
- Irritable, quarrelsome
- Aggressive
- Lacking concern for others

Systematic enquiries about personality

A standard method of enquiry should be employed to ensure that all relevant aspects of personality have been considered. The usual scheme is shown in Table 31.2.

When a patient asks advice for a problem, personality assessment is at first concerned with traits that can lead to difficulties and with those that could help to explain the presenting problem. It is, however, important to go on to assess traits that are actual or potential assets. Some traits are assets in one situation but cause problems in others. For example, to be orderly and precise may be an asset in certain kinds of work but a problem when faced with the uncertainties of physical illness.

The amount of detail required varies with the problem and the situation. This account indicates the full range of enquiries under each of the main headings. When time is short (e.g. an emergency) only the most important and relevant points can be covered, with those more relevant to further care being considered later.

Before starting the specific enquiries listed below, it is useful to ask a general question, to set the scene; for

Table 31.2 A scheme for assessing personality

- Relationships
- Usual mood
- Other traits (see Table 31.1)
- Attitudes, beliefs, and standards
- Usual habits: daily routine, smoking, alcohol, illicit drugs

example: 'How do you think your friends and family would . . . describe your personality?' or '. . . describe you as a person?'

1 Relationships. This section is concerned with (i) *relationships at work* (with colleagues, people in authority, and juniors), (ii) *relationships with friends*, and (iii) *intimate relationships*. The interviewer asks whether the patient makes friends easily, has few friends or many, has close friends in whom he or she can confide, and has lasting friendships. The interviewer also asks whether the patient is sociable and confident in company, or shy and reserved. Finally, ask about the nature of romantic relationships—their nature, quality, and sense of permanence or instability.

2 Usual mood. The aim is to discover the person's usual or habitual mood, not the present or recent mood. There are three elements. First, the general character of the person's mood; is it generally cheerful, middle of the road, or gloomy? Secondly, whether it is stable, changeable, or volatile. If mood is changeable, the interviewer asks how long the changes last, and whether they occur spontaneously or in relation to events. Finally, the interviewer asks whether the person shows his feelings or hides them.

3 Other traits. When enquiring about other traits it can help to keep in mind the list in Table 31.1. Each characteristic has a positive as well as a negative side and it is appropriate to ask patients where they lie between the extremes; for example:

'Some people are placid, others get into arguments—where do you fit in?';

or,

'Some people are very careful, and weigh up all the options at length before making a decision, whereas others make decisions very quickly, perhaps too quickly—which are you?'.

It is useful to check answers by asking for examples from the patient's recent life, and checking with a corroborant. Characteristics such as jealousy or lack of feeling for others may not be revealed because the person is ashamed of them or does not recognize their presence. Observations should be recorded objectively, avoiding value judgements. General terms such as 'immature' or 'inadequate' should not be used; instead, the interviewer should record in what ways the person has difficulty in meeting the demands of adult life.

4 Attitudes, beliefs, and standards. Relevant points include attitudes to illness, religious beliefs, and personal standards. Usually, these become apparent when the personal history is being taken, but they can be explored further at this point in the interview.

5 Usual habits. Although not strictly part of personality, the person's usual lifestyle is often relevant. What was their typical daily routine (timeline, structure, activities), and what was their typical daily use of tobacco, alcohol, and illicit drugs? These aspects of a person's life may help by (i) indicating possible aetiological factors in current mental illness, or (ii) indicating possible features of current mental illness. For example, a person whose usual alcohol habit was to drink half a bottle of wine on a Friday and Saturday evening with friends may start to drink more than half a bottle each evening on their own, as 'self-medication' to cope with their low mood.

Is there personality disorder?

Having built up a picture of the personality, the interviewer decides whether the personality is disordered. The criterion for disorder is suffering (distress or disability) by the patient or by others as a result of the patient's personality. The criterion requires a difficult judgement about the extent to which the patient's problems have been caused by personality and how much by circumstances.

■ Types of personality disorder

Psychiatrists classify abnormal personalities according to one or other of the detailed schemes set out in ICD-10 and DSM-IV. For other doctors, who treat people with highly abnormal personalities less often, a simpler scheme is usually adequate. Such a scheme is compatible with the specialist classifications (with one exception—lacking self-esteem), and is shown in Table 31.3. Each of the groups in this scheme will be described together with its relationship to the specialist classification, which is shown in outline in Table 31.4.

Note that:

- the category for personalities lacking self-esteem and self-confidence is included in neither DSM-IV nor ICD-10;
- cyclothymic and schizotypal 'personalities' are not included in the classification of personality disorder, but in 'bipolar mood disorder' and 'schizophrenia', respectively, due to their close epidemiological links to those disorders.

Table 31.3 A simplified classification of personality

- Anxious, moody, and prone to worry
- Lacking self-esteem and confidence
- Sensitive and suspicious
- Dramatic and impulsive
- Aggressive and antisocial

Table 31.4 Classification of personality disorders in DSM-IV and ICD-10 (generally, the same terms are used in DSM-IV and ICD-10; where there are differences the ICD term is shown in parentheses)

Anxious, moody, and prone to worry

- Avoidant (anxious)
- Obsessive-compulsive (anankastic)
- Dependent
- Affective (depressive, hyperthymic, cyclothymic)

Sensitive and suspicious

- Paranoid
- Schizoid
- Schizotypal (ICD-10: classified with schizophrenia)

Dramatic and impulsive

- Histrionic
- Borderline (emotionally unstable—impulsive)
- Narcissistic

Antisocial

- Antisocial (dissocial)

Anxious, moody, and worry-prone personalities

This group includes the dependent, avoidant (anxious), and obsessive-compulsive (anankastic) personality disorders (Table 31.5). We also mention the 'affective personality disorders' here, although this is an outmoded term—these important clinical problems are now thought of as closely related to the affective disorders, with which they have close epidemiological links.

Avoidant (anxious) personality disorder

These people are persistently anxious, ill at ease in company, and fearful of disapproval or criticism. They feel inadequate and are timid. They avoid taking new responsibilities at work and avoid new experiences generally. This tendency to avoid is the basis of the DSM term *avoidant*.

Table 31.5 Characteristics of anxious, moody, worry-prone personalities

- Persistently anxious
- Worried about day-to-day problems or health
- Inflexible, obstinate, indecisive (obsessional traits)
- Persistently gloomy and pessimistic *or*
- Unstable moods, mild elation, or overconfidence alternates with mild depression and/or self-deprecation

Obsessive-compulsive (anankastic) personality disorder

These people are inflexible, obstinate, and rigid in their opinions, and they focus on unimportant detail. They are indecisive, and having made a decision they worry about its consequences. They are humourless and judgemental, while worrying about the opinions of others. Perfectionism, rigidity, and indecisiveness can make employment impossible. They appear outwardly controlled but may well be irritated by those who disturb their carefully ordered routine, and may have violent feelings of anger.

Dependent personality disorder

These people are passive and unduly compliant with the wishes of others. They lack vigour and self-reliance, and they avoid responsibility. Some achieve their aims by persuading other people to assist them, while protesting their own helplessness. Some are supported by a more self-reliant partner; left to themselves, they have difficulty in dealing with the demands and responsibilities of everyday life.

Persistent mood disorders

These disorders represent a *lifelong* tendency to persistent gloom, elation, or varied mood which is abnormal, but not severe enough at any one time to constitute depressive or manic episodes. Because of the close epidemiological links that we now know exist between these disorders and the mood (affective) disorders, the 'affective personality disorders' are now classified among the mood disorders in both DSM-IV and ICD-10.

These people have lifelong abnormalities of mood regulation, as follows:

1 **Dysthymia** (ICD-10 and DSM-IV). Formerly depressive personality disorder. The person is persistently gloomy and pessimistic with little capacity for enjoyment.

2 **Cyclothymia** (ICD-10 and DSM-IV). Formerly cyclothymic personality disorder. The person's mood alternates between gloomy and elated over periods of days to weeks. This instability can be particularly disruptive to work and social relationships.

Personalities lacking self-esteem and confidence

This group is common and important in primary care and general medical practice (Table 31.6). These personality features are associated with recurrent depressive moods, eating disorders, and self-harm and are often seen among young people who seek help for these problems. Unfortunately, this group does not appear as a separate entity in the specialist classifications of personality disorder.

Table 31.6 Characteristics of personalities lacking self-esteem

- Lack confidence
- Feel inferior
- Expect criticism
- Strive to please others
- Shyness and social withdrawal/inappropriate efforts to please others

Sensitive and suspicious personalities

People in this group are difficult to engage in treatment and they may distrust their doctors (Table 31.7). This group includes paranoid, schizoid, and schizotypal personality disorders.

Paranoid personality disorder

These individuals are sensitive and suspicious; they mistrust others and suspect their motives, and are prone to jealousy. They are touchy, irritable, argumentative, and stubborn. Some of these people have a strong sense of self-importance and special ability, although they may feel that their potential has been stymied by others letting them down or deceiving them.

Schizoid personality disorder

These individuals are emotionally cold, self-sufficient, and detached. They are introspective and may have a complex fantasy life. They show little concern for the opinions of others, and pursue a solitary course through life. When this personality disorder is extreme, the person is cold, callous, and insensitive.

Schizotypal personality disorder

These individuals are eccentric and have unusual ideas (e.g. about telepathy and clairvoyance) or ideas of reference. Their speech is abstract and vague, and their affect may be inappropriate to the circumstances. In ICD-10

Table 31.7 Characteristics of sensitive and suspicious personalities

- Sensitive, touchy, irritable; see rebuffs where none exist
- Suspicious, mistrustful
- Cold, detached, show little concern for others, reject help when it is offered
- Eccentric, with unusual ideas about topics such as telepathy
- Self-sufficient
- Lacking concern

Table 31.8 Characteristics of dramatic and impulsive personalities

- Seek the limelight, dramatize their problems
- Vain, self-centred
- Demanding of others, to an unreasonable extent, perhaps using 'emotional blackmail'
- Act a part, self-deceiving, lack awareness of their image to others
- Impulsive, sometimes with harmful behaviours
- Short-lived enthusiasms but lack persistence
- Unrestrained emotional display

this disorder is classified with schizophrenia rather than as one of the personality disorders.

Dramatic and impulsive personalities

This group includes histrionic, borderline, and narcissistic personality disorders (Table 31.8).

Borderline personality disorder

People with borderline personality represent an important clinical group that presents frequently to healthcare, including A&E departments. The term 'borderline' refers to a combination of features seen also in histrionic and antisocial personalities, which are centred around impulsivity and poor self-control. The term originates in the now abandoned idea that the condition was related to (on the borderline with) schizophrenia. Note that ICD-10 uses the term *emotionally unstable personality disorder* for the same patient group. People with borderline personality disorder have intense but unstable relationships. They have persistent feelings of boredom and emptiness, with uncertainty about personal identity and a fear of abandonment. Their moods may be unstable, with unwarranted outbursts of anger, and low tolerance of stress. They are impulsive, and may engage in self-damaging behaviours, such as reckless spending or gambling, reckless sex, chaotic eating, and substance abuse. Threats or acts of self-harm may be recurrent.

Histrionic personality disorder

These people appear sociable, outgoing, and entertaining but at the same time they are self-centred, prone to short-lived enthusiasms, and lack persistence. Extreme displays of emotion may leave others exhausted while the person recovers quickly and without remorse. Sexually provocative behaviour is common but tender feelings are lacking. There may be astonishing capacity for self-deception and an ability to persist with elaborate lies long after others have seen the truth.

Narcissistic personality disorder

This disorder is not included in ICD-10. Narcissism is morbid self-admiration. Narcissistic people have a grandiose sense of self-importance and are preoccupied with fantasies of success, power, and intellectual brilliance. They crave attention, exploit others, and seek favours but do not return them.

Antisocial personalities

This group corresponds to the dissocial (ICD-10) or antisocial (DSM-IV) groups in the specialist classifications (Table 31.9). The difficulties are often increased by abuse of alcohol or illicit drugs.

■ Epidemiology

The overall prevalence of personality disorder in community surveys is between about 5 and 10 per cent. Overall rates are higher in men than women and decrease with age. Antisocial personality disorder, which is present in about 1–3 per cent in community surveys, is more common in men. Histrionic personality disorder (about 2 per cent) and borderline personality disorder (about 1–2 per cent) are more common in women. Personality disorders often coexist with mental disorders. A particularly important association is between antisocial personality disorder and alcohol and substance abuse. There is a strong association between borderline personality disorder and self-harm.

Table 31.9 Characteristics of antisocial personalities

- Impulsive behaviour, low tolerance of frustration, and lack of consistent striving towards goals, leading to, for example, an unstable work record
- Callous acts, inflicting pain, cruelty, or degradation on others
- Tendency to violence
- Lack of guilt
- Failure to learn from experience, leading to behaviours that persist or escalate despite negative social consequences and legal penalties
- Failure to sustain close relationships, including intimate relationships
- Disregard of the feelings of others
- Family problems, including violence towards partner, and neglect of or violence towards children; frequent separation and divorce
- Often lengthy forensic history, perhaps starting with petty delinquent acts but escalating to callous, violent crime

■ Aetiology

Personality and its disorders result from the interaction of genetic factors and upbringing. The relative contribution of these causes is uncertain and difficult to clarify because of the many factors involved in childhood upbringing and the difficulty of recording these accurately and relating them to personality features assessed many years later.

The little scientific knowledge that has been accumulated is mainly concerned with antisocial personality disorders and it is the only aspect that will be considered here. Despite this lack of scientific data concerning other kinds of personality disorder, it is sometimes possible to achieve an intuitive understanding of the possible childhood origins of some aspects of personality. For example, frequent criticism and lack of affection from parents may be the antecedents of a personality with low self-esteem.

Causes of antisocial personality disorder

Genetic factors. The children of parents with antisocial personality disorder have greater rates of antisocial behaviour than children of parents who do not have this personality. A similar excess has been reported also among adopted children whose biological parents have antisocial personality disorder and whose adoptive parents do not. These findings suggest a genetic contribution to aetiology.

Childhood experience. Separation from parents in early childhood is more frequent among people with antisocial personality disorder than among controls. This association could be due to (i) parental disharmony preceding separation, (ii) the separation itself, or (iii) a consequence of separation such as upbringing in care rather than in a family.

Injury to the brain at birth is sometimes followed by impulsive and aggressive behaviour. Such injury has been suggested as a cause of antisocial personality disorder but without convincing evidence.

Abnormal brain development has been suggested as a cause. The only evidence, which is indirect, is that some adults with antisocial personality have non-specific features in the electroencephalogram (EEG) of a kind found normally in adolescents, not adults. This suggests that these findings might reflect delayed brain maturation among people with antisocial personality.

Serotonin. Recent studies have found an association between aggressive behaviour and low levels of brain serotonin (5-HT), inferred from the results of neuroendocrine challenge tests. However, the association between serotonin and aggression is not confined to aggression in antisocial personality disorder.

■ Prognosis of personality disorder

Clinical experience indicates that some abnormal features of personality, such as aggressive traits, tend to become less marked as the person grows into middle age. There are, however, no reliable follow-up studies to confirm this observation. In old age, abnormal features of personality sometimes increase again, causing difficulties for patients and carers.

■ Management of personality disorder

Since personality is by its nature unchanging, it is not surprising that personality disorders are difficult to treat. There are, nevertheless, ways of helping patients with personality disorder, usually by dealing with any factors that exacerbate the problems. Since personality disorders lead to problems that may affect the management of any illness, all clinicians should be able to assess the problems and arrange appropriate management, either within their own clinical team or by referral to a psychiatric service.

Aims of management

Management focuses on ways of dealing with any recent exacerbations of problems associated with the personality disorder. This can be done in five ways.

1 Identify and treat any co-morbid psychiatric disorder(s).

2 Treat any associated substance misuse.

3 Help the patient to deal with or avoid situations that provoke problem behaviours.

4 Provide general support to reduce tension and increase self-esteem.

5 Support the family.

Help may be needed over a long period, often many years, and involved healthcare professionals need patience, the ability to accept repeated setbacks, and realistic goals.

Assessment

● **Diagnose the personality disorder and identify positive features.** The diagnosis of personality disorder focuses on unfavourable features of personality.

Management requires an assessment of the positive features as well because it may be possible to encourage and develop these. *Low self-esteem* is a frequent problem in all kinds of personality disorder. Self-esteem can sometimes be improved by identifying talents and skills, which can be developed by further education or training, leading to a greater sense of self-worth.

- **Identify any co-morbid psychiatric disorder.** Treatment of a co-morbid disorder can lead to an improvement in the problem behaviours associated with the personality disorder. Depression should be considered whenever the personality problems have increased recently without another obvious cause, even when the patient does not complain spontaneously of depression.

- **Assess any substance misuse.** Alcohol or other substances may be used by people with personality disorder to relieve tension, unhappiness, or feelings of inadequacy. However, they can exacerbate mood disturbance, and their disinhibiting effects can encourage histrionic or aggressive behaviour and self-harm.

- **Identify provoking factors** for problem behaviours by asking the patient to keep a *daily diary* of the behaviours and the situations in which they occur. Most patients cooperate with this practical approach and provoking factors can often be identified directly. Sometimes, however, the link between the provoking factor and the response is indirect. For example, aggression may be provoked by social rejection, which is the response of others to the patient's lack of social skills. Treatment would then include social skills training.

- **Assess the effects on the family,** particularly the effects on any children living with the patient. Although these enquiries are particularly important when the person is aggressive, the problems of people who are persistently anxious, histrionic, or suspicious may also affect their families.

- **Assess risk, both to self and to others** (see Chapter 9).

General aspects of management

The plan should be realistic, focusing on specific problems and not attempting personality change. The aims should be clearly understood by the patient, and carried out consistently. The general approach is to help patients:

- to take responsibility for their actions and be willing to solve their own problems;

- to agree modest aims and work to achieve them over time. Progress is usually by a series of small steps, punctuated by failures. Patience is needed in the management of personality disorders, which may have to be provided for many years;

- to gain confidence and learn from their mistakes. Setbacks are viewed as opportunities to learn more about the problem, not as signs of failure.

Specific therapeutic interventions are listed below.

- **Build the relationship between the patient and professional.** This relationship is particularly important when treating personality disorder. The patient should feel valued as a person, and be able to trust and confide in the healthcare professional. At the same time, the relationship should not be allowed to become too intense, nor should the patient become dependent or demanding. When more than one person is involved in treatment, their respective roles should be defined and made clear to the patient. Any attempt to play one off against the other should be discussed between the professionals and with the patient.

- **Agree a care plan.** Some patients with personality disorder make unreasonable demands on those caring for them. They may seek help at inappropriate times, attempt to impose unrealistic conditions on treatment, behave in a seductive way, or threaten self-harm if their demands are not met. Such problems are met especially with overdependent, borderline, histrionic, or aggressive personalities. Once established, these behaviours can be very difficult to control, so clinicians should be alert for their first signs. The practical limits on the help that can be offered should be agreed by all those involved in the patient's care and explained to the patient.

- **Build on strengths.** Management should not focus exclusively on defects in the personality. Whenever possible patients should be encouraged to recognize and develop their talents and skills by obtaining further training, changing to a job better suited to their skills or interests, or by developing more satisfying leisure activities.

- **Deal with or avoid provoking factors.** The patient should be helped to identify and find new ways of dealing with or avoiding any situations that regularly cause problems. These changes may require patients to give up some of their previous goals and accept new ones more in keeping with the structure of their personalities.

- **Reduce alcohol/illicit drug use.** When abnormal behaviour is provoked or made worse by the misuse of alcohol or drugs, help should be given to limit the use of these substances. Among prescribed drugs, benzodiazepines can have disinhibiting effects similar to those of alcohol. They should be avoided when prescribing for patients with abnormal personalities.

- **Help the family.** This may be needed especially when the personality disorder is of the aggressive or antisocial kind. If a mother has a personality disorder, the health and development of the children should be assessed and appropriate steps taken to alleviate any problems.

- **Drug treatment.** The main role for drug treatments is in the management of co-morbid mental illness. Outwith that role, they are often used in specific ways, although randomized evidence is limited almost entirely to borderline personality disorder. *Antipsychotic drugs* may be calming at a time of increased stress in several disorders, and may reduce depression and hostility in borderline personalities. *Lithium carbonate and other anticonvulsants*, such as carbamazepine, may be used when there is affective instability or impulsivity, such as in borderline personalities (and, of course, may be used in the persistent mood disorders dysthymia and cyclothymia). *Antidepressants*, such as the SSRI fluoxetine, may benefit mood in borderline personalities. In general, anxiolytic drugs such as benzodiazepines should be avoided because, although like alcohol and cannabis they may improve immediate well-being, they may produce disinhibition and dependency.

- **Psychological treatment.** This may be delivered through self-help in the first instance, if the patient is motivated to change, and has reasonable literacy. For example, people with low self-esteem may be helped by a cognitive behavioural intervention delivered by a self-help book (see this chapter's Further Reading).

Role of the psychiatric services

The general measures described above can be carried out by all clinicians, though it may be difficult for them to find time to deal with more complex problems. Referral to a psychiatrist is indicated:

1 for *assessment*;

2 to *stabilize* the patient at times of crisis;

3 when there is *co-morbidity* with another psychiatric disorder.

Psychiatric services adopt the same general approach, supplemented at times by one or more of the following special techniques.

- **Psychological treatments.** These may help some people with low self-esteem and difficulties in social relationships. *Cognitive behavioural methods* are generally more appropriate than dynamic therapy since they focus on current behaviour and the patient's own role in changing this. Sensitive–suspicious and antisocial–aggressive personalities seldom benefit from any form of psychotherapy.

- **Therapeutic community methods.** These can be used to assist people with antisocial personality to learn from experiences of their relationships within a community of patients with similar problems, and from frequent and intensive discussion of problems within the group. In therapeutic communities, the community itself is the primary therapeutic instrument and, through time, can reduce the expression and impact of negative aspects of personality, and increase the expression of positive aspects. Although traditionally the term 'therapeutic community' has been associated with group residential settings, it is increasingly being applied to more flexible arrangements including day programmes, such as the innovative Complex Needs Service in Oxfordshire (see Box 31.1).

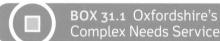

BOX 31.1 Oxfordshire's Complex Needs Service

This innovative service is funded by the UK's Department of Health, to develop new ways of working with people with 'personality disorder' or 'complex needs'. Traditionally, this group of people has been regarded as difficult to help, with the result that services have been difficult to find, and, where they exist, often poorly organized and poorly evidence based. The Complex Needs Service (CNS) emphasizes the person's own responsibility and they can, for example, self-refer to the service. They progress through several tiers, as follows:

- **Initial assessment and options group.** This provides informal support, and introduction to a group environment, while the person considers whether tier 2 is right for them.

- **Intensive group programme.** This comprises one of two different types of weekly group. For example, the patient may choose the larger structured group which meets for up to 3 hours weekly. The session starts and ends with a community meeting, chaired by a group member, and includes a therapeutic group using an integrative, multi-method psychotherapeutic model. Twenty-four-hour telephone support is available from other members.

- **Intensive day programme.** This is a 4.5 days per week commitment to a therapeutic community which uses several psychotherapeutic approaches, including psychodrama, CBT, dialectical behaviour therapy, and activity groups.

- **Post-therapy programme.** This aims to support patients as they take on new responsibilities and opportunities in work, education, and relationships—aspects of life which many of us take for granted, but which may be new and challenging to many Complex Needs Service patients.

Treatment according to personality type

Anxious, moody, and worrying types. These patients are generally helped most by a cognitive behavioural treatment designed to identify and change maladaptive ways of dealing with situations that the patient finds stressful, and to recognize the relationship between thinking and emotion. In this group, patients with obsessional traits may be least likely to change.

Sensitive and suspicious personalities. These patients seldom benefit from any kind of psychological treatment. The aim is to establish, often over considerable time, a gradually greater degree of trust with the patient. These patients may provoke strong negative feelings in healthcare professionals, who should learn to recognize these reactions at an early stage and ensure that such feelings do not affect their clinical judgement.

Dramatic and impulsive personalities. It is particularly important to set limits of engagement for this group. A problem-solving approach should be used to help the patient cope better with the stressful events that provoke abnormal behaviours. Emphasizing the individual's responsibility for their own actions is important. Dynamic psychotherapy is seldom effective and may lead to transference problems (see p. 133) that are difficult to manage.

Aggressive and antisocial behaviour. Usually the most practical aim is to prevent the accumulation of secondary problems resulting from rash decisions, unintentional antagonism of potential helpers, and the abuse of drugs and alcohol. The approach should be practical and take account of the patient's sensitivities. Rude or aggressive behaviour may need to be accepted tolerantly at times. Patients who are irritable and impatient should not be kept waiting without first explaining the reason. *Importantly*, patients who are potentially aggressive should be seen in a place where help can be called for easily, and will arrive promptly.

A *problem-solving approach* should be applied to situations that regularly provoke aggressive and antisocial behaviour. *Anger management techniques* (a form of cognitive behaviour therapy) may help some patients to respond more appropriately. As noted above, limited time is sometimes spent most usefully in *helping the family*, especially any dependent children.

Low self-esteem and confidence. These patients are helped by a trusting relationship in which they are encouraged to see the positive side of their personality and gain confidence. Taking time to take them and their problem seriously is implicitly supportive of their value as an individual. A cognitive behavioural approach can help these patients understand the relationship between their unrealistic ways of thinking and their response to situations in which they feel defeated or inferior, and may be delivered in a stepwise approach in which the first step is a self-help book (see Further Reading). Assertiveness training may help people who are unduly submissive.

 Further reading

Fennell, M. (2009). *Overcoming Low Self-esteem: A Self-help Guide Using Cognitive Behavioural Techniques*. Constable & Robinson, London.

Gelder, M., Andreasen, N., Lopez-Ibor, J, & Geddes, J. (2009). *New Oxford Textbook of Psychiatry*, 2nd edn. Section 4.12. Personality disorders, pp. 847–910. Oxford University Press, Oxford.

CHAPTER 32

Child and adolescent psychiatry: specific disorders

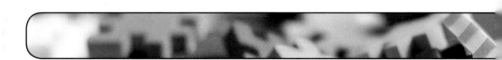

Chapter contents

■ Introduction

This chapter describes common and/or important mental health disorders seen in children and adolescents. More general information about classification, aetiology, assessment, and management is discussed in Chapter 17. The disorders are divided into those commonly seen in preschool children, developmental disorders, and those in older children. Many of the psychiatric problems seen in adolescence are the common disorders of adulthood; in the latter part of the chapter these are briefly covered, identifying adolescent-specific presentation or treatment with reference to the general information in relevant adult chapters. There are some specific points regarding the psychological well-being of children with physical illness; these are discussed at the end of the chapter.

■ Problems of preschool children

Common problems in preschoolers are shown in Table 32.1. Most problems are short-lived and whether they are reported to doctors depends on the attitudes of the parents as well as on the severity of the issue. The aetiology of these conditions is primarily related to individual variations in development and temperament, but family problems can play a large role in certain situations.

Temper tantrums

Temper tantrums are normal from 1 to 3 years, are mostly mild in nature, and improve with time. Only frequent or severe tantrums are abnormal. There are a number of

Table 32.1 Common disorders of preschool children

Common problems

- Attention seeking
- Disobedience
- Temper tantrums
- Breath holding
- Sleep problems: insomnia, nightmares, night terrors
- Feeding problems: food fads, food refusal, pica

Less common problems

- Excessive and indiscriminate attachment (especially in children raised in institutions)

Poor attachment to the carer (may be a sign of abuse, past or present)

different triggers to a tantrum: frustration at not being able to make themselves understood, desire for independence (e.g. strapping a child into a high-chair), hunger, tiredness, or wanting attention. Tantrums are often provoked by inconsistent discipline and reinforced unintentionally by excessive attention to the child when they take place. Temper tantrums usually improve when the parents set consistent limits to the child's behaviour, enforce these limits kindly but firmly, and pay less attention to the child during the tantrums. It is important to discover why the parents have been unable to achieve consistent discipline (e.g. there may be marital problems), and to give common-sense advice on setting and enforcing limits.

Breath holding

Periods of breath holding occur in 5 per cent of children aged 2–5 years. Breath-holding spells usually occur when a child is frustrated, upset, or angry. Often the child will throw what begins to look like a temper tantrum, but cut short the screaming or crying with a breath-holding spell. For several seconds it may look as though the child is still raging though no sound accompanies the actions. Children turn blue or purple during the spell and may pass out for a few seconds. Rarely a seizure ensues. This behaviour can be very alarming to parents, especially if the child loses consciousness, but it is extremely unlikely the child will be harmed by the episode. The nature of the attacks should be explained to the parents, and they should be helped to respond calmly, and to avoid reinforcing the behaviour with excessive attention. Managed in this way, the attacks usually disappear with time.

Sleep disorders

Sleep disorders affect one-third of young children and are usually a temporary phenomenon. It is important to differentiate between primary sleep disorders and sleep disturbance secondary to another physical or mental disorder (e.g. asthmatic nocturnal cough). Risk factors include poor bedtime routine, sharing a bedroom with a parent or older child, and physical or learning disability.

Insomnia

One-fifth of children aged between 1 and 2 years take at least an hour to fall asleep or are repeatedly wakeful for long periods during the night, thus disturbing their parents. Most of these problems resolve within a few months and reassurance is all that is needed. If the sleep problem is more severe or persistent, the parents' response to the problem should be studied. Often, they are inadvertently maintaining the behaviour by responding as soon as the child cries, spending long periods at the child's bedside, allowing the child to return to the living room, or taking the child into their own bed. The condition usually improves if the parents follow basic sleep hygiene rules:

- establish a regular bedtime routine;
- make sure the bedroom is cool, dark, and quiet;
- provide calming bedtime activities (soft music, reading);
- reduce or avoid daytime naps;
- reduce stimulating food, drinks, and activities in the evenings;
- do not reinforce the problem behaviour.

Hypnotic medication should be used seldom and then only briefly in conjunction with the above measures. At first, it may be difficult to persuade the parents to keep to the new rules, and continued support may be needed. When this simple approach fails, there may be a wider problem in the child or the family and specialist assessment may be required.

Feeding problems

Food fads and food refusal are common in preschool children, but only in a minority is the behaviour severe or persistent. When this happens it is often because the parents are unintentionally reinforcing behaviour that would otherwise be transient. Usually, children whose parents are concerned about their eating habits are healthy and growing well. Picky eating is more common in those who have had less chance to experience a wide range of foods, or when parents are very anxious about the correct amount and type of food the child should have. Some parents offer alternative (and sometimes unsuitable) food, or take other steps to persuade the child to eat, which reinforces the behaviour. Parents should be encouraged to ignore the feeding problem as far as possible, to refrain from offering the child alternatives when they do not eat what is first offered, and to stop using other special ways to persuade them to eat.

Pica is the eating of items that are not foods (e.g. soil, paint, and paper). It needs to be separated from the exploratory mouthing of objects in children aged 1–2 years. Pica is often associated with other behaviour problems, autism, or learning disability. Parents should be reassured that the problem is a recognized disorder that usually improves. They should take common-sense measures to keep the child away from non-edible items, and reduce stressful situations. With this approach the problem usually disappears; if it does not there may be a wider problem requiring specialist assessment.

■ Disorders of development

Pervasive developmental disorders

Pervasive developmental disorders (PDDs) are relatively common conditions characterized by deficits and delays in social and communicative development, which are associated with restricted patterns of interest and behaviour. The most widely recognized PDD is childhood autism, which was first recognized as a distinct clinical entity in the 1940s, but there are four other diagnostic categories within the classification systems. Therefore PDD is a term that includes the following conditions (DSM-IV term first, ICD-10 term in parentheses if different):

1 autistic disorder (childhood autism);

2 Rett's disorder;

3 childhood disintegrative disorder;

4 Asperger's syndrome;

5 pervasive developmental disorder not otherwise specified (PDD-NOS, atypical autism).

The phrase 'autistic spectrum disorders' (ASD) is widely used to describe all of the conditions above, but recognizes that the disorders may overlap to some extent and that within any category there is a wide variation in severity of symptoms. It takes into account the fact that a child with a PDD may have an IQ that is subnormal, normal, or above normal, and that family members of those with autism may show autistic-like traits in their behaviour. The clinical features of each of the five conditions will be individually described below, but the aetiology and management sections are common to all ASDs.

Autistic disorder (childhood autism)

Classical autism is characterized by difficulties in three areas, a 'triad of impairment'.

1 **Social deficits.** Examples include babies who don't like being held, and also reduced eye contact, unusual facial expressions, lack of gestures, poor understanding of others' feelings, lack of empathy, and few peer relationships. Frequently, the child does not respond to affection, and may not value the company of their parents over that of complete strangers.

2 **Communication deficits.** Speech in autistic children shows wide variety; it may be completely absent (30 per cent), or merely show unusual or asocial qualities. Common abnormalities of speech include echolalia, odd prosody (unusual pitch/stress/rhythm/intonation) and pronoun reversal (referring to themselves as he or she). These children have difficulty in two-way conversations, and some ask a string of questions instead.

3 **Restricted/repetitive interests and behaviours.** Autistic children often show a deep interest in things others regard as very mundane; for example, washing machines or licence plates. They often spend the majority of time with these objects, rejecting other toys or imaginative play with their peers. Stereotypies are repetitive movements often triggered by stress; examples include hand-flapping or head rolling. Autistic children may have elaborate routines of behaviour and almost inevitability show a resistance to change ('sameness') in daily routine. Self-harming is not uncommon, and may include biting or hitting.

The clinical features of autism must be present by 3 years in order for a diagnosis to be made. It is important to remember that only some of the characteristic symptoms are likely to be present in any given child. Box 32.1 shows the full diagnostic criteria for autistic disorder.

Prevalence

Some epidemiological statistics for PDDs are shown in Table 32.2.

Differential diagnosis

- **Asperger's syndrome** (see below).

- **Deafness.** This can be excluded by appropriate tests of hearing.

- **Specific developmental language disorder**, in which the child usually responds normally to people, but has deficits in speech and language.

- **Learning disability**, in which there is general intellectual retardation with relatively less language impairment than in autism and a more normal response to other people.

Aetiology

The cause of autism is poorly understood, but is likely to be multifactorial with a strong polygenic genetic component.

Genetic factors. Twin studies indicate that autism has 90 per cent heritability. The risk of autism in a sibling of an affected child is 2 to 20 per cent, a massive increase over the general population risk. There are also higher rates of social,

BOX 32.1 DSM-IV diagnostic criteria for autistic disorder

A

1 **Qualitative impairment in social interaction** as manifested by at least two of the following:

  (a) marked impairment in the use of multiple non-verbal behaviours;

  (b) failure to develop peer relationships appropriate to developmental level;

  (c) a lack of spontaneous seeking to share enjoyment, interests, or achievements with others;

  (d) lack of social or emotional reciprocity.

2 **Qualitative impairments in communication** as manifested by at least one of the following:

  (a) delay in, or total lack of, the development of spoken language;

  (b) in individuals with adequate speech, marked impairment of ability to sustain a conversation with others;

  (c) stereotyped and repetitive use of language or idiosyncratic language;

  (d) lack of varied, spontaneous make-believe play or social imitative play.

3 **Restricted repetitive and stereotyped patterns of behaviour, interests, and activities**, as manifested by at least two of the following:

  (a) encompassing preoccupation with one or more stereotyped and restricted patterns of interest that is abnormal either in intensity or focus;

  (b) apparently inflexible adherence to specific, non-functional routines or rituals;

  (c) stereotyped and repetitive motor mannerisms;

  (d) persistent preoccupation with parts of objects.

B Delays or abnormal functioning in at least one of the following areas, with onset prior to age 3 years: (1) social interaction, (2) language as used in social communication, or (3) symbolic or imaginative play.

C The disturbance is not better accounted for by Rett's disorder or childhood disintegrative disorder.

ICD-10 childhood autism

A type of pervasive developmental disorder that is defined by:

(a) the presence of abnormal or impaired development that is manifest before the age of 3 years;

(b) the characteristic type of abnormal functioning in all the three areas of psychopathology: reciprocal social interaction, communication, and restricted, stereotyped, repetitive behaviour.

In addition to these specific diagnostic features, a range of other non-specific problems are common, such as phobias, sleeping and eating disturbances, temper tantrums, and (self-directed) aggression.

---

language, and learning problems in relatives, suggesting that autism may represent the severe end of a general predisposition to developmental difficulties.

Table 32.2 Epidemiology of pervasive developmental disorders

Diagnosis	Prevalence	Gender ratio (male : female)
Overall pervasive developmental disorders	2 per 1000	4 : 1
Autism	13 per 10 000	4 : 1
Asperger's syndrome	1 per 2000	4–20 : 1
Rett's syndrome	1 per 12–15 000	Females only
Childhood disintegrative disorder	1 per 12 000	Unknown but males predominate

Organic brain disorder. The occurrence of seizures in about 20 per cent of patients at the time of adolescence suggests an organic brain disorder, at least in some cases. However, currently neuropathological, brain imaging, and neurochemical findings are inconsistent.

Cognitive abnormalities involve, in particular, symbolic thinking and language. An important deficit, present in many but not all of these children, is the inability to judge correctly what other people are thinking and to use this knowledge to predict their behaviour (lack of a 'theory of mind'). It is proposed that this deficit is the core abnormality underlying the ASDs.

Abnormal parenting has not been shown to be a cause.

Course and prognosis

About two-thirds of the children who meet the criteria for autism acquire some useful speech, although serious impairments usually remain. Most of the abnormal behaviours continue into adulthood, but may change and become less socially impairing with time. Only about 10 to 20 per cent of children are able to attend a mainstream school, and a minority (usually those with normal IQ) go on to live independently and obtain work.

Atypical autism

Atypical autism (PDD-NOS) is a diagnostic category for children who do not quite meet the diagnostic criteria for a specific PDD, but show many of the characteristics typical of them.

Asperger's syndrome

Asperger's syndrome is a condition in which a child has the characteristic impairments in social interaction and repetitive behaviours or restricted interests that are seen in autism, but has normal speech and intellectual abilities. Asperger's takes its name from the Austrian paediatrician who described it in 1944. The typical clinical presentation is of a child with the following characteristics:

- developmentally appropriate speech and language;
- unusual use of language (e.g. prosody, abnormal rate/ rhythm/volume, novel words);
- motor clumsiness;
- unusually deep interest in one particular topic;
- rigid behaviour and stereotypies;
- social awkwardness or an eccentric social style; the child fails to read the other person's feelings, and often does not understand humour or irony;
- difficulty in making close friends;
- the child often shows an enhanced ability to rote learn information about their special interests, or perform at a high level in one particular activity.

Asperger's frequently does not become obvious until around 4–8 years, whereas autism is by definition recognized earlier than this. The reason for this is usually that the expectations for social interaction by society only start to become relevant around this age, and that even small children without an ASD can have favourite toys and special interests. However, whilst a normal 5-year-old may love trains, it is less likely that a fascination with different types of light-bulb fitting is innocent. The diagnostic criteria for Asperger's syndrome are shown in Box 32.2.

Co-morbidities

The commonest co-morbidities are mood disorders and anxiety disorders, seen in 65 per cent of those with Asperger's by adulthood. Asperger's is also associated

---

☐ BOX 32.2 DSM-IV diagnostic criteria for Asperger's syndrome

I   Qualitative impairment in social interaction, as manifested by at least two of the following:

   (A) marked impairments in the use of multiple nonverbal behaviours;

   (B) failure to develop peer relationships appropriate to developmental level;

   (C) a lack of spontaneous seeking to share enjoyment, interests, or achievements with others;

   (D) lack of social or emotional reciprocity.

II Restricted repetitive and stereotyped patterns of behaviour, interests, and activities, as manifested by at least one of the following:

   (A) encompassing preoccupation with one or more stereotyped and restricted interests;

   (B) apparently inflexible adherence to specific, nonfunctional routines or rituals;

   (C) stereotyped and repetitive motor mannerisms;

   (D) persistent preoccupation with parts of objects.

III The disturbance causes clinically significant impairments in social, occupational, or other important areas of functioning.

IV There is no clinically significant general delay in language.

V   There is no clinically significant delay in cognitive development.

VI Criteria are not met for another specific PDD or schizophrenia.

ICD-10 Asperger's syndrome

A disorder characterized by the same type of qualitative abnormalities of reciprocal social interaction that typify autism, together with a restricted, stereotyped, repetitive repertoire of interests and activities. It differs from autism primarily in the fact that there is no general delay or retardation in language or in cognitive development. This disorder is often associated with marked clumsiness. There is a strong tendency for the abnormalities to persist into adolescence and adult life. Psychotic episodes occasionally occur in early adult life.

with tics, Tourette's syndrome, attention deficit hyperactivity disorder (ADHD), OCD, and bipolar disorder.

Course and prognosis

Currently, there are few long-term data on the prognosis of children with Asperger's syndrome. The core symptoms tend to remain stable with time, but many individuals are able to learn and cope with them better by adulthood. The majority of children can attend a mainstream school with some extra classroom support, but may be subject to bullying due to their social eccentricity. Most complete their education and can work, especially in areas of their particular interest!

Rett's syndrome

Rett's syndrome is a rare developmental disorder of females which bears more resemblance to a neurodegenerative disorder than a psychiatric condition. However, children with Rett's show many of the characteristic features of autism so it remains within the PDD classification. Rett's is thought to be caused by mutations in the *MECP-2* gene on the X-chromosome, which may occur either sporadically (95 per cent) or via phenotypically normal mothers who have a germline mutation. The exact genetics of inheritance and the reason for males not being affected are unknown, but it is likely that male fetuses with the mutation do not survive to term.

Girls with Rett's syndrome generally develop normally until 6 to 18 months, at which time they start to regress developmentally. They lose speech, purposeful hand movements, motor skills, and head growth. Stereotypies start to develop, especially hand washing, bruxism, and flapping. Breathing problems—hyperventilation, breath holding, and sighing—are common, and help to distinguish Rett's from autism. Mental retardation is invariably present by mid-childhood. Physical health problems are abundant, including epilepsy (80 per cent), constipation, poor growth, scoliosis, and cardiac and motor problems. The average life expectancy of females with Rett's syndrome is 30 years.

Childhood disintegrative disorder (CDD, Heller's disease)

This rare condition is characterized by entirely normal development for the first 2 years, followed by marked regression and loss of skills in multiple areas of development over a few months. The child develops the deficits in social skills, communication skills, and repetitive/restrictive interests and behaviour seen in the rest of autism. The course and prognosis of CDD are poorly understood. In about two-thirds of children the deterioration reaches a plateau, although skills are never regained. Outcome IQ is usually less than 50, and the majority of children develop severe epilepsy. Life expectancy is not reduced, but function remains extremely low and the individuals are never independent.

Assessment

An appropriate assessment of the child and their family should be carried out, including all of the general points outlined on p. 162. The gold standard diagnostic tools are the **Autism Diagnostic Interview** and **Autism Diagnostic Observation Schedule,** which are interviews carried out with the parents and child, respectively. A full examination should be undertaken to exclude an organic cause for the symptoms.

Management

Treatment of the PDD/ASDs will never be curative; it is therefore a question of providing appropriate skills and an environment in which the child can learn to interact with the rest of society in the best way possible. Table 32.3 shows an outline of the various treatment options.

General measures

Psychoeducation is best done by a specialist in PDDs. One of the most distressing decisions for the parents will be to choose an appropriate school for their child; the choice between mainstream and special schools can be very difficult. An individual decision is made, and this may be changed throughout the school-age years as the child or family's needs alter with time. Support for the family is extremely important; for example, putting parents in touch with the National Autistic Society or providing respite care.

Biological treatments

Several randomized controlled trials have demonstrated that atypical antipsychotics (especially risperidone) are effective in reducing aggression, tantrums, stereotypies,

Table 32.3 Treatment options for the pervasive developmental disorders

General
• Psychoeducation
• Finding an appropriate educational setting
• Treating psychiatric and physical co-morbidities
• Parental training courses

Biological
• Atypical antipsychotics
• Stimulants
• Antidepressants
• Melatonin

Psychological
• Speech and language therapy
• Social skills training
• Behavioural modification programmes

and self-injury. The side effects of these medications are troublesome, so they are reserved for use after behavioural modifications have failed. Stimulants or atomoxetine are effective in children with co-morbid ADHD, and SSRIs can decrease repetitive or obsessive behaviours. Recently, there has been much debate as to the worth of melatonin in affecting sleep cycles; some parents advocate the use of it in their autistic children who suffer from severe sleep–wake cycle disturbances.

Psychological treatments

The mainstay of treatment in any PDD is intensive, focused behavioural training programmes. Usually, the aim is to reduce antisocial or troublesome behaviours, whilst promoting more socially acceptable and productive ones. Children with PDDs cannot transfer skills easily, and need to be taught how to do this, although this is not always successful. It is helpful for therapy to be carried out in a multitude of settings; outpatient clinic, home, school, and social groups. Social skills training classes are appropriate for higher-functioning children (e.g. Asperger's), especially as this provides them with a sheltered opportunity for social interaction. Speech and language therapists are invaluable in the early years; they can help the child to achieve their verbal potential, which then to some extent defines what they can later achieve.

Specific developmental disorders of speech and language

Disorders of speech and language are common, affecting 3–5 per cent of children, and it is important to identify them early so that appropriate therapy can be given. There are a variety of factors needed for the development of normal speech: reasonable-quality hearing, the ability to understand what is being said, the ability to process what has been said, and the ability to form and verbalize a response. If any one part of this process is faulty, then a speech or language disorder may occur. For example, if a child is unable to understand spoken words as well as expected, they have a receptive language disorder. There is often a family history of speech problems.

- **Specific speech articulation disorder** is found in 2 per cent of 6–7 year olds, falling to 0.5 per cent of teenagers. These children have difficulty in using appropriate speech sounds, especially in substituting one sound for another.
- **Expressive language disorder** occurs when there is a delay in the ability to use spoken language appropriately, in the context of normal language comprehension.
- **Receptive language disorder** is a reduced ability to understand language. It is often associated with expressive disorders, but alone is relatively uncommon.

Speech and language disorders are more frequent in children with ADHD, oppositional defiance disorder, and conduct disorders. Approximately half resolve completely by adulthood, whilst the rest tend to improve to varying extents. Any child with a suspected speech disorder should be referred to a speech and language therapist. Treatment should start with psychoeducation, but speech therapy should be offered when the disorder starts to interfere with the child's everyday life, and is usually after 3 years of age. It is done in the child's usual environment (e.g. school) as this has proved more effective than the structured therapy sessions used for other conditions.

Specific reading disorder (dyslexia)

The child's reading age is significantly (two standard deviations) below the level expected from age and IQ and this is not due solely to inadequate education or poor vision. Writing and spelling are also impaired but the rest of development is normal. Compared with children with general backwardness at school, those with specific reading disorder are more often boys (2:1) and are more likely to have minor neurological abnormalities; they are less likely to come from disadvantaged families. The prevalence is 4 per cent of 4–10 year olds using diagnostic criteria, but studies report widely differing figures. By late adolescence, 25 per cent have caught up with their peers, but the rest have varying degrees of persisting difficulty with reading and spelling. The child may need special help with reading at school.

Stammering

Stammering is a disturbance of the rhythm and fluency of speech. It may take the form of repetitions of syllables or words, or of pauses in the production of speech. Stammering is four times more frequent in boys than girls and usually resolves by mid-childhood. Treatment is usually with speech therapy, but the long-term effects of this are currently unknown.

Gender identity disorder

Gender identity disorder (GID) is a condition in which a person experiences discomfort with the biological sex with which they were born to such an extent that it becomes clinically significant.

Children with GID typically behave as children of the opposite sex do, choosing to dress like them, play their games, prefer their toys, and use their verbal and physical mannerisms. All of the child's friends are usually of the opposite sex, and they may avoid playing with anything or anyone related to their own gender. Very young children may not verbalize the desire to be the other sex, but they usually do by mid-childhood. Boys tend to have a very effeminate manner, but it is harder to recognize in females, as tomboyish behaviour is relatively common

BOX 32.3 DSM-IV diagnostic criteria for gender identity disorder

A A strong and persistent cross-gender identification (not merely a desire for any perceived cultural advantages of being the other sex). In children, the disturbance is manifested by four (or more) of the following:

1 repeatedly stated desire to be, or insistence that he or she is, the other sex;

2 in boys, preference for cross-dressing or simulating female attire; in girls, insistence on wearing only stereotypical masculine clothing;

3 strong and persistent preferences for cross-sex roles in make-believe play, or persistent fantasies of being the other sex;

4 intense desire to participate in the stereotypical games and pastimes of the other sex;

5 strong preference for playmates of the other sex.

B Persistent discomfort with his or her sex or sense of inappropriateness in the gender role of that sex.

C The disturbance is not concurrent with a physical inter-sex condition.

D The disturbance causes clinically significant distress or impairment in social, occupational, or other important areas of functioning.

ICD-10 gender identity disorder of childhood

A disorder, usually first manifest during early childhood, characterized by a persistent and intense distress about assigned sex, together with a desire to be (or insistence that one is) of the other sex. There is a persistent preoccupation with the dress and activities of the opposite sex and repudiation of the individual's own sex. The diagnosis requires a profound disturbance of the normal gender identity; mere tomboyishness in girls or girlish behaviour in boys is not sufficient.

---

amongst non-gender-disordered children. The diagnostic criteria are shown in Box 32.3. The prevalence of GID is unknown. The mean age of presentation to psychiatric services is 7–8 years, typically when parents become concerned their child's behaviour is not just a passing phase. Five times as many boys as girls are diagnosed with GID.

Aetiology

The cause of this disorder is unknown. A number of factors have been shown to influence psychosexual development, but their relationship to GID is currently unclear.

- **Hormones.** Female children with congenital adrenal hyperplasia produce an excess of androgens, leading to virilization. These children tend to engage in more masculine games and behaviours from a young age, and often have male friends. However, they do not have the psychological wish to be the other sex. There have been several cases of male children who have undergone penectomy secondary to trauma and were reassigned to female before 2 years of life. These children, although brought up as females, tend to revert to their original sex in early adulthood, or become homosexual in orientation. This suggests a prenatal influence on gender identity.

- **Early differences in behaviour.** Children as young as 10 months are thought to be able to distinguish between those who are the same and opposite sex from themselves. By 12 months, children start to show a preference for toys associated with their sex, and start to prefer the company of the same-sex parent. Boys begin to be more assertive and

physically aggressive at about 18 months, whilst girls are more passive. At about this age, children become aware of sex stereotypes, believing that boys like to play with trucks and build things, whereas girls cook and play with dolls.

- **Parental influences.** There is robust evidence that parents tend to buy toys for their child that are gender related—dolls for girls and soldiers for boys. When mothers are presented with a young child call John and dressed as a boy, they treat them as a boy, even if the child is actually a dressed-up girl.

Prognosis and outcome

A large proportion of gender dysphoric children will improve significantly through adolescence and go on to live the rest of their lives as their biological sex. Approximately two-thirds of these individuals have a homosexual or bisexual orientation in adulthood. A minority of children with GID make the decision to change to the other sex, and spend the rest of their life living as the other gender. GID is associated with other psychiatric disorders, especially depression, anxiety disorders, and poor self-esteem.

Assessment and management

Assessment of a child with GID should include all of the elements of a basic assessment outlined in the previous chapter.

Psychoeducation is a key part of treating GID. Educating the whole family about gender identity, normal and abnormal, is very important and helps to establish that it is not necessary for boys to behave in one specific way, and that variation is normal.

Behaviour modification techniques can be used to help the child. Finding other children of their biological sex who are less stereotypical in their behaviours (e.g. sporty girls, non-physical more home-orientated boys) can assist the child in widening their peer group and interests. Individual therapy can be used in slightly older children, to address abnormal thought paths and associated psychological issues.

Cross-gender living. A small number of families make the decision to allow the child to live as the opposite sex. This is not a decision to be made lightly, and involves considerable discussion with all concerned, including the child's school. Once the child is a teenager, puberty can be a very distressing time. Physical changes are unwanted, and problems such as facial hair and menses are particularly difficult to contend with. Recently, a few clinicians have been experimenting with using GnRH analogues to block puberty in the early stages, and later (depending on the child's preferences) can either give cross-sex steroids or stop the GnRH to allow normal puberty to continue. Currently, surgical interventions are not recommended.

■ Disorders of school-age children and teenagers

Disorders in older children and adolescents are shown in Table 32.4; those of adolescence are fundamentally the same as the adult disorder and are discussed in their relevant chapters.

Table 32.4 Psychiatric disorders in older children and adolescents

Children aged 5 to (approximately) 13 years	Adolescents
• Anxiety disorders	• Depression
• OCD	• Bipolar disorder
• Mood disorders	• Anxiety disorders and OCD
• Attachment disorder	• Eating disorders
• Somatization disorders	• Schizophrenia and other psychoses
• Enuresis and encopresis	
• Eating disorders	• Deliberate self-harm and suicide
• Tics and Tourette's syndrome	• Somatoform disorders
• ADHD	• Substance abuse
• Conduct disorder	• Conduct disorder
• Sleep disorders	

Anxiety disorders (see Chapter 24)

Anxiety disorders are very common in childhood—10 to 20 per cent are affected—with separation anxiety disorder being the most common condition. Females are much more likely to be affected than males, as are those from lower socio-economic classes. Anxiety disorders tend to follow a stereotypical path; separation anxiety and phobic disorder usually start in preschool years, while social anxiety starts later. Panic disorder is usually only seen in adolescents. The general symptoms and co-morbidities associated with anxiety are shown in Table 32.5.

Aetiology

1 **Genetics.** Children with parents who have anxiety disorders are two to four times more likely to develop one than the general population. Heritability for anxiety disorders is estimated to be 40 to 50 per cent.

2 **Personality.** The child's temperament plays a large role—if they are shy or hesitant and fearful in new situations, they are at higher risk of an anxiety disorder.

3 **Parent–child attachment.** An insecure attachment to either parent is linked to anxiety disorders, as is a lack of reassurance and support being provided from parent to child. Overly strict parenting can also promote anxiety, as the child tends not to develop confidence to explore their environment.

4 **Parental anxiety disorder.** If parents or other people in the home are anxious, then aside from the genetic risk the child may also learn anxious behaviour from them.

Course and prognosis

The episode of anxiety itself is likely to remit, but leaves the child at very high risk of developing anxiety-related problems or depression in adulthood; 50 per cent of adults with depression have had an anxiety disorder in childhood or adolescence.

Table 32.5 Symptoms of childhood anxiety disorder

- Fearfulness and phobia
- Timidity
- Excessive worrying
- Poor concentration
- Poor sleep
- Physical symptoms: headache, nausea, vomiting, abdominal pain, bowel disturbance
- Overdependence
- Separation anxiety
- Co-morbidities: mood disorders, eating disorders, substance abuse

Table 32.6 Treatment of childhood anxiety disorder

General measures

- Psychoeducation: explain the nature of the problem to the parents and child
- Provide self-help materials
- Help the child to talk about their worries
- Reduce or avoid stressors

Psychological treatment

- Cognitive behaviour therapy
- Anxiety management therapy

Pharmacological treatment

- SSRIs

Treatment

The stages of treatment are summarized in Table 32.6. Psychological treatments—specifically cognitive behavioural therapy—are the first-line approach, as there is good evidence for their efficacy. If therapy does not provide an adequate response, an SSRI can be tried, but the number needed to treat for a clinically positive response is three in adolescents and four in children. Usually, a combination of a supportive approach, education, and CBT will be effective. Benzodiazepines are not recommended.

Separation anxiety disorder

Separation anxiety disorder occurs when the child fears that harm will occur to an attachment figure if they are apart, and is severe enough to interfere with daily activities and social development. It occurs in 3 to 5 per cent of primary school age children, and is more common in girls. Children with separation anxiety cling to their parents and are extremely distressed when parted from them. In severe cases it may present as school refusal, or avoidance of leaving the house. The condition may be initiated by a frightening experience such as admission to hospital, or by insecurity in the family; for example, when the parents are contemplating divorce. Separation anxiety is often maintained by overprotective attitudes of the parents and treatment is directed to changing these attitudes and reassuring the child.

Social anxiety disorder (social phobia)

The child experiences extreme anxiety in social situations where they perceive they are scrutinized, or could be embarrassed. It may present either as general shyness, or as anxiety produced by specific situations; for example, speaking in class, asking for something in a shop, speaking to strangers. Usually the child avoids these situations, which can interfere with their attending social functions, being included at school, and reaching their academic potential. CBT and social skills training are the best forms of management.

Generalized anxiety disorder, phobias and panic disorder are described in Chapter 24.

Somatic symptoms of emotional disorder

Children often communicate distress by complaining repeatedly of physical symptoms for which no physical cause can be found. The terms **functional or medically unexplained symptoms** are sometimes used, and the process is called somatization. The symptoms are usually associated with stressful circumstances or with parental anxiety. Common complaints are of abdominal pain, headache, limb pains, and sickness. Of these, abdominal pain is particularly frequent.

Treatment. The steps in treatment are summarized in Box 32.4. The doctor explains to the child and parents that the physical symptoms are undoubtedly real, and are treatable. The relationship to stress and anxiety is explained; the analogy with headache is often helpful. When the symptom is pain, the parents are advised to convey sympathy but not to focus attention on the pain. The child and parents are helped to find ways of reducing the experience of pain without taking analgesics, such as having distracting activities or relaxing music available.

Selective mutism

Selective mutism is a condition in which a person who is normally capable of speech is unable to speak in certain situations, or to specific people. It is classified as an anxiety disorder, and is a rare condition almost exclusively found in children. The person has a normal understanding of language and can often speak fluently at home with familiar people, but refuses to do so in some situation, for example at school or in the presence of strangers. It needs to have been present for at least 1 month and the child should not have a PDD or psychosis in order to make the

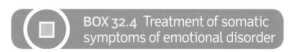

BOX 32.4 Treatment of somatic symptoms of emotional disorder

Explain that the symptoms real but have psychological rather than physical causes

Help the child to talk about the symptoms and worries

Reduce or avoid stressors

Psychoeducation for family members

Family therapy if there is unresolved conflict or relationship problems

CBT or behavioural therapy to modify the child's illness behaviour

Avoid using analgesics and anxiolytics

diagnosis. Selective mutism is reported to be present in 4 in 1000 children, but there have been no large epidemiological studies to date. The age of onset is usually 2–5 years, but it often does not become evident or a problem until the child starts school. It is more common in girls. A history of a speech disorder or abuse are the main risk factors.

Assessment and management

A general assessment of the child should be carried out, as on p. 162. It is important to exclude autism spectrum disorders or another developmental disorder. It is necessary to assess the child in a variety of settings—for example, home, school, outpatients—and with and without their carers. Treatment at an early age is important, as children with selective mutism rarely improve spontaneously. Referral should be made to a child psychiatrist.

Behavioural therapy is essential for successful treatment. The premise is that the mutism is a learnt behaviour. Stimulus fading is a common technique, where the patient is brought into an environment with someone else they are comfortable with. Gradually (in small steps) another person is introduced to the group, and the process continues slowly as the child gets used to it.

Play or art therapy is often used to try and examine the reasons underlying the child's mutism.

Family therapy helps to identify difficulties in family relationships that are contributing to the mutism, and to help the rest of the family cope with the mutism.

Speech and language therapy is often helpful, even if the child has no specific speech disorder.

There is currently no evidence for the use of medications in children with selective mutism.

Obsessive–compulsive disorder

Obsessive–compulsive disorder (OCD) is a condition characterized by obsessions and/or compulsions that the person feels driven to perform in order to prevent an imagined dreaded event. The general features of OCD in children are very similar to those seen in adults and are described on p. 299. The only diagnostic difference between adults and children is that whilst adults must realize that their thoughts are unreasonable or excessive to meet diagnostic criteria for OCD, in children this is not required. It is common for younger children not to have a clear idea of what they are trying to avoid whilst performing a ritual, and they may not be able to fully describe the obsessions they are experiencing. OCD is found in 0.5 per cent of adolescents and is more common in girls. It is highly associated with tic disorders, Tourette's syndrome, and mood and eating disorders.

Table 32.7 Management of OCD

Assessment
• Make a diagnosis and detect any co-morbidities
General measures for all patients
• Psychoeducation
• Problem-solving techniques and relaxation
• Guided self-help
Mild to moderate functional impairment
• Offer CBT
Severe functional impairment
• Combined treatment with CBT and an SSRI
• Family interventions
• Consider clomipramine

Management

The options for management of OCD are shown in Table 32.7. It is extremely rare for patients with OCD to need more intensive treatment than an outpatient programme, but if there is a high risk of suicide or deliberate self-harm then day- or inpatient treatment should be considered.

Medications

Medications are the second-line therapy, and should only be used if the child does not want or cannot engage with CBT, or has had a poor response to 12 weeks of CBT. The NICE guidance on OCD recommends the use of sertraline or fluvoxamine as the first-line option in children, with fluoxetine favoured if there is significant co-morbid depression. The second-line drug is clomipramine, which should only be used if SSRIs are not tolerated or ineffectual. Antidepressants should be continued for 6 months after cessation of symptoms, and the child should be followed up for at least a year.

Unipolar depression

Depression in childhood is relatively common, with the majority representing a normal response to distressing or adverse circumstances. Children tend to describe themselves as 'grouchy', 'empty', or 'unable to have fun' rather than low or depressed. Parents often present the child saying they are sad and tearful, or haven't been eating and sleeping well. The diagnostic criteria for depression in the diagnostic classifications include all ages (p. 223), although there are a number of slight differences in children.

• The core symptoms remain low mood, anhedonia, and fatigue; mood may also be irritable in children.

- Symptoms must be present for at least 2 weeks and have a negative effect upon functioning. In children the level of functioning in different settings may vary; for example, they may be very low at home but able to function slightly better at school.

- Sleep is often disturbed, but may not show the classical pattern of early morning awakening.

- Rather than weight loss, children may fail to gain weight or fall off of their growth centile.

- Occasionally, physical symptoms (e.g. abdominal pain, headaches, or fatigue) may be the only presenting complaint.

Prevalence

The prevalence of depression in prepubertal children is 1 to 2 per cent, and in adolescents is 3 to 8 per cent. In younger children the ratio of males to females is equal, but in adolescents it is 1:3.

Aetiology

The aetiology of depression is described in Chapter 21, but in childhood there is often a precipitating stressful event (e.g. bullying, a significant loss). Common environmental factors are shown in Box 32.5.

Course and prognosis

The majority of mild episodes of depression triggered by an identifiable event or situation will resolve in 2 to 6 months, but there is a high risk of relapse. About 5 per cent of episodes will become chronic, recurrent disorders that persist into adulthood. The risk factors for chronicity include severe depressive episode, ongoing adversities, personality disorder in child or parents, psychiatric illness in a parent, and poor psychosocial functioning. There is a 10- to 30-fold increased risk of suicide in young people with moderate to severe depression.

Management

The treatment of depression in children and adolescents within the UK is based on the National Institute for Clinical Excellence (NICE) guidelines issued in 2005. All but a very few children can be treated in the community as outpatients, and many will only need to see their primary care team. If any of the following features are present, the child should be referred to a child psychiatrist:

- moderate, severe, or psychotic depression;
- mild depression which has not responded to interventions in primary care;
- recurrence of depression after recovery from a moderate to severe episode;
- self-neglect;
- active suicidal ideation (these children may require day or inpatient treatment).

All children and their families should receive adequate psychoeducation, self-help materials, and advice about diet, exercise, and sleep hygiene.

Treatment of mild depression

Initially it may be appropriate to be supportive, undertake the general measures above, and arrange a follow-up in 2 weeks ('watchful waiting'). If the child has not improved, offer guided self-help or a short course of CBT.

Treatment of moderate to severe depression

The child should be given individual CBT, interpersonal therapy, or brief family therapy. If there is no improvement after 12 weeks, consider an alternative form of therapy or medications. In children aged 12–18 years, fluoxetine is the first-line medication for resistant depression. Start at 10 mg daily, increasing to 20 mg at 1 week unless there has been a good response. In adult-weight teenagers, higher doses may be used. Try to avoid using medication in children less than 12 years. If fluoxetine in

BOX 32.5 Environmental and social factors in the aetiology of childhood depression

Abuse at an early age	Neglect
Family discord	Family substance abuse
Criminality in the family	Traumatic life events
Losses or bereavements	Maternal–child conflict
Attachment difficulties	Good academic achievement
Bullying	Social isolation
Low-income family	Unstable or unpredictable family environment

combination with psychological therapy is not effective, consider changing to either sertraline or citalopram. Medications should be continued for at least 6 months after symptoms recede, and slowly tapered to avoid withdrawal symptoms. Children should be regularly reviewed for at least 12 months after their recovery.

Post-traumatic stress disorder (PTSD)

Post-traumatic stress disorder (PTSD) is severe psychological disturbance following a traumatic event, characterized by the involuntary re-experiencing of the event combined with symptoms of hyperarousal, dissociation, and avoidance. It is described fully in Chapter 23. Box 32.6 shows some frequent stressors in childhood, but specific traumatic events (e.g. war, earthquakes) may also play a role. The clinical features are similar to those in adults, and there is frequently co-morbid anxiety, depression, or ADHD. About 50 per cent of children develop PTSD after a major disaster (e.g. plane crash, volcanic eruption), and 25 per cent develop symptoms after lesser events such as road traffic accidents. However, more of these children will recover from the PTSD, with one-third of those diagnosed 1 to 3 months after a major disaster being symptom free at 1 year.

Management

General management should be carried out as in Table 32.5. The recommended first-line intervention is trauma-focused cognitive behavioural therapy (TF-CBT). Family therapy is usually offered alongside, and young children may benefit from formal art or play therapy. Medication is not recommended, unless there is significant co-morbid depression, in which case fluoxetine may be prescribed under close supervision.

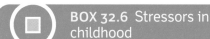

BOX 32.6 Stressors in childhood

Chronic

Poverty	Deprivation
Parental mental illness	Parental substance misuse
Chronic family conflicts	War
Refugee status	Social discrimination
Chronic physical illness	Physical, sexual, or emotional abuse

Acute

Accidents	Bereavement
Separation from carers	Bullying
Assault	Death of a pet
Change of school	Loss of friends
Physical illness	Illness of a relative

Somatization and somatoform disorders

Somatoform disorder is a syndrome of prolonged physical symptoms in the absence of an identifiable organic cause with associated functional impairment in the context of an identifiable stressor. These are described more fully in Chapter 25. It is extremely common for children to express their distress or unhappiness through physical symptoms, although a disorder fitting standard criteria is relatively rare. The commonest symptoms that children complain of are shown in Table 32.8, but by far the most frequent are abdominal pain and headaches. Co-morbid anxiety or depressive disorders are commonplace.

Prevalence

The prevalence of somatization disorder or somatic symptoms in children is unknown. Abdominal pain accounts for 10 per cent of new appointments with paediatricians, and in very few children is gastrointestinal pathology found. In 25 per cent of children presenting with headaches, somatization is thought to be a predominant factor. The peak age for unexplained symptoms is 8 to 12 years, and they are much more common in girls.

Table 32.8 Physical symptoms commonly relating to somatization in children

Cardiovascular
- Breathlessness
- Chest pain

Gastrointestinal
- Abdominal pain
- Nausea and anorexia
- Vomiting or regurgitation
- Diarrhoea or frequent bowel motions

Genitourinary
- Dysuria
- Frequency
- Copious vaginal discharge
- Odd sensations around genitalia

Neurological
- Headaches
- Tingling or numbness
- Amnesia
- Chronic fatigue

Musculoskeletal
- Aches and pains

Aetiology

There is no one cause of somatoform disorders, and their heterogeneous clinical presentation adds weight to the theory that they are multifactorial in origin. One theory suggests that somatization is merely the way in which children who are not mature enough to express themselves verbally communicate distress. It may also be that there are a group of individuals who tend to focus on physiological bodily sensations, and misinterpret their significance, thereby leading to a belief that something is wrong. There are many risk factors for somatization, which are shown in Box 32.7.

Assessment and management

The aims of assessing a child with a somatic complaint are threefold:

1 to gather information about the problem, the child's personality, family history and familial interactions, and home environment;

2 to exclude an organic cause for the symptoms;

3 to produce a management plan.

Assessment should be carried out in any child presenting with a psychiatric disorder. Whilst a thorough physical examination and basic investigations are appropriate, multiple and specialist investigations should be avoided.

Psychoeducation is the most important aspect of management. It is imperative to clearly explain to the child and family that a cause could not be found for the symptoms, but that this does not mean that they do not exist, and are probably linked to relevant psychological issues. It must be made clear that there is a very low probability of serious illness ensuing from the symptoms. Highlighting that improvements in family communication, environment, and relationships may help the child to recover more quickly is important. Teaching relaxation and problem-solving skills is often helpful, as are self-help or information leaflets about the relevant symptoms. Getting the child into school regularly and engaging in social activities is essential, and the family may need education and assistance in order to do this.

Family therapy can be extremely helpful in addressing problems such as unsolved conflict within the family, poor communication, and highly expressed emotions.

Individual CBT for the child can allow the links between thoughts, feelings, and physical sensations to be explored. Behavioural techniques may be used to help the child adjust their abnormal illness behaviour; for example, by increasing school attendance.

Physical interventions may be appropriate for some conditions. Basic approaches such as a hot-water bottle for a stomach ache or physiotherapy for joint problems are usually beneficial. Complex treatment regimes involving medications (especially long-term painkillers) should be avoided.

Antidepressants may be indicated in older children with co-morbid anxiety or depression. An SSRI (typically fluoxetine) would be the first-line choice.

Sleep disorders

The commonly encountered disorders of sleeping in children are **nightmares**, **night terrors**, and **sleep-walking**. These are all covered in detail in Chapter 28, so what follows are the specific points related to children and adolescents.

The physiology of sleep is very different in children and adults, and is complicated by the fact that it changes throughout development. Some of the differences include the following.

- The total amount of sleep needed is more than in adults (see Box 32.8).

- The circadian sleep–wake cycle does not become trained until 6–8 months.

 BOX 32.7 Risk factors for somatization in children and adolescents

Child factors
Previous physical illness
Oldest child in family
Low IQ
Experience of child abuse or neglect
Personality traits: perfectionism, anxiety, conscientiousness
History of depression or anxiety disorder

Family factors
Familial physical illness, especially chronic disease or disability

Psychiatric problems, especially depression or anxiety
Parental somatization
High expectations of the child
Poor intrafamily communication and relationships

Social factors
Lower socio-economic class
Poverty
Life stresses, e.g. bullying, academic pressures

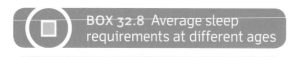

BOX 32.8 Average sleep requirements at different ages

Neonate	17 hours
2 years	13 hours
4 years	12 hours
10 years	10 hours
Adolescent	9 hours
Adult	5–9 hours

- Between 5 years and puberty, sleep is very sound at night and children are very alert during the day (there is less of a distinction in adults).

- Adolescents have increased daytime sleepiness compared with any other age; the sleep phase often becomes delayed, so that teenagers like to stay up late and lie in during the mornings.

It is important to recognize that sleep disturbance in childhood can have wide-ranging effects, including a direct negative effect upon mood, behaviour, and cognitive function. Adolescents are at particular risk of other psychiatric problems if they have continually inadequate sleep. Whilst adults tend to become slow in mental and physical activities when sleep deprived, children often show increased activity, irritability, agitation, and loss of temper control. Groups of children at particularly high risk of a sleep disorder are shown in Box 32.9.

Assessment of a child presenting with a sleep disorder

The general schedule for assessing patients with sleep disorders (p. 359) should be followed, but with a few

BOX 32.9 Groups at high risk of sleep disturbance

Anxious children or those with panic disorder
Traumatic experiences in early life
Depressive disorders
ADHD
Autism spectrum disorders
OCD
Tourette's syndrome
Parental mental illness
Chaotic household and disorganized daily routine
Homeless children
Children from lower socioeconomic households
Learning disorders
Neurodegenerative disorders
Acute physical illness (e.g. gastroenteritis)

alterations. It is important to get the parents to record a 24-hour sleep–wake pattern on at least one ordinary day, and then to keep a sleep diary for 2–4 weeks in order to determine the usual routine and sleep disturbances. A full developmental history should be taken and a physical examination done. Investigations can be carried out as for adults (p. 360); actigraphy is well tolerated and validated for use in children.

Insomnia

About 30 per cent of school-age children either have trouble getting to sleep or wake up repeatedly during the night. Common causes of sleeplessness in children include night-time fears (e.g. monsters), separation anxiety, daytime napping, worries, anxiety, depression, and in teenagers, caffeine, nicotine, and alcohol in the evenings. If a psychiatric or physical disorder is the cause, the best approach is to treat it. For many children, discussing their worries or fears can lessen them, and reassurance to the parents that the problem is likely to resolve by itself.

Nightmares

Nightmares are frightening dreams that cause the child to wake up, usually feeling slightly confused. The child may be distressed, and can take time to get back to sleep. They occur during REM sleep, and show a distinctive increase in activity on the EEG. Nightmares are common in childhood, especially around the ages of 5 or 6 years. Frequent nightmares may be accompanied by daytime anxiety. There is no specific treatment, so parents should be reassured that it is likely to improve with time and helped to reduce any stressful circumstances at home.

Night terrors

Night terrors are less common than nightmares. They are characterized by a sudden awakening in which the child sits upright, screams loudly, and has marked autonomic activation. Occasionally, there may be frantic motor activity which can lead to falling out of bed and injury. The episode occurs a few hours after going to bed, and usually lasts about 5 minutes. Afterwards the child goes back to sleep, and is unable to remember the events in the morning. There is no specific treatment, but it is important to reassure the family, make sure the child is safe at night, and ensure good sleep hygiene. Night terrors seldom persist into adult life.

Sleepwalking

Sleepwalking is characterized by complex, automatic behaviours occurring during sleep. In children this usually involves wandering around the house. The child's eyes are open and they avoid familiar objects. The child may appear agitated, does not respond to questions, and is often difficult to wake, although they can usually be led back to bed. Episodes usually last for a few minutes, although rarely they may continue for as long as an hour. It is most common between the ages of 5 and 12 years, occurring at least once in 15 per cent of children in this age group. Occasionally, the disorder persists into adult life. There is no specific treatment, but as sleepwalkers occasionally harm themselves, parents should protect the child from injury by fastening doors and windows securely, barring stairs, and removing dangerous objects.

Disorders of elimination

Functional enuresis

Functional enuresis is the repeated involuntary voiding of urine, occurring after an age at which continence is usual and in the absence of any identified physical disorder. The condition may be **nocturnal** (bed-wetting), **diurnal** (occurring during waking hours), or both. Nocturnal enuresis is referred to as **primary** if there has been no preceding period of urinary continence, and **secondary** if there has been a preceding period of urinary continence. There is no absolute period of continence needed to become secondary enuresis, but 6 months is a commonly used timeframe. Most children achieve regular daytime and night-time continence by 3 or 4 years of age, and *5 years is generally taken as the youngest age for the diagnosis.* Nocturnal enuresis can cause great unhappiness and distress, particularly if the parents blame or punish the child, and if the condition restricts staying with friends or going on holiday.

Prevalence

Nocturnal enuresis occurs in about 10 per cent of children at 5 years of age, 4 per cent at 8 years, 1 per cent at 14 years and 0.5 per cent in adulthood. The condition is more frequent in boys. Daytime enuresis has a lower prevalence and is more frequent in girls.

Aetiology

The majority of cases of nocturnal primary enuresis are idiopathic; there is simply a delay in maturation of the nervous system controlling the bladder. These children often have a family history of enuresis, as children who have either one or two parents who were enuretic have a 44 and 70 per cent chance, respectively, of being enuretic themselves. There are a range of other causes of enuresis, but these are more commonly associated with secondary nocturnal or diurnal enuresis (Table 32.9).

Assessment and management

Assessment should be undertaken as in any child presenting to psychiatry. It is important to determine if the enuresis is primary or secondary, any family history, and

Table 32.9 Aetiology of functional enuresis

Common causes of nocturnal primary enuresis

- Idiopathic developmental delay
- Genetics

Less common causes of enuresis (consider in secondary nocturnal or diurnal cases)

- Urinary tract infection
- Diabetes mellitus
- Abnormalities of the urinary tract (e.g. small bladder, vesicoureteric reflux)
- Structural abnormalities of the nervous system (e.g. spina bifida occulta)
- Chronic constipation
- Diuretics: caffeine, alcohol
- ADHD
- Learning disorders or syndromes of developmental delay
- Behavioural: being too engaged in play or 'leaving it too late'
- Psychological: a response to bereavement, stress, abuse, or bullying
- Obstructive sleep apnoea
- Epilepsy

if there are stressful situations at home or school. Many children will have already had some treatment—find out what this was and why it didn't work. It is essential to exclude a primary physical cause; do a full neurological examination, feel for a loaded colon, inspect for signs of spina bifida, and perform urinalysis.

The majority of children who are bedwetting at 5 years will outgrow it in the next 2 years—therefore, a watching and waiting approach is often the best option in this period. Many clinicians do not start to treat enuresis until 7 years unless it is causing functional, psychological, or social impairment. If a specific physical or psychiatric cause of the enuresis has been found, then it should be treated by a specialist in that field. Most cases of primary enuresis can be treated successfully in general practice. The treatment options are shown in Table 32.10.

Psychoeducation. The parents and their child should be reassured that enuresis is common and the child is not to blame. The parents should be told that *punishment and disapproval are inappropriate and ineffective*, and that they should *reward success* (e.g. with star charts), and *not focus attention on failure.* Reinforcing positives helps to increase self-esteem and also is a powerful tool in changing behaviour.

Table 32.10 Management of enuresis

General measures

- Treat any primary physical or psychiatric disorders
- Education and reassurance for parents and child
- Practical advice
- Basic behavioural measures—rewarding success
- Reduce stressors

For persistent cases

- Enuresis alarms ('bell and pad')
- Desmopressin
- Tricyclic antidepressants
- Bladder training and pelvic floor exercises

Practical advice

Parents can be advised to:

- restrict fluid intake before bedtime;
- wake the child to pass urine once during the night;
- use mattress covers;
- avoid pull-up nappies (these can prolong the problem).

Enuresis alarms. A sensor to detect urine is attached to the child's pyjama trousers and a miniature alarm is carried in the pocket or on the wrist. The child turns off the alarm and rises to complete emptying the bladder while the bed is remade if necessary. In the past, before the necessary sensors were available, the passage of urine was detected by two metal plates separated by a cotton pad. When the pad became wet, the current flowed and an alarm bell rang. The term *pad and bell method* is still in use to describe this approach to treatment. About 70 per cent of children improve within a month of this treatment, but a third relapse within a year.

Medication. The synthetic antidiuretic hormone analogue **desmopressin** (DDAVP) acts to reduce urine production whilst the child is asleep, and is effective at producing dry nights in 50 per cent of children. It is available as an oral tablet or as a nasal spray, which is preferred by most children. Unfortunately, desmopressin has only a short-term effect and most children relapse as soon as they stop taking it. However, it can be a useful method of allowing a child to attend a sleep-over or camp. Tricyclic antidepressants, especially **imipramine**, are effective at reducing bedwetting when given at a low dose. Most children improve partially on the drug, and about a third stop completely, although most relapse when the drug is stopped. Because of this high relapse rate, the side effects of tricyclics, and the potential danger of accidental overdose, the use of antidepressant drugs is limited mainly to enabling the child to be dry over a

short but important period, such as a school journey. It has a very limited longer-term role in those with persistent enuresis whose social, educational, or psychological development is being adversely affected by it.

Functional encopresis

Functional encopresis is an uncommon disorder in which the child passes faeces in inappropriate places after the age at which bowel control is usual. The age at which control is reached varies, but at the age of 3–4 years 94 per cent of children have control with only occasional accidents. Usually, encopresis would not be diagnosed in a child younger than 4, and it should have been taking place for at least once a month for at least 3 months. Encopresis occurs in about 1 per cent of children aged 4 and upwards, but after 5–6 years is much rarer. The condition is more common in boys than girls, by a factor of 6 to 1.

Aetiology

It is unusual to be able to identify a cause of encopresis, but some are listed below:

- idiopathic primary encopresis is more common in children with learning disabilities;
- chronic constipation and overflow incontinence;
- structural malformations of the colon (e.g. Hirschsprung's disease);
- anal fissures causing pain;
- traumatic or unsettling events;
- deliberate rebellion by the child against the parents (almost never the sole cause);
- associated with anxiety or mood disorder;
- associated with physical, sexual, or emotional abuse (extremely rare).

Treatment

The plan of treatment resembles that for enuresis.

- Treat any primary physical or psychiatric disorder.
- Reassure the parents that the problem occurs in other children and will improve in time.
- Avoid constipation with a high-fibre diet and adequate hydration. Empty the bowel with laxatives, and continue them as maintenance if necessary.
- Encourage normal bowel habits, starting by asking the child to sit on the toilet for 5 minutes after each meal.
- Encourage the parents to reward the child for opening his bowels in the appropriate place, and not to dwell on failure.
- Modify any stressful circumstances if possible.

Eating disorders

An eating disorder is *a disturbance of eating habits or weight control behaviour that results in clinically significant impairment of physical health and/or psychosocial functioning.* A full account of the major eating disorders can be found in Chapter 27, so what follows are specific points relating to children and adolescents.

Anorexia nervosa

Anorexia nervosa is a clinical syndrome characterized by extremely low body weight, amenorrhoea, distorted body image, and an intense fear of gaining weight. The average age of onset is 15 to 17 years, although increasingly prepubertal cases are being recognized. Prepubertal onset of anorexia nervosa is defined as the onset of the illness before menstruation has been established. Anorexia nervosa can have a devastating impact on the child's pubertal development and on family relationships. Children with anorexia nervosa are more likely to be male (15 per cent) and less likely to have other co-morbid psychiatric disorders than adults.

Clinical features

The features are similar to those found in adults. There is more often a definite precipitating event (e.g. change of school, bereavement, physical illness leading to weight loss) and a short illness course. The initial stages of the illness are usually symptoms of depression, irritability, social withdrawal, and sometimes school refusal. The child's parents then notice they are avoiding eating at mealtimes, and are engaging in all the anorexic behaviours seen in older patients (p. 335). Excessive exercise is common in young children, but laxative abuse and purging are less so.

Prepubertal children do not always show the typical extreme weight loss associated with anorexia nervosa; at first there is a failure to gain weight and a cessation of growth. Later there is weight loss and the usual symptoms and signs of starvation. Primary amenorrhoea is usual, and even in those who recover quickly, onset of menses may be delayed by several years. Other signs of secondary sexual maturation will be absent.

The core psychopathology of anorexia nervosa remains the same, but young children may express their anxieties in different ways. Even very young children will admit to being scared of becoming fat, but frequently don't express a distorted body image or definite valuation of themselves in terms of weight and shape. Occasionally, girls will say they are fearful of having menstrual periods, or that they do not wish to grow up. Depressive symptoms and obsessive–compulsive disorder are extremely common co-morbidities.

Assessment and investigations

Assessment should be carried out as for adults (p. 340), and the child should be referred to a child psychiatrist relatively urgently. Special attention should be paid to identifying any recent stressors at home or school, and to interaction and communication between family members. Weight and height should be carefully monitored, and recorded on a standard growth curve. BMI is not a reliable measure in the under-16s. Pelvic ultrasound monitoring of the uterus and ovaries is helpful in monitoring recovery in girls. At a low weight, the volume of the ovaries and uterus will be reduced compared with healthy girls, but this increases into the normal range with good nutrition and weight gain.

Management

The NICE guidelines published in 2004 relate to children and adolescents as well as to adults. Detail on the management can be found on p. 342, but the key points relating to young people are:

- Almost all children can be treated as outpatients, but more intensive treatment may be needed for severe emaciation, failure of outpatient treatment, or situations where the parents/guardians are unable to manage home re-feeding. Admissions should only be to facilities specifically for young people.

- First-line management is family therapy and home re-feeding—the Maudsley method. All members of the family should be involved.

- The child should also be offered individual therapy sessions based on the principles of CBT.

- If the child refuses treatment, either parental permission or use of the Mental Health Act 1983 can override their decision.

- Medication should not routinely be used, but may be indicated if there is significant co-morbid depression or anxiety.

The prognosis in children with a definite precipitating event for the illness, a short illness course, and rapid recovery is excellent. Those with a more insidious onset and resistance to recovery fare less well, with their illness often continuing into adolescence and early adult years.

Bulimia nervosa

Bulimia nervosa is an eating disorder characterized by recurrent episodes of uncontrolled excessive eating ('binges'), compensatory methods of weight control, and a fear of becoming fat. It is extremely rare in prepubertal children, with only a few case reports of children under 14 years having been published.

Attention deficit hyperactivity disorder (hyperkinetic disorder)

Attention deficit hyperactivity disorder (ADHD) is a persistent pattern of **inattention, hyperactivity,** and **impulsivity** that is more frequently displayed and more severe than is typically observed in individuals at a comparable level of development. Diagnosing and treating ADHD is important, because long term it may severely impact upon a child's ability to achieve their educational potential, cause difficulty in managing social and home environments, interfere with interpersonal relationships, and cause problems in finding employment.

Diagnostic criteria

The full diagnostic criteria for ADHD are shown in Box 32.10; ADHD is known as **hyperactivity disorder** in the ICD-10 classification. However, these are complex criteria so the key points are summarized below.

- The child must show core symptoms of **inattention, hyperactivity,** and **impulsivity**.
- Symptoms must have started before age 7.
- Symptoms are present in at least two settings (e.g. home and school).
- There must be definite evidence of impaired function.
- The symptoms are not caused or related to another mental health disorder.

Clinical features (see Table 32.11)

Children with ADHD have too much energy; they are restless, fidgety, and cannot sit still. They have difficulty

---

BOX 32.10 DSM-IV criteria for attention deficit hyperactivity disorder

I   Either A or B:

A   Six or more of the following symptoms of inattention have been present for at least 6 months to a point that is disruptive and inappropriate for developmental level:

- Inattentive:
1   Often does not give close attention to details or makes careless mistakes.
2   Often has trouble keeping attention on tasks or play activities.
3   Often does not seem to listen when spoken to directly.
4   Often does not follow instructions and fails to finish schoolwork, chores, or duties in the workplace.
5   Often has trouble organizing activities.
6   Often avoids, dislikes, or doesn't want to do things that take a lot of mental effort.
7   Often loses things needed for tasks and activities.
8   Is often easily distracted.
9   Often forgetful in daily activities.

OR

B   Six or more of the following symptoms of hyperactivity–impulsivity have been present for at least 6 months to an extent that is disruptive and inappropriate for developmental level:

- Hyperactivity:
1   Often fidgets with hands or feet or squirms in seat.
2   Often gets up from seat when remaining on seat is expected.

3   Often runs about or climbs when and where it is not appropriate.
4   Often has trouble playing or enjoying leisure activities quietly.
5   Is often 'on the go' or often acts as if 'driven by a motor'.
6   Often talks excessively.

- Impulsiveness:
1   Often blurts out answers before questions have been finished.
2   Often has trouble waiting one's turn.
3   Often interrupts or intrudes on others.

II   Some symptoms that cause impairment were present before age 7 years.

III   Some impairment from the symptoms is present in two or more settings (such as at school/work and at home).

IV   There must be clear evidence of significant impairment in social, school, or work functioning.

V   The symptoms do not happen only during the course of a pervasive developmental disorder, schizophrenia, or other psychotic disorder. The symptoms are not better accounted for by another mental disorder.

ICD-10 F90.0 Hyperactivity disorder

The ICD-10 criteria are more restrictive; the child must show hyperactivity, impulsivity, *and* inattention. All three must be present and impairing function in two or more settings.

Table 32.11 Clinical features of attention deficit hyperactivity disorder

- Extreme restlessness
- Sustained overactivity
- Poor attention
- Learning difficulty
- Impulsiveness
- Recklessness
- Accident proneness
- Disobedience
- Temper tantrums
- Aggression

in attending to one thing for long and in following instructions. Their school work is disorganized, never finished, and contains many careless errors. They are very impulsive and never think about the consequences of an action. The child tends to be forgetful, and is boisterous, reckless, and accident prone. Their behaviour exhausts their parents and their teachers, alienates other children, and disrupts their school work. All these problems lead to low self-esteem and sometimes to disobedience, temper tantrums, aggression, and other antisocial behaviour. Depressive mood is common. These behaviours vary in severity between places—for example, worse at school than at home—and from day to day.

Prevalence

Estimates of prevalence and incidence vary widely depending upon which criteria are used for diagnosis. DSM-IV criteria of ADHD have a prevalence of 3 to 5 per cent under 19 years, whereas ICD-10 criteria reduce this to 1 to 2 per cent. The ratio of males to females is 3:1. There has been a large increase in the percentage of the population diagnosed with ADHD in the past three decades; however, it is not entirely clear if this represents better diagnosis and easier access to treatment, or a genuine increase.

Co-morbidity

The following conditions are all frequently found in children with ADHD: depression, tic disorders, anxiety, oppositional defiance disorder, substance abuse, and PDDs.

Differential diagnosis

It is important to differentiate ADHD from a primary diagnosis of one of the conditions listed under co-morbidities, and from mania. Either condition presents as overactivity, talkativeness, fast thoughts, and irritable mood. In bipolar disorder these symptoms will be episodic, and there is usually euphoria and grandiosity—these can therefore be used to distinguish between the two conditions.

Aetiology

The aetiology of ADHD is undoubtedly multifactorial, but has a strong genetic component. Table 32.12 shows the factors that have so far been linked to ADHD.

Genetics. Twin studies have shown the heritability of ADHD to be very high; 75 to 90 per cent is reported in most studies. The risk of ADHD in a first-degree relative of a sufferer is five times the risk of the general public. ADHD has been linked to a variety of genes, the majority of which are related to the action of dopamine; for example, dopamine receptors, dopamine transporters, and the monoamine system.

Brain structure and function abnormalities. MRI scanning of patients with ADHD versus age-matched controls has repeatedly shown that the frontal lobes, striatum, and cerebellum are smaller in those with ADHD. The difference persists into adult life, and is greater in those who have not received stimulants. The restlessness and difficulty in concentration suggest an abnormality in the prefrontal cortex and related subcortical structures since these are involved in guiding and sustaining behaviour, and delaying responses. As these brain regions are rich in catecholamines this observation appears

Table 32.12 Aetiology of attention deficit hyperactivity disorder

Biological
- Genetics
- Structural brain abnormalities
- Catecholamine system dysregulation
- Abnormalities in executive and higher brain function
- Low birth weight

Psychological
- Severe early deprivation
- Physical, sexual, or emotional abuse
- Institutional rearing
- Poor family communication and interactions

Environmental
- Prenatal exposure to benzodiazepines, alcohol, cocaine, or nicotine
- Perinatal obstetric complications
- Brain injury in early life
- Exposure to high levels of lead
- Low socio-economic class
- Diet or food intolerances

to link with the genetic findings and with the observed therapeutic effect of stimulant drugs.

Psychological factors are clearly a much lesser player than genetics, but early deprivation (emotional, nutrition, stimulatory) has been clearly linked with an increased risk of ADHD. Romanian orphans who grew up in large-scale orphanages but were then adopted into Western European families before age 4 show extremely high levels of severe ADHD.

Environmental factors can be divided into prenatal and postnatal. Prenatally, maternal stress or use of various substances (benzodiazepines, nicotine, cocaine, alcohol, or anticonvulsants) predisposes the child to ADHD. It is unclear currently whether mothers with a tendency towards hyperactivity and impulsivity are more likely to use these substances,

and therefore the child would be at high risk anyway, or if it is a genuine association. Postnatally, head injuries or another brain disease (e.g. autism or Tourette's) have been strongly linked to ADHD. Some advocate dietary factors as being influential upon children's symptoms, and suggest excluding the problem substance (wheat/dairy/artificial sweeteners, etc.) from their diet (see Science box 32.1).

Prognosis

It was originally thought that ADHD was a condition confined to children, but longitudinal studies have now shown that 15 per cent of cases still meet diagnostic criteria in mid-adulthood, and a further 40 per cent still have subdiagnostic persisting symptoms. During adolescence overactivity tends to improve greatly, and a general increase in self-control

 Science box 32.1 Do food additives exacerbate hyperactivity in children?

The number of children diagnosed with attention deficit hyperactivity disorder (ADHD) has increased more than tenfold since the 1970s. In the USA, the prevalence is currently 4–5 per cent of children under 16 years; this represents 4.8 million children, half of whom are taking stimulants.[1] The reason for this change over such a short time period is clearly not genetics. One explanation is that we now have better detection, leading to more diagnoses. The other is that provocative environmental factors are causing or exacerbating hyperactivity in children. One area that has come under scrutiny has been childhood nutrition, specifically artificial food colours and additives (AFCA).

The association between diet and hyperactivity has been investigated since the early 1970s. In 1973, Feingold published a study claiming that half of all hyperactive children improved after eliminating all AFCA.[2] His 'elimination diet' required the removal of all processed foods and most fruit and vegetables, but it was surprisingly popular. Bateman *et al.* performed a double-blind cross-over study of 1873 4-year-olds to determine if AFCA affected their hyperactivity symptoms.[3] The sample included children with and without a diagnosis of ADHD, and included a 1-week AFCA-free period, 1 week of AFCA supplementation, and 1 week of placebo. A significant increase ($P < 0.007$) in hyperactivity on parental ratings occurred during the supplementation week. No difference was seen in impulsivity or inattention. In 2007, MacCann and colleagues published a randomized, double-blinded placebo trial of AFCA in 3 and 8/9-year-old children.[4] These were a sample of the general population, not children diagnosed with ADHD. For the first week all 153 children had an AFCA-free diet; then they were randomly allocated to weeks on supplementation and placebo. The results report

that supplementation of AFCA had a significantly adverse effect on behaviour compared with placebo ($P = 0.044$).

Taking the results above into account, the European Food Safety Authority (EFSA) reviewed the evidence linking AFCA with hyperactivity.[5] Out of 22 studies examined, 16 reported negative effects of AFCA upon behaviour. They concluded that whilst the aetiology of ADHD is clearly multifactorial, a comprehensive management plan for ADHD should include trials of dietary modifications.

Currently there is no definite answer as to the association between hyperactivity and food additives. It is likely that a subgroup of children are prone to develop hyperactivity with excessive intake of AFCA, and this appears to be primarily independent of whether they have been diagnosed with ADHD.

1 Newmark, S.C. (2009). Nutritional intervention in ADHD. *Explore* **5**: 171.

2 Feingold, B. (1975). *Why your Child is Hyperactive.* Random House, New York, NY.

3 Bateman, B. *et al.* (2004). The effects of a double blind, placebo controlled, artificial food colourings and benzoate preservative challenge on hyperactivity in a general population of preschool children. *Archives of Diseases of Childhood* **89**: 506–11.

4 McCann, D. *et al.* (2007). Food additives and hyperactive behaviour in 3 year old and 8/9 year old children in the community: a randomised, double-blinded, placebo-controlled trial. *Lancet* **370**: 1560–7.

5 AFC Panel (2008). Assessment of the results of the study by McCann *et al.* (2007) on the effect of some colours and sodium benzoate on children's behaviour. *European Food Safety Authority Journal* **660**: 1–54.

helps to reduce the inattention and impulsiveness. However, those who do not lose the overactivity are at high risk of conduct disorder, antisocial behaviour, and juvenile delinquency. It is currently unknown what the risk factors for continuation of the illness into adulthood are, but severity of initial ADHD symptoms, a family history, and co-morbid psychiatric disease are likely contenders. Taken across a lifetime, those given a diagnosis of ADHD in childhood are more likely than the general population to attain poor qualifications, become unemployed, be involved in multiple road traffic accidents, and serve a prison sentence.

Assessment

A full assessment should be carried out as for any psychiatric condition in a child (p. 162). Since the problem behaviours vary in different settings, information should be obtained from teachers and other adults involved with the child as well as from the parents and the child.

Management

Clinical management of ADHD in the UK is based upon the NICE guidelines published in 2008, which organize treatment into categories according to mild, moderate, or severe impairment of function. An overview of the available treatment strategies is shown in Table 32.13, and the structure of management recommended by NICE is outlined in Table 32.14.

Parental training courses and behaviour interventions within the family

Much of the required psychoeducation and training in behavioural techniques to modify behaviour are

Table 32.13 Treatment options for attention deficit hyperactivity disorder

General measures
- Psychoeducation
- Self-instruction materials
- Support groups

Psychological treatments
- Parent training and education courses
- Behavioural therapy at school or via family interventions
- Social skills training
- CBT: group or individual

Pharmacological treatments
- Stimulants: methylphenidate and dexamphetamine
- Non-stimulants: atomoxetine
- Unlicensed medications: clonidine, modafinil, imipramine

Table 32.14 NICE 2008 guidelines on management of attention deficit hyperactivity disorder

Diagnosis and advice
- Should only be made by a psychiatrist or paediatrician with specialist knowledge of ADHD
- GPs should refer to secondary services if the symptoms are moderate or severe
- Parents and child should receive psychoeducation and self-help materials

Mild impairment of function: management in primary care
- Watchful waiting for up to 10 weeks
- Offer referral to a parent training and education course
- Drugs are not recommended

Moderate impairment of function: management by a specialist team
- Offer a parent training and education course
- Offer the child a group social skills training course or group CBT
- Older adolescents may benefit from individual CBT
- Drugs should only be used if the above measures fail to improve symptoms

Severe impairment of function: management by a specialist team
- Offer drugs as the first-line intervention (methylphenidate, dexamphetamine, or atomoxetine)
- If drugs are not accepted or tolerated, consider CBT or social skills training
- If drugs fail to improve symptoms, add individual CBT or group social skills training
- Do not prescribe antipsychotics for children with ADHD
- Only consider unlicensed drugs in severe, resistant cases—they should be initiated by a specialist in tertiary care

effectively delivered to parents by taught courses. These are group sessions that allow the parents to meet with other families who have a child with ADHD, and to reinforce behavioural work being done at school and in therapy sessions. They help parents to identify and understand the exact problem behaviours, when they occur, what triggers them, and any effective strategies for reducing them. These courses are very effective at allowing parents to manage behaviour at home, and in mild to moderate cases of ADHD may be all that is needed. It is important that the parents monitor the child's behaviour and improvement, and help the child to do the same thing.

Behavioural modification at school

Most schools now have a special needs coordinator, who will arrange for appropriate classroom assistance for the child if necessary. The class teacher should be taught methods to identify particular problem behaviours in the classroom and to manage them. Examples include having the child sit near the teacher, setting shorter assignments for the child, and allowing the child to get up and run about at set intervals throughout the day. It is often helpful to have a similar reward and punishment system for behaviour to that in place within the home.

Psychological treatments for the child are useful for moderate or severe ADHD, and the recommended ones are group CBT or group social skills training. Individual sessions may be offered to adolescents, but provide no benefit in younger children. These are especially helpful for children with co-morbid depression, anxiety, or other psychiatric problems.

Medication

For unknown reasons, stimulant drugs such as methylphenidate and dexamphetamine have the paradoxical effect of reducing the overactivity in many cases. These drugs block monoamine transporters, inhibiting uptake of dopamine and norepinephrine (noradrenaline) from the synapse. Atomoxetine, a non-stimulant selective norepinephrine transporter inhibitor, has been shown to be as effective at reducing the symptoms of ADHD as the stimulants.

The indications for offering medication to a child are twofold:

1 failure of psychosocial interventions to reduce symptoms in ADHD with moderate functional impairment;

2 as a first-line therapy in ADHD with severe functional impairment.

The method by which a particular drug is chosen has historically been personal choice on the part of the clinician or from the best tolerance for the child, as all three drugs are equally efficacious. NICE recommends that the choice is made according to co-morbidities:

- Methylphenidate is the first-line choice for uncomplicated ADHD.
- Methylphenidate can also be used in children with co-morbid conduct disorder, tics, Tourette's, or anxiety disorders.
- Atomoxetine can be used in children with co-morbid tics, Tourette's, anxiety disorders, or substance misuse.
- Dexamphetamine should be reserved for children who do not improve on the maximum tolerated dose of methylphenidate or atomoxetine.

The main side effects of stimulants are nausea, appetite (and therefore weight) loss, reduced growth, insomnia, headaches, and stomach pains. It is important to record the height, weight, blood pressure, and pulse rate of the child at each follow-up appointment. Stimulants do lower the seizure threshold, but can be safely used in children with well-controlled epilepsy. There is a very small chance of liver injury, which parents should be warned about, but routine hepatic monitoring is not necessary. If there is no response to all three of the usual drugs, refer the child to a tertiary centre specializing in ADHD. Occasionally, further treatment with unlicensed drugs such as clonidine, imipramine, or bupropion may be considered.

Oppositional defiance disorder and conduct disorder

These two conditions are classed as **disruptive behaviour disorders**, and have many similarities; therefore, the clinical features will first be described separately; the rest of the section is common to both conditions.

Oppositional defiance disorder (ODD) is defined as a recurrent pattern of negativistic, defiant, disobedient, and hostile behaviour towards authority figures. It is one of the most common psychiatric disorders of childhood, and whilst a risk factor for the more serious conduct disorder, the majority do not progress to more serious psychopathology or psychopathy. The diagnostic criteria and clinical features of ODD are shown in Box 32.11.

Conduct disorder (CD) is defined as *a persistent pattern of antisocial behaviour in which the individual repeatedly breaks social rules and carries out aggressive acts*. CD is also a common condition, and together with ODD makes up the commonest reason for referral to child and adolescent mental health services (CAMHS) in Western countries. A proportion of children with ODD/CD will continue behaving in this way, and become adults with antisocial personality disorders. The diagnostic criteria for CD are shown in Box 32.12.

Prevalence

The prevalence of ODD is between 3 and 16 per cent of under 16s, and the prevalence of conduct disorder is 1 to 10 per cent. In both conditions the ratio of males to females is 4:1. The DSM-IV states that onset of ODD symptoms should usually have been before 8 years, and no later than early adolescence. CD is usually diagnosed from 10 to 15 years. Prevalence is significantly higher in lower socio-economic groups.

Co-morbidity

A thorough assessment of a child with ODD or CD is essential as they are commonly associated with other

BOX 32.11 Diagnostic criteria and clinical features of oppositional defiance disorder

Criterion	Examples
A pattern of negativistic, hostile, and defiant behaviour for at least 6 months, including at least 4 of the following oppositional behaviours:	1 Often loses temper 2 Often argues with adults 3 Often defies or refuses to comply with rules or requests 4 Deliberately annoys people 5 Blames others for their own behaviour 6 Is easily annoyed or 'touchy' 7 Is angry and resentful 8 Often spiteful and vindictive
The behaviour causes significant impairment in functioning:	Home, school, work
None of the following are present:	1 Behaviour only occurring during an episode of depression or psychosis 2 Criteria are met for conduct disorder 3 Criteria are met for antisocial personality disorder (> 18 years only)

conditions. Any of the following may be present: ADHD, learning disabilities, substance abuse, PTSD, anxiety disorders, depression, or psychoses.

Differential diagnosis

- **ADHD.** A child with hyperactivity, inattention, and impulsivity can be seen as being antisocial. However, those with only ADHD should not show any of the specific behaviours associated with ODD or CD. It is possible for the conditions to coexist.

- **Adjustment reaction to a specific stressful event.** Poor behaviour may occur in the first 3 months after a stressful event, but should resolve by 6 months.

- **Mood disorders.** Depression can present with irritability and oppositional behaviour in children, but mood is usually low, and there is associated disturbed sleep and anorexia.

- **Autistic spectrum disorders.** A standard autism diagnostic interview should be performed.

- **Learning disorders or specific developmental disorders.**

- **Dissocial/antisocial personality disorder.** This can only be diagnosed from 17 (ICD-10) or 18 years (DSM-IV). As CD may be diagnosed in adults, there is overlap between the conditions. Antisocial personality disorder refers to a pervasive, severe lack of regard for, and violation of, the rights of others dating back to mid-adolescence.

- **Psychosis.** A careful mental state examination should pick up hallucinations and/or delusions, often with associated disorganized behaviour.

Aetiology

At the current time there is a poor understanding of the aetiology of ODD and CD, although it is clearly a mix of genetics, adverse psychological experiences, and environmental factors. Table 32.15 outlines the potential aetiological factors, but these should be viewed more as risk factors until further research is available.

Genetics. Heritability is estimated to be 50 per cent; many children with ODD/CD have a positive family history, and twin and adoption studies have shown that children take their parental risk with them even when separated at a young age. The gene that has been most studied is a monoamine oxidase (MAO) promoter, in which polymorphisms have been linked to ODD/CD. The MAO enzyme metabolizes neurotransmitters which are said to relate to aggressive behaviour.

Psychological risks. Adverse early experiences such as neglect, abuse, poor parenting, and exposure to violence undoubtedly leave children vulnerable to disruptive behaviour. A pattern tends to be seen where children are ignored, they misbehave, and then the parent responds with negative approach, over-punishing the child. This results in an escalation of behaviour, and a vicious cycle which negatively reinforces the child's behaviour.

Environmental factors often provide the precipitating event to cause disruptive behaviour on a background of genetic and psychological vulnerability. A poverty-stricken, high-crime neighbourhood with poor schools and high unemployment leads to a much greater risk of CD/ODD. The influence of peers and adults around them may inspire

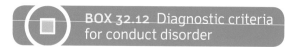

BOX 32.12 Diagnostic criteria for conduct disorder

A A repetitive and persistent pattern of behaviour in which the basic rights of others or societal norms or rules are violated.

B At least 3 of the following criteria have been present in the last 12 months, with at least 1 present in the last 6 months:

1 Aggression to people and animals
- Often bullies, threatens, or intimidates others
- Often initiates physical fights
- Has used a weapon
- Has been physically cruel to people
- Has been physically cruel to animals
- Has stolen while confronting a victim
- Has forced someone into sexual activity

2 Destruction of property and/or theft
- Has deliberately engaged in fire setting
- Has deliberately destroyed others' property
- Has broken into someone else's property
- Often lies to obtain goods or avoid obligations
- Has stolen items of non-trivial value

3 Serious violation of rules
- Often stays out at night despite parental prohibitions
- Has run away from home overnight
- Is often truant from school, beginning before 13 years.

C The disturbance in behaviour causes clinically significant impairment in social, academic, or occupational functioning.

D If over 18 years, criteria are not met for antisocial personality disorder.

children to behave in ways they would not otherwise have thought of, and lack of money can lead to adolescents having little to do but behave inappropriately.

Course and prognosis

Once ODD or CD is established, it is usually stable throughout the rest of childhood. Of those with early-onset CD (before age 8), 50 per cent will develop antisocial personality disorder in adulthood. Adolescent onset may be just as severe in the teenage years but 85 per cent only have minor problems by their mid-twenties. Box 32.13 shows factors predicting a poor

outcome in CD/ODD. CD is linked to many problems in later life, including unemployment and dependence on state benefits, divorce, domestic violence, completed suicide, substance abuse, and other mental health problems.

Assessment and management

Assessment should be undertaken as for any child presenting to psychiatry. The management options for children with ODD or CD are outlined in Table 32.16. In the past, treatment of a conduct disorder was mostly directed at the child; now involvement of the family is considered extremely important.

General measures

The usual scenario is that the child does not feel that their behaviour is unreasonable, and will be resistant to interventions from health services. In some situations it may also be difficult to engage their parents in the process. However, the basis of treatment is psychoeducation; each side needs to understand their own behaviour, how it impacts upon themselves and others, and how they could change it for the better. Providing written and self-help materials is useful, but only if the child is able to read them. Schools can be very helpful in providing remedial teaching if the child has specific difficulties with basic skills, or has dropped behind their peers. Teachers can also be trained in behavioural management techniques, which can reinforce work being done at home.

Pharmacotherapy

Medications should not be the first-line treatment for ODD or CD, but can be useful adjuncts. There is good evidence that appropriate use of stimulants or an SSRI decrease symptoms in children with co-morbid ADHD or depression. In adolescents with severe aggression, or violent outbursts, an atypical antipsychotic can reduce this behaviour considerably. Compliance with treatment can be a problem, and depot injections are often a good solution.

Psychological treatments

It is recommended that psychological therapies be the first-line management for ODD or CD. In children under 12 years there is good evidence for the efficacy of parental training courses. These are group sessions which teach the child's parents how to manage their child's behaviour in a more effective way. Skills learnt include promoting good behaviour and a positive relationship, setting clear rules and commands, remaining calm, and managing difficult situations. Systematic family therapy can also be beneficial, and may be a good option for older children. For the child themselves, the best approach

Table 32.15 Risk factors for disruptive behaviour disorders

Biological	Psychological	Social or environmental
• Genetics: family history of CD/ODD and twin studies	• Irritable temperament as a baby	• Maternal smoking in pregnancy
• Dysregulation of neurotransmitters	• Institutional care	• Low socio-economic class
• Low IQ	• Poor parent–child relationships	• Poor diet with lack of vitamins and minerals
• Language disorders or deficits	• Attachment difficulties	• Bad neighbourhood
• Minor physical anomalies	• Poor parenting: inconsistent rule setting, criticism, or hostility	• Crime in the family
• Low birth weight	• Low parental involvement with child	• Parental mental illness or substance abuse
• Brain injury or disease	• Physical, sexual, or emotional abuse	• Peer influences: associates with other children with OCD/CD
• Low resting heart rate	• Neglect	
	• Low self-esteem	
	• 'Unemotional' personality trait	

seems to be providing anger management and interpersonal skills training, rather than more traditional psychotherapies.

Tics and Tourette's syndrome

Tics are an important aspect of child and adolescent psychiatry for three main reasons.

1 Tics are extremely common; simple motor tics are found in 1–2 per cent of children.

2 Tics are associated with many other behavioural, learning, and psychiatric disorders.

3 Tics may cause great distress to both the child and their family, and can have a negative impact upon self-esteem, peer relationships, and school performance.

A tic is a sudden, *repetitive, non-rhythmic, stereotyped motor movement or vocalization involving discrete muscle groups.* They can be classified as either motor or vocal (phonic), or as simple or complex.

• **Simple tics** are typically sudden, brief, meaningless movements or sounds that usually involve only one group of muscles. Common examples include neck jerking, eye blinking, grunting, snorting, or throat clearing.

• **Complex motor tics** are typically more purposeful-appearing movements that last for rather longer. Examples include facial movements, jumping, touching, or even self-harming.

• **Complex vocal tics** involve words and phrases, and may include repetition of what was just heard or said (echolalia and palilalia) or socially inappropriate phrases (coprolalia).

It is also usual to define a tic as transient or chronic, the latter being when a tic has lasted for more than 12 months. The number of tics, their frequency, severity, and nature vary widely between patients, and can change over time. Usually, the patient is able to suppress the tic for a short period, but this causes a build-up of tension within the person which eventually can no longer be suppressed. Tics may be triggered or worsened by excitement, fatigue,

---

BOX 32.13 Risk factors predicting a poor outcome in ODD or CD

Male gender
Lower IQ
Parental alcoholism
Low-income family
Poor schools, low achievement
Severe, frequent antisocial acts

Co-morbid hyperactivity
Parental criminality
Harsh, inconsistent parenting
Troublesome neighbourhood
Lack of parental interest in child
Early onset

Table 32.16 Treatment of oppositional defiance disorder or conduct disorder

General measures

- Psychoeducation
- Provision of information and self-help materials
- Treat co-morbidities
- Reduce stressful circumstances
- School interventions

Psychological treatments (first line)

- Parental management training course
- Individual or group CBT
- Family therapy
- Anger management skills

Biological treatments (second line)

- Aggression: antipsychotics, lithium, or carbamazepine
- Co-morbid mood disorder: SSRI
- Co-morbid ADHD: stimulants

Table 32.17 Classification of tic disorders

Tourette's syndrome

- Multiple motor tics and at least one vocal tic have been present at some point in the illness
- Tics occur many times a day, nearly every day for more than 1 year
- Onset is before age 18 years
- The tics are not due to the direct effects of substances or a general medical condition

Chronic motor or vocal tic disorder

- Single or multiple motor or vocal tics, but not both, have been present during the illness
- Tics occur multiple times per day, nearly every day for more than 1 year
- Onset is before age 18 years
- The tics are not due to the direct effects of substances or a general medical condition
- Criteria are not met for Tourette's syndrome

Transient tic disorder

- Single or multiple motor and/or vocal tics
- Tics occur many times per day, every day for at least 4 weeks but less than 12 months
- Onset is before age 18 years
- The tics are not due to the direct effects of substances or a general medical condition
- Criteria are not met for Tourette's syndrome or chronic motor or vocal tic disorder

Tic disorder not otherwise specified

- Disorders characterized by tics that do not fit criteria for the above conditions, e.g. tics last less than 4 weeks or have an onset over 18 years

and visual cues, which tend to be specific to the patient. There are four main tic disorders, shown in Table 32.17.

Clinical features of Tourette's syndrome

The symptoms of Tourette's syndrome are worth a special mention because of the public perception of the condition. Typically, motor tics appear early in life (3–8 years) and are initially simple tics (e.g. blinking) which gradually evolve into more complex movements such as touching, licking, or making obscene gestures (copropraxia). Vocal tics such as grunting, sniffing, and throat-clearing are almost universal. The more antisocial tics of coprolalia, echolalia, and echopraxia are not seen in every patient, but when they are present represent a large burden for the patient to manage. The severity of the tics usually peaks at about 20 years and reduces somewhat after this. It is usual for the patient to report that they feel when a tic is about to happen, and that they may be able to suppress them for a short time. Tics are exacerbated by anxiety, boredom, fatigue, and excitement. They may be reduced by sleep, alcohol, and calming surroundings.

Prevalence

Ten to fifteen per cent of school-age children exhibit tics at some point, but only 1 to 2 per cent meet standard criteria for a tic disorder. The only large-scale study of Tourette's disorder was of recruits into the Israeli military, which gave a prevalence of 0.05 per cent. The mean age of onset of the first tic is typically 4 to 6 years, but they can occur as late as 15 years. Tics are more common in males than females (ratio 5:1), and do not seem to vary between races or socio-economic groups.

Co-morbidities

Tics are associated with many other psychiatric conditions, including ADHD, OCD, learning disorders, dyslexia, mood, and anxiety disorders.

Differential diagnosis

- **Abnormal movements due to neurological or neuropsychiatric disorder.** These include Sydenham's chorea, Huntingdon's disease, Wilson's disease, or tuberous sclerosis.

- **Abnormal movements caused by medications.** Antipsychotics and anti-epileptics may cause dystonic movements. Stimulants (e.g. methylphenidate, amphetamine) and opioids may cause or exacerbate tics.

- **ADHD.** Are the movements a failure of impulse control due to ADHD?

Aetiology

Biological factors

1 **Genetics**. The risk of developing Tourette's in a first-degree relative of a sufferer is 15 to 20 per cent. The figure for any tic disorder is much higher, approaching 50 per cent, although there appears to be incomplete expression and penetrance. There has been great debate as to whether Tourette's is an autosomal dominant disorder, but there is no definitive evidence of this yet. Twin studies of monozygotic twins show a 53 per cent concordance. The risk is also substantially increased in those with a family history of ADHD or OCD.

2 **Neuroimaging**. MRI studies have shown various anatomical abnormalities in patients with tic disorders. Imaging consistently shows a reduced volume of the caudate nucleus, and an increased volume of the prefrontal cortex. As tics are likely to be aberration of the cortico–striatal–pallidothalamo–cortical circuit which controls the suppression of unwanted movements and fine control of wanted movements, this would fit well.

3 **Dopamine dysregulation**. The efficacy of antipsychotics to reduce tics highly suggests that there is an excess of dopamine in the brain of those with tics. Post-mortem studies that have stained slices of the cerebrum to show dopamine have found increased numbers of dopamine-transporter sites in the striatum and prefrontal cortex. PET studies have demonstrated increased dopamine binding in these sites, and correlated the density of dopamine receptors to tic severity.

4 **Autoimmunity**. There has been some suggestion that tics and OCD may be caused by antibodies produced against streptococcus cross-reacting in the basal ganglia. This is further discussed in Science box 32.2.

Social and psychological factors

There is little evidence demonstrating that specific psychological vulnerabilities or events predispose to tics. However, tics often start or are exacerbated by a child undergoing life events—for example, moving house or starting school—suggesting that stress does play some role. Children who were of a low birth weight or exposed to high levels of caffeine, alcohol, or tobacco *in utero* are at higher risk of having a tic disorder. Adverse social circumstances (e.g. poverty) certainly increase the severity of tics, but do not appear to be a direct aetiological factor.

Course and prognosis

In the majority of children, tics are transitory phenomena, and vary in severity over 1–12 months before disappearing. In those with chronic tic disorders, the tics tend to peak in severity in middle children and then gradually reduce. Up to 30 per cent have tics remaining into adulthood, but they are usually simple motor tics. Children with severe tics or Tourette's syndrome often have substantial problems in childhood, but only a minority have long-term mental health problems. Risk factors for a poor prognosis include Tourette's syndrome, co-morbid OCD or ADHD, physical illness, unsupportive home circumstances, and substance abuse.

Science box 32.2 PANDAS: paediatric autoimmune neuropsychiatric disorders associated with streptococcal infections

PANDAS refers to a controversial condition and is used to describe a group of neuropsychiatric disorders that are said to have an autoimmune aetiology and to be related to infection with group A beta-haemolytic streptococcal infection. OCD, tic disorders, and Tourette's syndrome are all included in PANDAS. The mechanism of causation proposed is molecular mimicry, similar to that seen in Sydenham's chorea. In the latter, antineuronal antibodies are produced, which attack the streptococci but also cross-react with the basal ganglia, producing choreoathetoid movements. The basal ganglia are known to be the site of movement production control and suppression, classically demonstrated in Parkinson's disease. Various studies have attempted to isolate the specific antibodies involved, but as yet have been unsuccessful. The clinical criteria for PANDAS are as follows:

- presence of OCD and/or tic disorder;
- prepubertal onset;
- episodic course of symptom severity;
- abrupt onset or dramatic exacerbations associated with group A beta-haemolytic streptococcal infection (as shown by positive throat cultures and/or elevated anti-GABHS titres).

The prevalence of PANDAS is currently unknown, as are the factors rendering a child susceptible to developing it. A variety of treatment strategies have been used, including intravenous immunoglobulins, plasma exchange, and long-term prophylactic antibiotics. However, there is no robust evidence for the efficacy of any of these. Some argue that PANDAS does not exist, and further research is needed to prove the link between OCD/tics and GABHS.

Assessment

A full assessment should be undertaken of any child presenting with tics. In those with short-lived, non-functionally impairing tics no intervention may be necessary, but it is essential to check for and treat any underlying or co-morbid conditions and to educate and reassure the child and their family. Tics are inherently suppressible for short periods and usually fluctuate in severity throughout the day, so may not be seen in the interview. It may be helpful to ask the family to make a home video, which can be played to the assessment team. A formal examination of the child should occur, including a detailed neurological and ophthalmological survey looking for signs of other neurological conditions (e.g. Wilson's disease). The Yale Global Tic Severity Scale can be a useful index by which to measure symptom severity over time.

Management

There are currently no guidelines on the management of tics in the UK, but the principles are relatively simple. The most important aspect is appropriate education of the child, family, school, and everyone else involved. A general outline of treatment options is shown in Table 32.18.

Psychoeducation

It is crucially important to explain to everyone involved with the child that they cannot help making movements or sounds. Knowing that tics can be exacerbated by stress can help others to provide a stress-free environment for the child. Tics tend to fluctuate in severity over time and this should be discussed, and plans made for sudden deteriorations.

Pharmacological treatments

The most effective treatment for tics is medication, but because of the risk of adverse effects these should only be the first-line treatment in the following situations: severely disabling tics, interference with activities of daily living, risk to self or others, co-morbid ADHD/OCD, or learning disability making therapy impossible. The two effective groups of medications are antipsychotics and alpha-2 agonists. The former are the most efficacious, reducing tics by up to 60 per cent. However, the adverse effects associated with antipsychotics means that the safer alpha-2 agonists are the usual first choice. **Clonidine** and **guanfacine** are the most common drugs used, and they reduce tics by about 30 per cent. The most common side effects are sedation, headache, and irritability. Clonidine is available as a 48-hour transdermal patch, which can be useful in small children who can't swallow tablets. Atypical antipsychotics (risperidone and olanzapine have robust randomized controlled evidence) are a good choice, but they still come with the problems of sedation, weight gain, and the metabolic syndrome. Local injection of botulinum toxin has been used in older children and adults with isolated motor tics, and appears to be quite effective.

Psychological treatments

The most effective psychological therapy for tics is cognitive behavioural therapy (CBT). There is not much evidence that it is effective in disabling tics when used alone, but it is a helpful adjunct to pharmacotherapy, especially in children with co-morbidities. The best approach seems to be teaching exposure-response prevention techniques, similar to those used in treating phobias.

■ Disorders of adults also seen in adolescents

There are a variety of common psychiatric disorders of adulthood which may begin in adolescence (and occasionally childhood), and often the presentation is slightly differently to that in adults (Table 32.19). These differences

Table 32.18 Management of tic disorders

General measures

- Psychoeducation of child, family, and school
- Collaboration with the school
- Good treatment of co-morbidities
- Information about and referral to support groups

Pharmacological treatments

- Alpha-2 agonists
- Antipsychotics

Psychological treatments

- Cognitive behavioural therapy
- Exposure-response prevention
- Relaxation techniques
- Habit reversal training

Table 32.19 Psychiatric disorders in adolescents

- Depressive disorders (Chapter 21, see p. 438 in this chapter)
- Bipolar disorder (Chapter 21)
- Anxiety disorders (Chapter 24, see p. 436 in this chapter)
- Schizophrenia (Chapter 22)
- Eating disorders (Chapter 27)
- Suicide and deliberate self-harm (Chapter 9)
- Substance abuse (Chapter 29)
- Post-traumatic stress disorder (Chapter 23)
- Chronic fatigue syndrome (see p. 310)

are briefly outlined below, with references to further information in the chapter on each condition. Assessment of all young people should be carried out as outlined in Chapter 17, but also include the specific history/investigations used in adults with the condition.

Bipolar disorder

Bipolar disorder is rare before puberty, but increases in incidence rapidly in adolescence. The mean age for presentation is 20 years, meaning a large proportion of patients present to child and adolescent services. Diagnostic criteria remain as in adults, but young people frequently do not show the classical alternation between depression and manic episodes. Mixed episodes, where some symptoms of depression and mania are seen at the same time, are quite common, as is rapid cycling—switching between low and elevated moods over short periods. The symptoms of each state are usually allied to those found in older patients.

The prevalence of bipolar disorder in under-18s is approximately 1 per cent, although almost all of these are in postpubertal children. Males and females are equally affected. One specific tool widely used for assessment is the Young Mania Rating Scale, a questionnaire filled out by parents relating to their child's behaviour.

The younger the presentation of bipolar disorder, the poorer the prognosis; adolescent mania has a 50 per cent relapse rate within 5 years even with maximal treatment. Younger age at presentation, poor family relationships, psychosis, and a family history all carry a poorer prognosis.

Treatment of bipolar disorder in young people initially focuses on mood stabilization, as this is what tends to interfere with function, with emphasis moving towards psychoeducation and relapse prevention when this has been achieved. An outline of options is shown in Table 32.20. Most children will be treated as outpatients, but some (especially those with acute mania or severe depression) may need inpatient or day-patient care.

Psychoeducation of the child and their family is extremely important in achieving a good outcome. Compliance with medications and a non-provocative home environment can be achieved with good education and communication within the family. Many young people will need to take time out of school, so involvement of teachers is paramount. Relapse prevention can be formerly delivered within individual and family therapy, but is mostly education regarding compliance and recognizing the early signs of illness.

Pharmacotherapy is the mainstay of treatment. If the child is not on any antimanic drugs, an atypical antipsychotic is the first step, but most need a mood stabilizer (valproate or lithium) added in. Before starting medication, bloods should be done, as well as an assessment of height and weight, and

Table 32.20 Treatment of paediatric bipolar disorder

General measures
- Psychoeducation of child and family
- Self-help materials
- Appropriate educational setting

Pharmacotherapy
- Lithium (over 12 years)
- Atypical antipsychotics
- Sodium valproate (males)
- SSRIs (severe depression)

Psychological treatments
- Cognitive behavioural therapy
- Relapse prevention
- Family therapy

ECT: rarely used

an ECG. Sodium valproate should be avoided in women of child-bearing age, as it is teratogenic and can induce polycystic ovary syndrome. Lithium is only licensed over the age of 12. Medications should be continued for at least 18 months after stabilization, and many patients will need lifelong therapy.

Suicide and deliberate self-harm

This important topic is covered more fully in Chapter 9. Suicide is one of the top five leading causes of death in the 15–19 year group, and around 90 per cent of these individuals have underlying psychiatric disorders. Completed suicide is extremely rare before puberty, rising to 4–8 per 100 000 in the 15–19 age groups. About three-quarters of these are males, and young people who commit suicide are four times more likely than the general population to have a family history of suicide. The most common co-morbidities are mood disorders, alcohol and substance abuse, anxiety disorder, eating disorders, and chronic physical diseases. About one-third of completed suicides had made at least one previous attempt to end their life. Factors that are thought to be involved in the aetiology of suicide and attempted suicide are shown in Table 32.21. The strongest predictor of future suicide risk is past suicide attempts.

Deliberate self-harm (DSH) is any act with a non-fatal outcome, which is undertaken with the intention of causing harm to self. It is hard to obtain accurate figures of the prevalence and incidence of DSH as most young people never present to psychiatric services. Surveys of school-age teenagers suggest 10 per cent of 15–16 year olds have harmed themselves in the previous year, with the majority of these having done it more than once. Females are

Table 32.21 Aetiology of completed and attempted suicide

Biological	Psychological	Social or environmental
Family history of suicide or deliberate self-harm	Psychiatric disorders • Depression • Substance abuse • Conduct disorder • Anxiety disorder • Schizophrenia • Past suicide attempt	Stressful life events • Family discord • Parental divorce • Death of loved one
Self-harm in close friends		
Familial mental health problems		
Neurotransmitter dysregulation: low serotonin		Poor care or neglect
	Cognitive factors • Low self-esteem • Hopelessness • Guilt • Bullying • Confusion regarding sexual orientation	Imitation—exposure to real or fictional accounts of suicide
	Physical, emotional, or sexual abuse	

four times more likely to self-harm than males. The most common methods of self-harm are cutting and taking paracetamol overdoses.

Assessment

Assessment of a child who has attempted suicide or self-harmed has two aims: a risk assessment and an evaluation of the underlying psychopathology and context in which the act occurred.

A physical examination, routine blood tests, paracetamol, and salicylate levels, an ECG, and any special investigations related to the presenting complaint should be carried out immediately. Treatment of any physical effects of the DSH should be the first priority. The history should cover:

- circumstances leading up to the DSH;
- whether the child aimed to end their life;
- frequency, intensity, and severity of self-harm thoughts;
- was the act planned; if so, how?
- did the child seek help immediately, or try to avoid discovery of the act?
- are they still actively suicidal or thinking about self-harming again?
- background: previous DSH, mental, and physical disorders;
- current psychosocial functioning (home relationships, peer relationships, bullying, school performance, drug and alcohol abuse, conduct problems, abuse).

The child's parents and other relevant adults should be interviewed to provide a further background to the family situation and co-morbid psychiatric disorders, their account of the DSH event, and their reaction to the event.

Management

Keeping the child safe is paramount. A decision needs to be made as to whether they are at risk of acting upon suicidal thoughts, if there is a safe home environment, and if there is a responsible adult available to find help if the situation deteriorates. Most young people can be treated as outpatients (after any initial physical treatment for injuries); a few need to be admitted to acute psychiatric wards. The indications for inpatient treatment are active suicidal ideation and intent, young person not able to promise not to harm themselves, psychosis, impulsivity, and lack of a suitable home environment. Crisis teams who can provide intensive support at home are a good way of providing a safety net. Treatment options depend a lot on the underlying psychiatric diagnosis; specific conditions (e.g. depression, anorexia nervosa) should be treated by standard protocols. A written 'no suicide' contract is usually negotiated at the start of treatment; this usually involves the child promising not to engage in DSH behaviours without informing their parents or therapist. Individual therapy is usually offered; this may be CBT or dialectical behaviour therapy (DBT). The former is particularly useful in depressed teenagers, and the latter in those with borderline personality disorder. Family therapy is often a useful adjunct to address relationship problems and improve communication. There is no good evidence base for the use of medications in reducing suicidal behaviour in adolescents, but in adults both SSRIs and lithium reduce the risk of self-harm in depressed adults. There has been some concern that SSRIs increase suicidal ideation in young people, but as yet the issue remains controversial. If drugs are prescribed, regular monitoring of the patient's mental state is essential.

Schizophrenia

Schizophrenia is covered more comprehensively in Chapter 22, and is rare in children and adolescents. Childhood schizophrenia has been recognized since the condition was identified, but until the late 1970s included autism within its definition. The diagnostic criteria for schizophrenia are the same in children as in adults. Schizophrenia starting before age 18 is known as early-onset schizophrenia, and before 13 years as very-early-onset schizophrenia. The prevalence of all psychoses in one Scandinavian study was 0.9/10 000 at 13 years, rising to 17/10 000 at 18 years, the majority of which were schizophrenia. Positive symptoms are not pathognomonic of schizophrenia in young people, and the full differential diagnosis of psychosis should be considered. The aetiology of early-onset schizophrenia is similar to that in adults, but children are more likely to have a strong family history of psychosis. An overview of the assessment is shown in Box 32.14, and the differential diagnosis in Box 32.15.

Treatment of children with schizophrenia is very similar to that in adults. Early intervention in those with prodromal symptoms and/or a strong family history has been shown to reduce the likelihood of a poor prognosis. Medication use tends to be off licence, with an atypical antipsychotic used first line. After failure of two atypical antipsychotics, clozapine should be considered. It is important to monitor the child for side effects, especially weight gain and extrapyramidal movements. Psychological treatments are important in young people with schizophrenia. Psychoeducation, family therapy to reduce highly expressed emotion, and social skills and communication training have all been shown to improve outcome.

Early-onset schizophrenia has a poorer outcome than the adult-onset disorder. It is associated with a reduced IQ, increased cognitive deficits, increased negative symptoms, and less likelihood of independent living and holding down employment. Young people with schizophrenia often develop illnesses that are very hard to treat by the time they are in middle adulthood.

Substance abuse

Many adolescents take drugs, especially cannabis, and drink alcohol—but only a minority abuse these substances. Full details can be found in Chapter 29.

Juvenile delinquency

Parents sometimes ask general practitioners for advice about their delinquent adolescents. Delinquency is the failure of a young person to obey the law; it is not a psychiatric disorder, although psychiatric disorder, usually conduct disorder, is one of its causes. Delinquency is most common at the age of 15–16 years and in males. Up to a fifth of adolescent boys are found to have carried out an offence, albeit usually a trivial one (e.g. shoplifting). Of these adolescents, only a few continue to offend in adult life and parents can usually be reassured that a single act, especially if carried out as part of a group, is not likely to be of serious significance. Repeat offending

---

 BOX 32.14 Assessment of a child with suspected schizophrenia

Psychiatric history

- Symptoms at presentation, including course and co-morbid mood symptoms
- Previous psychiatric and medical history
- Family history
- Personal history and development
- Premorbid personality and level of functioning
- Substance use and abuse
- Self-harm, risk to self and others

Physical examination

- Examine respiratory, cardiovascular, and abdomen
- Neurology including extrapyramidal movements, tics, and abnormal involuntary movements

- Look for dysmorphic features, measure height/weight/head circumference

Investigations

- Blood tests (full blood count, urea and electrolytes, liver function tests, thyroid function tests, copper and caeruloplasmin)
- Electrocardiogram
- Urinalysis including drug toxicology
- Consider neuroimaging and EEG
- IQ testing
- Structured questionnaires for schizophrenia

BOX 32.15 Differential diagnosis of childhood schizophrenia

- **Organic conditions:** drug-related psychoses, Wilson's disease, temporal lobe epilepsy, SLE, thyroid disease
- **Developmental disorders:** autistic spectrum disorders
- **Other psychotic disorders:** mood disorders with psychosis, schizoaffective disorders, atypical psychosis
- **Other psychiatric disorders:** ADHD, conduct disorders, personality disorders, culture-bound syndromes

is associated with various socio-environmental factors (Table 32.22).

Management

Delinquency is dealt with by the courts, who generally obtain a social report about the young person's family and social and material environment, an educational report, and, in certain cases, a psychiatric report. Usually, the emphasis is on secondary prevention rather than punishment, with involvement of social, educational, and sometimes psychological or psychiatric services. Rarely, an individual may go to a young offender's institution.

Table 32.22 Risk factors for juvenile delinquency

Patient factors	Family-related factors	Environmental factors
• Poor education or school underachievement	• Parents divorced/ separated	• Low socio-economic class
• Hyperactivity	• Very large families	• Poverty
• Mental health disorders	• Parental criminality/ violence	• Poor housing
• Substance abuse	• Familial discord	• Peer group pressure

Further reading

Gelder, M., Andreasen, N., Lopez-Ibor, J., & Geddes, J. (eds) (2009). *New Oxford Textbook of Psychiatry*, 2nd edn. Section 9: Child and adolescent psychiatry, pp. 1587–816. Oxford University Press, Oxford.

National Institute of Health and Clinical Excellence (2008). *Attention Deficit Hyperactivity Disorder.* http://guidance.nice.org.uk/CG72.

National Institute of Health and Clinical Excellence (2005). *Depression in Children and Young People.* http://guidance.nice.org.uk/CG28.

National Institute of Health and Clinical Excellence (2009). *When to Suspect Child Maltreatment.* http://guidance.nice.org.uk/CG89.

Hawton, K. & James, A. (2005). Suicide and deliberate self-harm in young people. *British Medical Journal* **330**: 891.

Baird, G., Cass, H. & Slonims, V. (2003). Diagnosis of autism. *British Medical Journal* **327**: 488–93.

Psychiatry and you

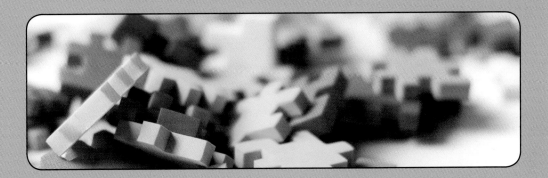

Psychiatry and you

■ Keeping yourself well

The problem

As a future doctor, your health and well-being are vital to that of your patients; if you are not functioning reliably, you will not be able to help your patients as much as you otherwise would. It is therefore vital that you look after your body and mind and, by implication, adopt a lifestyle that is both healthy and sustainable.

It is often said that doctors make bad patients. There is some evidence that doctors are slow to seek help for health problems, and comply poorly with advice given by other healthcare professionals. In addition, doctors' lives may be unhealthy, with high levels of stress, low levels of exercise, and excessive consumption of alcohol.

The mental health of doctors is a particular concern. Doctors are at relatively high risk of mental disorder, and female doctors appear to be at higher risk of suicide than women in the general population. The reasons are several, and include the following.

- **The nature of doctors.** Doctors are driven to succeed, and do not tolerate failure well. It is inevitable that some of our patients will die, some treatments will not be successful, and that, in a professional lifetime, some mistakes will be made. Our aim should be to reflect on and learn from these events, and then to move on positively.

- **The nature of doctors' work.** Doctors tend to work hard, work for long hours, and work in challenging, resource-constrained environments.

- **Poor help-seeking.** As we have seen, doctors are reluctant to seek help for their medical problems, and this is particularly likely when the problem is psychiatric.

- **Unsupportive and unsustainable lifestyle.** Many doctors have challenging careers and challenging home lives, and allow themselves little time to recharge their batteries away from these ever-present stressors.

- **Knowledge of and access to the means of suicide.** Doctors (and vets, farmers, and pharmacists, to whom the above factors also apply) have special expertise in the use of chemicals that are toxic in overdose.

Some solutions

The following points are intended to encourage you to think about how you will maintain your physical and mental health over your professional lifetime, which is likely to span several decades. As you accumulate responsibilities and commitments, both professional and personal, how will you manage the physical and emotional strains that they bring? Developing good habits now will stand you in good stead for the future.

- **Take some time off.** Even at your busiest, when you are working long shifts, or preparing for professional exams, make time to get away. Schedule regular breaks when you can unwind, and regain a sense of perspective.

- **Have interest(s) outside medicine.** As a person, are you defined entirely by your career? Having one or more non-medical interests can help to sustain your professional life.

- **Moderate your use of alcohol, and avoid using other substances.** It is easy to develop the habit of using alcohol to manage your stress or distress, but, as we have seen elsewhere, heavy or regular alcohol use has adverse health impacts and can impair coping.

- **Exercise regularly.** The physical benefits of exercise are clear, but there are emotional benefits, too.

- **Manage your thoughts and beliefs.** When we are tired or stressed, the thoughts that we have are less likely to be realistic than when we are rested or calm. These biases in our thinking can help to make our personal situation seem much worse than it actually is. Learning how to identify and challenge negative thoughts is a core self-management skill. When you have mastered it, you will be better equipped to teach your patients!

- **Cultivate stable and supportive relationships.** Don't neglect your friends and, of course, your boy/girlfriend, or life partner. Keeping in touch can help you to maintain a sense of stability, even when other aspects of your life feel 'out of control'.

- **Take holidays.** There is always time for these, despite what your negative automatic thoughts might be telling you. Planning a holiday or a short break in several weeks' time can help improve spirits and sustain you— and your partner—through a tough time.

- **Get yourself a GP! And use them. And don't self-medicate.** Many doctors, especially male doctors, are not registered with a GP or, if they are, they attend rarely. Make sure that you are registered with a GP, that they have up-to-date contact details, and that you change GP when you change location. Don't be tempted to self-diagnose or self-manage your illnesses; get a professional's objective advice and, if necessary, their prescription. Although registered medical practitioners are legally permitted to prescribe for themselves, the General Medical Council (GMC) states that 'doctors should, wherever possible, avoid treating themselves or anyone with whom they have a close personal relationship.'

- **Read more about looking after yourself.** Have a look at Butler and Hope's *Manage Your Mind* (2007), which is an excellent self-help book, written according to cognitive behavioural principles. It is excellent bedtime reading for stressed professionals, but also highly suitable for recommending to patients with common psychiatric disorders.

- **Prioritize looking after yourself.** Go on, do it!

■ Professional behaviours

As a medical student, you are in an unusual position. Your non-medical-student colleagues will have considerable flexibility in the way that they live their lives. If they turn up late to a teaching session, and are unable to concentrate due to a hangover, that is an educational matter. However, as a medical student, you need to develop and to demonstrate the kind of professional behaviours that will be expected of you as a qualified doctor. If you turn up late and with a hangover to a teaching session, this may pose a question mark over your ability to function consistently at a high level when you have qualified. Lateness keeps patients and your colleagues waiting, and adverse effects of substances such as alcohol may impair judgement and lead to medical errors.

The GMC provides comprehensive guidance on professional behaviours in *Medical Students: Professional Values and Fitness to Practise* (GMC and MSC, 2009), and this is an essential reference for every medical student. It should be read in conjunction with *Good Medical Practice* (GMC, 2006), which describes the duties of a doctor (Box 33.1).

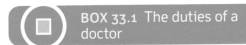

BOX 33.1 The duties of a doctor

Patients must be able to trust doctors with their lives and health. To justify that trust you must show respect for human life and you must:

- Make the care of your patient your first concern.
- Protect and promote the health of patients and the public.
- Provide a good standard of practice and care:
  - keep your professional knowledge and skills up to date;
  - recognize and work within the limits of your competence;
  - work with colleagues in the ways that best serve patients' interests.
- Treat patients as individuals and respect their dignity:
  - treat patients politely and considerately;
  - respect patients' right to confidentiality.
- Work in partnership with patients:
  - listen to patients and respond to their concerns and preferences;
  - give patients the information they want or need in a way they can understand;
  - respect patients' right to reach decisions with you about their treatment and care;
  - support patients in caring for themselves to improve and maintain their health.
- Be honest and open and act with integrity:
  - act without delay if you have good reason to believe that you or a colleague may be putting patients at risk;
  - never discriminate unfairly against patients or colleagues;
  - never abuse your patients' trust in you or the public's trust in the profession.
- You are personally accountable for your professional practice and must always be prepared to justify your decisions and actions.

■ Careers in psychiatry

Undergraduate medical training is dominated by training in general-hospital-based specialties. Yet the World Health Organization estimates that, in high-income nations, unipolar depressive disorders are greater contributors to disability than any other disorder, exceeding that arising from heart disease, diabetes, cerebrovascular disease, or respiratory disease. Alcohol misuse and dementia also feature among the top ten causes of disability. In low-income nations, psychiatric disorders are emerging as a major cause of disability as progress is made in conquering infectious disease. It follows that there is a great need for committed and capable psychiatrists, in all areas of the world, and that this need is likely to increase significantly in the coming years.

As you will have seen in these pages, mental disorder is wide-ranging in its manifestations, and challenging to treat. Psychiatry offers a stimulating career, not least because of the special skills and attitudes that psychiatrists need to develop, which include:

- being tolerant of, and able to manage, risk;
- being tolerant of, and able to manage, diagnostic and therapeutic uncertainty;
- being able to build relationships over long time periods with patients who lack insight;
- being able to work as part of a multidisciplinary team;
- being able to think in an integrated way about patients' problems;
- being realistic about goals of management.

If you are potentially interested in a career in psychiatry, you should endeavour to find out more, with two aims in mind: first, to help rule in or rule out psychiatry as your chosen career, and, secondly, to develop and sustain your interest until you enter postgraduate training in the field. Talk to your consultant, to one of the trainees, or to your course leader. What made them want to be a psychiatrist? What sustains them now? What do they like about the job? And not like? And what about their subspecialty? What advice would they give you? It is important to talk to more than one individual, to gather different opinions. You can also find out a lot more online, via the Student Associates section of the Royal College of Psychiatrists' website, at www.rcpsych.ac.uk/training/studentassociates.aspx. The website is extensive, and includes details of training pathways, summaries of the main subspecialties, and details of how to become a Student Associate of the College. This is available free of charge to any UK medical student and is highly recommended.

Options for continuing some exposure to psychiatry, after your standard clinical placement, include the following.

- **Undertaking special study modules or student-selected components.** These may be established modules, or modules which you arrange yourself.

- **Undertaking your elective, or part of your elective, in psychiatry.** This could be in the UK, at your or another medical school, or overseas.

- **Submitting entries for prize essay competitions.** In the UK, many are listed under 'Prizes and Bursaries' on the Royal College of Psychiatrists' Student Associates page.

- **Continuing occasional but regular contact with a mental health team.** For example, you might arrange to attend an outpatient clinic or ward round once a fortnight or once a month.

If you have a possible interest in academic medicine or psychiatry, it is worth considering:

- **Contributing to the work of a research team.** Research is challenging to complete, because it needs considerable time and expertise, and almost all medical research is now done in multidisciplinary teams. A feasible and effective way to learn about psychiatric research is to contribute to the work of a research team, in a modest way, but over a period of several months or more.

- **Helping to develop teaching materials for use by other students.** Working with your course organizer or another active teacher to help to develop materials for use by other medical students can be highly rewarding.

 Further reading

Butler, G. & Hope, T. (2007). *Manage Your Mind: The Mental Fitness Guide.* Oxford University Press, Oxford.

Index

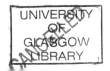